Green's Gynecology: Essentials of Clinical Practice
Fourth Edition

Daniel L. Clarke-Pearson, M.D.
Professor of Obstetrics and Gynecology,
Duke University School of Medicine;
Director, Division of Gynecologic Oncology,
Duke University Medical Center,
Durham, North Carolina

M. Yusoff Dawood, M.D.
Berel Held Professor and Director,
Division of Reproductive Endocrinology,
University of Texas Medical School at
Houston; Attending Obstetrician and
Gynecologist, Hermann Hospital, Houston

Foreword by
Charles B. Hammond, M.D.
E. C. Hamblen Professor and Chairman, Department of Obstetrics and
Gynecology, Duke University Medical Center, Durham, North Carolina

Little, Brown and Company
Boston/Toronto/London

To our wives, Katchy and Firyal,
and our children, Don, Emily, Mary, Mike, Fatimah, Fauzia, Firdaus, and Hassan
for their love and support of our endeavors

Contents

Foreword

Through three editions and for twenty-five years, the textbook *Gynecology: Essentials of Clinical Practice,* written by Thomas H. Green, Jr., M.D., has served to present concisely yet comprehensively the basic facts and principles of the specialty. While designed primarily for medical students and resident physicians, it has often been used by practitioners as a ready source of factual material. The text has served the useful role of providing data needed for a sound understanding and proper management of gynecologic disorders.

Because of Dr. Green's untimely death, the development of this fourth edition has been somewhat delayed. It has now been entirely rewritten and updated. Written and edited by Daniel L. Clarke-Pearson, M.D., and M. Yusoff Dawood, M.D., both outstanding academic physicians and educators, this new edition is even more useful and usable. The tradition of excellence established by Dr. Green has been upheld and expanded.

The fourth edition presents and updates the many changes seen in gynecologic practice during the last decade, yet continues an attention to detail with a strong clinical focus. Appropriately, it now includes sections not only on the major and common gynecologic disorders but also material on newer areas such as breast disease, sexual function and dysfunction, urinary incontinence, sexual assault, and contraception.

This is a needed textbook that will be of great use to the student of our specialty. I commend its use to all who practice gynecology and to all who desire to continue to improve those practice skills.

Charles B. Hammond, M.D.

Contributing Authors

Charles R. B. Beckmann, M.D., M.H.P.E.
Associate Professor of Obstetrics and Gynecology, University of Tennessee, Memphis, College of Medicine, Memphis

Daniel L. Clarke-Pearson, M.D.
Professor of Obstetrics and Gynecology, Duke University School of Medicine; Director, Division of Gynecologic Oncology, Duke University Medical Center, Durham, North Carolina

M. Yusoff Dawood, M.D.
Berel Held Professor and Director, Division of Reproductive Endocrinology, University of Texas Medical School at Houston; Attending Obstetrician and Gynecologist, Hermann Hospital, Houston

H. Alexander Easley III, J.D., M.D.
Associate Clinical Professor, East Carolina University School of Medicine; Attending Physician, Department of Obstetrics and Gynecology, Pitt County Memorial Hospital, Greenville, North Carolina

Jay J. Gold, M.D.
Clinical Professor of Medicine and Adjunct Professor of Obstetrics and Gynecology, University of Illinois College of Medicine, Chicago; Chairman, Section of Endocrinology, St. Francis Hospital, Evanston, Illinois

Erica Gold Sinsheimer, M.D.
Clinical Instructor of Medicine, University of Illinois College of Medicine, Chicago; Associate Attending, Department of Medicine, St. Francis Hospital, Evanston, Illinois

John T. Soper, M.D.
Associate Professor of Obstetrics and Gynecology, Duke University School of Medicine; Attending Physician, Division of Gynecologic Oncology, Duke University Medical Center, Durham, North Carolina

John F. Steege, M.D.
Associate Clinical Professor of Obstetrics and Gynecology, Duke University School of Medicine; Attending Physician, Department of Obstetrics and Gynecology, Duke University Medical Center, Durham, North Carolina

L. Lewis Wall, M.D., D. Phil.
Assistant Professor of Obstetrics and Gynecology, Duke University School of Medicine; Director, Bladder Function Clinic and Laboratory, Department of Obstetrics and Gynecology, Duke University Medical Center, Durham, North Carolina

I

General Considerations

1

Gynecologic History and Physical Examination

The importance of a thorough preliminary survey of the patient's overall background and current health status cannot be too strongly emphasized. An adequate general medical history, including a careful system review, and a thorough general physical examination are essential because of the frequency with which the gynecologic condition that prompts the patient to consult a physician is the first manifestation of a serious systemic disease. The menstrual irregularities that may be the first clue to latent diabetes are specific, frequently encountered examples of this relation. Furthermore, gynecologic disorders may be accompanied by significant, generalized disturbances, either directly related to and resulting from, or entirely incidental to, the primary pelvic disease. These disorders may have a marked influence on the overall plan of diagnosis and therapy. The systemic manifestations of the various primary pelvic disorders are discussed in more detail in the appropriate sections.

The presence of independent cardiovascular, renal, or pulmonary disease must also be determined, and this information often affects the choice of treatment where more than one alternative is available. The nature and details of past illnesses or operative procedures are also important, and it may be necessary to write to other physicians or hospitals to obtain accurate information on these points. If the patient is or has been receiving medications, it should be known. Certain hormones may cause abnormal bleeding; immunosuppressive chemotherapy drugs and broad-spectrum antibiotics may alter vaginal flora, allowing an overgrowth of *Candida,* causing vaginitis; certain cardiovascular medications, thyroid hormones, and cortisone compounds may have an important bearing on the preoperative preparations and choice of anesthesia should surgery be indicated. A history of allergy or sensitivity to any medications is important for obvious reasons.

Social and environmental factors that might have a bearing on pelvic symptoms should also be adequately explored. A general idea of the personality of the patient, her mental and emotional attitudes and problems, and the adequacy of her past and present adjustment to various life situations also prove helpful when evaluating her pelvic complaints, as symptoms arising in relation to the reproductive tract and its function may be partially contributed by nonorganic causes. The gynecologist must not only make sure to hear what the patient says but must listen with a "third ear" to what the patient does not say and must take note of nonverbal forms of communication such as body movements, evidence of inner tension or hesitation, and changes in attitude—all of which may help in understanding and dealing with the patient's problems.

Finally, inquiry should always be made regarding familial disorders, particularly if there is a family history of malignant disease, diabetes, tuberculosis, or allergies. A strong family history of any of these disorders should alert the physician to be on the lookout for similar conditions in the patient and may make it possible to detect them in an early, asymptomatic phase. For example, most patients with some form of pelvic malignancy show a tendency to a higher-than-normal incidence of malignancy in their family background.

The gynecologist must approach the care of the patient from a broad viewpoint. Although his or her principal function in the overall care of women has been and undoubtedly should remain that of a highly trained specialist-consultant in the field of gynecology, in practice the gynecologist has long served the important role of a primary care physician for women. This situation pertains because for a large number of American women the gynecologist is the principal source of medical supervision, advice, and occasionally initial care for nongynecologic problems. Thus the gynecologist often represents women's initial entrance into the total health care system and provides them continuity of care within this system. This primary care role of the gynecologist is likely to diminish with increasing provision of prepaid health care services.

GYNECOLOGIC HISTORY

The patient should initially be allowed to present her chief complaint and the story of her present illness in her own way and words. If necessary, the physician can eventually guide the conversation so as to avoid the presentation of repetitious or insignificant material. The present age of the patient should be noted. By judicious questioning the following points of information can be elicited, if they are not spontaneously reported by the patient, so as to complete the gynecologic history.

1. *Menstrual history:* age at menarche; length of cycle; regularity of cycle; premenstrual molimina (e.g., breast pain, tenderness and swelling, skin changes, cramps, headaches, tension, weight gain, edema); duration of flow; associated cramps or pelvic pain and time of occurrence; description of amount (number of sanitary pads required per day provides a rough index, with three to six as normal) and character of flow; dysmenorrhea, primary or secondary (characteristics of pain, location of pain, time of onset and subsidence, effective medications); dates of the last menstrual period and the previous menstrual period; description of any prior therapy for menstrual disorders; and if postmenopausal, age at menopause and description of menopausal symptoms.

2. *Sexual history:* age at first coitus; frequency of coitus; dyspareunia; satisfaction and orgasmic response; use of contraceptives, type and duration.

3. *Obstetric history:* number of pregnancies and dates (gravidity); number of deliveries and dates (parity) and whether births were normal, full term, or presented complications; type of delivery (normal, vaginal, forceps, section); episiotomy or other procedure; birth weight of babies; postpartum difficulties and complications; number of miscarriages (duration of pregnancy at the time, complications, need for curettage). The obstetric profile is recorded as gravida *x,* para *p-q-r-s,* where:

x = number of pregnancies
p = number of term pregnancies
q = number of preterm pregnancies (births)
r = number of aborted pregnancies
s = number of living children

Thus gravida 4, para 1-1-1-2 indicates that the patient is having her fourth pregnancy, with one previous term pregnancy, 1 preterm pregnancy, 1 abortion, and 2 living children (one full term and one preterm birth).

Special inquiries should be made concerning the following.

1. *Abnormal bleeding:* character and amount; any associated symptoms (e.g., pain, discharge); relation to periods (premenstrual, postmenstrual, intermenstrual, postmenopausal); frequency, duration, and onset (sudden or slow); if preceded by amenorrhea or other menstrual irregularities.

2. *Abnormal discharge:* amount, color (yellow, white, mucoid, brown), odor, and consistency (thin, watery, thick, cheesy, mucoid); relation to menstrual cycle (premenstrual or postmenstrual aggravation); associated symptoms (vulvovaginal burning and itching, urinary symptoms).

3. *Abnormal pelvic or abdominal pain:* type (sharp, dragging, aching, pressure or bearing-down, crampy, colicky, burning); sudden or gradual onset; duration; whether steady or intermittent; location and radiation; relation to menses or to phase of menstrual cycle; relation to position (upright versus recumbent); relation to function of other organ systems (gastrointestinal or urinary tract); associated symptoms (abnormal bleeding or discharge, gastrointestinal or bladder disturbances). Pain referred to the low back or buttocks is commonly associated with disease in the cervix, urethra, bladder neck, or lower rectum and often radiates into one or both legs. Discomfort due to uterine or vaginal disease or associated with inflammatory conditions of the bladder dome is usually localized in the lower abdomen. Ovarian pain and

pain due to disease of the fallopian tubes is most often referred to the lower abdominal quadrants just above the groin and often radiates down the medial aspect of the thighs.

4. *Back pain:* Backache of gynecologic origin is most commonly secondary to endometriosis, chronic pelvic inflammatory disease, large fibroids arising in the posterior uterine wall and wedged in the hollow of the sacrum, or posterolateral extension of carcinoma of the cervix. It is fair to say, however, that most backaches are of musculoskeletal rather than gynecologic origin.

5. *Infertility:* duration; prior use of contraceptives; type and duration of contraceptives used; frequency and timing of coitus; coital habits; dyspareunia (pain during coitus); prior studies; previous marriages of either partner and any resulting pregnancies.

6. *Abnormal symptoms of genital relaxation:* feeling of protrusion; dragging sensation; pressure; bearing-down discomfort; or sense of insecurity.

7. *Associated bladder symptoms:* frequency; nocturia; urgency; dysuria; difficult voiding; incontinence (stress, urgency).

8. *Associated bowel symptoms:* constipation; diarrhea; pain referred to region of the rectum; vaginal protrusion on straining during defecation.

9. *Miscellaneous:* history of any acute abdominal or pelvic illnesses or operations, especially of the pelvis or of a perforated appendix.

GYNECOLOGIC PHYSICAL EXAMINATION

A complete general physical examination should be carried out first, including determination of the height, weight, and blood pressure as well as a survey of the neck, breasts, heart, lungs, abdomen, inguinal and femoral regions, and lower extremities. A nurse or other female attendant should always be present for the physical examination if the gynecologist is male. The presence of another female in the room is comforting to female patients because for some the situa-

tion is a source of considerable apprehension and embarrassment. Furthermore, it affords complete protection to the physician against the possibility that a patient with an unsuspected psychotic tendency or ulterior motive may subsequently allege improper behavior on his part in the examining room. The patient should be warm, physically comfortable, and relaxed; she should be properly draped and have had an opportunity to void immediately prior to examination. The patient's mental ease and relaxation should also be ensured by a conscious effort to gain her confidence and cooperation while obtaining the history and by continued reassurance during the physical examination. If the patient is not comfortable and relaxed, examination is more difficult and maximum information cannot be gained from the examination.

The examination is conveniently begun with the patient in a sitting position on the edge of the table. The physician first checks the head and neck (including palpation of the thyroid and the cervical and supraclavicular nodes), breasts, axillae, back, and lungs. The patient then lies flat on the table for a further check of the breasts, heart, abdomen, groins, and lower extremities.

During examination of the breasts, it is well to inspect them first with the patient sitting erect, with her arms at her sides and again while she raises them. This maneuver frequently discloses breast asymmetry, nipple fixation, or a fixed mass underneath the areolar margin, any of which might go unnoticed in the recumbent position. A careful, methodical examination of all quadrants of the breasts and the adjacent axillary regions should then be carried out with the patient in both the erect and supine positions. Palpation is best performed and breast masses most readily appreciated if the flat, palmar surface of the hand and contiguous palmar surfaces of the apposed fingers are employed rather than the actual tips of the fingers. It is important to learn to distinguish the somewhat finely granular, irregular consistency of normal breast tissue from discrete masses that may represent either neoplasm or benign fibrocystic change. It is also important to be aware of the frequent existence of an axillary extension of normal breast tissue, the "axillary tail," and not to mistake it for a tumor; when present, it is almost invariably bilateral and symmetric. Finally, the areolar areas should gently be compressed to demonstrate the presence of any abnormal secretion or bloody fluid in the nipple glands and ducts.

Because nearly all breast irregularities or lumps are first discovered by the woman herself, it is well worth the effort to instruct patients about the proper method of breast self-examination. The patients can readily be shown the correct technique during the course of the physician's examination and should be urged to examine her breasts every month, just after completion of the menstrual period, at a time when normal premenstrual breast engorgement and tenderness are not misleading. She should be taught to inspect her breasts in front of a mirror, first with her arms at the side, then with arms overhead, looking for changes in size or contour or for dimpling of the skin. Next, lying flat, she can be shown how to palpate correctly with the right hand all four quadrants of the left breast, preferably with a small pillow under the left shoulder and with the left hand under the head while palpating the inner half of the breast, the left arm down at the side while palpating the outer quadrants. The procedure is then reversed to examine the right breast with the left hand. It is to be hoped that such instruction in proper self-examination of the breast will permit women to recognize any changes more promptly and hence will lead to the earlier detection of breast cancer.

Careful, detailed examination of the abdomen is obviously an integral part of the gynecologic physical examination. It is also particularly important never to neglect examination of both groins, as many gynecologic disorders affecting the vulva and vagina are accompanied by inguinal adenopathy, whether inflammatory or neoplastic in type.

The patient is then placed in the lithotomy position with her feet in stirrups and is suitably draped by the nurse. Rarely, the lateral Sims, knee-chest, or standing position is employed, as it is occasionally more suitable than the lithotomy position for determining specific points. The actual pelvic examination begins with inspection; the lower abdomen, the external genitalia (mons veneris, vulvar skin, and labia majora and minora, prepuce and clitoris, introitus, hymeneal or vaginal opening, visible portions of the anterior and posterior vaginal walls), the urethral meatus, and the anoperineal area are surveyed first for abnormal distribution or character of hair or pigmentation, clitoral hypertrophy, generalized or local skin lesions, visible subcutaneous or submucosal abnormalities (e.g., inflammation, leukoplakia, ulcers, tumors, atrophy), and gross displacement and relaxations. The external genitalia, including the labia majora and minora, mons pubis, and perineum, should be palpated next for any masses or swellings.

The examiner now sits directly in front of the patient with a suitable flexible lamp and carries out the speculum examination, introducing the previously warmed blades (holding the blades under running warm tap water) after separating the labia and depressing the perineal body with the opposite hand. If the introitus and vagina are dry, it is better to wet the speculum blades with warm water rather than a lubricant, which can interfere with obtaining cervical and vaginal cytology smears and specimens for culture of organisms. A Graves bivalve speculum of appropriate size—small (infant), medium ("regular"), medium with narrow blades (Pederson), or large, depending on the size of the introitus and the size and length of the vaginal canal—is inserted at the proper angle and with a slight rotary motion (Fig. 1-1). In most instances, even in the presence of an intact hymen, the hymeneal opening is sufficient to permit both one-finger bimanual vaginal and speculum examinations (usually employing the narrow-bladed instrument) without difficulty if they are properly and gently done. (If these examinations are not possible, information obtained by a bimanual rectal examination is often sufficient in a young girl; otherwise, examination under anesthesia is necessary.) The speculum is gently but firmly inserted its full length, and the blades are then opened, exposing the cervix for inspection, preparation of a Papanicolaou smear, cervical or endometrial biopsy, or any other office diagnostic procedure required (Fig. 1-2). A little manipulation may be necessary to expose the cervix if the uterus is retroverted or if the vaginal walls are lax and redundant. A cotton pledget grasped at the end of a curved uterine-dressing forceps may be used as a "pusher" to facilitate exposure. As the instrument is withdrawn,

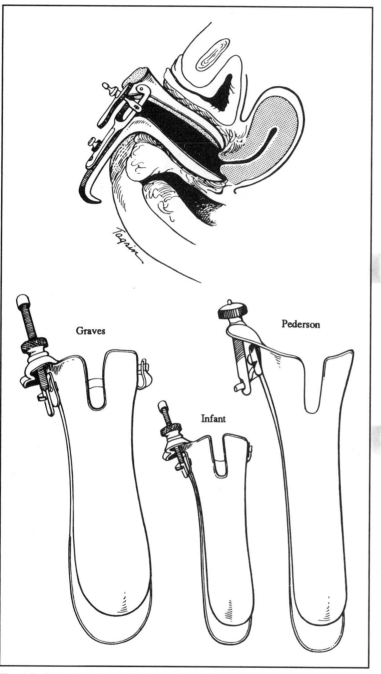

Fig. 1-1. Insertion of a vaginal speculum. Various speculum types are shown.

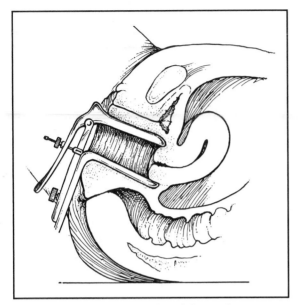

Fig. 1-2. Speculum examination of the cervix.

the vaginal wall, including the posterior fornix, and any secretions or discharge present are examined for evidence of vaginitis, atrophy, or other lesions.

After the speculum examination, bimanual vaginal examination is performed. Although it has long been taught that the left hand should be used to perform bimanual examination, it is not mandatory. The hand one is most accustomed to employ or with which one feels most natural and proficient during palpatory examination of any body region should be used consistently. The labia are gently separated and one or two well lubricated fingers of the gloved hand are introduced, depressing the perineum and posterior vaginal wall so as to avoid undue and uncomfortable pressure against the more sensitive anteriorly placed structures. With the finger depressing the perineum, the perineal body and pubococcygeal (levator) muscles are palpated. The patient is asked to strain or cough, or both, which further reveals any tendency to perineal relaxation, cystocele, rectocele, or prolapse of the uterus or vagina (Chap. 19). Abnormalities of the structures at the level of the introitus (urethra, Skene's glands, Bartholin's glands) are searched for between the thumb and forefinger. The fingers are then inserted at the proper angle (approximately 30 to 45 de-

grees above the horizontal) the length of the vagina, palpating the vaginal wall and exocervix and the external os as this maneuver is carried out.

Bimanual examination of the uterus and adnexal regions is then carefully done, checking on the size, outline, consistency, mobility, and position of the uterus, ovaries, and any palpable pelvic masses; the "vaginal" fingers serve to steady and elevate the cervix and uterus anteriorly where the "abdominal" hand can then perform the evaluation (Fig. 1-3). The vaginal vaults (lateral fornices or adnexal regions) are then palpated, feeling primarily with the vaginal fingers, the abdominal hand being used to sweep the adnexa down to them (Fig. 1-4). Anterior and posterior (cul-de-sac or pouch of Douglas) fornices are then explored bimanually in the same way, and the fingers are then turned and pressed laterally to feel the pelvic walls as well. Normal adnexa are frequently not palpable even under ideal conditions (normal fallopian tubes probably never), particularly if the patient is unrelaxed or obese. However, under anesthesia, normal-sized ovaries are nearly always palpable even in an obese patient. Unusually mobile adnexa (with relaxed and elongated infundibulopelvic and ovarian ligaments) may result in the ovaries being palpated in the cul-de-sac posteriorly at the time of rectal examination, rather than during vaginal examination. Palpation of "normal-sized" ovaries (e.g., 3.5 × 1.5 cm) in the premenopausal woman with active ovarian function is to be expected. However, palpation of ovaries of "normal size" in a woman 3 to 5 years after her menopause has been found not to be a normal or expected clinical finding; on the contrary, it suggests that the ovaries are not normal at all and may signify early ovarian cancer, which has its peak incidence between the ages of 45 and 60. (Serious consideration must be given to surgical exploration and removal of the gonads in this situation, as the normal postmenopausal ovary is usually one-third or less the size of the premenopausal ovary and is ordinarily not palpable.)

Finally, a rectovaginal examination (the index finger in the vagina and the middle finger in the rectum) is done to look for external and internal hemorrhoids, fissures, fistulas, or anorectal polyps or tumors; the uterus is palpated bimanually (only now is the fundus

to the many facets of the various psychosomatic mechanisms and disturbances that may be encountered in the gynecologic patient. Acute or chronic emotional disorders, by interfering with the normal, delicately balanced neuroendocrine control of the cyclic activity of the female reproductive tract, often cause fundamental disturbances in this cyclic function. The result is that distressing symptoms arise on a purely psychosomatic basis. Such psychosomatic mechanisms are almost invariably important in the comprehension and management of many of the functional gynecologic disorders discussed in Chapter 5 and elsewhere in the book: so-called hypothalamic amenorrhea, the premenstrual tension syndrome, the "pelvic congestion" syndrome and related types of functional pelvic pain, idiopathic pruritus vulvae, and so on. Undoubtedly, they also play an important etiologic role in many instances among the large group of women with recurring functional menstrual irregularities as well as in some patients suffering from infertility or habitual abortion. Certainly, the significance of psychological factors in the production of many of the disabling menopausal symptoms experienced by a few women is well recognized.

On the other hand, among the various manifestations of organic disease of the reproductive tract, there may be secondary symptoms that have a psychological basis. This situation arises because disturbed function of or complaints localized to the region of the pelvic viscera invariably are the source of considerable anxiety. They may raise the specter of premature loss of or failure to completely fulfill childbearing potential, cause concern over possible loss of sexual function, or arouse the fear that cancer or a "shameful social disease" is present. In fact, pelvic symptoms often suggest to the patient a serious threat to her integrity as a female person, either as a result of what the disease itself will do to her or as consequence of the treatment that may be required, e.g., hysterectomy. Thus the physician must also take into account emotional factors and sympathetically deal with them by explanation and reassurance for the patient with obvious organic disease as well as the woman who proves to have functional complaints.

Some of the more frequently encountered psychosomatic mechanisms and resulting gynecologic disturbances are considered more fully later in the appropriate chapters.

PROGRAM FOR EARLY DETECTION OF GYNECOLOGIC CANCER

Female genital cancer constitutes at least 25 percent of all malignant disease in women and is particularly susceptible to simple methods of early detection. Therefore the opportunity for early recognition of female genital tract cancer through the gynecologic history and complete gynecologic examination should never be neglected, regardless of the patient's chief complaint. Through the educational programs sponsored by a variety of medical and lay organizations, women (and their physicians) have become increasingly aware of the value of annual checkups and yearly Papanicolaou smears for the detection of early asymptomatic pelvic malignancy at a stage when cure rates are potentially good if treatment is prompt and adequate. From 1964 to 1974, an American Cancer Society survey showed that the percentage of women who had had a routine Papanicolaou smear rose from 48 percent to 78 percent, and the percentage of women who had a smear during the year immediately preceding this American Cancer Society study had risen from 23 percent in 1963 to 52 percent in 1974. Despite tremendous advances in surgical techniques, radiation treatment, and cancer chemotherapy, the only female malignancy to show a significant decline in mortality in the United States has been carcinoma of the cervix. The improvement in the cure rate for cervical cancer is largely due to earlier detection and prompt treatment of premalignant and early malignant lesions of the cervix. (Since the mid to late 1960s, a decrease in the death rate from cancer of the cervix by as much as 50 to 60 percent has been observed in several areas of the United States where long-term, ongoing Papanicolaou smear screening programs involving 90 to 95 percent of the local population have been in existence.)

The habit now adopted by many women of reporting for a vaginal smear each year has had equally important secondary dividends in the form of opportunities to carry out a complete medical examination. Thus a neoplasm arising elsewhere in the pelvis (e.g., ovary) or in other body regions (e.g., breast, thyroid, rectum), as well as significant benign disorders in the pelvis and other body regions or systems can also be discovered early and dealt with expeditiously and often successfully. It was noted in a 1970 study that when a cervical cancer screening program was extended to include a complete gynecologic examination as well as clinical examination of the breasts, 26 new, unsuspected malignant tumors (including seven breast cancers) were found in 4000 patients seen, and 23 percent of all patients examined were thought to be in need of treatment or further investigation of other, nonmalignant abnormalities. Because it has been the obvious value of the yearly vaginal smear that has made women "checkup-conscious," much of the responsibility for carrying out routine annual examinations has fallen on the shoulders of the gynecologist. This burden can, should, and will be shared by other physicians if the benefits of annual checkups are to be extended to a larger segment of the female population and as prepaid health care programs (health maintenance organizations, preferred provider organizations) emerge in larger numbers.

Yearly pelvic cancer detection procedures should probably be offered to all women over the age of 18 or 20 (the teenager should certainly be included if she is sexually active) and are particularly feasible on a broad scale in obstetric patients, nearly all of whom are now under regular medical supervision and thus readily available for a routine screening program. Any physician's office may be simply and inexpensively equipped to carry out a complete gynecologic cancer detection study. The only materials needed are the following.

1. Bivalve vaginal specula, preferably of assorted sizes.
2. Cervical biopsy punch.
3. Small endometrial biopsy curet.
4. Uterine tenaculum.
5. Uterine sound.
6. Endometrial aspiration cannula (optional).
7. Curved glass pipets and a rubber suction bulb for obtaining vaginal cytologic smears.
8. Throat sticks (or a special spatula) for securing cervical cytologic smears.

9. Small bottles of 10% formalin solution to be used as tissue biopsy fixative.
10. Small bottles of Papanicolaou fixative (equal parts of ether and 95% alcohol; as an alternative, pure 95% alcohol may be employed), which serves as the fixative for cytologic smears. Smears may be submitted in the original bottle of fixative; or if more convenient, the glass slides may be left in the fixative for at least 30 minutes, then air-dried and forwarded to the laboratory in simple cardboard mailing containers.
11. Bottle of Schiller's solution, which may be required as an additional procedure at colposcopy (Chap. 2).
12. Glass slides, paper clips, a diamond marking pencil for labeling glass slides.

Routine screening of the patient with no apparent symptoms referable to the pelvic organs should include the following.

1. Inquiry regarding abnormal bleeding or discharge (particularly significant if the occurrence is post-coital, intermenstrual, or postmenopausal); menstrual irregularities, pelvic or lower abdominal discomfort; change in or abnormalities of bowel or bladder function; pruritus or lesions of the vulvar skin.
2. Cytologic examinations: Papanicolaou smear; vaginal vault smear in women without a uterus and cervix.
3. Pelvic examinations (a careful general examination including a survey of the neck, breasts and axillae, abdomen, groins, and legs should of course be done prior to the vaginal and rectal examinations), which involves:
   a. Inspection and palpation of the external genitalia.
   b. Bimanual abdominal-vaginal examination.
   c. Speculum examination of the cervix and vagina.
   d. Rectal examination, including a rectovaginal examination.
4. Stool for occult blood in women over 40 years of age.

The following additional office procedures are indicated in patients in whom any of the abnormal symptoms are elicited during the interview, in whom examination reveals any suspicious findings (e.g., cervical "erosion," a questionable adnexal mass, a vulvar lesion of unknown nature), or for whom doubtful or positive vaginal or cervical smears are reported.

1. Cervical and endocervical smears (scrapings), if not previously obtained.
2. Schiller's test of the cervix (Chap. 2).
3. Cervical biopsy of grossly abnormal areas or grossly normal areas that do not stain with Schiller's solution.
4. Colposcopy if available and colposcopically guided biopsies of the cervix if indicated; endocervical biopsy (curettage).
5. Endometrial biopsy; endometrial-aspiration cytologic smears (optional).
6. Biopsy of any suspicious vulvar or vaginal lesion; toluidine blue test of vulvar skin (Chap. 2).
7. Careful, repeated follow-up observations in all patients with presumed fibroids, physiologic ovarian enlargements, benign vulvar lesions, and so on.

If the source of suspicious symptoms or the abnormal vaginal smear remains undetected, or if the nature of any abnormal finding is not completely clarified by the office diagnostic survey, further gynecologic evaluation becomes essential and may involve pelvic ultrasound, computed tomography, magnetic resonance imaging, hysterosalpingography, examination under anesthesia, fractional curettage of the endocervix and endometrial cavity, more extensive cervical biopsies or cold-knife total cone biopsy of the cervix, laparoscopy, hysteroscopy, or exploratory laparotomy if an ovarian tumor is suspected. If some of the less invasive tests yield positive results and disclose definite malignancy, a more complete evaluation of the exact extent of the disease may be immediately carried out and subsequent treatment planned.

The value of such routine cancer detection programs, whether carried out by the individual physician or within the framework of large medical institutions or special cancer detection clinics, has been amply demonstrated.

PREMARITAL EXAMINATION

The original purpose of the premarital examination was simply to determine that both the prospective bride and groom were free of venereal disease. It is now an established requirement for obtaining a marriage license in many states. Certification by the physician that a serologic test for syphilis is negative is all that is required, since the law does not precisely stipulate that a physical examination should also be done. However, many couples realize the importance of obtaining the full benefits of premarital counseling. Such benefits can only be secured through a complete examination, preferably of both partners, and, in particular, an adequate opportunity during the interview with the woman for a discussion of the basic facts of feminine physiology and hygiene. Unsuspected anatomic or endocrinologic abnormalities that might seriously interfere with normal marriage or childbearing functions will occasionally be discovered in this way. Even more important, misinformation and misapprehensions concerning the sexual aspects of marriage can be corrected by providing proper information, general guidance, and reassurance. Finally, the premarital examination offers the couple an opportunity to obtain information and advice concerning conception control and family planning, information often vital to their happiness and success with respect to both their marriage and careers.

An adequate premarital examination should, first of all, include the taking of a complete history and the performance of a complete physical examination, including a pelvic examination. In addition to a serologic test for syphilis, premarital serologic testing for rubella is available and is mandatory in some states. Depending on the result, the patient can then elect immunization against rubella at her convenience. In some states, a blood test such as the HIV test for acquired immune deficiency syndrome (AIDS) is required.

Information and help regarding family planning should be provided. If the couple wishes to use contraception, this is a convenient time to discuss the various methods available, their specific advantages, disadvantages, side effects, as well as the couple's own preferences, if any. If use of a diaphragm is elected, it is usually possible to fit it properly and instruct the patient in its use during the pelvic examination that follows the interview. For those few wishing to use a diaphragm in whom a snug hymenal orifice precludes premarital fitting, either a vaginal spermicidal jelly alone or an oral contraceptive may be temporarily prescribed, with the patient returning a month or two following initial sexual intercourse for permanent fitting and instruction in the use of a diaphragm. Details of the various methods of conception control and the manner in which the patient is to be instructed and supervised in their use are discussed in detail in Chapter 22.

Only occasionally does the pelvic examination reveal a hymenal orifice so small that the question of whether or not to perform premarital hymenectomy or dilatation of the hymen need be considered. In general, the premarital hymenal surgery should be avoided. Rarely does the presence of an abnormally thick, fibrous hymen or an extremely tiny opening definitely indicate the advisability of preliminary dilatation or hymenectomy under anesthesia. Dilatation is done initially in the office and continued at home by the patient using a few simple tubular dilators graduated in size. If a formal hymenectomy is deemed necessary, it should preferably be done at least six weeks prior to sexual intercourse to allow adequate time for complete healing and freedom from any local sensitivity.

One other question frequently asked during the premarital examination concerns the matter of douching as part of the routine program of feminine hygiene for the sexually active woman. Regular periodic douching is entirely unnecessary, and the healthy female of any age need never douche. However, those women who still feel impelled to douche occasionally should be assured that it will do them no harm.

EXAMINATIONS FOR SPECIAL GYNECOLOGIC SITUATIONS

Further attention to details in the history or physical examination of the women in special gynecologic situations, such as the rape victim, or in specific gynecologic disorders are given in the subsequent respective chapters. The examination of the rape and sexual assault victim presents not only medical but legal challenges, which are discussed in detail in Chapter 20.

2

Laboratory Tests and Diagnostic Surgical Procedures in Gynecology

A complete, thoughtfully elicited history and thorough physical examination, with obvious emphasis on the recognition and proper interpretation of significant findings demonstrated by abdominal, pelvic, and rectal examinations, are the two basic and most important elements in the diagnosis of pelvic disorders. The information obtained may be all that is necessary to arrive at an exact diagnosis. At the least, the broad outlines of the clinical problem posed by the chief complaint have been narrowed considerably, so that further investigation of a limited number of more likely possibilities may now be effectively undertaken. Only in this way can the wide variety of laboratory tests and special procedures that are useful for establishing a diagnosis be cost-efficiently applied, avoiding delay in diagnosis and treatment and reducing to a minimum the number of unnecessary studies performed. A conflict in clinical care arises between the need to reduce and contain health care costs and the medical-legal climate in which the diagnosis and treatment may be questioned without adequate testing or radiographic confirmation. These diagnostic evaluations (which for the purposes of this discussion include laboratory serum evaluation, cultures, radiographs, and diagnostic surgical procedures) are often expensive and, in some instances, invasive procedures. Therefore the emphasis of the next two chapters is to delineate the utility of these tests along with discussion of the risks and costs. A few special procedures, commonly employed only in connection with a specific problem (e.g., urinary incontinence or cervical dysplasia) are described in more detail elsewhere in the appropriate chapter.

The diagnosis of gynecologic pathology may be aided by surgery. Compared to the medical history, the physical and pelvic examination discussed in Chapter 1, and the routine laboratory tests discussed in this chapter, diagnostic surgery is expensive and may put the patient at risk for major complications or even death. Therefore before subjecting the patient to the diagnostic surgical procedures discussed in this chapter, the clinician should clearly understand the goals of these procedures and their value to the patient, as well as their risks and benefits.

Several invasive surgical procedures are performed primarily to diagnose or stage gynecologic conditions. Several of these procedures may also be therapeutic or may be performed in conjunction with a therapeutic surgical procedure. The diagnostic aspects of these operations are discussed in this chapter.

BASIC OFFICE DIAGNOSTIC TECHNIQUES

Cytopathology

The diagnosis of gynecologic conditions based on microscopic study of single cell morphology owes its greatest debt to Papanicolaou, who pioneered the recognition of characteristics associated with cervical cancer, as detected by exfoliative cytology of the cervix and vagina. This single diagnostic screening technique has had the largest impact on the reduction of mortality from cervical cancer over the last five decades. The Papanicolaou (Pap) smear is now used routinely for screening all sexually active women and all women over age 18. The principles and methods for performing a Pap smear are discussed in detail in Chapter 25. A pertinent point when obtaining a Pap smear is that sampling of the transformation zone and endocervix by the Pap smear spatula must be adequate (Fig. 2-1). The gynecologist must prepare the specimen appropriately on the microscope slide and have it fixed immediately to obtain the best material for cytopathologic interpretation. The Pap smear not only diagnoses cervical carcinoma, it also reveals preinvasive changes of the squamous cells of the exocervix (dysplasia or cervical intraepithelial neoplasia). The increasing incidence of human papilloma virus (HPV) infections in the female population and the link

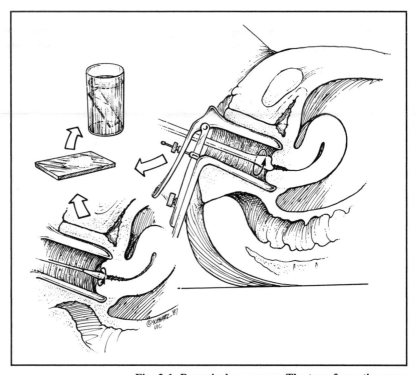

Fig. 2-1. Papanicolaou smear. The transformation zone and the squamocolumnar junction of the cervix are scraped in a circular motion using the Ayre spatula. The material obtained is immediately smeared on the glass slide and then fixed in absolute alcohol. A second specimen from the endocervix is obtained using a saline-moistened Q-tip or small brush. This sample is fixed immediately on a separate slide, then submitted to the pathologist.

between HPV and the development of invasive carcinoma suggest that cervical dysplasia (intraepithelial neoplasia) must be carefully detected and eliminated to reduce the incidence of cervical cancer. Genital cytopathology may also suggest endometrial carcinoma or carcinoma arising from the ovary, fallopian tube, or elsewhere in the peritoneal cavity. Cytopathology obtained from the vulva is less accurate and is not considered a routine screening diagnostic method today. Many times cytopathology of the cervix and vagina also suggests the etiology of a vaginitis such as that caused by *Candida,* herpes, or *Trichomonas.* On the other hand, the Pap smear is not as sensitive and specific for diagnosis of these infections as are culture techniques, which are readily available.

Cytologic study of vaginal smears may also serve as a qualitative estimation of estrogen levels. By studying the type of vaginal cells obtained from smears of the lateral midvagina, parabasal, intermediate, and superficial cells may be identified. After counting several hundred of these vaginal cells and distinguishing their three types, a maturation index may be reported. For the maturation index, three numbers are recorded, with the first number representing parabasal cells, the middle number the intermediate cells, and the third number the superficial cells. For example, in a patient with adequate marked estrogen effect, the index might be 0/10/90; poor estrogen effect might be 20/75/5; complete absence of estrogen might be 100/0/0; and maximum progesterone effect in the presence of adequate estrogen might approach 0/100/0. As a rough guide, the significance of the percentage of superficial cells is as follows.

SUPERFICIAL CELLS (%)	ESTROGEN EFFECT
1–10	Slight
10–30	Moderate
> 30	Marked

If 50 percent or more of the cells are basal cells, low estrogen effect is also indicated. The relative percentage of intermediate cells is highly variable and not significant, except when more than 90 percent of the cells are of this type: Either pregnancy (suppression of estrogen effect by progesterone) or relative estrogen lack is then indicated. The presence of inflammation (e.g., chronic cervicitis or vaginitis) disturbs the cornification pattern and renders it unreliable as an index of estrogen effect.

In a postmenopausal woman not receiving estrogen replacement therapy, the vaginal smear should show a low maturation index. Therefore evidence of marked estrogen effect in such a patient suggests the possibility of an estrogen-secreting granulosa cell or theca cell tumor of the ovary. However, it should be noted that an abnormal estrogen-like effect on vaginal cy-

tology has also been observed in postmenopausal women taking digitalis and related cardiac glycosides, and a markedly elevated maturation index is regularly seen in most of the women who have been on digitalis two years or more.

Endometrial Cytology

With the success of cervical-vaginal cytology for the detection of malignant and premalignant changes of the cervix, several investigators have attempted to develop techniques by which the endometrial cavity might also be sampled. Several methods, including aspiration, brush, spiral helix, and lavage (Fig. 2-2) have been evaluated in an attempt to obtain cells from the endometrial cavity. All of these methods successfully obtain endometrial cells. However, the cytopathologist has reasonable difficulty identifying premalignant changes of the endometrial cells on cytopathologic material. To date, the routine criteria for cytologic diagnosis makes it difficult to differentiate between secretory endometrium, hyperplastic endometrium, and adenomatous atypical hyperplasia. Therefore the sensitivity and specificity of endometrial cytology is less than desirable, and it certainly cannot be recommended as a routine screening technique. In fact, in the patient who has signs or symptoms of endometrial pathology, endometrial biopsy or dilatation and curet-

Fig. 2-2. Endometrial cytology. Several methods for obtaining endometrial specimens for cytology are available. Here a Gravlee Jet Washer obtains an endometrial cytologic specimen through a negative-pressure lavage technique. The material is collected in the syringe and submitted to the cytopathologist for interpretation.

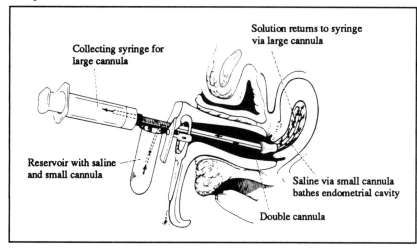

tage (D&C) remain the gold standard for diagnosis and cannot be replaced or supplanted by endometrial cytology.

Microscopic Evaluation of Vaginal Smears and Cultures

Vaginitis and cervicitis are the most frequent complaints evaluated by gynecologists. Simple microscopic examination of the vaginal discharge diluted with saline (wet preparation) may identify the offending organism (Fig. 2-3). The addition of a few drops of potassium hydroxide (KOH preparation) makes *Candida* hyphae more easily recognizable. KOH dissolves the epithelial cells and white blood cells, thereby unmasking the hyphae and budding yeast forms.

Culture techniques are also available to more precisely identify an offending organism. They are especially helpful in situations where the clinical diagnosis based on wet preparations and KOH preparations is unclear or in cases resistant to what was thought to be adequate therapy. *Trichomonas* may be cultured on either Feinberg-Whittington medium or Diamond's medium. *Candida* is best cultured on Nickerson's medium. Cultures for herpes and *Chlamydia* must be handled specially with the proper media and transport vials. Gonococcus is best cultured on Thayer-Martin plates. Culture techniques are also available for the routine identification of anaerobes that commonly inhabit the lower genital tract. Cultures of the normal vagina identify several anaerobes and aerobes that are usually found living in symbiosis. Some of these organisms, when grown in excess, can be pathogenic. However, routine bacterial culture of the vagina is many times misleading and of no diagnostic value, as many bacteria are identified. Anaerobic and aerobic cultures therefore should be obtained in the face of an abscess of the vulva, groin, or pelvis, or to further delineate the etiology of apparent salpingo-oophoritis. The details of these culture techniques and their application to the diagnosis of vaginitis, cervicitis, and upper genital tract infections are further discussed in Chapters 14 and 15.

DETERMINATION OF CHROMOSOME PATTERN

Nuclear Sex Chromatin

The oral or buccal smear is commonly employed for determining the presence of nuclear sex chromatin, and the test can also be carried out easily and rapidly on a blood smear or a biopsy specimen. Vaginal smears are less satisfactory. The test is based on the recognition of a chromatin mass (sex chromatin body) in the cell nucleus adjacent to the nuclear membrane in females. It is absent or virtually absent in the cell nuclei of tissue or desquamated cells in males (Fig. 2-4). The sex chromatin body is present in about 65 to 75 percent of all nuclei in suitably prepared histologic sections (e.g., skin) of female tissues and in 20 to 80

Fig. 2-3. Vaginal smear preparations. A. Microscopic appearance of *Trichomonas vaginalis* organisms. B. Microscopic appearance of candidal vaginitis.

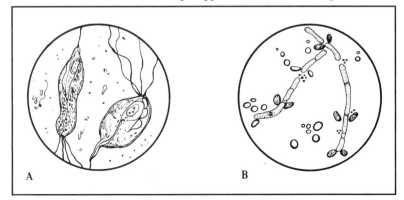

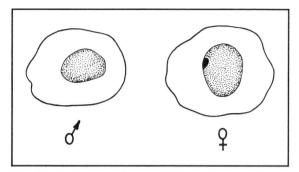

Fig. 2-4. Nuclear sex chromatin determination. Note that the chromatin mass (Barr body) adjacent to the nuclear membrane represents the inactive X chromosome material and is present only in the normal female nucleus, or cells with at least two X chromosomes. The sex chromatin mass is absent in the normal male nucleus.

percent of satisfactorily preserved nuclei in buccal smears from genetic females. In buccal smears from normal males, less than 4 percent of nuclei have sex chromatin bodies. However, in the case of genetic disorders involving sex chromosome mosaicism such as XO,XX (Chap. 8), the nuclear sex chromatin count may be in an intermediate range, e.g., 10 to 15 percent, which should raise the suspicion of some form of gonadal dysgenesis with mosaicism. (In some of the sex chromosomal disorders described in Chapter 8, more than one chromatin body may be present.) Discovery of an abnormality of nuclear sex chromatin should be followed up with chromosome analysis.

Nuclear sex chromatin determination can be performed on fetal cells obtained from amniotic fluid by amniocentesis performed at midtrimester of pregnancy. This method can successfully predict fetal sex prenatally. If the nuclear chromatin is less than 3 percent, the fetus is likely to be male, but if it is 12 percent or more (usually 20 to 40 percent) it is definitely female. However, this method is now supplanted or should be checked with the chromosome karyotype of the fetal cells from the amniotic fluid. The increasing use of chorionic villi biopsy, which can be carried out during the first trimester, adds to the rapid eclipse of nuclear sex chromatin determination for prenatal sex determination, which is usually carried out for deter-

mining risk of sex-linked disorders rather than just for knowing fetal sex.

The following clinical situations are indications for determining nuclear sex chromatin.

1. Primary amenorrhea in apparent females
2. Presence of ambiguous external genitalia at any age
3. Prepubertal girls with pronounced shortness of stature
4. Male infertility
5. Mental retardation and/or psychotic or antisocial behavior in either females or males
6. Aggressive, antisocial behavior in males of excessive height

An outline of the technique for buccal smear is as follows.

1. A large area of buccal mucosa is firmly scraped with a wooden or metal spatula, and the material is transferred to a small area of a slide coated with a thin film of egg albumin.
2. The slides are immediately fixed in Papanicolaou fixative (equal parts of 95% alcohol and ether) for a half-hour or more and then immersed for 5 minutes each in 70% alcohol, 50% alcohol, and distilled water (two changes).
3. Staining is done in 1% cresyl violet for 5 minutes, 95% alcohol (two changes) for 5 minutes, and absolute alcohol until cleared (check with microscope).
4. The slides are cleared further in two changes of xylene and mounted in balsam.

Some cytology laboratories prefer to employ Feulgen's reaction, using Schiff's reagent (basic fuchsin), which stains nuclear detail more specifically than either cresyl violet or hematoxylin.

For the nuclear sex chromatin test to be positive, usually at least two X chromosomes must be present, with one of them showing its material as the Barr body. If there are three X chromosomes, two Barr bodies may be seen; of four X chromosomes, three Barr bodies; and so forth. The results of the buccal smear is reported simply as *chromatin-positive* (when Barr bodies are present and therefore at least two X chromosomes) or *chromatin-negative* (when the Barr body is absent and therefore no more than one X chromosome is present). The results usually have to be supplemented with the definitive results of chromosome karyotyping. Unlike the latter, a buccal smear for sex chromatin material cannot provide information about the Y chromosomes, sex chromosome mosaicism, breakage in the X chromosome, or other chromosomes. Thus Turner's syndrome, various forms of gonadal dysgenesis, a variety of ambiguous genitalia, and recurrent or habitual aborters require chromosome karyotyping.

Chromosome Karyotyping

The technique, indications, and interpretation of chromosome karyotyping, which is a highly specialized laboratory investigation, is described in Chapter 8, as it is often used in the field of reproductive endocrinology and infertility.

TESTS FOR EVALUATION OF HEMORRHAGIC TENDENCY

For about 10 to 20 percent of all serious hemorrhagic disorders in women, the earliest, most significant, or sole manifestation is excessive menstrual flow or prolonged uterine bleeding. Therefore it is important to keep this possibility in mind when studying and managing women suffering from menorrhagia, particularly when there is no response to the usual measures for control of dysfunctional bleeding on a hormonal basis and when local uterine abnormalities that might cause excessive bleeding have been excluded. In this situation, investigation of the possible existence of an abnormal bleeding tendency is clearly indicated.

A useful, simplified approach to the study of these possible hemorrhagic disorders assumes that serious organic disease with secondary hemorrhagic tendencies has been ruled out. The approach is outlined below.

Evaluation of Platelets (Platelet Count and Blood Smear)

If the platelet count is low (thrombocytopenia), bone-marrow aspiration and further hematologic studies are done to determine the etiology of the thrombocytopenia. If the platelet count is normal, the bleeding time is determined.

It should also be mentioned that several even more sophisticated platelet function tests are now available that can aid in the detection of thrombotic disorders and abnormalities of the hemostatic mechanism. These tests include techniques to demonstrate reduced platelet coagulation capacity as well as to identify abnormally increased platelet adherence and platelet aggregations characteristic of the presence of intravascular thrombotic processes and tendencies.

Bleeding Time

If the bleeding time is also normal, the chances that any fundamental hemorrhagic disorder is present are remote in the female. If the bleeding time is prolonged, a diagnosis of von Willebrand's disease is strongly suggested. Approximately 75 percent of all women with this disorder have menometrorrhagia as a prominent symptom.

Jacobson Method

1. With the patient reclining and one forearm supported at the level of the heart, an area of the volar aspect of the forearm (avoiding superficial veins) is sterilized by placement of a sponge soaked in acetone (no rubbing).

2. A blood pressure cuff placed on the upper arm is inflated and maintained at 40 mm Hg during the test.

3. Employing a new No. 11 sterile Bard-Parker blade, a longitudinal incision 3 mm deep and 3 mm long is made in the previously prepared area on the forearm (a 3-mm longitudinal ink mark is made on the forearm, and a transverse ink mark is also made 3 mm from the tip of the scalpel blade to ensure complete accuracy and uniformity in the dimensions of this incision). Today, a disposable lancet device with two small blades is used. Pressing a lever on the lancet instantly releases the blades, which are automatically ejected onto the skin surface, producing two parallel 3 mm long × 3 mm deep incisions.

4. The arm is tilted to allow blood to flow away from the incision, and the blood is picked up by filter paper every 30 seconds until the bleeding ceases, taking care not to allow the filter paper to touch the incision. Bleeding ordinarily does not begin for 30 to 60 seconds. If an immediate flow of dark, venous blood occurs, a superficial vein has been entered, and the test is invalid; the incision should then be repeated elsewhere on the forearm.

5. At the conclusion of the test, the edges of the incision are approximated by an adhesive bandage that is left in place for 48 hours. The average bleeding time by this method is 3½ to 5½ minutes, with the upper limit of normal at 6½ minutes. [*Note:* Certain medications, especially aspirin but also chlorpromazine and related phenothiazines, phenylbutazone, and glycerylguaicolate (an ingredient of most cough syrups and cold remedies) may prolong the bleeding time; hence the test is not valid or reliable if any of these drugs has been taken by the patient within the preceding 10 days.]

Partial Thromboplastin Time

Finally, if a coagulation disorder rather than an abnormality of platelets or vascular fragility is suspected, a partial thromboplastin time (PTT) can be determined. This test is a sensitive, reliable indicator of the integrity of the entire so-called intrinsic pathway of normal blood coagulation and is vastly superior to the clotting time as a screening test for the presence or absence of a coagulopathy. The PTT has a normal range of 22 to 37 seconds. It is abnormally prolonged in patients with clotting disorders due to liver disease or vitamin K deficiency, in those receiving heparin or coumadin anticoagulants, and in those in whom a "consumption coagulopathy" develops in association with defibrination-fibrinolysis syndromes secondary to disseminated intravascular coagulation. Of special interest to the gynecologist among the disorders that can produce the latter situation are gram-negative endotoxemic shock (as is encountered with septic abortion), retained dead fetus syndrome, and incompatible blood transfusion reaction. Rarely, the PTT is slightly elevated in patients with von Willebrand's disease.

Comment

If these three screening tests are normal, the likelihood of a general hemorrhagic disorder is completely ruled out. The other commonly employed battery of tests (e.g., capillary fragility test, clotting time, clot retraction, prothrombin time) rarely if ever add any useful information and are often unnecessary.

(*Note:* The prothrombin time remains useful for monitoring anticoagulant therapy with either heparin or coumadin. Rarely, clotting time determinations are helpful for monitoring heparin therapy in patients with disseminated intravascular coagulopathy, as with this disorder the PTT and prothrombin times are abnormal and are useless as monitoring indexes.)

TESTS FOR EVALUATION OF ENDOCRINE STATUS

From the standpoint of gynecologic diagnosis, determination of the steroid hormones normally produced by the ovary, i.e., estrogen and progesterone (or their urinary metabolites), is obviously of greatest concern. However, because disorders of adrenal function frequently have a profound effect on ovarian physiology as well, and because the ovary under certain circumstances can also be the site of formation of both adrenal steroids and androgens, it is usually important to be able to obtain as complete a measurement of the steroid hormone pattern as possible. It is particularly true when abnormalities of steroid metabolism in either ovary or adrenal, or both, are suspected. Currently available assays of steroid hormones for routine use have become increasingly useful and valuable for both the diagnosis and the clinical management of patients, as well as in the research investigation of the various diseases and biochemical mechanisms involved.

Although biochemically separable, the four principal types of steroid compounds—estrogens, progesterone, androgens, corticoids—are interrelated in a somewhat complicated fashion. Interpretation of the results of urinary steroid hormone assays is therefore sometimes fraught with difficulty and often provides only limited information about the exact nature of the physiologic disturbance in the patient. These difficulties result from the facts that (1) only one of the four main steroid-secreting glands (ovary, testis, adrenal cortex, placenta) may produce any or all of the four principal types of steroid hormone; and (2) interconversion among the four principal and chemically separable types of steroid compound frequently takes place during their catabolism and excretion. Thus simple measurement of the urinary excretion products is not invariably an index of the original nature and biologic activity of the steroid hormones being secreted or of the organ or type of glandular tissue in which they were initially produced. Combined with these factors are the difficulty of obtaining a complete 24-hour urine collection and the ready availability of specific radioimmunoassays for estrogens, progesterone, and androgens and glucocorticoids in serum or plasma.

Cervical Mucus Arborization Test (Fern Test)

Arborization or the formation of fern patterns in dried cervical mucus depends on the presence in cervical secretions of sodium chloride and other electrolytes, together with various protein substances in certain definite proportions. Because control over these proportions appears to be exerted exclusively by ovarian steroid hormones through their effects on the secretory activities of the endocervical glands, the presence or absence of fern patterns at any given moment is directly dependent on the ovarian hormonal status of the patient at that particular time. Cervical mucus ferning is seen in its typical form only when adequate amounts of estrogen are available. Maximum ferning is seen after exposure to adequate estrogens and when their levels reach a peak, usually during the preovulatory estrogen rise prior to ovulation. Progesterone inhibits or completely abolishes cervical mucus ferning even in the presence of sufficient estrogen. Minor variations (atypical fern patterns) are also recognizable in the presence of fluctuations in the relative amounts of estrogen and progesterone that may occur during a normal menstrual cycle, in patients with ovarian dysfunction, and during pregnancy. Because of its direct correlation with ovarian hormone levels, particularly estrogen, the fern test has proved useful for qualitative evaluation of ovarian function.

The test, easily performed in the office or clinic, is carried out as follows: After the cervix is exposed and gently swabbed clean, a sample of endocervical mucus is obtained with a dry sterile plastic cannula or glass pipet and is spread on a clean glass slide. If the secretion is spread too thinly or if blood is present, arborization does not occur, even when adequate estrogen levels exist. The slide is air-dried for at least 10 to 20 minutes (drying must be absolutely complete) and then is read under both low- and high-power magnification on the microscope. If true arborization with crystallization is present, it is indicative of a predominant estrogen effect, and the test is positive (Fig. 2-5, left). If a cellular pattern without crystallization and arborization is seen (Fig. 2-5, right), the test is negative and indicates either little or no estrogen effect or, more commonly, suppression of estrogen activity by progesterone. As an indirect quantification of the extent and intensity of estrogen effect, the cervical ferning can be graded according to the branching of the ferning pattern upon crystallization: grade 1 for primary branching, grade 2 for secondary branching, grade 3 for tertiary branching, and grade 4 for quarternary branching, the maximum observable.

Diagnostic Uses

OVULATION. Within a few days, ovulation and the production of progesterone by the corpus luteum normally result in a shift from the positive fern test characteristic of the preovulatory phase to a negative test typical of the latter half of the menstrual cycle. Therefore this simple office procedure can be employed as an index of ovulation and normal corpus luteum function. Because both low estrogen levels and chronic endocervicitis may lead to a continually negative test throughout the cycle, at least two tests must be done, one during each half of the cycle, for a valid conclusion to be reached.

POSTCOITAL TEST. Cervical mucus ferning is an integral part of the postcoital test (Chap. 13), as it is carried out around ovulation. A characteristically positive ferning test with adequate amount of cervical mucus indicates not only good estrogen effects but also correct timing of the postcoital test.

PREGNANCY. A positive fern test in a woman who has recently missed her period would strongly favor

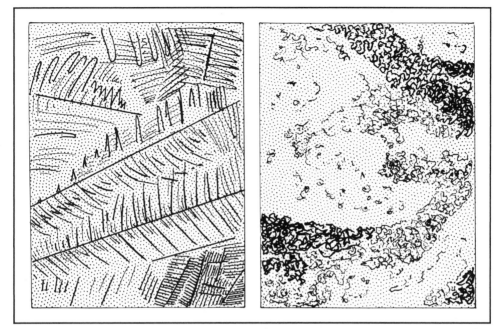

Fig. 2-5. Cervical mucus arborization tests (Fern test). The Fern phenomenon indicates good estrogen effect on the left; a progesterone effect (or lack of, or failure of the cervix to respond to estrogen) is shown at the right.

an anovulatory cycle (predominant estrogen effect) with a delay in onset of flow and would argue against the existence of pregnancy. A negative test can be consistent with pregnancy but not absolutely diagnostic unless a previous test showing arborization had been done during the first half of the same menstrual cycle.

DISORDERS OF EARLY PREGNANCY. Patients with persistence or reappearance of cervical mucus ferning during early pregnancy were found to have a high incidence of abortion. Such a change in the fern test may reflect the development of a progesterone inadequacy, but dependence on such a qualitative test has been rapidly replaced with more direct measurements of hormones (human chorionic gonadotropin, estrogen, progesterone) and ultrasonography.

Endometrial Biopsy

The ease with which a sample of endometrium can usually be obtained for histologic study is of tremen-

dous help in the office evaluation and management of a variety of pelvic disorders. With menstrual disturbances and infertility, two outstanding examples, endometrial biopsy nearly always proves useful and informative. When performing endometrial biopsy, one should ensure that the patient is not pregnant and that she does not have active pelvic inflammatory disease. The biopsy is performed after bimanual examination, which has ascertained the size, shape, and position (anteverted versus midplane or retroverted) of the uterus.

The cervix is exposed by speculum, and the external os is swabbed free of mucus and painted with povidone-iodine (Betadine) solution. The anterior cervical lip is then grasped with a tenaculum a slight distance from the external cervical os. A uterine sound is passed to determine the length and direction of the cervical canal and endometrial cavity. The patient is warned to expect slight discomfort similar to a menstrual cramp. To obviate or reduce the discomfort from the uterine contraction and cramp, the patient can be given a prostaglandin synthetase inhibitor such as ibuprofen 400 mg or sodium naproxen 275 mg orally 15 to 20 minutes before the procedure. A curved

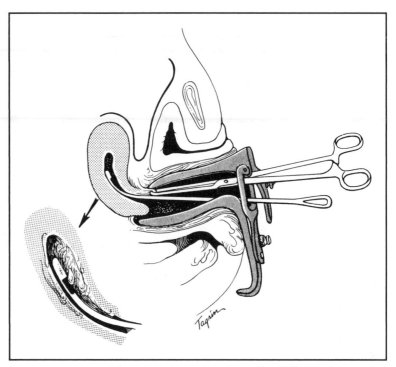

Fig. 2-6. Endometrial biopsy. A small curet is passed into the endometrial cavity, after which samples of the endometrium may be obtained by curettage or aspiration (inset).

endometrial biopsy curet, e.g., a Novak's curet, is introduced to the top of the fundus (Fig. 2-6). The curet is pressed firmly against the wall of the fundus anteriorly, posteriorly, or laterally and is then withdrawn, the cupped, spoonlike end removing a strip of endometrium.

A variety of endometrial sampling devices are available that provide a portion of endometrium. This sample is then fixed in formalin and processed routinely as a surgical pathology specimen, allowing evaluation of tissue architecture. These endometrial sampling devices function either as a small sharp curet or as a suction aspirator of endometrial tissue. The two methods are equal in terms of accuracy of diagnosis and are similar in potential for risks and complications. Therefore gynecologists usually select one method of endometrial biopsy for their office procedures and perform it routinely.

Details of the recent menstrual history should always accompany the pathology laboratory requisition, which should request endometrial dating if it is for evaluation of infertility. A histologic diagnosis of

proliferative or secretory endometrium by the pathologist is only partially informative because on the basis of certain histologic criteria the endometrium can be reliably dated during the luteal phase of the cycle. This "dating" must then be compared against the known day of the patient's current cycle, which should, however, be calculated backward from the actual day of the forthcoming menstrual flow.

Endometrial biopsy is most often utilized as an index of ovulation and progesterone effect in the course of an infertility investigation or as an aid in the diagnosis and further management of dysfunctional (anovulatory) bleeding. Obviously, biopsy must be performed during the immediate premenstrual phase or on the first day of menstruation to be of any help in either situation. Endometrial biopsy is also diagnostically useful in patients suspected of harboring endometrial cancer; a positive report facilitates the diagnosis, but a negative report is of little value and does not alter the need for diagnostic curettage in women with symptoms suggestive of this lesion.

Spotting after an endometrial biopsy may be present for a day or so but is usually not severe. A more serious complication of endometrial biopsy is uterine perforation. If the uterus is perforated in the midline, the myometrium of the uterine wall usually contracts and minimizes bleeding. Observation without surgical intervention is usually all that is necessary. Because of the potential for bacteremia induced by endometrial or endocervical biopsy, patients with cardiac valvular disease should receive prophylactic perioperative antibiotics to reduce the possibility of subacute bacterial endocarditis.

Fertility Evaluation

The postcoital cervical mucous test and the basal body temperature (BBT) chart are discussed in Chapter 13.

OFFICE TESTS FOR EARLY PREGNANCY

There are several office tests useful for the *presumptive diagnosis of early pregnancy* during the month immediately following the first missed period, at a time when the diagnosis is usually impossible on the basis of physical examination alone. Not all the tests are diagnostic.

Basal Body Temperature Chart

If the basal body temperature chart shows a typical biphasic ovulatory temperature curve, the temperature remains elevated after the first missed period, and an anovulatory cycle has been completely ruled out as a cause of the delayed period, pregnancy is essentially certain. This method probably represents the earliest means by which a diagnosis of pregnancy can be made with certainty. Conception while the patient is maintaining a record of her basal body temperature curve occurs fairly often during the course of an infertility investigation.

Cervical Mucus Test

Although the cervical mucus test yields indirect or circumstantial evidence only, as previously noted in this chapter, it can be fairly reliable. It is highly so if a preovulatory test in the same cycle had been done and showed a typical fern pattern that subsequently disappeared completely and remained suppressed.

Progesterone Withdrawal Test

The progesterone withdrawal test was once frequently used to distinguish between a pregnant and a nonpregnant cycle, but potential medical-legal problems have caused it to be used mainly in conjunction with a negative pregnancy (human chorionic gonadotropin) test. The progesterone test involves the administration of progesterone, either orally (10 to 20 mg daily for five days) or intramuscularly (100 mg in a single dose) in women with a history of normal, regular cycles whose regular period is overdue. If the missed period is not due to a pregnancy and there has been adequate exposure of the endometrium to estrogen, the administration of progesterone results in the onset of flow, usually within the next two to four days, the progesterone acting to produce endometrial maturation followed by withdrawal bleeding as the progesterone effect subsides. If the missed period is due to early pregnancy, no progesterone withdrawal flow occurs. Because the woman could be in early pregnancy, it is prudent to use the intramuscular progesterone injection rather than synthetic oral progestins.

SPECIAL LABORATORY PROCEDURES

Pregnancy Tests

Laboratory tests for pregnancy are based on the detection of chorionic gonadotropin in urine or serum. Human chorionic gonadotropin (hCG) is secreted by the syncytiotrophoblasts of the placenta mainly into the maternal circulation. Previously, a variety of bioassay techniques employing laboratory animals (mice, rats, rabbits, frogs, toads) were widely used. The biologic tests depended on the response of the ovaries or testes in immature animals (e.g., frogs, toads, and rats) to hCG. An increase in gonadal weight or hyperemia, or a response observed in the secondary sex organs due to increased gonadal steroidogenesis, were measured as endpoints. However, these tests have been replaced by immunologic tests that directly detect hCG.

Most previous immunologic tests involved use of a latex particle preparation sensitized to hCG, together with a standardized hCG antiserum. Based on an agglutination inhibition reaction, the test is carried out on a freshly voided morning urine specimen, and the results of the standard laboratory test-tube procedure are usually available within 2 to 3 hours. Simple and fairly accurate latex agglutination inhibition immunologic slide tests that can be performed in 2 minutes in the physician's office are commercially available, e.g., Gravindex Slide Test for Pregnancy (Lederle Diagnostics) and UCG-Slide Test (Wampole Laboratories). These slide tests are not as accurate as the 2-hour test-tube laboratory procedures, however. The immunologic tests for pregnancy have a precision and reliability equal to, if not greater than, that of any of the biologic tests and are much more easily and rapidly performed. The sensitivity of the immunologic test is such that it is often positive as early as four to five days after the first missed menstrual period. With the newer tests available employing more specific anti-hCG antiserum, including monoclonal antibodies, positive results are obtained even earlier, at the time of the expected period. Currently, a radioimmunoassay method for detecting and quantifying the hCG levels present in the plasma or serum is usually employed in most major medical centers for determination of early pregnancy and its viability, monitoring threatened abortion, evaluation and management of a suspected ectopic pregnancy, and diagnosis and monitoring of therapy of patients with trophoblastic disease (hydatidiform mole and choriocarcinoma).

Radioimmunoassay. The radioimmunoassay method is based on the competition for antiserum to hCG between a known amount of radioactive iodine-labeled hCG and the unlabeled hCG present in the sample (serum or urine) to be tested. By plotting a standard curve in which the sample to be tested is replaced with fixed increasing amounts of unlabeled standard hCG, the actual amount of hCG present in the sample

(serum) tested can be calculated. Thus with the radioimmunoassay of hCG, the actual hCG titers can be determined in the biologic fluid tested. The specificity of the test is further increased by the use of antiserum raised against the beta-subunit of hCG, which has an amino acid sequence distinctly different from those of follicle-stimulating hormone (FSH), luteinizing hormone (LH), and thyroid-stimulating hormone (TSH). It provides further reliability to the radioimmunoassay using the antiserum to beta-subunit of hCG for detecting low levels of hCG, which must be discriminated from the normal menstrual cycle levels of FSH and LH. The test is sensitive, with the reliable limits of detection for hCG currently down to about 3 to 5 mIU/ml when the specific antiserum is used. The development and availability of monoclonal antibody (see below) to the beta-subunit of hCG has further accentuated the specificity of the radioimmunoassays for hCG.

During the 1970s the radioreceptor assay of hCG seemed full of promise. This test is essentially similar to the radioimmunoassay but with the antiserum to hCG replaced by bovine luteal cell membrane receptors to hCG-LH. Because the radioreceptor assay of hCG could be rapidly performed (around 2 hours or so) and antiserum specific to hCG was in limited supply for routine clinical use, the radioreceptor assay offered a reliable and rapid method of determining hCG. However, the widespread commercial availability of antiserum specific to hCG, the improvement in radioimmunoassay methods, and the relative lack of specificity for hCG by the radioreceptor assay have rendered the radioreceptor assay for hCG no longer a method of choice for clinical practice.

When interpreting the results of these tests and applying them to specific clinical problems, it is important to note the following points.

1. The standard immunologic latex agglutination inhibition tests can be relied on for definitely positive or negative evidence of pregnancy ten to fourteen days after the first missed menstrual period. However, the hCG radioimmunoassay using the antiserum against the beta-subunit of hCG detects hCG in the blood nine to eleven days after the LH peak or seven to nine days after ovulation, corresponding to the time

shortly after implantation. At the time of the missed period, the serum hCG level is about 100 mIU/ml. Therefore radioimmunoassay for hCG is almost 100 percent accurate at around the time of the missed period, whereas most agglutination inhibition tests performed at this time carry a high rate of false-negative and inconclusive results. The latex agglutination inhibition test is a *qualitative* test for hCG, giving a positive or negative result, whereas the radioimmunoassay test is a *quantitative* test for hCG and therefore gives the actual level or titer of hCG present.

2. The chorionic gonadotropin level rises rapidly after implantation until a peak level of about 100,000 mIU/ml is reached at the tenth or twelfth week of pregnancy, when it may again fall rapidly, reaching levels only one-tenth of its peak titers, after the twentieth week. Therefore, depending on the sensitivity of the test employed, negative results are obtained occasionally after the fifth or sixth month of pregnancy.

3. Quantitative determination of hCG using radioimmunoassay can provide endocrine information on the viability or even abnormality of a gestation. During the first or second trimesters of pregnancy: (a) Abnormally low levels may indicate the likelihood of impending abortion; early in pregnancy, they may indicate the possibility of an ectopic gestation. (b) Abnormally high levels suggest the presence of hydatidiform mole, choriocarcinoma, or occasionally multiple pregnancy.

4. A urinary pregnancy test may still be positive three weeks after abortion. Prolonged persistence of positive tests four to six weeks after delivery or abortion indicates the likelihood of either retained placental tissue, mole, or a chorionic tumor of some type; and it requires determination of serum hCG titers, serially if necessary.

5. False-positive biologic and rarely even false-positive immunologic pregnancy tests are occasionally observed in patients who have pelvic inflammatory disease or who are receiving phenothiazine compounds such as chorpromazine, promethazine hydrochloride, and similar tranquilizers and antidepressants. It is believed that the neuroendocrine effects of these drugs result in increased production of pituitary gonadotropins, which cross-react with the antiserum for hCG. This situation can be avoided if a specific or monoclonal antibody raised against the beta-subunit of hCG is employed.

Serum hCG titer measured by radioimmunoassay using specific antiserum raised against the beta-subunit of hCG has proved to be a valuable adjunct for the diagnostic evaluation and management of ectopic pregnancy and for monitoring therapy for trophoblastic disease. Almost all patients suspected of having an ectopic pregnancy have a positive serum hCG titer by radioimmunoassay, albeit low for the gestational age, whereas those not having an ectopic pregnancy and who are not pregnant have a negative hCG level. In normal pregnancies and in some initially viable ectopic pregnancies, hCG titers may be normal but increase at different rates. In a normal viable intrauterine pregnancy, serum hCG titers double every two to three days. A serum hCG titer above 6000 mIU/ml is usually associated with an intrauterine pregnancy.

Serum hCG titers combined with ultrasonography have aided decision-making about proceeding to laparoscopy in a woman suspected of having an ectopic pregnancy but with a negative culdocentesis for nonclotting blood. Failure to identify an intrauterine pregnancy on abdominal sonography and a serum hCG titer well below 6000 mIU/ml but doubling every two days indicates that expectant management is appropriate; if the hCG does not double every two days, laparoscopy is indicated. With transvaginal ultrasonography (Chap. 3), the intrauterine gestational sac is visible at hCG titers of 1000 to 1600 mIU/ml usually around 5 weeks from the last menstrual period and certainly by 6 weeks. Again, failure to double the hCG titer warrants laparoscopy in the absence of an intrauterine sac. It should be remembered that the absolute levels of hCG used for such discrimination should be derived for each particular laboratory as values may differ slightly from one laboratory to another.

The increased sensitivity of and earlier detection by transvaginal sonography combined with sensitive, specific radioimmunoassays for hCG titers have enabled earlier and earlier detection of ectopic pregnancy. Both test methods are increasingly being used for nonoperative, medical treatment of ectopic pregnancy using methotrexate (Chap. 16). With such medical treatment, serial serum hCG titers are monitored to observe the reduction in and final nondetectability of hCG titers.

Serial measurements of serum hCG titers, especially when they fall to low levels, have become possible in the management of patients with trophoblastic disease, as the radioimmunoassay employing specific antiserum to beta-subunit of hCG became available. Such increased sensitivity and specificity of hCG titers have assisted in deciding when to stop chemotherapy and pronounced remission or cure. It is the rate of regression of serum hCG titers as well as the pattern that indicate the response of the disease to therapy and when to intervene (Chap. 30).

Monoclonal Antibodies. Produced by the B lymphocytes of bone marrow, spleen, and lymph nodes, monoclonal antibodies are highly specific and homogeneous in contrast to the heterogeneous antibodies found in antiserum from regular immunization. The latter is sometimes referred to as polyclonal antibodies. Monoclonal antibodies are produced by injecting an animal (usually the rat) with the antigen. Cells from the spleen or B lymphocytes of the animal after it has formed antibodies are then fused with a tumor cell line (e.g., a myeloma cell line) to form hybridoma cells. Because the tumor cell line can continue to grow in culture indefinitely, monoclonal antibodies continue to be produced by the hybridoma clones and can be continuously harvested from the culture medium. Although monoclonal antibodies are highly specific and therefore useful for hormone assays when great specificity is required to distinguish structurally almost identical hormones or substances, this property is a limitation in some situations. Monoclonal antibodies are not only being used for diagnostic measurements of hormones and tumor markers, they also offer promise as a potential "specific bullet" on which chemotherapeutic agents can be launched in the therapy of malignancies in a directed and targeted manner.

Enzyme-Linked Immunosorbent Assay. To obviate the need for expensive radioactive counters, large laboratory spaces, and handling of radioactive compounds, other assay techniques that are sensitive are being developed. The enzyme-linked immunosorbent assay (ELISA) is a "sandwich" technique that does not require use of radioactive tracers and can be employed for measuring many hormones. It is being used increasingly for measurement of hCG and other hormones. Instead of the radioactive tracer, an enzyme (often horseradish peroxidase) is employed that provides a color endpoint read by a spectrophotometer. For hCG and other glycopeptide hormones (FSH, LH, TSH), two monoclonal antibodies are employed, one against the alpha-subunit (coupled to a bead or plastic tube) and the other against the beta-subunit (coupled to the enzyme). The alpha-subunit end of the intact glycopeptide hormone molecule binds to the alpha-subunit antibody–bead complex. The beta-subunit antibody–enzyme complex then binds the exposed end of the beta-subunit of the glycopeptide hormone, which is now completely sandwiched. This action results in the bead or the plastic tube having enzyme connected to it via the sandwich. The color change is then read. Such assays can be safely performed in a small space or laboratory in a physician's office or in the clinic with little equipment. However, precision and meticulous care are necessary to avoid spurious or undependable results.

Pituitary Gonadotropins

Pituitary production and secretion of LH and FSH are responsible for development of the graafian follicles in the ovary and secretion of estrogen by the follicular cells. Development of radioimmunoassays for determining FSH and LH levels in tiny amounts of blood have provided data of increasing significance to our understanding of the normal and abnormal menstrual cycles as well as for identification and management of specific disturbances in the pituitary-gonadal axis of both women and men.

The radioimmunoassay method for the quantitative measurement of LH is similar to the one developed for hCG (see above), except LH replaces hCG for each of the reagents. The antiserum used is usually raised against LH and therefore cross-reacts and detects hCG as well. Consequently, if the antiserum employed is against LH, caution must be exercised if a high level of LH is detected in a woman who has amenorrhea, as she could be pregnant (early). In the nonpregnant woman, the LH levels obtained are reliable. The specificity of the LH radioimmunoassay can be further greatly improved if the antiserum is raised against the beta-subunit to LH. This immunologic test is specific and accurate, and its increasing use has served to confirm its simplicity, reliability, and accuracy for routine clinical use. Its sensitivity and precision appear to be considerably greater than reported for all other methods that detect and quantitate LH.

Similarly, the FSH radioimmunoassay employs an antiserum raised against FSH and radioiodine-labeled FSH. Because antisera to LH and FSH are now highly specific for their individual polypeptide hormones, chromatographic separation of the sample to be measured is not necessary, and whole serum can be used directly for the assay. The normal levels for serum FSH and LH in women and the clinical states that give rise to elevated or depressed levels are summarized in Table 2-1.

Prolactin

Prolactin, a polypeptide hormone with 191 amino acids and 161 of the amino acids similar to those of growth hormone, is produced and secreted by the lactotrophs situated in the ventrolateral aspect of the lobes of the anterior pituitary gland. Prolactin secretion in women is under the control of dopaminergic tone in the hypothalamus and thyrotropin-releasing hormone (TRH). Unlike the gonadotropins, prolactin secretion is under the inhibitory control of prolactin-inhibiting factor (PIF) from the hypothalamus. In the absence of isolation of PIF in women, it appears that dopamine acts as a PIF, whereas TRH stimulates not only thyrotropin but also prolactin. With the availability of specific radioimmunoassays, prolactin can be readily measured in the plasma or serum.

The mean normal serum prolactin level in nonpregnant women is about 20 ng/ml. It is slightly lower in prepubertal children, with a progressive rise during sleep and a modest rise following ingestion of food, especially a protein-laden meal. Pregnancy, lactation, stress, and massaging the breasts can also produce elevated prolactin levels. Therefore repetitive or stressful venipuncture to obtain blood or taking blood samples following breast massage can potentially elevate the levels of prolactin obtained.

Serum prolactin determinations are especially useful and indicated in women with amenorrhea, oligomenorrhea, ovulatory dysfunction, galactorrhea, suspected pituitary tumors, hypothyroidism, and elevated serum thyrotropin (TSH). Women with galactorrhea and amenorrhea have as much as a 70 percent incidence of elevated serum prolactin, and in those with amenorrhea alone it is as high as 40 to 50 percent. Ingestion of a wide variety of medications, especially the tricyclic antidepressants, chlorpromazine, haloperidol, reserpine, and the phenothiazines, can elevate serum prolactin. Because of some of the physiologic factors that can elevate serum prolactin, it is best to obtain blood for this test in the morning with the patient fasting or, at most, having had only clear liquids. With properly obtained samples and properly performed prolactin measurements, elevated levels indicate the need to rule out a prolactinoma (prolactin-secreting pituitary tumor) in the absence of a physiologic cause. The serum prolactin level is also used to monitor response to therapy in the management of prolactinomas or pituitary tumors pressing on the hypothalamohypophyseal portal circulation.

Table 2-1. Serum Levels of FSH and LH in Normal Women and Those with Disturbances of the Pituitary-Gonadal Axis

Specific clinical diagnosis	Serum FSH (mIU/ml)	Serum LH (mIU/ml)
Normal adult women		
Follicular or luteal phase	5–20	5–20
Midcycle surge	15–40	15–40
Hypergonadotropic women		
Menopause		
Bilateral oophorectomy	>40	>40
Ovarian failure		
Hypogonadotropic stage		
Prepuberty		
Hypothalamic dysfunction	< 5	< 5
Hypopituitarism		

Blood Steroids

Because of the problems of hormone determination in the urine, it is preferable to measure these hormones by radioimmunoassay in small volumes of blood. Almost all steroid hormones—including the three principal estrogens (estrone, estradiol, estriol), progesterone, 17α-hydroxyprogesterone, androgens (testosterone, free testosterone, dihydrotestosterone, androstenedione, dehydroepiandrosterone sulfate, and dehydroepiandrosterone), cortisol, aldosterone, and deoxycorticosterone—can be measured by radioimmunoassay with specificity and sensitivity. Most of these steroids have antisera that are highly specific. Unlike the larger peptide hormones, e.g., gonadotropins and prolactin, the steroids are small, nonprotein, and not immunogenic.

When conjugated to a larger protein such as bovine serum albumin, steroids become antigenic and are then able to stimulate an antibody response. Depending on where the protein is tagged onto the steroid molecule, as well as the structural similarity or differences of the steroid molecule, the antibody is either highly specific with little or no cross-reaction or it has considerable cross-reaction to structurally similar steroids. If the antiserum is highly specific, chromatographic separation of the steroids extracted in the plasma or serum is not necessary; otherwise the plasma extract is chromatographically separated, usually on Sephadex or Celite minicolumns, prior to actual measurement of the steroid. The radioimmunoassay of most steroids can detect as little as 5 pg per milliliter.

Most of the radioactively labeled steroids are tritiated (^{3}H); and because tritium counting requires liquid scintillation, the assay cannot be performed directly on unextracted plasma or serum. Many of the steroids, particularly estrogens, progesterone, and testosterone, have now been successfully radiolabeled with iodine, making it possible to measure these hormones in plasma or serum without extraction because many of the antisera employed are highly specific. Thus the radioimmunoassays of steroid hormones are not only highly specific but also sensitive.

The radioimmunoassay of plasma estradiol has replaced the urinary estrogen determination in the nonpregnant woman, and the plasma estriol assay has replaced the urinary estriol assay in pregnant women.

Plasma 17-hydroxyprogesterone assay has replaced urinary pregnanetriol determinations, and the plasma progesterone assay has supplanted the assay for urinary pregnanediol, the main urinary metabolite of progesterone. Similarly, measurement of plasma dehydroepiandrosterone sulfate (DHEAS) has replaced that for urinary 17-ketosteroids for evaluation of adrenal androgen production, and direct assays for plasma testosterone provide direct data. Plasma cortisol can be assayed in place of urinary cortisol, but the 24-hour urinary free cortisol assay remains a useful test, providing information regarding the total output from an endocrine gland in which there is diurnal rhythmicity. This diurnal variability is better demonstrated by measuring plasma cortisol or plasma free cortisol at 8 AM and 8 PM.

The normal levels for plasma estradiol, progesterone, 17-hydroxyprogesterone, and testosterone in women are summarized in Table 2-2. Of particular note are the differences in normal ranges during the various phases of the menstrual cycle with respect to estradiol, progesterone, and 17-hydroxyprogesterone.

Estradiol

Plasma estradiol assay is usually performed for evaluation of ovarian function and is therefore indicated in women suspected of having premature gonadal failure; during the menopause if diagnostic confirmation is needed; monitoring of follicle recruitment and timing of hCG administration during ovulation induction with human menopausal gonadotropin, human follicle stimulating hormone, or gonadotropin-releasing hormone; amenorrhea with a negative progesterone withdrawal test; patients with clinical evidence of inappropriately normal or excess estrogen levels that could be coming from an estrogen-producing ovarian tumor (granulosa cell tumor; Chap. 18).

Progesterone and 17-Hydroxyprogesterone

Progesterone is produced primarily by the corpus luteum after ovulation and during early pregnancy until the end of seven weeks from the last menstrual period when the placenta takes over and becomes the

Table 2-2. Normal Sex Steroid Hormone Levels in Women: Determined by Radioimmunoassay

Condition	Estradiol (ng/ml)	Progesterone (ng/ml)	17-Hydroxy-progesterone (ng/ml)	Testosterone (ng/ml)	Dehydroepi-androsterone sulfate (ng/ml)
Menstrual cycle					
Follicular phase	35–100 pg/ml	<1	0.15–0.70	0.2–0.8	1250–1950
Midcycle peak	200–600 pg/ml	1–2	0.15–0.70	0.2–0.8	1250–1950
Luteal phase	90–220 pg/ml	5–25	0.4–3.0	0.2–0.8	1250–1950
Pregnancy					
First trimester	1–5	25–40	2–3		
Second trimester	1–15	50–100	2–3		
Third trimester	10–40	100–300	3–6		
Postmenopausal women	5–30	<1	0.2–0.7	0.1–0.4	230–370
Children (female)	5–30	<1	0.03–0.90	0.1–0.4	

Note: Variations in the normal ranges may vary from laboratory to laboratory, the assay kits employed, and the specificity of the antisera used.

principal source. The urinary metabolite of progesterone is pregnanediol. Urinary pregnanediol assays have been completely replaced by radioimmunoassay of progesterone in the plasma or serum. The principal indication for measuring plasma progesterone is to evaluate ovulation during the luteal phase and less frequently to evaluate early pregnancy. A plasma level of 4 to 5 ng per milliliter indicates the presence of a corpus luteum and is therefore presumptive evidence of ovulation. For assessing the luteal phase and specifically the luteal phase defect, plasma progesterone performed on days 19, 21, and 23 (midluteal phase) should have individual levels well above 10 ng per milliliter (it may vary from laboratory to laboratory). Alternatively, equal volumes of plasma from each of the three days, when pooled, reduce it to a single test, thereby reducing cost. The progesterone level should still be more than 10 ng per milliliter. Because of the large day-to-day variability in plasma progesterone and a subnormal level in the presence of threatened abortion, plasma progesterone by itself does not have much to offer for the diagnosis of early pregnancy disorder. A normal value would certainly be reassuring, but a low value is not clinically conclusive.

Plasma 17-hydroxyprogesterone is secreted by the corpus luteum in adult cycling women but is clinically not used to assess luteal function. It is used to evaluate congenital adrenal hyperplasia and specifically to diagnose 21-hydroxylase deficiency, when plasma 17-progesterone levels are 5 to 50 times those obtained during the luteal phase (Table 2-2). In patients suspected of having a genetic variant or the heterozygous form of this enzyme deficiency, the ACTH test (see below) can be employed with plasma 17-hydroxyprogesterone replacing plasma cortisol; plasma 17-hydroxyprogesterone is significantly elevated compared to that in normal women. Plasma 17-hydroxyprogesterone assay has largely supplanted the assay for urinary pregnanetriol.

Androgens

The three principal androgens measured in plasma are testosterone, androstenedione, and dehydroepiandrosterone sulfate (DHEAS), all measured today by radioimmunoassay. Plasma androgen assays are indicated in women presenting with hirsutism or virilization, ambiguous external genitalia, or testicular feminization syndrome (elevated testosterone levels). In women, testosterone is derived from the adrenals (25 percent) and the ovaries (25 percent), and the rest from peripheral conversion of the weaker androgen, androstenedione. As a rule, androstenedione is largely of ovarian origin and DHEAS of adrenal origin in the premenopausal women. In cases of elevated levels of plasma testosterone, androstenedione, and DHEAS, the source of the increased androgen can be rapidly but not invariably narrowed to the ovary or the adrenal. With the dexamethasone suppression test (see below), suppression of testosterone and DHEAS markedly suggests an adrenal source, whereas an absence of suppression suggests an ovarian origin. Like plasma cortisol, there is a diurnal variation in plasma DHEAS, and blood is therefore obtained preferably at 8 to 9 AM. Normal levels of DHEAS and androstenedione are given in Table 2-2.

Plasma testosterone may be elevated in patients with hirsutism; but irrespective of any elevation, clinical evidence of hirsutism or virilization clearly indicates either current or recent exposure to high levels of androgens, increased end-organ sensitivity to androgens, or both. Nevertheless, the purpose of measuring plasma testosterone and other androgens is to rule out an androgen-producing tumor (Chap. 18). Plasma testosterone levels of 2 ng per milliliter are suggestive of a testosterone-producing tumor (arrhenoblastoma, lipoid cell tumor, hilar cell tumor), but high levels are also seen with severe polycystic ovarian disease. Levels below 2 ng per milliliter are less likely to be due to a tumor.

**Urinary 17-Ketosteroids and
17-Hydroxycorticosteroids**

Urinary excretion of the various metabolites of 17-ketosteroids, 17-hydroxycorticosteroids, testosterone, and other related androgens constitute the basis for measurement of 24-hour urinary 17-ketosteroids and 17-hydroxycorticosteroids. These assays have been largely supplanted by assays for plasma testosterone, androstenedione, and dehydroepiandrosterone sulfate, and for plasma cortisol and deoxycorticosterone, respectively. Nevertheless urinary 17-ketosteroids, 17-ketogenic steroids, and 17-hydroxycorticosteroids can provide useful and essential clinical information occasionally not provided by the direct plasma hormone assays.

Urinary 17-ketosteroids are measured by a colorimetric assay not involving radioactivity that detects the major urinary androgenic metabolites (usually the neutral 17-ketosteroids) but not testosterone itself. Therefore patients with elevated plasma testosterone levels can still have normal 24-hour urinary 17-ketosteroids. The normal level of urinary 17-ketosteroids in women is 10 ± 3 mg per 24 hours, but it changes with age. Measurement of urinary 17-ketosteroids reflects and has been largely replaced by plasma DHEAS assay.

Assays for urinary 17-ketogenic steroids and 17-hydroxycorticosteroids measure urinary metabolites of glucocorticoids, but the assay for 17-ketogenic steroids measures more metabolites. Mineralocorticoids such as deoxycorticosterone and aldosterone are not picked up by these two urinary tests. The normal levels of urinary 17-hydroxycorticosteroids is 7 ± 3 mg per 24 hours. The assay for urinary 17-hydroxycorticosteroids is similar to and has been largely replaced by the plasma cortisol assay.

Urinary 17-ketogenic steroids assay measures steroid compounds that are oxidized to 17-ketosteroids by sodium bismuthate. The resulting total 17-ketosteroids measured minus the initial 17-ketosteroids measured gives the 17-ketogenic steroids determined. The normal urinary levels of 17-ketogenic steroids is 10 ± 3 mg per 24 hours. The urinary 17-ketogenic steroids assay approximates and has been replaced by plasma cortisol and 17-hydroxyprogesterone assays.

ADRENAL FUNCTION TESTS

In addition to plasma 17-hydroxyprogesterone, which is markedly elevated with some forms of congenital adrenal hyperplasia and plasma androgens, several other tests are useful for evaluating the adrenal gland as it affects the practice of gynecology.

Urinary Free Cortisol

The 24-hour urinary free cortisol assay reflects the daily production and secretion rate of free cortisol, which is not protein-bound and is therefore the active and readily available form. The normal 24-hour urinary excretion of free cortisol is 20 to 90 μg. An increase in this urinary free cortisol output is seen with Cushing's disease, cortisol-secreting adrenal tumors, and adrenocortical hyperactivity. Conversely, a decrease in 24-hour urinary free cortisol levels suggests adrenal hypofunction, as is seen with Addison's disease, hypopituitarism, or bilateral adrenalectomy.

Blood Cortisol

Plasma cortisol (both bound and free) and free cortisol levels can be readily measured by specific radioimmunoassays. Cortisol in the blood is bound to corticosteroid-binding globulin (CBG), which is increased by estrogen administration, oral contraceptives, and pregnancy. Thus free cortisol is a more sensitive and reliable marker of cortisol activity because it reflects only the active and available form in the circulation and is therefore not affected by changes in CBG levels. Free cortisol comprises 5 to 8 percent of the total cortisol. Normal levels of plasma free cortisol are 0.12 ng per deciliter at 8 AM and 0.02 ng per deciliter at 8 to 10 PM. Plasma free cortisol is elevated in Cushing's disease, but so is plasma total cortisol. However, because of the confounding variability introduced by CBG, the plasma free cortisol level is even more reliable. Because ACTH, which stimulates adrenal cortisol secretion, is secreted episodically with more frequent pulses of greater magnitude in the morning, blood levels of both ACTH and cortisol are highest in the early morning and lowest in the evening (diurnal variation). Normal levels of plasma cortisol at 8 AM is 10 to 25 μg per deciliter, at 8 PM about 5 to 12 μg per deciliter, and at 10 PM usually less than 12 μg per decliter. In Cushing's syndrome, there is loss of this diurnal variation or rhythmicity in plasma cortisol even before absolute levels of plasma cortisol are elevated. Therefore this test of diurnal variability of plasma cortisol (morning and evening, usually 8 AM and 8 PM) is especially useful in early cases of Cushing's syndrome when the symptoms may be bizarre.

ACTH Stimulation Test

The responsiveness of the adrenal glands to ACTH can be assessed by measuring plasma cortisol before and after the administration of ACTH. If the adrenal glands are functioning normally, there is an increase in plasma cortisol two to three times over the basal level 30 and 60 minutes after 250 μg of synthetic ACTH (Cortrosyn).

A subnormal response to the ACTH stimulation suggests poor adrenal reserve. Some cases of borderline Addison's disease may be detected this way. However, it should be noted that the ACTH stimulation test gives a subnormal response if the adrenals have not been exposed to ACTH for a long period of time (as in panhypopituitarism) or if the ACTH used was of poor quality and ineffective.

Dexamethasone Suppression Test

Glucocorticoids suppress ACTH secretion and thereby reduce the secretion of cortisol and its by-products. Therefore in the normal situation the adrenal and the anterior pituitary gland control each other through ACTH–cortisol–ACTH regulation. Temporary suppression of the adrenals by exogenous glucocorticoids has been employed as a test of adrenal function to evaluate the pituitary-adrenal system and to assess the contribution of the adrenal glands in the evaluation of hirsutism. Dexamethasone, a biologically potent glucocorticoid, is used to suppress pituitary secretion of ACTH.

Normally 0.5 mg dexamethasone is given every 6 hours for 48 hours. The plasma cortisol level falls to less than 5 μg per deciliter and the urinary 17-hydroxycorticosteroids fall to less than 2.5 mg per day. Similarly, if the source of androgens is predominantly the adrenals, testosterone and DHEAS are markedly suppressed. A modified and more rapid test is the overnight dexamethasone suppression test, when only 0.5 mg dexamethasone is given at 8 or 10 PM. Blood is obtained for the plasma cortisol assay before the dexamethasone is taken and at 8 AM the following day. Failure to suppress cortisol production with dexamethasone suggests adrenal hyperactivity due to hyperplasia or a functioning adrenal tumor.

Metyrapone Test

Metyrapone inhibits 11β-hydroxylase enzyme activity in the adrenal glands, thereby interfering with cortisol production. If the hypothalamo-pituitary-adrenal axis is intact and the hypothalamus and pituitary are functioning normally, metyrapone administration induces an increase in ACTH secretion, leading to a secondary rise in urinary 17-hydroxycorticosteroids and plasma 11-deoxycortisol. The test is an evaluation of ACTH reserve.

Metyrapone 750 mg is given orally every 4 hours for six doses. Normally, urinary 17-hydroxycorticosteroids at least double, compared to baseline, during the next day. Alternatively, plasma 11-deoxycortisol may be measured at 8 AM, 4 hours after the last dose of metyrapone; the level should not exceed 10 μg per deciliter. If the urinary 17-hydroxycorticosteroids response is reduced or plasma 11-deoxycortisol is not suppressed with metyrapone, the adrenocorticotropic hormone (ACTH) reserve is reduced.

Plasma ACTH

Plasma levels of ACTH can now be determined by radioimmunoassay. The normal levels in healthy adults is usually less than 50 pg per milliliter. There is a diurnal pattern of plasma ACTH, with the lowest levels between 6 and 11 PM, a rise during the morning hours, and a peak at 6 to 8 AM. Because ACTH is secreted in a pulsatile fashion, interpretation of the normal value is difficult. However, plasma ACTH levels (more than 1000 pg per milliliter) are useful for diagnosing primary hypoadrenocorticism, ectopic production of ACTH by tumor, and Cushing's disease after adrenalectomy.

THYROID FUNCTION TESTS

Thyroid dysfunction is most common in women during the reproductive years and can interfere with the normal functioning of the pituitary-ovarian axis. Therefore the gynecologist often encounters thyroid disorders through their presentation affecting the menstrual cycle and fertility. Hence an understanding of thyroid function tests is essential if one is to choose appropriate tests and then to interpret such tests.

For adequate thyroid hormone synthesis and therefore function, an adequate dietary supply of iodine is necessary. Absorbed as iodide in the small bowel, plasma iodide enters the thyroid gland under the regulation of thyroid-stimulating hormone (TSH) secreted by the anterior pituitary gland. TSH in turn is controlled by the tripeptide thyrotropin-releasing hormone (TRH), secreted by the hypothalamus. In the thyroid gland, iodide is oxidized back to iodine and bound to tyrosine. Combination of mono- and diiodo-

tyrosines produce thyroxine (T_4) and triiodothyronine (T_3). T_3 and T_4 are stored as part of thyroglobulin in a colloid form. TSH induces proteolysis of the stored complex, which releases iodothyronines as T_3 and T_4 into the blood, where thyroid hormones are then bound to thyroid-binding globulin (TBG).

Excess estrogen (as with estrogen therapy or during pregnancy) produces a rise in thyroid-binding globulin capacity. This point is important when evaluating thyroid function tests. Nevertheless, it is not the protein-bound thyroid hormone but the free thyroxine that is the critical determinant of the biologic effects of thyroid hormone and therefore normal function.

Interestingly, although T_4 is secreted 20 times faster than T_3—which is three to four times more potent, however, T_3 is responsible for most of the action of the thyroid hormones on target tissues. Because T_4 is more tightly bound to serum proteins and has a tenfold lesser affinity for nuclear receptors in the cells than T_3, T_4 accordingly exerts less effect than would be expected for its serum concentration. One-third of T_4 secreted daily is converted to T_3, mainly by the liver and kidneys, and 40 percent to the inactive reverse T_3. Therefore T_3 is not a true reflection of thyroid gland secretory function. Because T_4 plays a more critical role in TSH regulation, T_4 and TSH continue to be more reliable indices of thyroid gland function. Thus T_3 levels may be normal in a woman with goiter, whereas TSH levels are elevated and T_4 levels are depressed.

Although many thyroid function tests were done in the past and continue to be done at present, many are not necessary and add little to the evaluation and management of most patients seen by gynecologists. The current status of screening and evaluation of thyroid function revolves essentially around assays of free T_4, TSH, and T_3, each of which is measured by radioimmunoassay.

Thyroxine

Total thyroxine (T_4) (both free and protein-bound) and free T_4 determinations by radioimmunoassay have completely replaced the protein-bound iodine (PBI) and butanol-extractable idoine (BEI) assays because T_4 and free T_4 assays are not affected by changes in intake of inorganic iodides, mercurial diuretics, or iodine-containing contrast media used in diagnostic radiology. Nevertheless, total T_4 is still affected by changes in concentrations of thyroxine-binding globulin (TBG), just as in the case of both PBI and BEI; therefore it may be elevated (1) during pregnancy; (2) in patients taking estrogens, oral contraceptives, or phenothiazines; (3) in patients who have liver disease; and (4) in rare cases of congenital excess of TBG. Conversely, the T_4 level may be abnormally low in: (1) patients with severe liver failure, nephrotic syndrome, or congenital TBG deficiency; (2) patients receiving androgen or corticosteroid therapy; or (3) patients who are on large doses of diphenylhydantoin. Therefore free T_4, which is unaffected by these factors, is a more reliable test. Nevertheless, drugs taken orally for cholecystograms inhibit the peripheral conversion of T_4 to T_3 and can elevate T_4 levels for up to 30 days after administration. In the absence of any of these situations in which the TBG level is abnormal, the T_4 assay is elevated only in hyperthyroidism and depressed only in hypothyroidism. Abnormal levels of free T_4 are encountered only in the presence of either hyper- or hypothyroidism. The normal range for the free T_4 assay is 0.8 to 2.4 ng per deciliter. The normal range for total T_4 assay is 4 to 11 mg per deciliter.

Triiodothyronine

Triiodothyronine (T_3) is currently also measured by radioimmunoassay. Normal serum concentrations in adult nonpregnant women are 80 to 180 ng per deciliter. T_3 secretion correlates with T_4 secretion, except in certain situations. In some forms of thyrotoxicosis, only T_3 is elevated (T_3 hyperthyroidism). T_3 is normal in patients with dietary iodine deficiency, in patients with Hashimoto's thyroiditis, or after medical or surgical treatment of thyrotoxicosis, despite low T_4 levels.

Thyroid-Stimulating Hormone

The normal range of serum TSH is 0.5 to 4.0 μU per milliliter, with 10 percent of normal individuals and essentially all hyperthyroid patients having undetectable levels. In patients with primary hypothyroidism

or in those with diminished thyroid reserve due to Hashimoto's thyroiditis, previous radioiodine therapy, or surgery for hyperthyroidism, the serum TSH is invariably elevated. Conversely, with secondary hypothyroidism due to pituitary or hypothalamic disease, the serum TSH is low. Serum TSH determinations are thus most useful for diagnosing hypothyroidism, differentiating primary from secondary hypothyroidism, the early detection of diminished thyroid reserve, and monitoring thyroid replacement therapy for hypothyroidism. The normal values of serum TSH by radioimmunoassay are usually fairly similar in most laboratories, as shown above, but may be slightly higher in some. With the use of more recently available, highly specific monoclonal antibodies to TSH, the levels detectable can be measured to even below 0.5 μU per milliliter.

Thyrotropin-Releasing Hormone Stimulation Test

The TRH stimulation test, which involves administration of the hypothalamic tripeptide TRH, is useful for distinguishing secondary hypothyroidism due to pituitary or hypothalamic disease from primary hypothyroidism originating in the thyroid. With both types of hypothyroidism, serum TSH levels are low. TRH is given as an intravenous bolus dose of 400 μg. In normal women, serum TSH rises rapidly to reach a peak 20 to 30 minutes later followed by a slow decline to basal levels within 2 to 3 hours. Usually the test involves measuring serum TSH just before and 30 minutes after TRH administration.

With primary hypothyroidism, TRH induces an accentuated TSH response, with the peak levels markedly increased. With secondary hypothyroidism, the basal TSH levels are not increased, indicating a diagnosis of suprathyroid (trophoprivic) hypothyroidism; thus the fault is at the pituitary or hypothalamic level. Although the test is diagnostic, it is also academic, as treatment for both types of hypothyroidism is thyroid hormone replacement.

Antithyroid Antibodies

The antithyroid antibodies assay is a tanned red cell agglutination test that is particularly helpful for confirming the diagnosis of Hashimoto's thyroiditis, in which considerably elevated antibody titers are the rule.

Other Thyroid Tests

Other thyroid tests, which were once performed often and are still used by some, are less reliable and therefore are of little value compared to T_4, T_3, and TSH assays. These previously popular thyroid function tests included basal metabolic rate, serum PBI, BEI, T_3 resin uptake, and radioactive iodide uptake test. Because they are of little value and no longer clinically useful, they are not described here.

DIAGNOSTIC SURGICAL PROCEDURES

Examination Under Anesthesia

Although evaluation of the pelvis through complete pelvic and abdominal examination can identify pelvic disease in most instances, examination under anesthesia adds to the clinician's information in some instances. It is particularly true in patients who are uncooperative or in such pain as to not allow a thorough examination. Such patients include some children and adolescents and patients with pelvic pain caused by pelvic inflammatory disease, endometriosis, or malignancy. Patients who are obese may also be difficult to examine while awake. Examination under anesthesia often adds to the diagnostic capabilities for identifying pelvic disease. Therefore prior to undertaking any pelvic surgery, examination should be performed under anesthesia, as the findings may alter surgical technique or strategy.

Examination under anesthesia may be combined with cystoscopy and proctosigmoidoscopy when evaluating the patient with gynecologic cancer. In addition, areas of suspicion may be biopsied at this same time using standard punch biopsy forceps or a scalpel or needle biopsy technique. The examination under anesthesia should include careful visual inspection of the vulva, vagina, and cervix. Bimanual and rectovaginal examinations are performed in the same sequence as discussed in Chapter 1.

Fractional Dilatation and Curettage

Fractional D&C is the gold standard diagnostic technique for evaluating the endometrium and endocervix. However, with the advent of smaller biopsy devices and the risks and expenses of a surgical procedure requiring anesthesia, most patients may be evaluated and managed based on endometrial (see above) and endocervical biopsies, discussed previously. Fractional D&C should be performed in situations where the biopsy is inconclusive, in the patient who has not responded to therapy that was based on endometrial biopsy results, or in the patient in whom endometrial biopsy could not be performed because of cervical stenosis or low pain threshold.

Fractional D&C requires adequate anesthesia levels to perform dilatation and sharp curettage of the endocervix and endometrium. It is usually accomplished with general or spinal anesthesia. Some patients tolerate a fractional D&C with only local (paracervical) anesthesia. As the term connotes, fractional D&C obtains a fraction from the endocervix as well as a sample of the endometrium. These specimens are submitted separately so that the exact location of pathologic process may be more fully identified. This technique is particularly important for distinguishing between endocervical and endometrial adenocarcinoma and for staging endometrial adenocarcinoma.

After obtaining adequate anesthesia, the endocervical canal is curetted sharply. The uterine cavity is then sounded to determine the depth and direction of the canal. The cervix is grasped with a tenaculum to stabilize it and to pull down (and thereby straighten somewhat) the uterine cavity. The cervical canal is dilated with blunt dilating instruments that are graduated in size. The cervix should be dilated only to the size adequate to introduce the appropriate endometrial curet. Thorough curettage of the endometrial cavity is then performed and the tissue submitted to a pathologist. Following sharp curettage, stone forceps are passed into the endometrial cavity, and attempts are made to grasp any endometrial polyp that may not have been removed by the curet.

Complications of fractional D&C include uterine perforation. If the perforation occurs on the lateral aspects of the uterus and a vein or artery is injured, a broad ligament and retroperitoneal hematoma may form. If bleeding is uncontrolled, hysterectomy may be required to achieve hemostasis. In most instances, however, uterine perforation occurs in the uterine fundus and is of no consequence. Sharp curettage, especially in an infected uterus, may result in intra-uterine synechia with subsequent problems with oligomenorrhea and infertility (Asherman's syndrome) (Chap. 13).

Cold Knife Conization

Surgical excision of a cone-shaped portion of the cervix may be used for diagnosis and treatment of cervical dysplasia. Prior to considering conization for diagnosis, the patient with an abnormal Pap smear should undergo colposcopy with directed biopsies of the exocervix and endocervical curettage. In most cases the patient with dysplasia may be managed without conization. Cold knife conization is required in the following circumstances: (1) when the lesion cannot be seen on the exocervix; (2) when the lesion extends into the endocervix and cannot be fully evaluated by colposcopy; (3) when the endocervical curettage shows dysplasia in the endocervix; (4) when biopsy shows microinvasive carcinoma (less than 3 mm of invasion); (5) when the Pap smear suggests invasive carcinoma that cannot be detected by colposcopy and directed biopsies; (6) when the Pap smear is two or more grades higher than the dysplasia found on biopsy.

The goals of conization are to excise entirely the cervical lesion with an adequate surgical margin. Colposcopic evaluation can be used to individualize the size of the conization so that an excessive amount of normal tissue is not removed. For example, if the exocervix appears normal on colposcopy and there is a suspicion of disease in the endocervical canal, a "long, narrow" cone can be designed to excise the cervical canal but not an extensive amount of exocervix. Similarly, when performing a conization during pregnancy for a lesion that has been found to have microinvasion on a colposcopically directed biopsy, a superficial but wide conization around the area detected by colposcopy would be satisfactory for diagnosis with no attempts to extend high into the endo-

cervical canal where disease is not suspected. The individualized cone should minimize complications.

Conization is usually performed in an outpatient room under general or spinal anesthesia. After excision of the conization specimen, curettage of the remaining endocervical canal is usually performed. In premenopausal women the addition of a fractional D&C is not necessary or advised unless endometrial pathology is suspected.

Immediate complications of conization include intraoperative or postoperative hemorrhage. Bleeding can occur approximately 1 week after surgery when the absorbable suture placed in the surgical bed reabsorbs. Infection of the conization bed may occur, although it infrequently requires antibiotic therapy. Long-term complications of conization include cervical stenosis with subsequent infertility or difficulty of cervical dilatation at the time of labor and delivery. Additionally, excessive excision of the cervical stroma may lead to an incompetent cervix with premature dilatation of the cervix during the second trimester or a subsequent pregnancy. These complications of cervical stenosis and incompetent cervix occur in approximately 1 to 2 percent of patients who undergo conization. Because conization requires operating room time and expense and is associated with some significant complications, it should be avoided unless absolutely necessary. In approximately 90 percent of evaluated patients with abnormal Pap smears, the patient can be fully treated without performing a conization.

The carbon dioxide laser can be used in place of cold knife cone biopsy. Laser conization of the cervix is carried out the same way as the cold knife procedure. The cervix is injected with vasopressin (Pitressin) to reduce hemorrhage and promote vasoconstriction, and laser conization is then carried out. Bleeding is minimal both intraoperatively and postoperatively, and the cervix heals well.

Second-Look Laparotomy

Because ovarian cancer metastatic to peritoneal surfaces is often clinically occult, assessment of the patient who is being treated with chemotherapy for ovarian cancer may be difficult. Unless a palpable pelvic mass or mass noted by radiography can be followed, there remains uncertainty as to tumor status. Therefore decisions as to whether to continue, change, or discontinue chemotherapy are difficult to make based on clinical assessment alone.

The serum antigen CA-125 has been helpful for evaluating the status of ovarian cancer in patients undergoing treatment. Nonetheless, CA-125 may be normal when the patient has persistent cancer.

Because of these uncertainties of tumor status in patients clinically free of disease, second-look laparotomy is often recommended. The primary goal of this surgical procedure is to assess tumor status. On occasion it is accomplished by laparoscopy; but in situations where significant adhesions have formed or laparoscopic visualization is limited to a small area, tumor may be overlooked.

In the process of performing the laparotomy, a midline incision is made, all peritoneal surfaces are inspected, and any suspicious lesions are biopsied. If no lesions are noted, random biopsy specimens are obtained from normal-appearing tissues (especially peritoneum) where it is known that tumor was left at the completion of the initial surgical procedure. Additionally, adhesions are resected, peritoneal washings are obtained from the pelvis and upper abdomen, and selective pelvic and paraaortic lymphadenectomy is performed.

The goal of the operation is to assess as completely as is technically possible the status of the patient's disease. After reviewing all pathology, decisions may then be made as to discontinuation or a change in therapy. The value of second-look laparotomy in terms of the patient's long-term survival is debatable, especially in patients who have failed first-line chemotherapy because, at the writing of this textbook, there is no uniformly effective second-line systemic therapeutic agent. Intraperitoneal chemotherapy may effectively treat small residual disease (less than 5-mm nodules) and intraperitoneal ^{32}P or whole-abdomen radiation therapy may achieve cures in patients who have microscopic disease at second-look laparotomy.

Retroperitoneal Lymphadenectomy

In patients with advanced cervical cancer, evaluation of retroperitoneal lymph nodes, especially in the common iliac and paraaortic chains, is suggested so that radiation therapy may be directed to involved areas. Initial staging studies for advanced cervical cancer usually include a pelvic and abdominal CT scan looking for distant metastases. Because the CT scan may be falsely negative in 10 to 30 percent and falsely positive in 10 percent of patients, surgical excision of the lymph nodes is sometimes advised for more complete and accurate staging information.

A retroperitoneal approach is recommended for assessing these lymph nodes. The prime reason for proceeding through the retroperitoneal space without violating the peritoneal cavity itself is to minimize postoperative adhesions. It is clear that radiation therapy complications are increased when intraperitoneal and especially intrapelvic adhesions form, thereby trapping small bowel in the pelvis. This trapped bowel receives a full dose of radiation and so is more likely to be injured, leading to obstruction, enteritis, or fistula formation. Because the retroperitoneal staging laparotomy is a major operation, it is usually reserved for selected patients in whom aggressive extended radiation therapy would be considered in the setting of treatment considered curative.

Endometrial Biopsy

The endometrial biopsy was discussed earlier in this chapter.

Endocervical Biopsy

Endocervical biopsy (curettage) is performed as part of the routine outpatient evaluation of patients with an abnormal Pap smear. It may also be combined with endometrial biopsy for evaluating patients with abnormal uterine bleeding. At the time of a fractional D&C, the specimen from the endocervix should be submitted separately from the endometrial specimen so as to be able to distinguish the site of pathology.

Endocervical curettage is performed with a small, sharp curet that is introduced into the endocervical canal. Using a curetting motion, the endocervical canal is then sampled. Care is taken to avoid trauma to the exocervix, as dysplasia arising in the transformation zone may be scraped off along with the endocervical specimen, thus confusing the true location of the dysplastic squamous epithelium. As with endometrial biopsy, endocervical curettage induces some uterine cramping, which can usually be managed with nonsteroidal antiinflammatory agents. Endocervical curettage should not be performed during pregnancy because of the possibility of rupturing the amniotic membranes.

Vulvar Biopsy

Biopsy of the vulva is critically important to the diagnosis and management of many conditions noted grossly on the vulva. If the lesion is small enough, it may be entirely excised (excisional biopsy). On the other hand, many lesions are large enough that excisional biopsy cannot be achieved in the office, and definitive therapy may require more than excisional biopsy. In this setting punch biopsy of the vulvar lesion (lesions) may be performed using the Key's punch and local anesthesia.

After preparation of the vulvar skin with an antiseptic solution such as povidone-iodine, 1% lidocaine is infiltrated into the region to be biopsied. The Key's punch (usually 3 or 4 mm in diameter) is used to obtain a punch biopsy specimen of the skin and superficial subcutaneous tissue. Using a rotating motion, the circular punch incises the area of interest, and the base is excised using sharp Iris scissors or a scalpel. The specimen should be oriented on a slice of cucumber or filter paper so that appropriate perpendicular cuts may be made through the tissue at the time of sectioning in the pathology department. Hemostasis is achieved with silver nitrate or a single absorbable suture. This procedure is not associated with any significant major side effect. Because vulvar lesions are not necessarily pathognomonic on general examination, vulvar biopsy is encouraged when any lesion is encountered.

Vaginal Biopsy

Vaginal biopsy is usually performed in the office to evaluate a patient with an abnormal Pap smear in whom a lesion can be seen in the vagina. Colposcopy may aid in locating the vaginal lesion. Dysplasia may

occur at any portion of the vagina, although it is frequently located near the vaginal apex. Vaginal biopsy can usually be performed using the same biopsy forceps employed to biopsy the cervix. Local anesthesia with injectable 1% lidocaine or topical analgesia using benzocaine is usually sufficient to allow comfortable biopsy. Hemostasis may be achieved with silver nitrate or a suture. There are no untoward side effects of vaginal biopsy.

Colposcopy

The lower genital tract may be evaluated with the aid of magnification provided by the colposcope. The colposcope is essentially a binocular dissecting microscope, usually used with a magnification power of approximately 15×. Colposcopy has found its widest application in the evaluation of patients with abnormal Pap smears suggesting cervical intraepithelial neoplasia or invasive carcinoma. Because it is expensive, time-consuming, and skill is required to perform it, colposcopy is not a routine screening technique. Nonetheless, when used appropriately in the situation requiring further evaluation of the cervix, colposcopy and directed biopsy eliminate the need for diagnostic surgical procedures such as cold knife conization. The details of the colposcopy technique are discussed in Chapter 25.

Biopsy of the Cervix

Biopsies of suspicious cervical lesions identified with the naked eye or with colposcopic magnification can usually be performed in the office or outpatient setting with the use of little or no anesthesia. An endocervical biopsy is usually performed in conjunction with biopsy of the exocervix. The details of cervical biopsy technique are discussed in Chapter 25.

Schiller's Test

Schiller's test was used much more extensively prior to the advent of colposcopy. It is still used today in several clinical situations, however, especially when colposcopy cannot identify an abnormal lesion on the cervix or vagina, or when correlation with colposcopic findings is advantageous so that surgical biopsies or conization may be performed without the repeated use of the colposcope in the operating room. Schiller's test is based on the observation that glycogenated squamous epithelium (of the cervix and vagina) takes up an iodine-based stain.

Schiller's solution (1 part iodine, 2 parts potassium iodide, 300 parts water) is applied to the vagina and upper cervix with a cotton pledget. Normal squamous epithelium usually takes up the stain, and a homogeneous mahogany-brown color is noted. In many patients with cervical dysplasia, in whom the nuclear/cytoplasmic ratio is increased (and therefore glycogen in the squamous epithelial cytoplasm is diminished), Schiller's stain is not taken up, and the epithelium appears light yellow. This area of unstained epithelium is considered a positive Schiller's test. Unfortunately, a cervix that has undergone trauma that has deepithelialized the tissue, tissue with cervicitis, and columnar epithelium do not take up the stain, which may lead to a false-positive test. Schiller's test is clearly not as sensitive or specific as colposcopy for identifying cervical intraepithelial neoplasia.

Culdocentesis

Access to the peritoneal cavity may be helpful for recognition of intraperitoneal bleeding (such as might be associated with an ectopic pregnancy), purulent material from the pelvis associated with tuboovarian abscess or salpingo-oophoritis, or peritoneal fluid that might be studied cytologically for the identification of malignant cells such as is noted with ovarian cancer. The easiest access to the peritoneal cavity to accomplish any of these goals is through the posterior cul-de-sac. The distance between the peritoneum of the posterior cul-de-sac (pouch of Douglas) and the vaginal mucosa is less than 1 cm in most women. Therefore it is relatively easy to introduce a needle across the posterior vaginal mucosa just behind the cervix into the pouch of Douglas.

Culdocentesis may be performed under a local (1% lidocaine) or topical (benzocaine) anesthesia. After preparation of the vagina with povidone-iodine and obtaining adequate anesthesia, a 22-gauge spinal needle attached to a syringe may be passed across the mucosa and peritoneum (Fig. 2-7). Blood obtained at culdocentesis (especially if more than 1 ml) suggests intraperitoneal bleeding, especially if the blood does not clot after 5 to 10 minutes. (In this setting, especially with a clinical history and symptom complex compatible with possible ectopic pregnancy, intraperitoneal bleeding must be strongly considered.) Nonclotting blood obtained during culdocentesis is considered a "positive" culdocentesis. On the other hand, obtaining blood that clots may simply mean that the needle at the time of culdocentesis actually performed a venipuncture.

Culdocentesis is neither sensitive nor specific for ectopic pregnancy but may be used in combination with clinical, ultrasound, and laboratory results (Chaps. 2, 3, and 16). Purulent material obtained on culdocentesis should be cultured for anaerobes and aerobes, the results of which may guide specific antibiotic choices for a pelvic infection. In patients treated for ovarian carcinoma, culdocentesis may be performed to obtain a small amount of peritoneal fluid; or if no fluid is present, the cul-de-sac may be lavaged with 10 ml of saline and then aspirated. This fluid should then be submitted for cytopathology, searching for the presence of malignant cells, which may be an early indicator of recurrent disease.

Pelvic Endoscopy

Culdoscopy and laparoscopy enable the gynecologist to inspect the pelvis and pelvic viscera and thus avoid exploratory laparotomy when confronted by puzzling diagnostic problems that may or may not require surgical intervention. Laparoscopy has replaced culdoscopy in most clinics because it provides superior visualization of the entire pelvis, especially the cul-de-sac, and permits more complete visualization of the abdominal cavity. Laparoscopy is not only more accurate than culdoscopy but offers the ability to do operative procedures as well, such as tubal ligation (Chap. 22), lysis of adhesions, oocyte retrieval (Chap. 13), and cauterization or laser vaporization of endometriosis (Chap. 12). Thus laparoscopy is both a diagnostic and a therapeutically definitive surgical

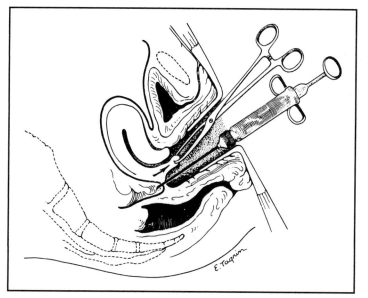

Fig. 2-7. Culdocentesis. A 22-gauge needle is introduced across the posterior vaginal fornix and into the peritoneal cavity (cul-de-sac of Douglas). Fluid (blood, peritoneal fluid, ascites, or pus) can then be aspirated for diagnosis.

procedure. Although laparoscopy usually requires general anesthesia (but can be done under local or regional block such as epidural or spinal anesthesia), it is less unpleasant than culdoscopy, where the patient is placed in the knee-chest position and is given sedation and local anesthesia. The presence of pathology or disease in the pelvis, especially with adhesions or fixation of organs or structures in the cul-de-sac, makes it impossible to perform culdoscopy. For these reasons, culdoscopy has been abandoned as a *diagnostic* surgical procedure in most centers and by newly trained gynecologists, who are often technically competent with laparoscopy.

Laparoscopy

There are several indications for gynecologic laparoscopy.

1. Reproductive failure—assessment of tubal factor such as peritubal adhesions, tubal occlusion, hydrosalpinges, and postoperative evaluation of tuboplasty and appraisal of the ovaries and ovarian function.
2. Pelvic pain and dysmenorrhea—searching for causes such as endometriosis, pelvic adhesions, and other responsible pelvic pathology.
3. Acute lower abdominal pain—searching for ruptured and unruptured ectopic pregnancy, tubal abortion, leaking corpus luteum, differentiation between these conditions and salpingitis, and translaparoscopic surgical treatment of ectopic pregnancy.
4. Pelvic mass—establishing the presence, source, origin, and nature of a mass (fibroids, ovarian cysts, hydrosalpinx, pelvic malignancy).
5. Known or suspected endometriosis—establishing the diagnosis, extent of disease, suitability of treatment forms, and follow-up of therapy.
6. Pelvic cancer—staging and second look to appraise the chemotherapy of ovarian cancer.
7. Endocrinopathies and anomalies—evaluation of uterine and ovarian development in primary amenorrhea and premature ovarian failure in secondary amenorrhea.
8. Control of vaginal surgery—prevent or evaluate uterine perforation at curettage.

9. Foreign bodies and trauma—looking for a displaced intrauterine device or pelvic hematomas.

The principal contraindication to laparoscopy is serious cardiac or pulmonary disease with impaired cardiopulmonary reserve. Previous lower abdomen surgery is only a relative contraindication depending on the technical skill of the laparoscopist. However, if bowel is suspected to be adherent, especially near the umbilicus or along most parts of the anterior abdominal wall, as occasionally occurs with small bowel endometriosis or after previous surgery, it is prudent not to perform laparoscopy. Nonetheless, an *open* laparoscopy (see under technique section below) can safely be performed and is recommended.

The procedure is almost always carried out as outpatient surgery. General anesthesia is usually given, and the patient is placed in the Whitmore position (modified lithotomy) combined with steep Trendelenburg positioning. The procedure can be performed under local anesthesia with sedation, but it is often uncomfortable for the patient owing to the pneumoperitoneum needed. If the laparoscopy is performed for infertility evaluation or when chromopertubation (instillation of dye transcervically into the uterus) is required, it is better to perform any endometrial biopsy or D&C after the chromopertubation; otherwise the D&C can be performed first to evaluate the curettings. The bladder should be catheterized and completely emptied to avoid possible injury. If the laparoscopy is expected to be prolonged (e.g., operative laparoscopy), an indwelling catheter can be left in place throughout the procedure.

The cervix is then grasped with a tenaculum and the uterine cannula inserted into the cervical canal and uterus after having sounded it. Other devices or manipulations for moving the uterus around transvaginally can be alternatively employed. To perform the laparoscopy, the peritoneal cavity must be insufflated with gas, usually 3 to 4 liters of carbon dioxide (other gases have been used) to create a pneumoperitoneum for adequate visualization, getting the bowel out of the way, and avoiding injury to the bowels. The pneumoperitoneum is created through a Verres needle inserted usually through a small sub-

umbilical, semilunar incision. The operator watches the pressure gauge carefully; the initial pressure should be only 10 to 20 cm (if higher, the Verres needle has either failed to enter the free peritoneal cavity or is partly occluded by omentum or an adjacent abdominal viscus), and the pressure should not rise more than a few centimeters during the insufflation. Percussion of the lower abdominal wall during the insufflation should evoke easily recognizable tympany if the pneumoperitoneum is developing properly, and liver dullness should disappear.

The laparoscopy trochar-cannula is then introduced through the skin incision, running down under the skin for 2 to 3 cm before penetrating the rectus fascia and underlying peritoneum (this maneuver prevents gas leaks around the cannula later on). When penetration has been accomplished, the cannula is connected to the carbon dioxide reservoir tubing, setting the dial on "Automatic" to maintain a steady flow of carbon dioxide, as needed, to replace any leak; the trochar is then removed. The laparoscope, prewarmed in hot saline to prevent fogging of the lens by exposure to intraperitoneal temperature and moisture, is then inserted through the cannula (the latter has a built-in air lock to minimize gas leakage) into the peritoneal cavity. Visualization of the pelvis and lower abdomen and the visceral contents thereof is then carried out in detail (Fig. 2-8).

If the procedure is being done as part of an infertility investigation, methylene blue dye can be instilled through the intrauterine cannula while the surgeon watches through the laparoscope for spillage of dye from the fallopian tubes. A second incision, 0.5 cm wide, can be made in the midline suprapubically just at the superior edge of the pubic hair line or the right or left lower quadrant of the abdomen (avoiding the epigastric vessels by first transilluminating the abdominal wall with the laparoscope); a small, secondary trochar can then be inserted. The tubal ligation instrument or a special probe to manipulate the tube and ovary or other intraperitoneal structures for better inspection (a biopsy forceps or an aspiration cannula) is introduced through this trochar. A third puncture can be employed through any of the above-mentioned sites for additional instruments if needed.

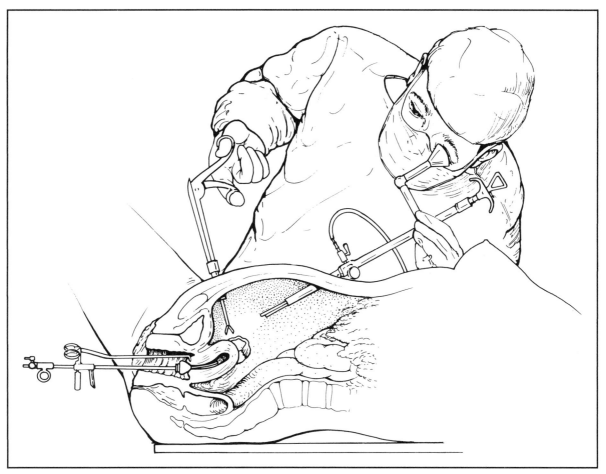

Fig. 2-8. Laparoscopy. The patient is undergoing laparoscopy with a two-puncture technique. Note the second puncture instrument in the lower abdomen. This instrument is used to move pelvic organs to allow better visualization. Similarly, instruments needed for lysing adhesions, grasping, biopsy, or cauterizing may be introduced through this puncture site and cannula.

Laparoscopy is inadequate for evaluating the retroperitoneal lymph nodes or other retroperitoneal structures. The laparoscope may be directed to survey the remainder of the peritoneal cavity, however, including the appendix (unless it is located in a retrocecal position), gallbladder, liver, and diaphragms. If careful inspection of all surfaces of the bowel serosa and mesentery is required (as when searching for persistent ovarian carcinoma), laparoscopy is inadequate, as it cannot see all surfaces of the bowel. Biopsy specimens may be obtained from suspicious lesions through the laparoscope to confirm the visual diagnosis.

Diagnostic laparoscopy carries with it the risks associated with inserting instruments into the peritoneal cavity, especially viscus perforation (bowel, bladder), vascular injury (mesenteric vessels, aorta, inferior vena cava, and other pelvic vessels), electrical burns of the skin, abdominal incision of internal structures (intestine, ureters, bladder) if the electrocoagulation instrument has been used, and bleeding from biopsy sites or wound.

Hysteroscopy

Although the hysteroscope has been available since at least the 1970s, it has become widely used only during the 1980s, especially after the design of the instrument, its availability, and its diagnostic capabilities were markedly improved. The original instrument was similar to a cystoscope in design and use, permitting an endoscopic view of the interior of the uterus and using continuously running water as the observation medium. However, the apparatus was cumbersome to use and the view frequently unsatisfactory and difficult to interpret. A further modification was developed employing a saline-filled, transparent rubber balloon mounted on the endoscope and inflated after its insertion in the uterine cavity; this instrument was thought to provide a superior view without the trauma and bleeding caused by the old model. Nevertheless, this modification made direct biopsy of visualized lesions impossible and has largely been abandoned.

Modern hysteroscopes are equipped with a fiberoptic lighting system and employ either 5% glucose in water, highly viscous dextran solutions (e.g., 30%

dextran 70), or carbon dioxide as the uterus-distending medium. Because adequate dilatation and distention of the uterine cavity are absolutely essential to obtain a clear view of the endometrial surface, pressures of 50 to 100 mm Hg or higher are usually necessary. Rinsing the uterine cavity is also frequently required to clear away blood and secretory debris that tend to obscure the field. To use the hysteroscope effectively and to obtain maximum information, extensive special training and experience are required. In addition to direct visualization, the operating hysteroscope allows visually directed biopsies as well as resection of abnormalities confined to the endometrial cavity or submucous wall of the uterus (Fig. 2-9).

The use of the hysteroscope has also permitted intrauterine occlusion of the fallopian tube ostia by chemical cauterization with quinacrine, electrocauterization, cryosurgery, and latex and metal plugs. These

Fig. 2-9. Diagnostic hysteroscopy. The hysteroscope is inserted into the uterine cavity, which is distended by carbon dioxide or dextran (Hyskon). There is an operating channel in the telescope, through which biopsies or other intrauterine surgical procedures can be performed.

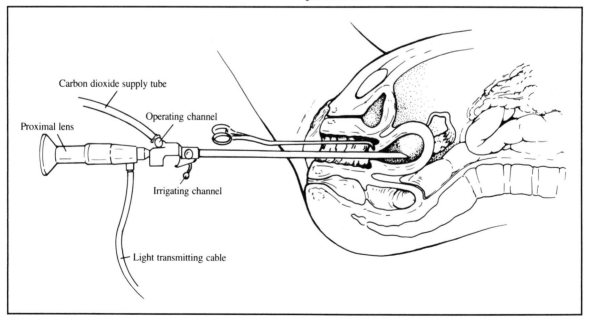

Carbon dioxide supply tube

Proximal lens

Operating channel

Irrigating channel

Light transmitting cable

methods of sterilization are far from perfect, however, compared to the conventional methods (Chap. 22) that have been established. Nevertheless, with advances in bioinstrumentation this hysteroscopic approach could be further refined with metallic microstents as occlusive devices that could potentially be removed and therefore offer a reversible form of sterilization performed in the office or outpatient surgicenter. Hysteroscopy is indicated and commonly used for the following conditions.

1. Abnormal uterine bleeding to rule out an organic cause
2. Suspected submucous leiomyomas or polyps
3. Uterine cavity anomalies due to congenital uterine malformations such as a septate or subseptate uterus
4. If an intrauterine device string is missing and cannot be visualized
5. Postmenopausal bleeding to rule out an organic cause
6. Primary or secondary infertility with hysterosalpingographic abnormalities
7. As a surgical technique for lysis of intrauterine adhesions, septate uterus, or resection of submucous myomas

Currently, with the availability of lasers, the hysteroscope has been employed to deliver the laser beam into the uterus. It has been used to stop endometrial bleeding as well as to cause endometrial ablation to induce a complete uterine cavity occlusion through synechiae formation, thereby rendering women with bleeding diathesis amenorrheic. It is a simpler, shorter procedure than hysterectomy. Finally, the hysteroscope is now being employed to open up proximal tubal occlusion using a balloon tuboplasty technique. The balloon catheter and cannula are introduced into the proximal end of the tube through the uterine cavity via the hysteroscope.

Hysteroscopy and hysteroscopic surgery offer a shorter but skillful procedure that can be done in the office or outpatient surgical suite with sedation. With extensive intrauterine excisions, the hysteroscopic procedure is usually done under laparoscopic guidance, and general anesthesia is often necessary. However, such endoscopic procedures offer shorter recovery, lower morbidity, and less absenteeism.

Hysteroscopy can produce complications, including bleeding, uterine perforation, infection, and even bowel injuries.

SELECTED READINGS

Bast, R. C., Klug, T. L., St. John, E., et al. A radioimmunoassay using a monoclonal antibody to monitor the course of epithelial ovarian cancer. *N. Eng. J. Med.* 309:883, 1983.

Berek, J. S., Hacker, N. F., Lagasse, L. D., et al. Second-look laparotomy in stage III epithelial ovarian cancer. *Obstet. Gynecol.* 64:207, 1984.

Borten, M. *Laparoscopic Complications: Prevention and Management.* Toronto: Decker, Inc. 1986.

Creasman, W. T., and Weed, J. C., Jr. Screening techniques in endometrial cancer. *Cancer* 38:436, 1976.

Einerth, Y. Vacuum curettage by the Vabra method. *Acta Obstet. Gynecol. Scand.* 61:373, 1982.

Fortier, K. J., Clarke-Pearson, D. L., Creasman, W. T., et al. Fine needle aspiration in gynecology: evaluation of extrapelvic lesions in patients with gynecologic malignancy. *Obstet. Gynecol.* 65:76, 1985.

Gomel, V., Taylor, P. J., Yuzpe, A. A., Roux, J. E. *Laparoscopy and Hysteroscopy in Gynecology Practice.* Chicago: Yearbook Medical, 1986.

Grimes, D. A. Diagnostic dilatation and curettage: a reappraisal. *Am. J. Obstet. Gynecol.* 142:1, 1982.

Hulka, J. F. *Textbook of Laparoscopy.* Orlando: Grune & Stratton, 1985.

Iversen, O. E., and Segadal, E. The value of endometrial cytology: a comparative study of the Gravlee jet-washer, Isaacs cell sampler, and Endoscan versus curettage in 600 patients. *Obstet. Gynecol. Surv.* 40:14, 1985.

Kaplan, E. B., Sheiner, L. B., Boeckmann, A. J., et al. The usefulness of preoperative laboratory screening. *J.A.M.A.* 253:3576, 1985.

Lagasse, L. D., Creasman, W. T., Shingleton, H. M., et al. Results and complications of operative staging in cervical cancer. *Gynecol. Oncol.* 9:90, 1980.

LaPolla, J. P., Schlaerth, J. B., Gaddis, O., et al. The influence of surgical staging on the evaluation and treatment of patients with cervical carcinoma. *Gynecol. Oncol.* 24:194, 1986.

Lewis, B. V. Hysteroscopy in gynaecological practice: a review. *J.R. Soc. Med.* 77:235, 1984.

Romero, R. New criteria for diagnosis of gestational trophoblastic disease. *Obstet. Gynecol.* 66:553, 1985.

Saleh, J. W. *Laparoscopy.* Philadelphia: Saunders, 1988.

Semm, K. *Operative Manual for Endoscopic Abdominal Surgery.* Chicago: Yearbook Medical Publishers, Inc., 1987.

Siegler, A. M., and Lindemann, H. J. *Hysteroscopy, Principles and Practice.* Philadelphia: Lippincott, 1984.

Symonds, E. M., and Zuspan, F. P. *Clinical and Diagnostic Procedures in Obstetrics and Gynecology.* New York: Marcel Dekker, 1984.

3

Diagnostic Imaging in Gynecology

The discovery of x-rays led to the development of radiographic methods for diagnostic imaging of body tissues and structures. Initially such radiographic imaging took advantage of the differences in density of tissues, fluid, and air. Thus the lungs, bones, fluid, and gas could be readily visualized with little difficulty. Further developments led to the use of radiopaque contrast material, which permitted the tissues or channels of interest to be outlined clearly by the contrast. Such methods of imaging included intravenous pyelography, arteriography, venography, lymphangiography, and hysterosalpingography.

With refinements in radiographic equipment and a reduction of the ionizing radiation used, tomograms that allowed multiple radiographic sections of a tissue area with a suspected lesion enabled three-dimensional localization of the lesion. Fluoroscopy added a dimension of real-time radiologic visualization of the tissue under study, especially with contrast material. The advent of ultrasonography together with rapid advances in microchip development and microprocessing have revolutionized diagnostic imaging by eliminating exposure to ionizing radiation, thereby opening up a safe, noninvasive way of studying early gestation as well as the reproductive organs. Still in its diagnostically developing stages in gynecology, magnetic resonance imaging (MRI) is promising; it complements some of the other imaging techniques and appears to offer better image resolution. With developments in superconductivity, MRI equipment is likely to become smaller and probably more affordable. Potentially, diagnostic imaging in gynecology is likely to develop to a stage where the tissues under study are visualized in color, with greater clarity and capability for magnification. Such diagnostic imaging advances can offer

stereotactic surgery that is less invasive than incisional approaches.

Currently the methods in use for diagnostic imaging in gynecology are (1) radiologic imaging with or without the use of contrast material, (2) radioisotope scanning, (3) computed tomography, (4) ultrasonography, (5) MRI, and (6) bone densitometry. These techniques and their application in gynecology are described in this chapter (Table 3-1).

RADIOLOGIC IMAGING

Every effort should be made to avoid the unwitting use of elective diagnostic pelvic and abdominal x-ray studies in the presence of an early and unsuspected, normal intrauterine pregnancy. Bearing this point in mind, the following roentgenologic studies are frequently of great value for evaluating many gynecologic disorders.

Chest Radiograph

Routine radiographs of the chest are obtained for most gynecologic surgery patients as part of the preoperative workup. However, it is increasingly common not to do it in young, fit patients with no significant past illness who are undergoing only day surgery, e.g., dilatation and curettage (D&C), laparoscopy, and tubal ligation. Anteroposterior and lateral chest radiographs allow evaluation of pulmonary and cardiac disease. The chest radiograph is important for the initial staging and evaluation of patients with all gynecologic malignancies.

Metastasis may be identified as parenchymal metastasis, pleural effusions, or mediastinal adenopathy. The presence of a pleural effusion in association with a pelvic mass and ascites may not necessarily represent advanced ovarian carcinoma but may be Meigs' syndrome (Chap. 18). An upright chest radiograph is also the best radiographic method to detect free air in the peritoneal cavity, which would gather under the diaphragm (suggesting bowel perforation as the cause of pneumoperitoneum). Free air is also noted under the diaphragm for up to seven to ten days after abdominal or vaginal surgery. The chest radiograph, on rare

Table 3-1. Preferred Methods of Imaging Common Gynecologic Conditions in Female Tissues

Organ or tissue and pathology suspected	Preferred method
Pituitary	
Tumors	CT scan or MRI
Adrenals	
Tumors	Radionuclide scan or CT scan
Hyperplasia	Radionuclide scan
Ovaries	
Follicle growth	
Tumors	Vaginal ultrasound
Ectopic pregnancy	
Uterus	
Fibroids	Vaginal ultrasound or MRI
Early pregnancy	Vaginal ultrasound
Congenital anomalies	Hysterosalpingography or possibly vaginal ultrasound
Uterine synechiae	Hysterosalpingography
Carcinoma	MRI
Trophoblastic disease	Ultrasound or MRI
Fallopian tubes	
Tubal occlusion	Hysterosalpingography
Ectopic pregnancy	Vaginal ultrasound
Cervix	
Incompetent cervix	Hysterosalpingography (cervicogram) or vaginal ultrasound
Thyroid	
Goiters	
Tumors	Radionuclide scan
Nodules	
Bone	
Puberty disorders	Radiograph bone age
Osteoporosis	CT scan, dual-photon densitometry
Postmenopausal osteopenia	CT scan, dual-photon densitometry, single-photon densitometry
Metastasis	Radionuclide bone scan

occasion, also suggests the etiology of pelvic pain and nodularity as evidenced by pulmonary tuberculosis.

Kidney, Ureter, and Bladder

A plain radiograph of the abdomen—kidney, ureter, and bladder (KUB)—may show the following: a pelvic mass; calcified fibroids; a dermoid cyst with recognizable teeth (see Fig. 18-2) or the characteristic layering pattern of the cyst's contents of liquid sebaceous material; calcified ovarian tumors (occasional psammoma bodies); fetal skeletal structure after 4½ months of pregnancy; lithopedions; or bony changes characteristic of osteoporosis or metastatic cancer. It may reveal or confirm the presence of ascites or intestinal obstruction secondary to disease of the pelvic organs.

Bone Age

In patients with growth and sexual development disorders, the hormonal effects on bone maturation can be assessed by radiographs of the epiphyseal centers, usually of the hand and wrist. The "bone age" of the patient is determined by comparing her radiographs with those of normal children at different ages. If the bone age is more than two standard deviations outside normal, abnormal delay or advancement of growth is probable. Retarded bone age is seen with hypothyroidism, Cushing's syndrome, hypopituitarism, and gonadal dysgenesis if these signs occur prepubertally and around puberty. Advanced bone age is seen with hyperthyroidism and congenital adrenal hyperplasia during the prepubertal years.

Intravenous Pyelogram

The intravenous pyelogram (IVP) is frequently used for evaluating patients with gynecologic disorders. This radiographic technique requires intravenous administration of an iodinated radiographic contrast material that is excreted from the kidneys. Over the course of excretion, the kidneys and their upper collecting systems may be visualized along with the ureters draining urine to the bladder; the bladder is also outlined. The IVP is particularly helpful for evaluating the kidneys and the course of the ureters. Although information may be gained regarding the shape and position of the bladder, other more specific tests, such as cystoscopy and cystography, are more specific for evaluating the bladder itself. Tomograms may be made through the kidneys during the course of an IVP to assess more fully the upper collecting systems and kidney anatomy.

With regard to the evaluation of common problems associated with gynecologic disease and urologic abnormalities, the following conditions are most frequently studied.

1. Evaluation of a patient with apparent congenital müllerian anomalies should include evaluation of the urologic system (Chap. 8). Congenital anomalies of the kidneys or ureters with duplicate or absent collecting systems are frequently found.

2. Prior to undertaking gynecologic surgery for benign gynecologic conditions, it is frequently helpful for the surgeon to be sure that the urinary tract is normal or to be able to identify abnormalities. Common abnormalities that might alter the surgical approach include the identification of duplicate collecting systems or absent collecting systems. Furthermore, on rare occasions a pelvic mass is a pelvic kidney (Fig. 3-1). Deviation of the ureter by a pelvic mass or obstruction of the ureter may also be identified (Fig. 3-2). Further evaluation and treatment at the time of gynecologic surgery may be necessary. A pelvic mass arising from the pelvis and attaining the size of a 16-week gestation often causes extrinsic compression of the ureters at the pelvic brim, leading to a variable degree of hydronephrosis and proximal hydroureter. Likewise, endometriosis may invade the retroperitoneal space and lead to ureteral deviation or obstruction.

3. During evaluation for gynecologic malignancy, the urinary tract should be inspected as well. It is frequently found that carcinoma of the cervix deviates or obstructs the ureter in the pelvis, especially if parametrial extension has occurred. Likewise metastatic disease to the lymph nodes, as is seen with cervical, endometrial, and ovarian carcinomas may lead to ureteral

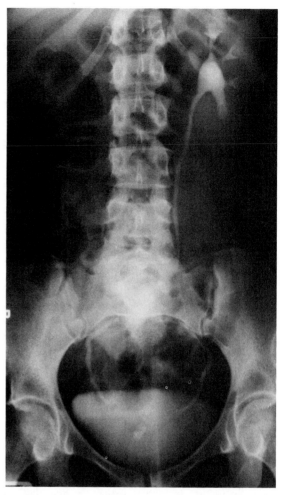

Fig. 3-1. IVP of an adult woman presenting with a pelvic mass that turned out to be a pelvic kidney.

obstruction or deviation. Abnormalities seen by IVP are incorporated into the staging system for carcinoma of the cervix.

4. IVP may be helpful for evaluating the patient with a possible urinary tract fistula. It is particularly helpful for identifying ureteral injury or ureterovaginal fistula. Other methods for evaluating the bladder and urethra are more specific.

5. Potential surgical injury to the ureter may be assessed postoperatively with an IVP. Evidence of ure-

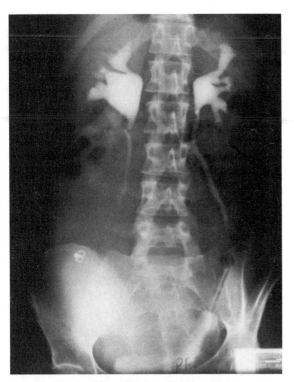

Fig. 3-2. Preoperative IVP in a 39-year-old woman with a pelvic mass the size of a 24-week pregnancy but due to multiple fibroids. The IVP shows an irregularly shaped soft tissue pelvic mass compressing the bladder, with the ureters displaced laterally in the pelvis, and bilateral hydronephrosis.

teral obstruction or deviation may be identified by IVP. On the other hand, other modes of evaluation, such as cystoscopy with retrograde pyelogram or passage of ureteral stents, may be helpful in further evaluation and treatment.

A pelvic mass often compresses or deviates the dome of the bladder, as noted in the cystogram phase of an IVP (Fig. 3-2). On the other hand, a normal anteflexed uterus causes indentation of the dome of the bladder that is entirely normal.

The risks of an IVP are primarily related to reactions noted in patients who have iodine allergies, usually manifested by urticarial reaction or wheezing. More severe reactions may lead to respiratory arrest. Because the contrast material is excreted from the

kidneys, patients who have underlying renal disease (e.g., diabetes or hypertensive renal disease) or patients who have taken nephrotoxic drugs (e.g., cisplatin) are at risk for further renal compromise. Therefore assessment of the patient's history of iodine allergy (e.g., a sensitivity to shellfish or a previous reaction to IVP dye) and an assessment of renal function (serum creatinine) should be undertaken before performing an IVP.

Other methods for assessing the urinary tract, including a retrograde pyelogram, cystogram, and cystourethrogram, are discussed in more detail as they specifically related to the abnormalities of the lower urinary tract discussed in Chapter 19.

Barium Enema

Barium enema is performed primarily to evaluate the colon and terminal ileum. Barium is injected as an enema and observed under fluoroscopic control as it fills the colon and terminal ileum. Radiographs are obtained during the filling and evacuation phases, with detailed films made of areas of interest. Air may also be injected into the colon to obtain more detail of mucosal lesions (air contrast barium enema) (Fig. 3-3). Details of the rectum are poorly evaluated by barium enema and are probably better studied by proctosigmoidoscopy.

Barium enema may reveal involvement of the colon by gynecologic disease. A large pelvic mass may cause extrinsic compression or deviation of the colon (Fig. 3-4). Ovarian carcinoma, in more advanced stages, not only may cause extrinsic compression but may actually invade the colon and its mesentery. This situation is most frequently noted in the sigmoid colon, although the cecum and transverse colon may also be involved. Preoperative barium enemas in patients with an adnexal mass may give some suggestion as to colonic involvement and thereby allow adequate preparation for colonic surgery. Benign conditions, especially endometriosis, may also invade the colon and lead to intestinal obstruction or perforation. Conversely, pelvic disease may have as its primary etiology colonic disease, particularly colon cancer, which may be detected as a pelvic mass either as a palpable rectosigmoid lesion or as an enlarging ovarian metas-

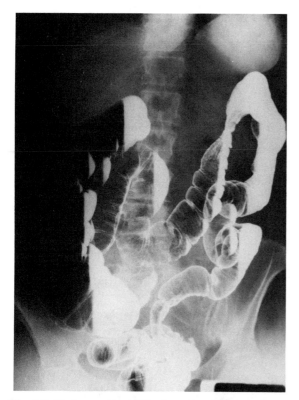

Fig. 3-3. Barium enema with air contrast shows an essentially normal large bowel.

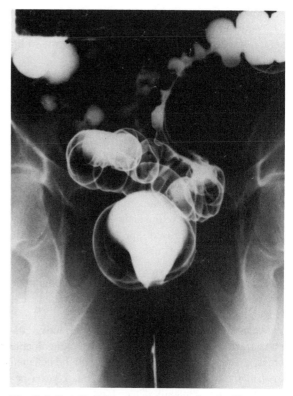

Fig. 3-4. Detail of the rectosigmoid colon (in Figure 3-3) showing compression and deviation of the sigmoid colon by an extrinsic mass that was ultimately found to be a mucinous cystadenoma of the left ovary.

tasis (Krukenberg tumor). Diverticulitis or a diverticular abscess may be the etiology of a pelvic mass, which would be suggested by barium enema. Colonic obstruction, stricture, and fibrosis caused by radiation therapy may also be diagnosed. Rectovaginal fistula is often diagnosed by a barium enema; and multiple fistulous tracts, such as are associated with advanced ovarian carcinoma or severe radiation injury, may be more clearly delineated. Barium enema is also indicated in cases of rectal bleeding or a guaiac-positive stool. Rectal bleeding may be caused by colonic carcinoma, polyps, or other associated conditions such as radiation proctitis.

The primary risks and side effects of barium enema are patient discomfort and exposure to additional radiation. Perforation caused by barium enema is infrequent (probably less than 1 in 1000), although in situations such as diverticulitis or colonic carcinoma

perforation may be increased. Barium spilling into the peritoneal cavity may cause barium peritonitis, which unless managed appropriately with prompt evacuation, fecal diversion, and peritoneal lavage may be fatal. Finally, barium allowed to remain in the colon after a barium enema study may become an inspissated hard mass leading to impaction.

Mammography

Conventional mammography using ordinary soft-tissue radiographic techniques was first attempted during the 1930s; but it was not until the 1960s, with improved methodology and greater experience, that this approach to the diagnosis of breast disease became reliable and more frequently used. Radiographic instrumentation is now sufficiently developed that radiation exposure during screening mammography is minimal, seldom exceeding 1 rad per breast with a two-view bilateral study.

Xeroradiography has gradually begun to replace conventional mammography; it is probably even more accurate, the films are easier to interpret, and the radiation exposure to the breast is lower. Xeromammography involves a photoconductive imaging process that uses routine radiography equipment but a special cassette that is dry-developed (no film is involved) to produce a paper radiograph. All the image densities occur on the paper in sharp contrast and are easy to interpret. Further developments in sensitive intensifying screens, improved specialized radiographic films, microfocal spot tubes, and radiographic grids for mammography have dramatically improved film screen mammography. Thus both xeroradiographic and film screen mammography are accurate and sensitive diagnostic imaging techniques.

Screening mammography is the most effective current method available for diagnosing nonpalpable breast cancer. Breast cancer can generally be detected by screening mammography up to about 2 years before it becomes clinically detectable by the patient or her physician. Data from the Breast Cancer Detection Demonstration Project indicate that mammograms were positive or suspicious for nearly 90 percent of all cancers detected. Mammography not only was responsible for breast biopsy being performed in 42 percent of cancers detected but was able to detect early disease (infiltrating breast cancer of less than 1 cm). Undoubtedly such early detection carries a better prognosis and may require less mutilating surgery for effective therapy.

Because of the above benefits and the low radiation involved with current mammography instruments, screening mammography should begin in all women probably from age 40 to 45, when the incidence of breast cancer begins to rise. The American Cancer Society guidelines call for a baseline (first) mammogram at 35 to 40 years of age and earlier for patients at highest risk. Although annual mammography has been recommended for women over 50 years of age, repeat mammograms for those at 40 to 50 years

should be carried out at intervals determined by their physicians based on the initial study, risk factors, and clinical examination findings. Mammography is an invaluable aid for the evaluation and management of women with diffuse, bilateral irregularities due to fibrocystic disease of the breast (Fig. 3-5) in whom random biopsy obviously cannot exclude the possibility that one of the palpable "irregularities" is an early cancer. In a patient with a single, dominant lump, biopsy or needle aspiration is indicated, even though the lesion may appear benign on mammography. Mammography is not necessary to make that decision; nevertheless, it is useful, even in this situation, for

Fig. 3-5. Mammogram of a patient with generalized lumpiness of the breast showing fibrocystic disease (fibrocystic change) of the breast, with no single discrete mass.

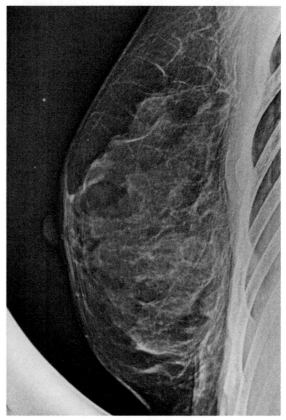

screening the opposite breast and other areas of the breast containing the palpable lump for occult cancer.

Interpretation of mammography is improved, and accuracy of diagnosis is enhanced by correlation of radiographic observations with physical findings. Important signs of breast carcinoma visualized on mammograms are (1) the presence of a mass lesion and (2) identification of clustered microcalcifications. Mass lesions are most significant if the density is irregular or the margins are spiculated. If microcalcifications are also present with the mass lesion, the probability of malignancy is greatly enhanced. However, even without a mass lesion, clustered microcalcifications (less than 0.5 mm in size) that are often irregular must be carefully searched for—if necessary, with a magnifying hand lens (Fig. 3-6A). Suggestive of benign disease are smooth, smudged, rounded calcifications of uniform size. Irregular, branching, and uneven microcalcifications usually signify malignancy. The coarse calcification of degenerating fibroadenoma (Fig. 3-7), the tubular calcifications of benign secretory disease, and vascular calcifications should not be cause for concern. Indirect signs such as asymmetry of the breast tissue and vascular structures, focally dilated ducts, and architectural distortion of varying degrees, when correlated with clinical findings, warrant further studies or suspicion of potential malignancy. Follow-up mammograms should always be compared with previous ones, especially when there is inexplicable interval change, at which point biopsy becomes necessary.

It is important to note that about 10 percent of breast cancers cannot be detected by mammography alone, especially when there is minimal radiographic change, dense breast tissue, abundant cystic changes, or implanted prostheses.

Breast lesions can be preoperatively localized with placement of a special needle with coaxial wire hooks under radiographic control at or adjacent to the lesion, with little risk of displacement before excision (Fig. 3-6B and C). Thus radiographic imaging of the breast is also a therapeutic aid. Such a technique enables precise but minimal (cosmetically more attractive) breast tissue excision if the growth is benign.

Ultrasound examination of the breast is valuable diagnostically when combined with mammography. Ultrasound can be employed to differentiate a cystic from a solid mass in the breast with accuracy (Fig. 3-8). Ultrasonography also plays a limited role for evaluating radiographically dense breasts, reducing the value of mammograms. Nevertheless, ultrasonography of the breasts cannot yet be employed as a sensitive screen technique for occult neoplasms.

Hysterosalpingography

Hysterosalpingography is radiographic delineation of the uterus and fallopian tubes using a contrast material introduced into the uterus via the cervical canal. The contrast outlines the uterine cavity, the lumen of the fallopian tubes and their patency, and the cervical canal. Hysterosalpingography should be carried out under fluoroscopic monitoring, as this method provides maximum information with respect to the manner and rate with which the dye fills the uterine cavity and the fallopian tubes and the actual spill of dye from each fallopian tube if it is patent. This dynamic relation between the müllerian tract system and the instilled dye cannot be readily appreciated from the static spot films alone, but the latter are taken at the appropriate moment of relevant clinical interest seen by fluoroscopy for subsequent review and reading. It is probable that the fluoroscopic screening itself can be recorded on videotape and replayed for study purposes.

A diagnostic procedure commonly employed for evaluation of female infertility and recurrent abortion, hysterosalpingography is also helpful for the management and treatment plan of gynecologic disorders such as abnormal uterine bleeding, intrauterine adhesions (Asherman's syndrome), congenital anomalies and diethylstilbestrol exposure in utero, and preoperative evaluation prior to myomectomy and tubal reconstruction. Hysterosalpingography is often used for postoperative assessment of uterine and tubal integrity, after tubal reconstruction without pregnancy occurring, and after tubal ligation with questionable histologic documentation that the tubes were ligated. Although pregnancies have occurred after hysterosalpingography for evaluation of infertility, there is no

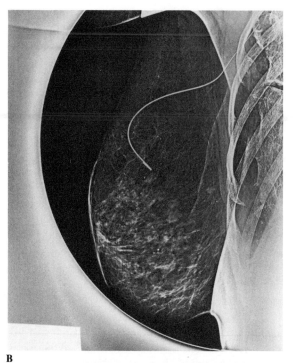

A

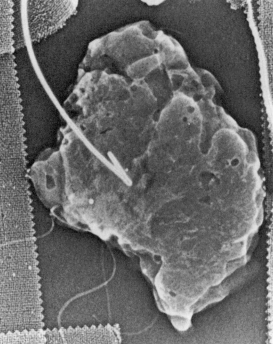

B

C

Fig. 3-6. A. Mammogram of the left breast of a 53-year-old postmenopausal woman showing a small cluster of microcalcifications of irregular appearance in the upper outer quadrant. The breast generally shows fibrocystic change (fibrocystic disease). B. Needle localization mammogram of the patient showing the area to be biopsied, with the hook-wire positioned directly in the center of the microcalcification cluster. C. Biopsy specimen from the patient showing a cluster of microcalcifications within the specimen and partially hidden by the localizing wire. Histology showed multiple small foci of intraductal carcinoma in an area of fibrocystic change with the tumor not extending to the resected margins.

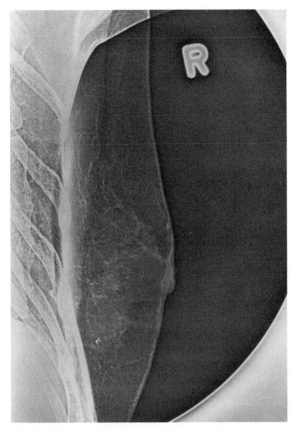

Fig. 3-7. Mammogram shows a fibroadenoma with calcifications in a woman with a clinically discrete, freely movable breast lump. The condition remained unchanged clinically and in repeated mammograms over many years.

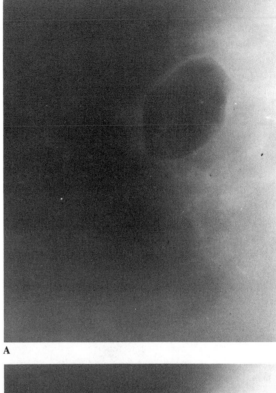

A

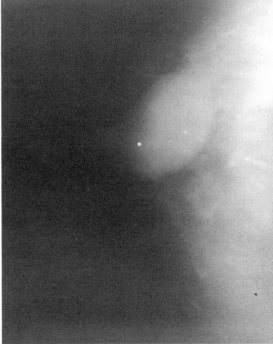

B

Fig. 3-8. Ultrasound of the breast. A. Breast cyst. B. Same cyst after needle aspiration of the cyst fluid and replaced with air.

conclusive proof that the procedure is therapeutic. It is possible that the mechanical flushing effect of the dye instillation may wash out debris in the tube and therefore subsequently facilitate spontaneous pregnancy; however, hysterosalpingography is best not advocated as therapy. The diagnostic value of hysterosalpingography is greatly enhanced by laparoscopy and can sometimes be replaced by the latter procedure. However, for abnormalities within the uterine cavity and the cervical canal, hysterosalpingography provides additional information.

Contraindications to hysterosalpingography include pregnancy or suspected pregnancy, active uterine bleeding, menstruation, acute pelvic inflammatory disease, and hypersensitivity to iodine or iodine-containing dyes. Complications of hysterosalpingography are relatively infrequent, 0.3 to 1.7 percent. The complication seen most often is pelvic infection following the procedure. Other less frequent complications include allergy to the contrast material injected, vasomotor reactions including flushing, dizziness, transient hypotension (all of which are self-limiting and not serious), and allergic reaction to the contrast material. Oil embolism and tubal and peritoneal granulomatous reactions are complications associated with the use of oil-based contrast medium. For these reasons, the use of a water-soluble contrast medium is preferable. The risk of radiation exposure to the ovaries is small. The amount of radiation to the ovaries depends on the fluoroscopic unit employed, the duration of fluoroscopy (a time limit is set for most machines for this procedure so as not to exceed the maximum dose of radiation), and the size of the patient. For usual hysterosalpingography examinations, the amount of radiation is small (less than 750 mrad).

The hysterosalpingography procedure is as follows. A pelvic examination is first performed. After inserting the vaginal speculum, the vagina and cervix are cleaned with povidone-iodine (Betadine) solution; excess cervical mucus is removed, and the cervix is grasped with a tenaculum. Either a Foley balloon catheter (No. 8 French), polyethylene catheter (No. 5 French), polyvinylchloride catheter, or regular metal cannula with a rubber cone or a metal cannula to which is attached a plastic cone with a plastic cannula tip is inserted into the cervix. Occasionally, in patients with uterus didelphys bicollis (two cervices and two uteri), two cannulas must be inserted to inject the dye separately into each cervix and uterus. The Foley catheter has the distinct disadvantage of the balloon obstructing the view of the lower uterine segment, makes examination of the incompetent cervix (internal os) difficult, and not being sufficiently rigid does not permit adequate mobilization of the uterus and surrounding structures. Insertion of the Foley catheter with a metal introducer is not simple and often is painful compared to the regular uterocervical cannula. (This author has never had to resort to a Foley catheter.) After inserting the cannula tip into the cervix and applying adequate countertraction on the tenaculum on the cervix, fluoroscopy is started to visualize and locate the tip of the cannula in the lower uterine segment. The speculum should be removed so that the patient may straighten her legs and be comfortable. A metal speculum in the vagina not only hurts the patient upon straightening the legs but blocks (radiopaque) visualization of the cervix and upper part of the vagina.

The whole delivery system through which the contrast medium is injected should be primed with the medium initially so that trapped air in the dead space is not delivered into the uterus, as air bubbles give rise to spurious filling defects and temporarily even block the uterotubal opening. The dye is then instilled slowly at first to visualize how the uterine cavity and fallopian tubes are filled. Any delay in filling or any filling defects should be noted; and if necessary, a radiograph is obtained to demonstrate such abnormalities. Spillage of dye from both fallopian tubes should also be noted and a film taken to show it. If the tubes do not fill at both uterotubal junctions, cornual spasm must be ruled out. Amyl nitrite can be given as an inhalation, or currently glucagon 1 mg is given intramuscularly to relieve the spasm; injection of the contrast is then continued after a few minutes. The tenaculum should be moved around to mobilize the uterus and to straighten it so as to appreciate the movement of the tubes in relation to the uterus. Lateral or oblique view films are necessary in some cases to obtain a three-dimensional reconstruction of the location of some intrauterine abnormalities but are not necessary for all cases. Common problems relating to the hysterosalpingography procedure are an inadequate amount of contrast material used and reflux of the contrast into the vagina because of poor cervical occlusion.

Normal Findings. The normal uterine cavity outline is a triangle with the base at the fundus and the apex inferiorly meeting and extending into the endocervical canal. However, many normal variations to this basic simplified outline are seen in normal uteri. The internal os is usually well demonstrated. If there is extreme uterine anteflexion, the fundal part of the uterine cavity is superimposed end-on with the inferior part of the cavity. This problem can be overcome by "straightening" the uterus with tension on the cervical tenaculum or taking an oblique view if the uterus does not straighten. The tubes emerge from the uterine cornua outward and can be identified as the interstitial segment, isthmus, ampulla, and infundibulum.

Abnormal Findings. Abnormalities detectable on hysterosalpingogram include those of the fallopian tubes, uterus, and cervix. Cervical incompetence can be readily demonstrated by the wide internal os and cervical canal. Abnormalities of the fallopian tubes seen on hysterosalpingograms include (1) obstruction with no further filling of the dye beyond the point of obstruction; (2) observation of the fimbrial end with no contrast material spillage (Fig. 3-9); (3) some contrast material spillage with a loculated, confined, well circumscribed collection, suggestive of adhesions between the distal tube and ovary into a kind of pocket but a fimbrial opening still present; and (4) complete fill and spill of the contrast from the tubes, which, however, show a "fixed" or "rigid" pattern in relation to the uterus suggestive of peritubal adhesions. Obstructed tubes can be due to pelvic inflammatory disease, endometriosis, previous sterilization, salpingectomy, or previous unsuccessful tubal reconstruction. Salpingitis isthmica nodosa shows a characteristic circoid, stippling pattern usually present at the isthmal region. Tuberculosis of the tubes may appear similar to salpingitis isthmica nodosa on hysterosalpingograms. Tubal polyps and tumors are also demonstrable. Although an ectopic pregnancy can be localized, hysterosalpingography is not employed as an imaging technique to diagnose it.

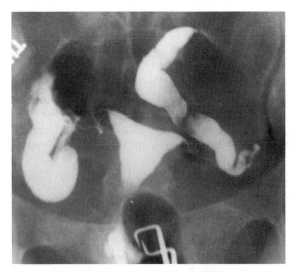

Fig. 3-9. Hysterosalpingogram of an adult woman with primary infertility demonstrates bilateral hydrosalpinges and no dye spillage from the distal end of either tube.

Acquired uterine abnormalities detected by hysterosalpingography include (1) myomas, which, if submucous, show distortion or enlargement of the uterine cavity; (2) endometrial polyps, which appear as well circumscribed filling defects often with a base from the uterine wall; (3) endometrial carcinoma appearing as round filling defects, either single or multiple; (4) uterine synechiae or Asherman's syndrome appearing as filling defects of varying extent, often with a craggy border (Fig. 3-10); and (5) early disruption of a cesarean section scar, appearing as a slight protrusion of dye along the scar line. Congenital anomalies of the uterus identified by hysterosalpingography include (1) arcuate, subseptate, septate, and bicornuate uterus, all of which show changes in the superior aspect of the uterine cavity outline ranging from a mild heart-shaped intrusion to a complete septum (Fig. 3-11); (2) unicornuate uterus with only one tube emerging from the superior end of a cylindrically shaped uterine cavity; (3) uterus didelphys showing two separate uterine cavities; and (4) T-shaped uterine cavity or a constricted lower segment in women who were exposed to diethylstilbestrol in utero.

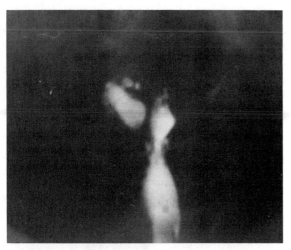

Fig. 3-10. Hysterosalpingogram shows an irregular, large filling defect in the uterine cavity due to uterine synechiae (Asherman's syndrome). The patient presented with amenorrhea and infertility.

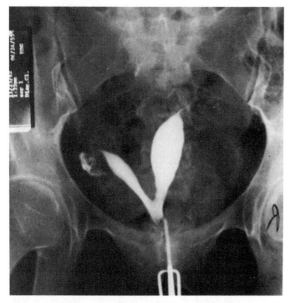

Fig. 3-11. Hysterosalpingogram shows a bicornuate uterus that was confirmed at surgery. The appearance of the uterine cavity shows bifurcation at the upper end that may be due to a bicornuate uterus or a subseptate uterus.

Pelvic Venography

Venography of the pelvic veins may be helpful for evaluating patients suspected of having pelvic or ovarian vein thrombosis and patients who have lower extremity edema that may be secondary to either thrombosis or extrinsic venous obstruction caused by retroperitoneal adenopathy. Because of the various drainage routes from the pelvis, there are three potential routes of access to the pelvic veins: (1) Ascending venography from the foot or femoral vein visualizes the external and common iliac veins and the vena cava. Occasionally, if there is venous obstruction, collateral circulation through the pelvis is also noted. However, in general, the internal iliac venous system is not visualized through this route. (2) Retrograde catheterization from the femoral vein into the common or external iliac vein down into the hypogastric vein followed by dye injection to visualize the internal iliac venous system. This invasive vascular radiology procedure is rarely performed. (3) The ovarian veins also drain from the pelvis and may be the source of thrombosis, flank pain, or pulmonary embolism. To visualize the ovarian vein, retrograde venography of the ovarian veins must be performed. It must be remembered that the left ovarian vein drains into the left renal vein, and the right ovarian vein drains into the vena cava.

The retrograde studies noted above are rarely performed today. In some instances, ovarian vein and pelvic vein thrombosis has been imaged by a noninvasive method such as computed tomography (CT) or magnetic resonance imaging (MRI). Likewise, CT and MRI may be more helpful for evaluating the potential for retroperitoneal masses obstructing veins. Therefore pelvic venography has little value today in patient management. The risks of venography are similar to those of the IVP in that the patient receives an iodinated contrast material intravenously that may cause an allergic reaction or a renal injury.

Pelvic Arteriography

Arteriography of the internal iliac artery with its myriad collaterals and branches plays a role in the management of several gynecologic conditions. To perform pelvic arteriography, a catheter must be inserted (usually into the femoral artery) and then the internal iliac trunk cannulated. Selective arteriography of the anterior or posterior division of the internal iliac artery may be accomplished through catheter manipulation and positioning. Arteriogram dye is injected rapidly, and rapid-sequence radiographs are obtained of both the filling and the drainage of the arterial and venous systems, respectively.

Pelvic arteriography plays a role in the management of the following conditions: (1) Pelvic arteriography may be helpful for locating the site of uncontrolled pelvic bleeding. It is particularly useful in postpartum patients, postoperative patients, the patient with a pelvic malignancy, or the infrequent patient who has radionecrosis of the pelvis. In each of these circumstances, arteriography may be used to identify the site of bleeding; and in conjunction with arterial embolization, bleeding may be controlled by obstruction of the particular segment of hypogastric artery contributing to the bleeding. Of course, pelvic bleeding may arise from other arteries, such as the inferior mesenteric or the ovarian arteries, neither of which can be visualized or controlled by embolization of the hypogastric artery. (2) Arterial venous malformations may occur congenitally or after gynecologic surgery. The pain, pressure, and potential for hemorrhage has been recognized with arteriovenous malformations, which are best visualized by arteriography. When the specific artery contributing to the vascular malformation is identified, it may also be embolized to partially control symptoms. (3) Patients with gestational trophoblastic disease who have become resistant to therapy may benefit by having a hysterectomy performed to excise a resistant focus of trophoblastic disease invasive to the myometrium. On occasion, arteriography assists in the confirmation of invasive gestational trophoblastic disease of the uterus, thereby confirming potential benefits of hysterectomy in excising occult disease. MRI of the uterus may be more helpful for identifying invasive disease in the future. (4) Infusion of chemotherapy agents through the pelvic vascular bed is experimental but may have some role in the future treatment of advanced gynecologic malignancy.

Pelvic arteriography requires the skill of a trained vascular radiologist and is associated with some risk. Aside from the risks associated with the iodinated contrast material previously noted for IVP and venography, complications arise from cannulation of the femoral and external iliac arteries. Arterial thrombosis as well as hematoma at the arteriotomy site may occur. Most hematomas resolve spontaneously, although arterial thrombosis may require embolectomy or even arterial bypass surgery. Occasionally, a lower extremity has been lost owing to extensive arterial thrombosis.

Gynecography

Gynecography employs air to provide contrast for radiographic imaging of the pelvic region. The technique of gynecography is as follows: Approximately 1000 cc of carbon dioxide is introduced through a culdocentesis needle with the patient in the knee-chest position, allowing air to enter the peritoneal cavity directly via the needle. Films made with the patient either in the knee-chest or the prone Trendelenburg position permit identification of the soft-tissue shadows of the pelvic viscera of any abnormal pelvic masses adjacent to them, which are outlined by the surrounding pelvic pneumoperitoneum. Further contrast can be obtained by performing simultaneous hysterosalpingography. Used in the past primarily for the demonstration of enlarged bilateral polycystic ovaries and for differentiating fibroids from ovarian tumors, gynecography has been largely replaced by laparoscopy, sonography, CT, and MRI. Presacral pneumoretroperitoneum for adrenal pneumogram employing carbon dioxide as the contrast medium is likewise replaced by the less invasive but more informative CT and MRI.

Lymphography (Lymphangiography or Lymphangioadenography)

Perfected during the 1960s, lymphography (the technique for radiographic demonstration of lymph vessels and lymph nodes) was used for evaluating the presence or absence of lymphatic spread in patients with pelvic cancer. The method has since proved to be

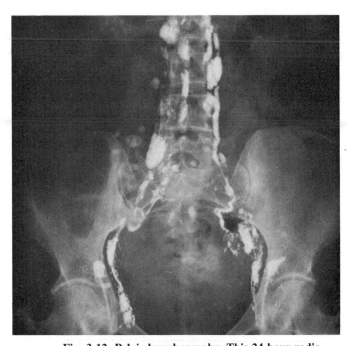

Fig. 3-12. Pelvic lymphography. This 24-hour radio-graph of a patient with cervical cancer shows the excellent visualization of the pelvic wall and paraaortic nodes usually obtained. A filling defect in the right pelvic wall node at the level of the pelvic brim is clearly demonstrated. This node was subsequently proved at laparotomy to contain metastatic disease.

less accurate and reliable than had been hoped. In several reported series of cervical cancer, there was a 25 to 30 percent rate of error in the attempt to make an early diagnosis of lymph node metastases. It is significant that false-positive results were just as frequent as false-negative results.

To perform pelvic lymphography, the four inter-metatarsal dorsal web spaces of both feet are given a preliminary intradermal injection of 2 ml of an aqueous solution of Patent Blue V-F dye; this step permits ready identification of lymph vessels when small transverse incisions are made on the dorsum of each ankle an hour later. One lymph vessel on each side is cannulated with a small needle connected by a polyethylene catheter to a syringe containing the radiopaque medium. Ethiodized oil (Ethiodol) has proved to be a satisfactory medium, and approximately 12 ml is injected slowly, over a period of an hour, into each lower extremity. Anteroposterior roentgenograms are then obtained of the legs, thighs, pelvis, abdomen, and chest, demonstrating not only the lymph channels but the lymph nodes as well (inguinal, femoral, exter-

nal and common iliacs, and paraaortic chains). Additional radiographs obtained 24 to 48 hours later frequently show the architecture of the lymph nodes to even better advantage (Fig. 3-12).

When lymph nodes contain metastatic tumor, a characteristic marginal filling defect is seen, and the nodes are usually readily differentiated from normal nodes or from lymphadenitis or lymphoma. The technique has been useful for diagnosing lymph node metastasis in patients with cervical carcinoma. It can also be used to determine the completeness of pelvic lymphadenectomy by a comparison of pre- and postoperative films. Furthermore, it is now possible to add an effective color dye to the radiopaque medium used for injection, a feature that may prove helpful for visualizing and identifying the lymphatic channels and nodes during the actual performance of radical pelvic operations.

RADIONUCLIDE SCANNING

The method of imaging body structures called radionuclide scanning employs injection of a radioactive isotopically labeled substance that is preferentially taken up by the organ or structure of interest. Radionuclide scanning is an effective diagnostic procedure, especially with the availability of the newer imaging radiolabeled agents. Hyperfunctioning tissues take up more of the radiolabeled agent than do normal functioning tissues.

Adrenal Glands

Radionuclide imaging of the adrenal glands employs ^{131}I-6β-iodomethylnorcholesterol (^{131}I-6-iodocholesterol) for visualizing the adrenal cortex and ^{131}I-meta-iodobenzylguanidine (^{131}I-MIBG) for the adrenal medulla. Radionuclide scanning of the adrenals provides information on adrenal structure as well as function.

Indications for radionuclide scanning of the adrenals include adrenal tumors (adenomas, carcinomas) and adrenocortical hyperplasia. Requiring a high radiation dose and several days between injection of the imaging agent and imaging, the procedure is relatively noninvasive and free of complications.

If the adrenals are normal, both glands show fairly symmetric uptake, which can vary from patient to patient. Because ^{131}I-iodocholesterol is metabolized in the liver and excreted in the intestines, these two structures are also visualized. Cortisol-producing adenomas show unilateral increased uptake, with suppression of the normal gland, as early as 2 days after the injection. Bilateral cortical hyperplasia shows diffuse increased bilateral uptake. Scanning can be combined with functional endocrine suppression by dexamethasone in patients with hyperandrogenism strongly suspected to be adrenal in origin. Such suppression with unilateral increased uptake suggests a localized functioning adrenal tumor (e.g., adrenal adenoma),

whereas diffuse increased bilateral uptake is indicative of hyperplasia.

Bone Scan

Radioisotope bone scanning is a helpful supplement to and usually more sensitive than a routine metastatic skeletal radiographic survey in patients known to have or who are suspected of having skeletal metastases. Various radioisotopes have been employed for this purpose, including sodium fluoride (^{18}F), strontium, and technetium (^{99m}Tc)-labeled phosphate compounds. A clearly visible increased radioisotope uptake is seen in areas of bone involved by metastatic tumor. There is also increased uptake with increased vascularity or increased calcium metabolism, so that results of the scan must be interpreted carefully and correlated with the clinical picture. In gynecologic cancer patients without symptoms or signs of skeletal metastases, a bone scan is not indicated as a routine screening procedure because the yield of positive scans is low. Routine skeletal radiographs sometimes reveal lesions not demonstrated by radioisotope skeletal imaging and vice versa, and in the initial stages some lesions escape detection by either method.

Brain Scan

A similar procedure employing ^{99m}Tc pertechnetate is available for brain imaging with the high-performance gamma scintillation camera. Again, this scan should be employed only in gynecologic cancer patients who have signs or symptoms suggestive of cerebral metastases, as the incidence of cerebral metastases from primary cancers of the pelvic organs is low. This technique has been largely replaced by the CT scan.

Liver Scan

Liver scanning has been used clinically since 1955. The current procedure provides imaging of both liver and spleen, and it employs ^{99m}Tc sulfur colloid as the radioisotope. Liver–spleen scanning is potentially more useful in the overall evaluation and screening of patients with gynecologic cancer, as liver metastases are more likely to occur as cancer of the reproductive tract becomes more extensive and begins to spread. Despite technical advances in the procedure, the number of patients with small hepatic metastases not visualized by liver scanning remains high (20 to 25 percent false-negative results). There is also a significant incidence (10 to 15 percent) of false-positive results.

Gallium Citrate Scanning

Gallium 67 is a radiopharmaceutical that accumulates in inflammatory tissues and in some tumors as well. Hence radionuclide scans of the abdomen 48 hours after the administration of gallium 67 can be helpful for establishing the presence and location of an intraabdominal abscess, either secondary to underlying pelvic inflammatory disease or occurring in a postoperative patient. Occasionally used to supplement the standard bone, liver–spleen, and brain scans, a gallium scan may contribute additional information in patients with known or suspected metastatic disease because it is often picked up by metastastic tissues, not only in liver and bone but also in lymph nodes, as well as in more obscure, nonosseous sites.

COMPUTED TOMOGRAPHY

Computed tomography is a computerized imaging technique involving ionizing radiation. With the newer generation CT scanners, thin slices of 1-mm tomograms of the structure or organ under study are obtained. CT is becoming increasingly useful for the diagnosis and evaluation of intraabdominal and pelvic lesions, intracranial pathology, and intrathoracic conditions as they relate to the practice of gynecology. However, the technique is more complex and expensive than sonography and exposes the patient to ionizing radiation. Particularly useful for evaluating pelvic and pituitary neoplasms, CT offers the ability to assess parietal soft tissue planes, including muscle and fat as well as bones, vessels, lymph nodes, and other retroperitoneal structures. CT imaging can be further enhanced with the use of contrast medium. If an oral contrast medium is ingested before the CT imaging, intraabdominal tumors can be delineated in sharp contrast to the dye-filled loops of bowel. CT scanning is useful for the following conditions: (1) enlarged pelvic and paraaortic lymph nodes; (2) retroperitoneal diseases; (3) assessment of a previously irradiated pelvis, the examination of which is otherwise seriously hampered by extensive fibrosis and scarring; (4) pituitary microadenomas and their suprasellar extension, empty sellar syndrome; (5) secondary metastases in the brain from gynecologic malignancy (e.g., choriocarcinoma); (6) CT-directed thin-needle biopsies of CT-visible lesions in the pelvis and elsewhere, obviating a major operative procedure to obtain tissue diagnosis; and (7) assessment of bone mineral mass particularly in the thoracolumbar vertebra (T12–L4) of postmenopausal and hypogonadal women.

Because CT can image many organs, it may replace or eliminate the need for several other studies. For example, CT may be used to evaluate patients with gynecologic malignancies in the search for distant metastases. This single test may be used to evaluate the lungs, liver, upper abdomen, urinary tract, retroperitoneal lymph nodes, and pelvic structures. Therefore in the setting of staging of gynecologic malignancy, CT may replace chest tomography, liver scanning, pelvic ultrasound, IVP, and lymphangiography.

The broadest application of CT today is for the staging of gynecologic cancers. CT imaging may be helpful for identifying local extension of cervical carcinoma, involvement of lymph nodes, and identification of distant metastases. The identification of metastatic disease in pelvic or paraaortic lymph nodes depends on the size of the lymph node. The CT scan cannot differentiate an enlarged hyperplastic lymph node due to hyperplasia from those containing metastases. Lymph nodes of 1.5 to 2.0 cm are considered suspicious, and nodes larger than 2.0 cm are considered abnormal. When evaluating local extension of gynecologic malignancies, such as cervical carcinoma, CT is not entirely accurate and is not necessarily more sensitive or specific than a careful gynecologic pelvic examination. In this setting MRI may be more accurate. Identification of distant metastases in the liver, lungs, or brain may be detected more accurately by CT scan than other scanning techniques. CT may also provide information similar to that of an

IVP identifying normal kidneys and patent ureters. Detailed evaluation of the urologic system, however, is better performed by IVP.

The role of CT scanning of the pelvis for evaluating a pelvic mass is limited. The CT scan cannot distinguish between the benign and malignant pelvic mass (Fig. 3-13). CT may be helpful for evaluating the characteristics of the mass (solid versus cystic or mixed components) and may be helpful for identifying cyst content especially if it is fat. Because nearly all cases of a pelvic mass require surgical exploration, excision, and pathologic study, CT scan information does little to help the clinician establish a diagnosis and rarely changes the need for surgical exploration and excision. When evaluating ovarian carcinoma, CT is more sensitive for identification of ascites than is the clinical examination, and it may also identify metastases at other peritoneal sites such as the omentum, liver, or bowel mesentery. However, the sensitivity and specificity of CT scanning for evaluating intraperitoneal disease is limited, and rarely are metastases smaller than 2 cm identified, primarily because of the varying consistency of the abdominal cavity, with

Fig. 3-13. CT scan of the abdomen and pelvis shows a pelvic mass (cystic ovarian neoplasm) in a 75-year-old woman.

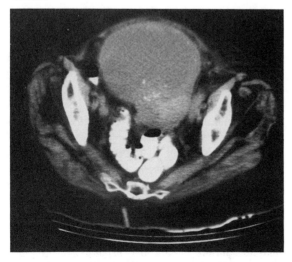

loops of bowel, omentum, and intestinal mesentery making up parts of the CT cuts.

In order to identify loops of small bowel, the intestines are usually filled with radiographic contrast material. Likewise, in the retroperitoneal space, differentiation of vessels from retroperitoneal lymph nodes is aided by the use of intravenous iodinated constrast material. Without these contrast techniques, CT scanning has a reduced capability to identify intraperitoneal and retroperitoneal disease. Evaluation of depth of invasion of endometrial carcinoma is poorly defined by CT scan; MRI appears to be more accurate.

The CT scan may be helpful in the identification of distant metastasis in lymph nodes, liver, or elsewhere in the peritoneal cavity in patients completing treatment for their gynecologic malignancy or who are suspected to have a recurrence. CT identification of a suspected metastasis can usually be confirmed by fine-needle aspiration and cytopathologic diagnosis (Fig. 3-14).

The CT scan is also helpful in the search for intraabdominal abscesses that may follow gynecologic surgery for patients with pelvic inflammatory disease and lymphocysts after pelvic lymphadenectomy. Abscesses and lymphocysts may be drained by CT-guided needle aspiration and catheter placement. Thus CT scans and CT-guided procedures could be used to avoid major surgical procedures in many patients. In a few cases, CT scanning has been helpful for the identification of ovarian vein and pelvic vein thrombosis.

Computed tomography is also helpful in the identification and follow-up of patients with pituitary adenomas. CT has a better sensitivity and specificity than, and has replaced, serial polytomography of the sella turcica. A CT scan of the pituitary can distinguish an empty sella syndrome from a true pituitary adenoma. Therefore CT is useful for evaluating patients with hyperprolactinemia and their follow-up.

Scanning of the abdomen and pelvis takes about 45 minutes and has as its major risks radiation exposure and exposure to intravenous contrast material. On the other hand, one of the major advantages of CT scanning is its ability to replace several other diagnostic radiographic techniques.

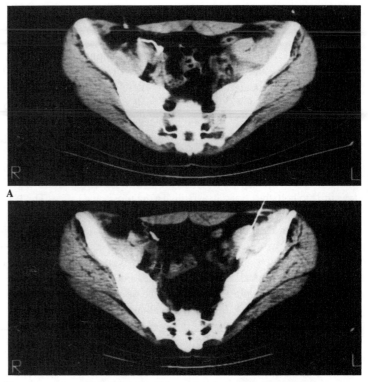

A

B

Fig. 3-14. A. CT scan of the pelvis demonstrates recurrent cervical carcinoma in lymph nodes and the left pelvic sidewall. B. Using CT scanning for guidance, fine-needle aspiration is performed. Cytopathology confirmed malignant squamous cells in the lymph node.

SONOGRAPHY

The use of diagnostic ultrasound has been well established in obstetric practice. However, until recently, abdominal ultrasound for imaging in gynecology did not have the clarity and accuracy needed to aid clinical decision-making. With improvement in the technology (e.g., high-frequency transducers, magnification of the image, real-time sonography, and transvaginal sonography), ultrasound imaging of the nonpregnant reproductive tract and during early pregnancy is rapidly gaining dependability.

For maximum effectiveness of using ultrasound imaging and because it is often carried out by the gynecologist in the clinic or office, it is necessary to understand some of the basic principles involved in this method of imaging. Ultrasound refers to high-frequency sound waves exceeding 20,000 Hertz (Hz), with most sonogram instruments usually having a sound frequency range of 2 to 10 mega-Hertz (MHz) (1 Hz is sound with a frequency of one cycle or one

peak per second). In the ultrasound machine, the ultrasound energy is produced by a transducer containing crystal structures that convert electrical energy to ultrasound waves and the returning echoes back to energy. Thus each crystal in the transducer acts both as the transmitter and receiver. Most diagnostic equipment generates a sound pulse every *millisecond* with a pulse duration of 1 *microsecond*. Thus the duration of exposure of the tissue to the high-frequency sound wave is brief. The returning echo is converted to an electrical signal by the transducer and displayed on an oscilloscope screen (what is visualized). The electrical signal is directly proportional to the intensity of the returning echo, which in turn depends on the density of the medium (e.g., tissues) through which it passes. The speed of the returning echo is faster and its signal on the screen brighter after reflection off bone than off less dense tissues such as muscle, fat, brain, or water. A coupling medium, or gel, is applied between the transducer and skin or vagina to obviate air interface, as air decreases transmission of sound waves and therefore gives a poorer image on the screen.

The diagnostic images can be produced in several ways.

A mode (amplitude modulation), when the returning echo is displayed as a *spike* proportional to the returning echo amplitude

M mode (motion mode), when the returning echo is displayed as a *spot* generating a horizontal line on a moving display

B mode (brightness modulation), when the returning echo is displayed as *signals of varying brightness* proportional to the returning echo amplitude

In gynecology the B mode is usually employed with a real-time array transducer. A storage oscilloscope creates a compounded image of the target to produce a two-dimensional picture; and combined with the real-time array transducer systems, the image is created so rapidly (fraction of a second) that movement of structures in real time can be visualized.

Vaginal Sonography

Transvaginal sonography has two major advantages over abdominal sonography. First, no acoustic window is required for transvaginal scanning; therefore a full bladder to push the female reproductive organs out of the pelvis, necessary for abdominal sonography, is not required. Second, the transvaginal transducer is closer to the pelvic structures than the abdominal probe, thereby increasing the spatial resolution. Because there is little adipose tissue at the vaginal apex, the problem of increased signal attenuation through tissues, with the use of a high-frequency transducer, can be overcome by moving the transducer probe closer to the object. At present, transvaginal transducers have frequencies up to 7.5 MHz compared to abdominal scanning, which is usually carried out with 3.5- or 5.0-MHz transducers.

Abdominal sonography for gynecology requires a full bladder to draw the reproductive organs up and out of the true pelvis. Satisfactory visualization of the pelvis is also difficult in obese women. However, the increased beam intensity and gain required to visualize distant structures reduces image clarity because high-frequency sound waves are absorbed with tissue penetration. The image cannot be significantly magnified during abdominal scanning in order for the posterior pelvis to be also visualized. These disadvantages or shortcomings of abdominal scanning of the pelvis are overcome with vaginal ultrasonography.

A transvaginal scan is usually best done with an empty bladder, for which the patient is grateful. A preliminary abdominal scan may infrequently be indicated. Vaginal scanning is carried out with the patient lying in the lithotomy position on a gynecologic examination table, slightly in the reverse Trendelenburg position to pool free peritoneal fluid in the pelvis to enhance visualization. The transducer is covered with a condom or a rubber glove into which some sonograph coupling gel has been placed; additional gel is placed on the outside for lubrication. The probe is then inserted into the vagina up to the vaginal apex, and pelvic structures are visualized in the sagittal or coronal plane. Usually it is helpful to identify the uterus first on the scan so that the adnexal regions can be scanned and structures identified in relation to it. The iliac vein and artery are convenient landmarks for the pelvic sidewalls, and the ovary is usually medial to these vessels. Withdrawing the transducer slightly from the vaginal apex allows the cervix to be scanned. Transvaginal sonography has been employed or is useful for the following gynecologic conditions or situations.

Ovary. Because of its posterolateral location, the normal ovary is difficult to visualize in detail with abdominal scanning. Abdominal scanning of the ovaries requires extensive bladder filling; but even with this maneuver, the ovary sometimes tends to displace deep into the posterior pelvis. Under such circumstances and also with obese patients, the resolution of the sonogram scan is limited. Transvaginal sonography provides a definite improvement in sonographic visualization and scanning of the ovary and has therefore become the method of choice for sonographic scanning of the ovaries. With this technique, there is improved visualization of ovarian follicles in as many as 85 to 90 percent of patients who had suboptimal abdominal ultrasound examination of the ovaries.

Transvaginal sonographic scanning of the ovaries is currently carried out for: (1) routine follicle scanning and monitoring of follicle recruitment and rate of growth (Fig. 3-15); (2) ultrasound guidance of follicle aspiration transvaginally for in vitro fertilization; (3) examination of the ovary for ovarian enlargement or adnexal mass; (4) routine measurement of ovarian size and volume in the postmenopausal woman to determine its potential value for early detection of ovarian neoplasm. With transvaginal ultrasonically guided oocyte retrieval, fertilization and pregnancy rates are similar to those obtained with laparoscopic recovery; but this method has the added advantages of requiring only local or regional anesthesia, being done readily in the office or clinic, and reducing the cost of in vitro fertilization. More and more centers doing in vitro fertilization are employing this method of oocyte retrieval, so that transvaginal ovarian sonographic imaging is not only diagnostic but can be employed as an adjunct for surgical therapy. Vaginal sonography of the ovaries is also employed for detecting cysts and ovarian tumors. With cysts single or multiple fluid-filled cavities are easily detected; the homogeneous echogenicity is higher in dermoid cysts than in single cysts. Endometrial chocolate cysts also have homogeneous echogenicity, resembling dermoid cysts. Solid ovarian tumors have irregular echogenicity.

Tubes. The normal fallopian tube cannot be readily seen on sonography for a variety of technical reasons, unless the tube is surrounded by or distended with some kind of fluid. Transvaginal sonographic scanning is particularly useful for visualization of diseased fallopian tubes and the ovaries. Ectopic pregnancy in the fallopian tubes and ovaries can be readily detected, and any free fluid in the cul-de-sac due to a hemoperitoneum can also be immediately visualized. It then allows culdocentesis to be carried out, if necessary, under vaginal ultrasound guidance. Because of the closeness of a tubal pregnancy examined with a vaginal probe and the high-frequency transducer employed, resolution of the image of the ectopic pregnancy is clearer and better. With an acute disease such as inflamed tubes or a tubal gestation, the walls are widened and the longitudinal endosalpingeal folds can be seen. With ectopic pregnancy, blood clots may fill the tubal cavity, or an unruptured pregnancy sac with or without active heartbeat is seen.

Fig. 3-15. Transvaginal sonograms of the ovary in a woman undergoing induction of ovulation with human menopausal gonadotropins. The scan of the left ovary shows follicles with the two leading follicles measuring 14 × 23 mm and 13 × 18 mm in diameter.

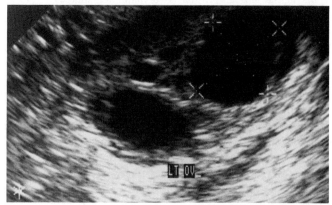

Cervix and Uterus. The cervix appears first on the screen upon scanning in a transverse plane if the uterus is anteverted; if the uterus is retroverted, the fundus appears first and is close to the sacrum. The exact poisition of the uterus and cervix is best displayed when scanning in the longitudinal plane. The internal and external cervical os as well as the length of the cervical canal can be measured in the longitudinal views. With this view, cystic structures of the cervical canal representing probably endocervical gland structures must be differentiated from very early ectopic cervical pregnancy. The uterine artery and veins can be recognized together with blood flow at the level of the internal os on a real-time scan. On the exocervix, nabothian cysts are recognized as translucent thin-walled structures.

The position of the uterus is examined, and common pathology of the uterine wall (e.g., myomas or polyps) should be sought. Sonographically, myomas display variable echogenicity, arranged in bundle-like "turbulent" structures interspersed with acoustic shadows produced by the dense fibroid tissues (Fig.

Fig. 3-16. Transvaginal sonogram (transverse scan) of a uterine myoma in the left cornual region. The calculated size of the myoma was 2.7 × 2.8 cm. At myomectomy the location and size of the myoma were confirmed.

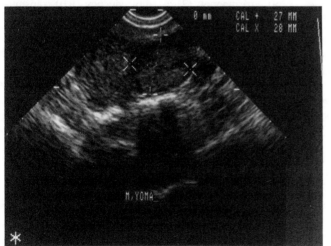

3-16). Unlike ovarian masses, solid masses on the uterus usually move in the direction in which the vaginal probe is pushed; and if the sonographic appearance is similar to the uterine texture, the mass is likely to be a fibroid. The postmenopausal uterus tends to be significantly smaller but has a uniform echogenicity if it is disease-free. The uterine cavity and its endometrial lining should be carefully scanned. The appearance of the endometrium changes throughout the menstrual cycle, and an empty uterus shows a regular, thin, obvious "cavity line." If bleeding is present, the blood-filled uterine cavity is readily outlined. Malformations of the uterus can be detected.

Early Gestation. Transvaginal sonography can detect an intrauterine gestational sac earlier than abdominal sonography, and it may be a potential technique for studying pregnancy as early as the periimplantation period. An intrauterine gestation has been visualized on vaginal sonography, showing a 4-mm sac as early as 4 weeks and 1 to 6 days from the last menstrual period. At this stage, the serum human chorionic gonadotropin (β-hCG) is usually only 400 to 800 mIU/ml. More often the pregnancy sac is readily seen by 5 weeks, and a yolk sac is seen in the gestational sac at 5 weeks 2 days. By 6 weeks the diagnosis of

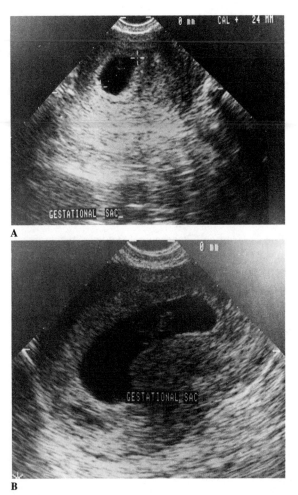

A

B

Fig. 3-17. Transvaginal sonograms of early intrauterine pregnancy. A. Transverse scan showing a pregnancy sac (24 mm) with a second internal ring (4 mm) at 43 days from the last menstrual period in a woman given clomiphene citrate to induce ovulation. The basal body temperature chart indicated a rise in temperature 15 days from the last menstrual period. B. Transverse scan of the same patient but at 55 days from the last menstrual period shows the intrauterine gestational sac with the early fetus in it.

intrauterine pregnancy with vaginal sonography becomes easy (Fig. 3-17). Characteristically, the gestational sac appears as a double line, which is a different picture from that produced by other intrauterine elements, such as bleeding and decidual reactions.

MAGNETIC RESONANCE IMAGING

Magnetic resonance imaging measures the magnetic properties of hydrogen nuclei. Using no ionizing radiation and with no moving parts on the equipment, MRI produces images similar to those obtained by CT scan. Not only can MRI provide anatomic delineation of various body structures, it provides data about molecular concentration and relaxation. MRI techniques are being used increasingly to study the structure and function of intact organs and organisms under physiologic and pathophysiologic conditions.

As indicated above, MRI is based on measuring the magnetic properties of hydrogen nuclei. Some elements or tissues have nuclei possessing magnetic moments as a result of the motion or spin of charged subnuclear particles, e.g., protons and neutrons. Magnetic properties become evident only in those nuclei that have uneven numbers of protons or neutrons. When these nuclei are put in a magnetic field, they become aligned either parallel or antiparallel to the main field. Two properties—the gyromagnetic ratio and the field strength of the magnet being used to measure magnetic properties—determine the characteristic frequency at which each nuclear species spins. Used clinically, MRI employs the proton nucleus.

The MRI systems consist of: (1) a large-bore (50 to 60 cm) magnet; (2) a radiofrequency (RF) transmitter-receiver; (3) a gradient coil system; and (4) a computer. Most MRI systems now use resistive, permanent, or superconducting magnets with field strengths of 0.15 to 1.50 Tesla. With further advances in superconductivity, smaller magnets with similar or greater power could be used, thus making the MRI units smaller. The RF transmitter-receiver is for stimulating and recording RF responses. The gradient coils provide spatial localization. The computer coordinates and organizes RF stimulation reception and image production. MRI equipment used for clinical purposes focuses on the proton (H^1) nucleus. The images obtained are composites of *proton concentration* (density) and *proton relaxation* (T1, T2) values. T1 is the longitudinal or spin-lattice relaxation. It is the result of stimulated nuclei losing their kinetic energy because of retarding forces of adjacent nuclei. T1 is dependent on the *temperature, viscosity,* and *strength of interaction of protons.* T2 is the spin–spin or transverse relaxation. It is an *exponential time constant* at which the nuclear magnetic resonance signals decay following excitation. Because proton density (concentration) is relatively homogeneous throughout biologic tissues owing to little variation in water content, delineation of different image intensities reflects essentially T1 and T2 information. Thus current MRI used clinically provides anatomic dissemination based on *proton relaxation* rather than *proton concentration.*

To obtain the magnetic resonance images, the patient is placed inside the bore of a powerful magnet, and a second, oscillating magnetic field is applied to the patient. This second field causes the hydrogen nuclei to move out of alignment with the first, thereby generating the signals discussed above.

The technical advantage of MRI includes the ability to obtain images in any dimension; moreover, the absence of magnetic resonance signal by calcium renders bone with its high calcium content transparent to the imaging method. Whereas these characteristics enable good imaging of the brain and spinal cord, absence of a calcium signal renders the technique incapable of picking up calcium deposits in a soft-tissue malignant tumor, of which CT is capable. MRI is not hazardous to the patient because, unlike CT, ionizing radiation is not used for MRI. Animal studies indicate that there is little or no risk to fetuses exposed to MRI in the womb, but currently it is preferable not to use this imaging technique for early pregnancy because ultrasound is available. Patients going through MRI studies may feel claustrophobic and anxious as they are delivered and are alone in the bore of the powerful magnet for the duration of the imaging studies. A serious hazard of MRI is "flying projectiles" if metal objects are brought too close to the strong magnets used in the instruments. Because of the heat that could possibly be generated during MRI studies, caution should be exercised when examining the patient who has fever or a disturbed thermoregulatory system, such as the elderly or those taking certain drugs.

Magnetic resonance imaging can be used for imaging the head, thorax, musculoskeletal system, and abdomen and pelvis. MRI continues to undergo evaluation, and its full role, advantages, and limitations for evaluating gynecologic disease have not been defined.

Therefore the imaging of patients with MRI should take place in the setting of careful study and assessment so that information may be gained pointing to the proper role of this technique. Because these imaging methods are reasonably expensive and resources are limited, neither MRI nor CT scanning should be used or considered part of routine gynecologic evaluation.

Head

Of particular relevance, MRI of the head region is valuable in gynecologic oncology for detecting and locating metastases of tumors such as choriocarcinoma and other pelvic tumors as well as in gynecologic endocrine and infertility practice. In patients with hyperprolactinemia and galactorrhea-amenorrhea syndrome, Cushing's disease, and some forms of primary amenorrhea, MRI is as good as or eventually better than CT scans of the pituitary for demonstrating the presence of or ruling out a pituitary adenoma or prolactinoma.

Chest

Imaging of the thorax by MRI is useful for demonstrating small pulmonary metastases of gynecologic malignancies and is potentially useful for imaging endometriotic lesions in the thorax.

Abdomen and Pelvis

It is in the abdomen and pelvis that MRI is currently used in gynecologic practice and probably more so in the future as the procedure does not use ionizing radiation. It is useful in gynecologic endocrinology for viewing the adrenals in patients suspected of Cushing's disease, patients with severe hirsutism of perhaps adrenal origin, or those with an adrenal tumor.

MRI has also been used for imaging the uterus and ovary. The normal uterus appears to have three layers of varying intensity when studied by MRI (Fig. 3-18). In the center of the uterus is a high-intensity area consistent with the endometrium. Proceeding outward, there is a low-intensity "band" that is thought to be the stratum basale, or innermost myometrium, sepa-

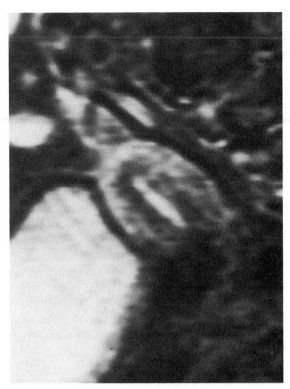

Fig. 3-18. MRI of an adult female pelvis shows the normal three layers of the uterine wall. (Illustration courtesy of Charles E. Spritzer, M.D., Department of Radiology, Duke University Medical Center.)

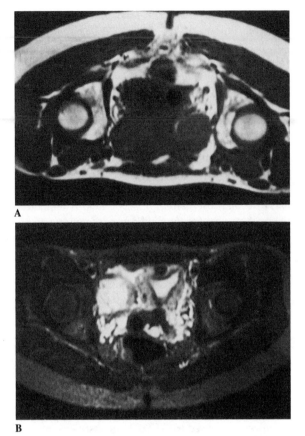

Fig. 3-19. MRI of the pelvis (axial) shows a uterine myoma. A. A T1-weighted spin echo image shows the uterus. B. Cross axial T2-weighted spin echo image shows zonal anatomy and a fibroid in the uterus. (Illustration courtesy of Charles E. Spritzer, M.D., Department of Radiology, Duke University Medical Center.)

rating the endometrium from a zone of moderate intensity, which represents the myometrium. The cervix also has three zones identified by MRI. In the center of the cervix is a high-intensity zone correlating with cervical mucus, whereas the stroma and glands of the cervix are of low intensity, and the outer muscularis layer is of intermediate intensity. Studies of the uterus in different phases of the menstrual cycle or in patients receiving oral contraceptives show varying imaging characteristics of the uterus induced by fluctuating hormone levels.

For the evaluation of uterine pathology, MRI appears to have more sensitivity than CT. MRI of the uterus has been used for benign tumors such as fibroids (Fig. 3-19) as well as for malignant tumors such as molar pregnancy, choriocarcinoma, and endometrial cancer, where the tumor location, depth of myometrial invasion, and extent of cervical invasion and myometrial invasion can be readily determined. However, a degenerating myoma may be impossible to distinguish from a uterine sarcoma or other malignancies. Although the quality of images and the assessment of myometrial involvement are improved with MRI compared to other radiographic techniques, its clinical application remains somewhat limited for *managing* uterine lesions. For example, the depth of myometrial invasion, although of prognostic significance, does not necessarily alter the treatment course, which would include surgical exploration with total abdominal hysterectomy, bilateral salpingo-oophorectomy, and consideration of selective pelvic and para-aortic lymphadenectomy. Likewise, management of a uterine myoma that is symptomatic or that requires surgical resection by myomectomy or hysterectomy would be little influenced by the MRI findings. As with other radiographic techniques, MRI does not absolutely confirm histology and may only suggest the distinction of benign from malignant conditions. Whenever there is a serious concern regarding malignancy, further diagnostic methods including biopsy must be obtained.

When evaluating adnexal pathology, MRI is probably of little more value than the CT scan. Normal ovaries are often difficult to identify by MRI because they may not be separated from adjacent loops of small intestine. Small cysts on the ovaries can be seen, and fat included in a dermoid cyst is easily identified. On the other hand, MRI may not detect calcification in dermoid cysts. The value of MRI for diagnosing pelvic endometriosis, particularly with nonbleeding or small foci, is not established and may be less promising. Implants of endometriosis in the peritoneum and especially in the posterior cul-de-sac may be identified by MRI, but distinguishing these implants from those of ovarian carcinoma is not yet possible by this imaging technique. MRI may be less accurate than CT for the evaluation of patients with ovarian carcinoma because a longer scan time is required by MRI for each "cut," and bowel peristalsis, vascular pulsation, and respiration blur the abdominal contents and their images. These technical factors render MRI less sensitive than CT scanning for detection of abdominal carcinomatosis and evaluation of lung lesions. For detection of metastases in lymph nodes, MRI may have sensitivity and specificity similar to those of the CT scan. Both techniques show enlargement of nodes, with biopsies required to differentiate between enlarged hyperplastic nodes and nodes containing metastatic carcinomas. On the other hand, neither diagnostic technique appears to be sufficiently sensitive for detecting microscopic metastases in normal-sized lymph nodes. Because MRI distinguishes clearly between blood vessels and other retroperitoneal structures, it may be more accurate for detecting lymph nodes, especially when intravenous radiographic contrast material cannot be used at the time of CT imaging.

BONE DENSITOMETRY

Imaging for determining bone mineral mass has gained increasing attention because of the concern for accelerated bone mineral depletion following menopause and the increasing numbers of postmenopausal women with increased longevity. The exact value of routine screening bone densitometry after menopause is not yet established. In practice, routine screening may not be necessary other than for research or epidemiologic purposes. Selective screening may be useful in women at high risk for developing osteoporosis, women who may not be on postmenopausal estrogen replacement therapy, and as an added indication for postmenopausal estrogen replacement therapy if the bone mineral mass is already low.

Major risk factors for osteoporosis in women include hyperparathyroidism, Cushing's syndrome, gastric or small bowel resection, chronic immobilization, prolonged amenorrhea, premature menopause, thyrotoxicosis, chronic alcoholism, and chronic treatment with anticonvulsant drugs, glucocorticoids, or thyroid hormones. When several general risk factors for osteoporosis are present, bone density measurements could be useful; such factors include a reduced weight/height ratio, positive family history for osteoporosis, smoking, social alcohol use, nulliparity, and low calcium intake.

Currently three practical bone densitometry methods are available: (1) single photon absorptiometry (SPA); (2) dual photon absorptiometry (DPA); and (3) quantitative computed tomography (QCT) of the spine.

Single Photon Absorptiometry

Developed by Cameron and Sorenson in 1963, SPA is applicable only to appendicular bones, e.g., those in the arms and legs. It is a practical, easy, noninvasive method for measuring bone mineral mass at cortical bone sites. The site usually scanned is the lower forearm (distal radius and ulna) or the radius alone, as these sites have an increased number of fractures in postmenopausal women.

The forearm, placed under water, is scanned with a collimated ^{125}I source (200 mCi or 7.4 GBq), and the transmitted beam intensity is picked up and measured with a scintillation detector on the other side of the arm. In many SPA units the scintillation detector and the ^{125}I source move together. The thickness of the bone mineral in the path of the photon beam is then registered. Using a mathematic formula for deriving the bone mineral mass and a computer program, the data are then printed out as grams per centimeter and as a plot of the percentile to which this patient belongs when matched for age. The precision of this method of measurement is 2 to 3 percent.

Dual Photon Absorptiometry

The DPA technique allows measurements of bone mineral in the axial skeleton, especially in the lumbar spine and hips, where relatively more trabecular bone is present than in other sites. Trabecular bone is rapidly affected by prolonged hypogonadism, as after menopause.

With DPA, two photon energies are transmitted through two materials, bone and soft tissue. The radioactive energy source is gandolinium 153 ([153]Gd; 1.5 Ci or 55.5 GBq), which produces two energy peaks, seen in the NaI detector. The region of the bone or bones under study is subjected to a rectilinear scan, and a point-by-point determination of bone mineral is made. Again using a mathematic formula to account for differential energy absorption and transmission between the soft and osseous tissues, the bone mineral content is obtained. With most current instruments the data are calculated in a microprocessor; and the results are then printed together with a computer-generated printout of the mineral image of the bone under study showing the distribution of the mineral intensities. For the spine the bone mineral content is derived from lumbar vertebrae 1 through 4 (L1–L4), and for the hip the mineral content is calculated for the femoral neck, trochanter, and shaft. The precision of DPA is 3 to 5 percent for the vertebrae.

Quantitative Computed Tomography

The QCT method measures purely trabecular bone. Because the vertebrae have a proportionally higher percentage of trabecular bone than most other bone sites, QCT is carried out on the thoracolumbar vertebrae and the bone density calculated from the twelfth thoracic vertebrae (T12) through the fourth lumbar vertebrae (L4). The density is expressed as grams per milliliter, and it is therefore a true volume measurement. The precision of this method of bone densitometry is 2 to 5 percent, and its sensitivity is high. It can detect early significant loss of trabecular bone mass.

SELECTED READINGS

Bandy, L., Clarke-Pearson, D. L., Silverman, P. M., et al. Computed tomography in evaluation of extrapelvic lymphadenopathy in carcinoma of the cervix. *Obstet. Gynecol.* 65:73, 1985.

Bassett, L. W., and Gold, R. H. *Mammography, Thermography, and Ultrasound in Breast Cancer Detection.* New York: Grune & Stratton, 1982.

Beljan, J. R., Bohigian, G. M., Dolan, W. D., et al. Early detection of breast cancer: a council report from the Council on Scientific Affairs. *J.A.M.A.* 252:3008, 1984.

Clarke-Pearson, D. L., Bandy, L., Dudzinski, M., et al. Computed tomography in evaluation of patients with ovarian carcinoma in complete clinical remission: correlation with surgical pathologic findings. *J.A.M.A.* 255:627, 1986.

Council on Scientific Affairs. Magnetic resonance imaging of the abdomen and pelvis. *J.A.M.A.* 261:420, 1989.

Dawood, M. Y., Lewis, V., Ramos, J. R. Cortical and trabecular bone mineral content in women with endometriosis: Effect of gonadotropin-releasing hormone agonist and danazol. *Fertil. Steril.* 52:21, 1989.

Dietemann, J. L., Portha, C., Cattin, F., et al. CT follow-up of microprolactinomas during bromocriptine-induced pregnancy. *Neuroradiology* 25:133, 1983.

Feig, S. A. Radiation risk from mammography: Is it clinically significant? *A.J.R.* 143:469, 1984.

Gross, B. H., Moss, A. A., Mihara, K., et al. Computed tomography of gynecologic diseases. *A.J.R.* 141:765, 1983.

Hubbell, F. A., Greenfield, S., Tyler, J. L., et al. The impact of routine admission chest x-ray films on patient care. *N. Engl. J. Med.* 312:209, 1985.

Johnson, I. R., Symonds, E. M., Worthington, B. S., et al. Imaging ovarian tumors by nuclear magnetic resonance. *Br. J. Obstet. Gynaecol.* 91:260, 1984.

O'Brien, W. F., Buck, D. R., and Nash, J. D. Evaluation of sonography in the initial assessment of the gynecologic patient. *Am. J. Obstet. Gynecol.* 149:598, 1984.

Rucker, L., Frey, E. B., and Staten, M. A. Usefulness of screening chest roentgenogrms in preoperative patients. *J.A.M.A.* 250:3209, 1983.

Sabbagha, R. E. *Diagnostic Ultrasound Applied to Obstetrics and Gynecology* (2nd ed.). New York: Lippincott, 1987.

Sack, R. A. The value of intravenous urography prior to abdominal hysterectomy for gynecologic disease. *Am. J. Obstet. Gynecol.* 134:208, 1979.

Sickles, E. A., Filly, R. A., Callen, P. W. Benign breast lesions: Ultrasound detection and diagnosis. *Radiology* 151:467, 1984.

Sommer, F. G., Walsh, J. W., Schwartz, P. E., et al. Evaluation of gynecologic pelvic masses by ultrasound and computed tomography. *J. Reprod. Med.* 27:45, 1982.

Timor-Tritsch, I. E., Rottem, S. *Transvaginal Sonography.* New York: Elsevier, 1988.

Walsh, J. W., Amendola, M. A., Konerding, K. F., et al. Computed tomographic detection of pelvic and inguinal lymph-node metastases from primary and recurrent pelvic malignant disease. *Radiology* 137:157, 1980.

Walsh, J. W., and Goplerud, D. R. Prospective comparison between clinical and CT staging in primary cervical carcinoma. *A.J.R.* 173:997, 1981.

Yoder, I. C. *Hysterosalpingography and Pelvic Ultrasound: Imaging in Infertility and Gynecology.* Boston: Little, Brown, 1988.

4

Preoperative Evaluation, Preparation, and Principles of Gynecologic Surgery

Surgical intervention is required to diagnose and treat many gynecologic disorders. Successful outcome of this surgery rests on the careful evaluation and preoperative preparation of the woman. Many comments referable to preoperative preparation are also appropriate to patients undergoing general surgical procedures and are touched on only briefly in this chapter. The specific evaluation and preparation needed for the surgical procedures specific to the gynecologic organs are discussed more fully.

PREOPERATIVE EVALUATION

Medical History and Physical Examination

Complete medical evaluation of a patient is necessary to achieve a successful outcome. Surgery undertaken without a thorough understanding of a patient's medical history and a complete physical examination carries the hazard of developing otherwise preventable complications. The historical information to be carefully obtained includes any significant medical history or medical illnesses that might be aggravated by or complicate anesthesia or surgical recovery. Inquiry should be made about current medications taken, even those discontinued within the months prior to surgery. Specific inquiries should be directed at the possibility of nonprescription drugs taken and the use of oral contraceptives, as many patients consider these agents a routine part of their lives rather than a medication. Use of a nonprescription medication such as aspirin may lead to bleeding complications intraoperatively and postoperatively. Oral contraceptives should be discontinued six weeks prior to elective surgery to reduce the risk of postoperative venous thrombosis. Specific instructions must be given to the patient

about the need to discontinue or continue (e.g., cardiac or antihypertensive) medications prior to surgery.

The patient should be questioned about known allergies to medications (e.g., sulfa drugs and penicillin), as well as other allergies to foods or environmental allergens. Because iodinated intravenous contrast material is used for the intravenous pyelogram (IVP), enhanced computed tomography (CT) scanning, and venography/arteriography, the patient should be questioned about her tolerance of other iodinated substances. A history of hypersensitivity to previous intravenously administered iodine-containing compounds should be clearly noted, and the patient should not undergo further exposure to iodine-containing compounds unless absolutely mandatory. In these critical settings, corticosteroid preparation should be instituted to prevent life-threatening anaphylactic reactions. A history of sensitivity to shellfish may be the only clue to iodine sensitivity.

Inquiry should be made about previous surgical procedures, including such minor procedures as dilatation and curettage (D&C) or tonsillectomy. The patient's course following those surgical procedures should be reviewed to identify potential complications that might be avoided in the subsequent operation. Reaction and response to anesthetic techniques should be identified and thoroughly evaluated with the anesthesiologist in charge. Inquiries should be made about other complications, including excessive bleeding, wound infection, or deep vein thrombosis. Previous pelvic surgery should alert the gynecologist to the possibility of distorted surgical anatomy and possible preexisting injury to adjacent organ systems, such as small bowel adhesions in the pelvis or ureteral stenosis from previous periureteral scarring. An IVP in such a setting is wise to establish bilateral patency of the ureters or to identify any preexisting abnormality. Operative notes from previous pelvic operations should be obtained and reviewed to determine precisely the extent of the surgical procedure and other surgical findings. Many times a patient is not clear about the extent of the procedure or the details of the intraoperative findings. This point is particularly important in patients who have had surgery for pelvic inflammatory disease or a pelvic abscess, endometriosis, or a pelvic malignancy.

Family history should be reviewed to minimize the possibility of familial traits that might complicate planned surgery. A history of excessive intraoperative or postoperative bleeding, malignant hyperthermia, and other potentially inherited conditions should be sought. General review of systems should also be included in the questioning, searching for any other co-existing medical or surgical conditions. Inquiry about gastrointestinal and urologic function is particularly important prior to undertaking pelvic surgery, as many gynecologic diseases involve adjacent nongynecologic viscera.

A thorough physical examination must be performed preoperatively. Although many women undergoing gynecologic surgical procedures are otherwise healthy, with pathology identified only on pelvic examination, other major organ systems must not be neglected in the physical examination. Identification of abnormalities such as a heart murmur or pulmonary compromise should lead the surgeon to undertake additional testing and consultation to minimize intraoperative and postoperative complications.

Laboratory Evaluation

Preoperative laboratory work to be obtained depends on the extent of the anticipated surgical procedure and the patient's general health evaluation. As a minimum for patients undergoing general anesthesia, a blood count including hematocrit, white blood cell (WBC) count, and platelet count should be obtained. Serum chemistries and liver function testing are rarely abnormal in the asymptomatic patient who is not taking other medications. In women under age 35, a chest radiograph and cardiogram are likewise of low yield for identifying asymptomatic cardiopulmonary disease and may not always be necessary, especially in patients undergoing short surgical procedures of a minor nature. On the other hand, women over age 35 and those undergoing major gynecologic surgical procedures should have a chest radiograph, cardiogram, and serum electrolytes as a minimum evaluation—if only to serve as baseline data for comparison to other studies should complications develop. Further evaluation of adjacent organ systems should be undertaken in individual cases. For example, an IVP is indicated

to delineate ureteral patency and course in such cases as a pelvic mass, gynecologic cancer, or congenital müllerian anomaly. An IVP may identify a duplicate collecting system or an absent collecting system. Furthermore, it may identify an obstructed ureter in a case of gynecologic cancer that might be totally asymptomatic. An IVP is also part of the primary staging of most gynecologic cancers.

Similarly, a barium enema or upper gastrointestinal (GI) series with small bowel follow-through might be of significant value when evaluating patients prior to undergoing pelvic surgery. Because of the proximity of the female genital tract with the lower gastrointestinal tract, the rectum and sigmoid colon may be involved with benign (endometriosis or pelvic inflammatory disease) or malignant gynecologic conditions. Conversely, a pelvic mass could be from gastrointestinal origin, e.g., a diverticular abscess or a mass of inflammatory small intestine (Crohn's disease). Clearly, any patient with gastrointestinal symptomatology should be further evaluated including the above-mentioned radiographs as well as proctosigmoidoscopy (or flexible sigmoidoscopy or colonoscopy).

Patients with pulmonary disease should have baseline assessment of pulmonary function and arterial blood gases. Chronic obstructive pulmonary disease may be improved significantly by preoperative preparation with antibiotics and bronchodilators. Identifying such patients and providing several days or weeks of preoperative preparation often optimizes the anesthetic and surgical recovery.

The results of other preoperative studies that may have been obtained immediately prior to surgery should be checked. It is especially important to know the results of an endometrial biopsy or a Papanicolaou (Pap) smear that may have been obtained only a few days prior to surgery. In all patients undergoing major or minor gynecologic surgical procedures, the results of a Pap smear should be known prior to surgery.

The potential for blood transfusion should be discussed with the patient. In cases where the probability of intraoperative or postoperative blood transfusion is real, consideration should be given to donor-directed blood transfusion or preoperative banking of the patient's own blood. This method is especially feasible prior to elective surgical procedures, which may be anticipated weeks in advance. Discussion between the patient and the surgeon as to his or her philosophy regarding blood transfusion is appropriate and allows the patient to have an understanding of the potential risks associated with such transfusion. It may only be during such discussions that the surgeon learns of a patient's religious preference that blood not be transfused.

During the history and physical examination a careful search should be made for cardiovascular disease. Although it is unusual that cardiovascular disease contraindicates surgery, further preparation is often necessary to minimize complications. With a large number of older women having essential hypertension, this history should be sought as well as noted when the blood pressure is obtained during physical examination. Patients with diastolic blood pressures between 100 and 110 mm Hg must be controlled preoperatively to minimize complications. On the other hand, patients with hypertension that is controlled medically are at minimal additional risk during general anesthesia and major surgery. The specific antihypertensive drugs used should be recorded and in general should be continued throughout the perioperative period. Monoamine oxide inhibitors should be discontinued at least two weeks prior to surgery. Because many patients with mild to moderate hypertension are taking a diuretic, the serum potassium should be checked and corrected should the patient be hypokalemic.

The presence of valvular heart disease may be recognized during preoperative cardiac auscultation and examination. Cardiology consultation should be obtained, and echocardiography or cardiac catheterization may be required for full preoperative evaluation. Patients with moderate to severe valvular heart disease often benefit from preoperative Swan-Ganz monitoring to allow complete assessment of cardiovascular status intraoperatively and throughout the immediate critical postoperative period. Prophylactic antibiotics (e.g., a combination of ampicillin and gentamicin) are usually recommended for patients with valvular disease to reduce the risk of subacute bacterial endocarditis.

As the female population ages, coronary heart disease is becoming a more frequent problem. A history

of angina or atypical chest pains should be fully evaluated, and the patient may require correction or intraoperative invasive monitoring to have a successful postoperative outcome. Patients with a recent myocardial infarction are clearly at high risk to have subsequent postoperative infarction. In general, a six-month period should intervene between a recent myocardial infarction and elective general gynecologic surgery. Perioperative monitoring with cardiogram and serial cardiac enzyme evaluation is recommended for patients with significant coronary artery disease. Careful perioperative management of fluid volumes, blood replacement, and serum electrolytes (especially potassium) is important to the successful recovery of these patients. Likewise, surgery performed on the patient with congestive heart failure is fraught with postoperative complications and potential mortality. Congestive heart failure should be reversed with appropriate cardiac medication and diuretics, and any cardiac pathology corrected. These patients too may significantly benefit by careful monitoring of central venous pressure and other cardiac parameters.

A variety of other medical illnesses that may predispose to complications should be corrected or managed appropriately, and medical consultation should be sought liberally. Complications of surgery are most often prevented by thorough preoperative evaluation and management and astute, careful intraoperative and postoperative surgical and medical care.

PREOPERATIVE PREPARATION

Specific preoperative preparation of patients undergoing major gynecologic surgery is intended to prevent complications most frequently associated with pelvic surgery. These complications include infection, hemorrhage, venous thromboembolism, and injury to adjacent viscera. Although myriad other complications may also be encountered, they are usually common to general anesthesia and other major surgical procedures and are not discussed in this chapter. The reader is referred to any one of a number of more lengthy general surgical textbooks regarding other complications.

Infection following pelvic surgery is a frequent complication and was a major hazard to patients prior to the advent of adequate antibiotic therapy. Because the vagina and lower genital tract cannot be thoroughly sterilized, there is always potential and real contamination by bacterial pathogens in the operative field, especially with vulvar and vaginal surgery or pelvic surgery performed through the vagina. Infectious complications may be subdivided into infections of the abdominal incision or the pelvic or vaginal surgical site, and other infectious complications of urinary or pulmonary origin.

The risk of wound infection is increased by a variety of factors. Surgery in an infected field (e.g., pelvic inflammatory disease) or entry into the gastrointestinal tract significantly increases the risk of wound infection. Wound infection is also increased in the obese patient, patients undergoing prolonged surgery, patients who have had previous radiation therapy in the operative field, and those with poor nutritional status. Although removal of abdominal and pubic hair may be necessary to have a clean operative field and facilitate wound closure, prospective studies have demonstrated that shaving the night before surgery actually increases the risk of postoperative wound infection. It is currently recommended that skin preparation be achieved with a chemical depilatory, hair clipping, or shaving the hair immediately prior to surgery. Prior to the abdominal incision the skin is prepared with an aseptic solution, and sterile technique is maintained throughout the surgical procedure.

Infections in the pelvic surgical field were once frequent, and often serious infections resulted in a pelvic abscess that required secondary drainage. Clinical investigation into the role of prophylactic antibiotics has clearly shown that perioperative prophylactic antibiotics offer a significant advantage in patients undergoing vaginal surgery, cesarean section, and abdominal hysterectomy. Key to such usage is that the antibiotic be given prior to surgery such that effective circulating tissue levels are present at the time of the surgical incision and throughout the surgical case. That is, the antibiotic must be present in the operative field tissues during the time of maximum contamination and tissue trauma. The duration of use of prophylactic antibiotics is debatable, although it is clear that there is no advantage to using prophylactic antibiotics beyond 24 hours postoperatively. Some studies have suggested that a single dose of antibiotic prior to surgery sig-

nificantly reduces the incidence of postoperative infection. Prolonged use of "prophylactic" antibiotics, however, may lead to bacterial overgrowth of a resistant pathogen and increased hospital expense.

If colonic surgery is anticipated in the treatment of pelvic malignancy, oral prophylactic antibiotics should be given the day before surgery. A combination of oral erythromycin and neomycin has been found to significantly reduce the risk of pelvic infection, wound infection, and anastomosis breakdown. Because the gastrointestinal tract is immediately adjacent to the gynecologic organs, most patients undergoing major gynecologic surgery should at least undergo mechanical bowel preparation with cathartics and enemas during the 24 hours prior to elective surgery. This preparation eliminates fecal material and gas from the gastrointestinal tract that might otherwise occupy more space and compromise surgical exposure. Additionally, should gastrointestinal tract injury occur, there is a higher probability of successful repair in a field that is not contaminated with fecal material.

Because the pelvis is a highly vascular region of the body, intraoperative and postoperative hemorrhage are significant complicating factors of pelvic surgery. Preoperative preparation to minimize hemorrhagic complications should include a search for potential coagulopathies and a history of bleeding after surgical procedures. Should any suspicion of existing coagulopathy be entertained, appropriate coagulation parameters should be studied and a bleeding time test performed. Extended surgery for pelvic malignancies, severe pelvic inflammatory disease, or extensive endometriosis may also be associated with bleeding, which might be anticipated preoperatively. The surgeon should be prepared in these circumstances and have appropriate blood products available at the time of surgery in these higher risk surgical procedures. Poor exposure in the pelvis is also associated with more frequent bleeding complications. It is therefore important when operating on a patient who is obese or in whom difficult exposure is anticipated (e.g., reoperation for pelvic cancer) that adequate assistance be available to offer appropriate retraction and exposure.

Deep venous thrombosis and pulmonary embolism is another significant complication associated with gynecologic surgery. Identification of risk factors associated with deep vein thrombosis and pulmonary embolism may allow effective use of prophylactic measures to prevent these serious and sometimes fatal sequelae. Forty percent of deaths following gynecologic surgical procedures are attributed to pulmonary embolism, which is also the leading cause of death after surgery for gynecologic cancer. The long-term sequelae of deep vein thrombosis is postphlebitic syndrome, which leads to significant morbidity and disability from leg edema and ulceration.

Factors associated with the occurrence of deep vein thrombosis following surgery have been clearly identified and include advanced age of patients. This point is especially true for patients over age 40 and becomes significant in women over age 60. A history of deep vein thrombosis, varicose veins, or venous stasis changes of the lower extremity found on preoperative physical examination should alert the surgeon to a patient who is at high risk for subsequent venous thrombosis following major gynecologic surgery. Other factors associated with postoperative deep vein thrombosis include obesity, malignancy, history of pelvic radiation therapy, preoperative oral contraceptive usage, and extended surgical procedures.

A variety of strategies have been advanced to prevent deep vein thrombosis and pulmonary embolism following gynecologic surgical procedures. Low-dose heparin (5000 units given preoperatively and then every 8 to 12 hours postoperatively) has been demonstrated to effectively prevent deep vein thrombosis in general surgery and gynecologic surgery patients. This regimen carries a minimally increased risk of intraoperative and postoperative bleeding and is well tolerated by most patients. Dihydroergotamine added to heparin in an attempt to augment venous return by constricting the veins has also been shown to be an effective combination prophylactic method. Other methods to prevent venous stasis after surgery include early ambulation of the postoperative patient and mechanical methods such as compression stockings or pneumatically inflated sleeves that provide a pulsatile return of venous blood from the legs. All of these methods have been documented to reduce the incidence of deep vein thrombosis and therefore pulmonary embolism following surgery. At least one of

these active prophylactic methods should be used in patients who carry any of the risk factors previously noted.

Prevention of injury to adjacent viscera (bladder, ureters, pelvic vessels, rectum) primarily relies on good surgical technique and established anatomic planes. Preoperative evaluation with radiographic identification of abnormal anatomy (as documented by barium enema or IVP) prepares the surgeon for unexpected anatomic anomalies. The use of appropriate bowel preparation, mechanical evacuation, and antibiotics reduces the risk of complications should adjacent viscera be injured intraoperatively.

Preoperative Discussion and Informed Consent

The verbal and nonverbal rapport and trust that exist between the patient and her gynecologist begins on the initial office visit and should be built on at each subsequent visit. When surgery is deemed advisable by the gynecologist, the initial discussion should explain in sufficient detail to the patient the findings on examination and the results of testing, the natural history of the disease process, and the goals of the surgical procedure. This discussion should be carried out in an unhurried manner and be sufficiently detailed that the patient may decide to go ahead with the preoperative preparation, as described above. Because most gynecologic surgery is elective, the gynecologist has the opportunity to thoroughly evaluate the patient from a medical point of view as well as allow her to develop psychological coping mechanisms and ask questions that may not have been initially discussed. The surgeon should be available to discuss in person or by phone these questions prior to actual hospital admission.

On the day prior to anticipated surgery, another preoperative discussion should be carried out with the patient and key family members, perhaps including the spouse or significant other of an adult woman or the parents should a minor be undergoing surgery. Privacy should be ensured to allow thorough and frank discussion; it is particularly important when delicate questions regarding sexuality and sexual function may be raised by the patient. Discussions in hallways or office waiting rooms are to be condemned. A discussion should be carried out in a relaxed, quiet setting. Likewise, large group discussions with many members of the family and concerned friends should be avoided. To facilitate eye contact and an unhurried manner, the physician should sit down during this discussion.

The goals of this preoperative discussion should serve to allay anxiety and fears the patient may have and to answer any questions that may have developed during the preoperative period. The discussion should serve to further expand on issues relative to the surgery, its expected outcome, and its risks; it is the basis for obtaining the signed informed consent. This period is clearly an educational process for the patient and her family, and explanations by the physician must be made in understandable terms. The following items should be discussed at length, and after each area has been covered the patient and family should be invited to ask questions.

1. Nature and extent of the disease process
2. Extent of the actual operation proposed and potential modifications of this operation, depending on unexpected intraoperative findings
3. Anticipated benefits of the operation, with a conservative estimate of successful outcome
4. Risks and potential complications of the surgery
5. Alternative methods of therapy and the risks and results of those alternative methods of therapy

The nature and the extent of the disease process should be rediscussed prior to surgery with an explanation in layman's terms about the significance of the disease process. Is it life-threatening, or does it result in significant disability or dysfunction? To what extent does the disease process alter the patient's daily living? If left untreated, could the disease spontaneously resolve, or could it potentially worsen? What are the time course and natural history of the disease?

The goals of the surgery should be discussed in detail. Some gynecologic surgical procedures are performed purely for diagnostic purposes (e.g., D&C, cold-knife conization, diagnostic laparoscopy, staging laparotomy), whereas others are clearly aimed at correcting an anatomic defect or a specific disease process. The extent of the surgery should be outlined, in-cluding which organs will be removed. Most patients wish to be informed about the type of surgical incision and the expected duration of anesthesia.

The expected outcome of the surgical procedure must also be explained. If the procedure is being performed for diagnostic purposes, the outcome depends on surgical or pathologic findings that may not be anticipated. If no clear answer is known, truth and honesty by the surgeon saying "I do not know" is appreciated by most patients and their families. When treating anatomic deformity or disease, the expected success of the operation should be discussed as well as the potential for failure. This phase should include a discussion of the probability of failure of tubal sterilization or the possibility that stress urinary incontinence may not be alleviated. Likewise, the possibility of finding more advanced carcinoma should be included in the discussion as well as the potential need for unforeseen adjunctive therapy (e.g., postoperative irradiation or chemotherapy). Other issues of importance to the patient include loss of fertility or loss of ovarian function. These issues should be raised by the physician to make sure the patient understands adequately the pathophysiology that may result from the surgery and to allow her to express her feelings regarding these emotionally charged issues.

The risks and potential complications of the surgical procedure should be discussed with the patient. This area is probably the most difficult part of informed consent, in the sense that there are clearly innumerable potential complications associated with general anesthesia and major or minor surgery. The extent to which the surgeon must present this information to the patient is difficult to discuss from a legal standpoint, although some general principles can be outlined.

The most frequent complications of the exact surgical procedure should be discussed and mentioned to all patients. In general, they could include intraoperative and postoperative hemorrhage, postoperative infection, venous thrombosis, and injury to adjacent viscera. The potential of death from any anesthetic or surgical procedure should be mentioned. There are also specific risks that are increased for certain patients. For example, the patient with morbid obesity should be informed that the frequency of wound infection and dehiscence is increased, and that additional complications such as pneumonia are an increased risk because of her habitus. The potential requirement for intensive care monitoring postoperatively should be discussed with the patient who has significant medical problems and may require invasive monitoring or respiratory support with a ventilator. An offer should be made to the patient to review the additional, infrequent complications that may be encountered, although most patients do not wish to have such a lengthy discussion. The usual postoperative course should also be discussed in enough detail that the patient understands what to expect during the days following surgery. The information as to the need for a suprapubic catheter or prolonged central venous monitoring helps the patient accept her postoperative course and avoids surprises that may be disconcerting. Finally, the expected recovery period, both inside and outside the hospital should be mentioned. The patient may be able to return to work the day after minor surgical procedures, whereas she might require six weeks or more recovery at home before being able to return to her job after major abdominal or pelvic surgery.

Alternative methods of therapy are also mentioned as part of the preoperative discussion. Other medical management or other surgical approaches should be discussed, along with their potential benefits and complications. It should be clear to the patient after this discussion why the proposed surgery is the appropriate next step in her care.

The course of the final preoperative preparation the day before surgery should be outlined to the patient and her family so they understand the necessary interventions by the nursing staff, anesthesia staff, and house staff the evening and morning prior to surgery. This additional information continues to allay anxiety and avoid surprises that might not have been anticipated by the patient or her family. Finally, arrangements to meet the family immediately after operation should be established so that the surgeon and family may discuss the surgical findings and the patient's status as soon as she has been moved to the recovery room. Witnesses to the preoperative discussion and signing of the consent form should include a family member and another member of the health care team.

The discussion itself, however, should be performed by the responsible surgeon and not delegated to nursing staff or house staff, who may not have full understanding of the patient's disease process or the rapport or responsibility for her ultimate care.

Unanticipated findings at the time of surgery should also be mentioned. For example, should both ovaries be found to be diseased, they may require removal, which might have been unanticipated by the patient or her surgeon based on the preoperative physical examination and laboratory findings. The mention of these unanticipated findings and the judgments the surgeon must make intraoperatively alleviates many instances of surprise following surgery and unhappiness on the part of the patient or her family.

The anesthesiologist responsible for the surgical procedure should also have the opportunity to examine the patient, review her laboratory findings, and discuss the proposed anesthetic method with her. In many institutions the consent to the administration of anesthetic is included in the surgical consent form, whereas in others it is a separate form that should be obtained by the anesthesiologist after appropriate preoperative discussion. The anesthesiologist and gynecologist should come to agreement as to the type of anesthetic to be used for the particular surgical procedure.

GENERAL PRINCIPLES OF GYNECOLOGIC SURGERY

The purpose of this section is not to detail the variety of surgical procedures performed by the gynecologist but to allow the reader insight as to some general concepts and approaches to gynecologic surgery. There are a variety of surgical textbooks and atlases that detail the specifics of gynecologic surgical operations to which the interested reader is referred.

Examination Under Anesthesia

Following the induction of general or regional anesthesia, the surgeon should perform a careful pelvic examination. Despite the fact that an examination may have been done with the patient awake in the surgeon's office the day before surgery, a repeat examination is highly recommended to confirm the preoperative impression. With adequate levels of anesthesia, an optimal pelvic examination including careful inspection of the vulva, vagina, and cervix as well as complete bimanual and rectovaginal examination may be performed. It is not unusual to find additional pathology, which may alter the course of the surgical procedure. Furthermore, a pelvic mass that may have been noted in the office the day before occasionally has "disappeared," and a laparotomy incision in such an instance is not only embarrassing but carries medical-legal ramifications. The findings at the time of examination under anesthesia may also suggest the need for further diagnostic studies such as cystoscopy or proctosigmoidoscopy, which should be performed before undertaking a major surgical procedure. After examination under anesthesia but before final preparation and draping, the patient should be positioned appropriately on the operating room table for the surgical operation anticipated. Care must be taken when positioning the anesthetized patient to avoid musculoskeletal or nerve injury.

Positions for Gynecologic Surgery

Several patient positions are used when performing abdominal and vaginal surgery for gynecologic conditions. The choice of position primarily depends on whether the surgeon will be utilizing an abdominal route or a vaginal route, or if a combined approach from "above and below" is necessary to accomplish the particular surgical procedure. In rare instances it may be necessary to reposition the patient after portions of the operation, although this technique should be used infrequently. For most pelvic surgery performed through an abdominal incision (celiotomy), the supine position is satisfactory. With the patient draped in such a position, however, there is no sterile access to the vagina or perineum. When vulvar, anal, or vaginal surgery is planned, the dorsal lithotomy position is most frequently used. When positioning the patient in the lithotomy position, care must be taken not to injure the legs as they are brought up into the stirrups. Excessive flexion of the thigh can lead to femoral nerve injury or sciatic nerve injury. This position allows excellent exposure to the external genitalia, anus, lower rectum, and vagina.

With some surgical procedures it is necessary to have access to both the abdomen and vagina, and at such times the Whitmore position may be used. Some call it a modified lithotomy position, where the legs are abducted and the knees flexed somewhat. In this position the patient may be prepared and draped so that access can be gained to the vagina and perineum, as well as the abdomen, by the same surgical team. The Whitmore position is particularly useful when performing Marshall-Marchetti-Kranz cystourethropexy, radical hysterectomy, radical vulvectomy with en bloc inguinal lymphadenectomy, and pelvic exenteration. Because of potential injury of the perineal nerve and subsequent "foot drop" by pressure on the lateral knee, care must be taken when positioning the patient in this position.

Any of these positions may be altered somewhat by the modified Trendelenburg position. Many surgeons find the latter position helpful for gaining better exposure in the pelvis. The Trendelenburg position inclines the head downward and thus elevates the feet, which allows gravity to pull the intestines out of the pelvis, gaining better exposure. In the steep Trendelenburg position, often used during laparoscopy, shoulder supports should be attached to the table so the patient does not slide in this exaggerated inclined position. These braces should be adequately padded so as to avoid a brachial nerve injury.

It is important to do everything possible to avoid neurologic injuries because, although eventual recovery of motor and sensory function is usually the rule, the period of disability may last many months. Additionally, femoral nerve injury has been noted after abdominal laparotomy and has been attributed to the direct pressure of self-retaining retractors on the femoral nerve. When positioning the retractor, the surgeon must be careful that it is not pushing on the lateral pelvic wall. This mistake is especially common in slender patients, where the retractor blades are too deep and the patient is undergoing laparotomy through a transverse incision, which allows the retractor blades to push more laterally on the pelvic wall.

After positioning the patient, the surgical field

should be prepared with a surgical solution such as povidone-iodine and the patient draped sterilely. For most major abdominal and pelvic surgical procedures an indwelling urethral Foley catheter is placed for intraoperative drainage of the bladder as well as drainage postoperatively for a period of time. A suprapubic catheter is sometimes selected, especially if a urologic procedure is to be performed or if it is anticipated that the patient will require a long duration of postoperative bladder drainage, such as after radical hysterectomy with pelvic lymphadenectomy.

Abdominal Incision

The choice of the abdominal incision must rest primarily on the surgeon's judgment as to the amount of exposure necessary to safely accomplish the surgical procedure. This choice may be modified by the patient's habitus.

The *vertical midline* or *paramedian incision* usually extends from the pubis to the umbilicus. Excellent access and exposure to the pelvis is provided, and the incision may easily be extended cephalad in cases where a large mass is present or when it is found that additional surgery is required in the upper abdomen. Such circumstances might include a large abdominal and pelvic mass or known ovarian carcinoma. This incision may be used in essentially all patients. At other times the surgeon may choose a *low transverse incision* to gain entrance into the pelvis.

The *Pfannenstiel incision,* which does not cut the rectus muscles, is usually adequate for surgery on a slightly enlarged uterus or to perform surgical procedures on the adnexa. Because of its low orientation, surgery in the upper abdomen cannot be accomplished safely through this incision, and therefore it is not advised in patients who may require omentectomy or paraaortic lymphadenectomy for gynecologic malignancies.

The *Maylard incision* is also a transverse incision, but it allows additional exposure in that the rectus muscles are cut. It is often adequate for extended surgical procedures in the pelvis, such as radical hysterectomy with pelvic lymphadenectomy, or for removing a moderate-sized uterus. Transverse incisions in general tend to heal better and to be associated with a lower incidence of incisional hernias and dehiscence. In addition, they are more cosmetic and often can be reasonably well hidden along the pubic hair line.

Principles

Upon opening the abdominal cavity, it is important that a thorough *intraoperative exploration* be performed on every patient. Despite the surgeon's desire to proceed immediately with the planned operation, a few minutes must be taken to carefully explore the upper abdomen and exclude other coexisting pathology. Careful palpation and visualization (if the incision allows) of the diaphragms, liver, gallbladder, kidneys, stomach, small and large intestines, and omentum should be performed. In addition, the paraaortic and pelvic lymph nodes should be palpated. By performing this examination routinely in every case prior to initiating pelvic surgery, it is unlikely that the surgeon will miss rare but important coincidental pathology. This point is especially important during surgery for gynecologic malignancy, as the extent of the cancer may be more advanced than had been anticipated by preoperative examination and radiography. The findings of enlarged lymph nodes or metastases in the upper abdomen may change entirely the planned pelvic surgical procedure.

No matter what the planned surgical procedure, there are basic principles of pelvic surgery that should be employed to achieve optimal surgical outcome.

1. *Adequate exposure* must be established before initiating pelvic surgery. To achieve adequate exposure, the proper incision of the abdomen must have been performed. Because the full bladder may occupy over half of the pelvic space, a bladder catheter should be placed prior to beginning surgery. Likewise, mechanical bowel preparation should evacuate stool and gas from the small intestines and colon, thereby allowing more room for the surgeon to operate. The intestines should be pushed out of the pelvis and retained behind laparotomy packs and retractors. Availability of adequate assistants and equipment is paramount to the successful operation and is especially important

when operating on obese patients or those in whom extensive pathology is likely to be encountered. Adequate lighting must also be available.

2. The surgeon must be thoroughly familiar with *pelvic anatomy* and should strive to establish and identify that anatomy prior to undertaking the planned surgical procedure. In patients with extensive adhesions from previous operations, pelvic inflammatory disease, endometriosis, or carcinoma, the adhesions should be lysed and the pelvic viscera freed from adjacent vital structures. Care must be taken to identify the pelvic vessels, ureter, bladder, and rectum. Most major pelvic surgical procedures can be facilitated by use of the avascular pelvic spaces (Fig. 4-1). Most gynecologic disease does not extend into the retroperitoneum, and therefore these spaces may usually serve as a reference to normal pelvic anatomy. Furthermore, mobilization of the bladder and rectum away from the uterus, cervix, and upper vagina is usually necessary for a procedure such as an abdominal or vaginal hysterectomy.

3. The surgeon must observe the usual basic principles of *good surgical technique* outlined for any general surgical or gynecologic surgical procedure. It includes adequate hemostasis, gentle tissue handling,

and minimal trauma. Selection of appropriate instruments and suture materials is also key to a successful uncomplicated surgical outcome. These issues are discussed at length in surgical textbooks and are mentioned here only to emphasize their importance.

Because gynecologic surgery is performed in a relatively small, enclosed field (the pelvis), and because adjacent vital structures are in close proximity, the surgeon must be constantly vigilant and know the location of these structures. It is particularly important to visualize and know the location of the pelvic ureter and bladder. Injury to the ureter or its ligation in the course of gynecologic surgery is a major complication. There are three locations where the ureter is most commonly injured during pelvic surgery: (1) The ureter may be injured as it courses close to the ovarian vessels (the infundibulopelvic ligament) near the pelvic brim. The surgeon who ligates the ovarian vessels without identifying the ureter is courting postoperative disaster. (2) When clamping the vascular supply to the uterus, it must be recalled that the ureter is ap-

Fig. 4-1. Pelvic spaces and ligaments. Axial view of the pelvis demonstrates the supporting ligaments through which vascular and nerve supplies run. When performing pelvic surgery, the avascular spaces are often developed to facilitate surgical resection.

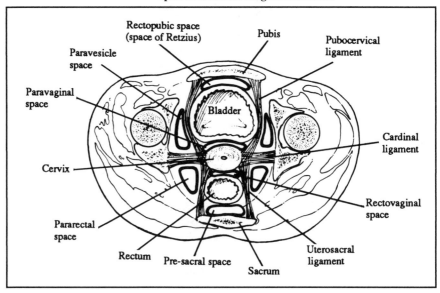

proximately 1.5 cm lateral to the uterus. Clamps placed wide of the uterus or ligatures taken out lateral to clamps to control arterial or venous bleeding are at risk to also ligate the ureter in its distal 5 cm. The ureter at this point in the pelvis is entering the paracervical tunnel and is not easily identified without more extended dissection. (3) Finally, the ureter may be injured as the vagina and cervix are divided from each other at the completion of abdominal hysterectomy or the beginning of a vaginal hysterectomy. At this juncture the ureter is within 2 cm of the trigone. The risk of ureteral injury at this point can be minimized by carefully advancing the bladder from its attachment to the cervix and upper vagina prior to clamping or incising the vagina.

Hysterectomy is the most commonly performed major gynecologic surgical procedure in the United States, and most of the procedures are performed using an abdominal approach. The decision as to whether the abdominal or vaginal approach is chosen should be dictated by the size of the uterus, the disease being dealt with, the need for upper abdominal or other pelvic surgery, and to some extent the philosophy and skills of the surgeon. There are clearly regional preferences in the United States as to which approach should be taken if all other issues are equal.

In general, the abdominal hysterectomy is performed in cases where vaginal hysterectomy is inappropriate. This situation might include inadequate exposure through the vagina because of an undilated introitus and vagina (as in a nulliparous patient) or the uterus that cannot be removed through the limited space of the vagina (e.g., large leiomyomas), or when there is known or presumed adnexal pathology (e.g., endometriosis, pelvic inflammatory disease, ovarian neoplasm). Whenever there is the potential that upper abdominal exploration and surgery may be necessary, the abdominal approach should be taken from the start.

Vaginal hysterectomy has the significant advantage in that an abdominal incision is not made, and therefore the duration of surgery (and anesthesia) is usually shorter. There is also no pain and no other complications (infection, disruption) of an abdominal incision. The patient therefore is usually able to ambulate sooner after surgery, and postoperative hospitalization is usually shorter. The vaginal approach is also neces-

sary when performing repairs of pelvic floor defects, e.g., anterior or posterior colporrhaphy, or when correcting enterocele. The abdominal and vaginal approaches both have advantages and disadvantages. It is the complete gynecologic surgeon who uses each appropriately and effectively.

Total hysterectomy denotes complete removal of the uterine fundus and cervix (usually as a single surgical specimen). Historically, *subtotal hysterectomy* was performed, removing the uterine fundus but leaving the cervix. The subtotal (or supracervical) hysterectomy was performed routinely until the early 1950s. The advantage of this technique was a reduction in surgical blood loss and infection, which increased when the vagina was opened. However, with the advancement of blood banking techniques, antibiotics, and surgical skill, complete removal of the uterus and cervix can now be safely performed with no additional morbidity and with the assurance that the patient will not subsequently develop pathology of the residual cervix.

The most commonly performed abdominal hysterectomy today is an *extrafascial hysterectomy,* where the fascia of the cervix is removed along with the surgical specimen (Fig. 4-2). An *intrafascial hysterectomy* is sometimes performed, which leaves the cervical fascia attached to the bladder and rectum while the cervix is cored out. The intrafascial hysterectomy may be advantageous in situations where the bladder cannot be separated from the cervix because of extensive previous scarring, although this situation is rarely seen.

Radical hysterectomy is most often performed in patients with early-stage cervical carcinoma. The radical hysterectomy includes resection of the parametrial, paracervical, and paravaginal tissues at the lateral pelvic sidewall. The goal of this surgical procedure is to remove the tissue lateral to the cervix along with lymphatic channels and lymph nodes that may contain metastatic carcinoma (Fig. 4-3). When performing this procedure, the ureter must be carefully dissected out of its normal anatomic location, which runs through the parametria. The ureter is retracted laterally to completely resect the desired parametrial and vaginal tissues. Radical hysterectomy does not imply removal of the fallopian tubes and ova-

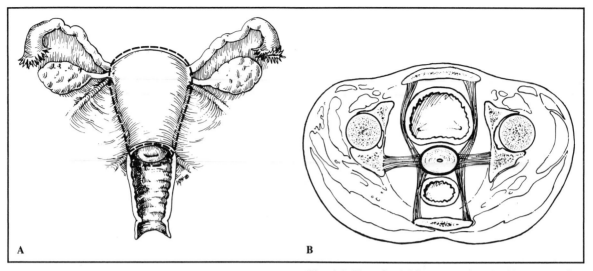

Fig. 4-2. Extrafascial hysterectomy. A. The extent of tissue removed when performing an extrafascial hysterectomy (whether it is vaginal or abdominal) is shown by the dotted line. B. The solid line around the cervix shows the extent of resection of ligaments.

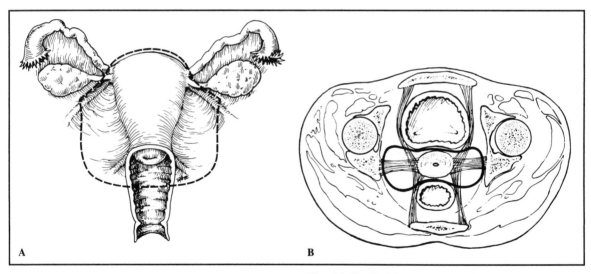

Fig. 4-3. Radical hysterectomy. This operation is usually performed for the treatment of cervical carcinoma. Therefore the goals include resection of the parametria and upper vagina to achieve a clear surgical margin around the cancer. A. Radical hysterectomy does not imply removal of the tubes and ovaries, which may often be preserved in young women. B. The cardinal ligament and major portions of the uterosacral and vesicouterine ligaments are resected as part of the radical hysterectomy.

ries, nor does it necessarily imply that pelvic and para-aortic lymphadenectomy has been performed in the treatment of early stage cervical carcinoma.

Removal of the ovaries at the time of pelvic surgery, especially in conjunction with hysterectomy, varies depending on the patient's age and the results of the preoperative discussion between the patient and the surgeon. It is strongly advised that patients who are postmenopausal should have their ovaries removed at the time of hysterectomy. This technique leads to no significant increase in surgical morbidity and may be viewed as a potential prophylactic measure to avoid ovarian carcinoma or other ovarian neoplasm in the years ahead. At the moment there is no clear-cut evidence that leaving the ovaries in place in the postmenopausal woman offers any physiologic benefit. In the premenopausal woman who has normal-appearing ovaries, the ovaries may be left in place with removal of the diseased (but not malignant) uterus. These ovaries usually continue to cyclically produce ovarian hormones and thus avoid the need for hormone replacement therapy in the young woman. In general, ovarian function diminishes at about the same time that the patient would have otherwise gone through normal menopause during her early fifties. The area of unclear decision-making is with the woman between age 40 and 50 who may have one to ten years of ovarian function remaining before she reaches natural menopause. Most gynecologists today recommend that a patient have her ovaries removed if she is age 45 or over, although this issue must be clearly discussed, with the patient making the final decision after weighing the pros and cons. There is no exact age at which the ovaries should be left in place or removed, and some patients because of cancerphobia, especially with a family history of ovarian cancer, may wish to have ovaries removed at a younger age than other women. Women who have had their ovaries removed before menopause should be given hormone replacement therapy to alleviate menopausal symptoms, prevent osteoporosis, and potentially offer protection from coronary vascular disease (Chap. 23).

Although the ovaries may always be removed through an abdominal incision, a vaginal approach may not allow adequate exposure or mobility of the ovaries to have them removed. The skilled pelvic surgeon is able to remove normal ovaries through a vaginal approach approximately 80 percent of the time. Therefore if the ovaries *must* be removed, it is advisable to take the abdominal approach from the outset.

Other general considerations of surgical concepts and strategies for specific gynecologic diseases are noted in appropriate chapters of this book. The interested reader is encouraged to use the Selected Readings noted at the end of this chapter for more details of gynecologic surgery techniques.

SUGGESTED READINGS

Cartwright, P. S., Pittway, D. E., Jones, H. W., et al. The use of prophylactic antibiotics in obstetrics and gynecology: a review. *Obstet. Gynecol. Surv.* 39:537, 1984.

Clarke-Pearson, D. L., Chin, N., DeLong, E. R., et al. Variables associated with postoperative deep venous thrombosis: a Prospective study of 411 gynecology patients with creation of a prognostic model. *Obstet. Gynecol.* 69:152, 1987.

Clarke-Pearson, D. L., Synan, I. S., Hinshaw, W. M., et al. Prevention of postoperative venous thromboembolism by external pneumatic calf compression in patients with gynecologic malignancy. *Obstet. Gynecol.* 63:92, 1984.

Cruse, P. J., and Foord, R. A 10 year prospective study of 62,939 wounds. *Surg. Clin. North Am.* 60:27, 1980.

Easterday, C. L., Grimes, D. A., and Riggs, J. A. Hysterectomy in the United States. *Obstet. Gynecol.* 62:203, 1983.

Garcia, D. R., Mikuta, J. R., and Rosenblum, N. G. *Current Therapy in Surgical Gynecology.* Toronto: B. C. Decker, 1987.

Hamod, K. A., Spence, M. R., and King, T. M. Prophylactic antibiotics in vaginal hysterectomy: a review. *Obstet. Gynecol. Surv.* 37:207, 1982.

Kaplan, E. B., Sheiner, L. B., Boeckmann, A. J., et al. The usefulness of preoperative laboratory screening. *J.A.M.A.* 253:3576, 1985.

Kaser, O., Ilke, F. A., and Hirsch, H. A. *Atlas of Gynecological Surgery.* Stuttgart: Georg Thieme Verlag, 1985.

Kursh, E. D., Morse, R. M., Resnick, M. I., et al. Prevention of the development of a vesicovaginal fistula. *Surg. Gynecol. Obstet.* 166:409, 1988.

Jewell, E. R., and Persson, A. V. Preoperative evaluation of the high-risk patient. *Surg. Clin. North Am.* 65:3, 1985.

Levinson, C. H., and Swolin, K. Postoperative adhesions: etiology, prevention and therapy. *Clin. Obstet. Gynecol.* 23:1213, 1980.

Mattingly, R. F., and Thompson, J. D. *TeLinde's Operative Gynecology* (6th ed.). Philadelphia: Lippincott, 1985.

Nichols, D. H., and Randall, C. L. *Vaginal Surgery* (2nd ed.). Baltimore: Williams & Wilkins, 1983.

Panton, O. N. M., Atkinson, K. G., Crichton, E. P., et al. Mechanical preparation of the large bowel for elective surgery. *Am. J. Surg.* 149:615, 1985.

Porges, R. F. Changing indications for vaginal hysterectomy. *Am. J. Obstet. Gynecol.* 136:153, 1980.

Shapiro, M., Munzo, A., Tager, I. B., et al. Risk factors for infection at the operative site after abdominal or vaginal hysterectomy. *N. Engl. J. Med.* 307:1661, 1982.

Versichelen, L. Physiopathologic changes during anesthesia administration for gynecologic laparoscopy. *J. Reprod. Med.* 29:697, 1984.

Wheeless, C. R., Jr. *Altas of Pelvic Surgery* (2nd ed.). Philadelphia: Lea & Febiger, 1987.

5

Complications of Gynecologic Surgery and Radiation Therapy

Complications following gynecologic surgery are in many ways similar to those encountered during other general abdominal operations. Problems unique to gynecologic surgery and the complications that occur with some frequency are discussed in this chapter. Postoperative complications may be reduced by careful patient selection and preparation (Chap. 4). The technical skills of the surgeon, excellent intraoperative execution of the planned procedure, and attention to details during postoperative care are key to the successful surgical outcome.

Even in the hands of the best surgeon, however, complications arise and must be managed promptly and carefully to ensure the best possible outcome. A thorough awareness of potential problems and early recognition of complications with proper management minimize poor outcomes. It is the surgeon who allows his or her ego to deny the occurrence of a possible complication or who is inattentive to the postoperative patient who is most likely to suffer serious and irreversible problems.

Today's medical-legal climate has pushed many surgeons to practice defensive medicine, fearful of litigation because of a complication of the surgical procedure. Nonetheless, it must be recognized that most complications are not the result of malpractice, and the best defense in these circumstances is careful attention to detail at every turn.

Communication with the patient is obviously important, beginning prior to hospital admission and continuing through the process of obtaining informed consent. Postoperatively, the patient must also be informed as to her status; and should a complication be suspected or recognized, a frank discussion of the problem and plans for management should be shared with the patient so that she may fully understand and cooperate.

POSTOPERATIVE FEVER

A fever (temperature higher than 38°C) following gynecologic surgery is a frequent problem that may resolve spontaneously within the first 48 hours of surgery or may herald a serious postoperative infection. Because of the seriousness of postoperative infection, all patients with a febrile course following surgery must be thoroughly evaluated. Low-grade fevers (38.0° to 38.5°C) during the first 48 hours after surgery are frequent and usually resolve spontaneously. These fevers occur most often during the evening hours and are usually attributed to microatelectasis of the lung following general anesthesia. Inflammatory reaction to suture material or devitalized tissue in the operative site is another explanation for these transient fevers.

Despite the fact that most fevers during the first 2 days after surgery resolve spontaneously, the patient should be carefully examined and appropriate laboratory tests obtained to exclude the possibility of a more serious cause of the fever. Usually the patient appears reasonably well and is not in distress. The white blood cell (WBC) count may be only minimally elevated (less than 10,000 per cubic millimeter) with an insignificant differential count. Management should be directed at increasing pulmonary expansion by ambulating the patient; turning, coughing, and deep breathing her; and performing incentive spirometry. In uncomplicated cases, respiratory therapy with intermittent positive-pressure breathing, bronchodilators, or percussion is not necessary.

Because the vagina cannot be made sterile, any patient who has undergone a gynecologic operation that enters, or is performed through, the vagina carries the increased risk of developing postoperative pelvic cellulitis. Untreated, cellulitis may progress to peritonitis, a pelvic abscess, or an ovarian abscess. Part of the differential, then, of an early or late postoperative fever should always entertain the possibility of pelvic cellulitis with later abscess formation. Early in its course, the patient may have minimal signs, and it may be difficult to distinguish lower abdominal pain or pelvic pain from the discomfort expected immediately postoperatively. Likewise, a pelvic examination following a hysterectomy is usually associated with normal induration and some tenderness. Clearly, palpation of a mass or fluctuance is abnormal and raises concern of a possible abscess or hematoma.

Prophylactic perioperative antibiotics (Chap. 4) have significantly reduced the occurrence of postoperative pelvic and wound infections; nonetheless, these problems continue to plague the gynecologic surgeon. Patients at high risk to develop postoperative pelvic infections include those with acute and chronic pelvic inflammatory disease, those undergoing extended pelvic dissection such as for cancer or endometriosis, those with diabetes, and those with immunosuppressive disorders.

The fever may initially be low grade (less than 38.5°C) but, left untreated, gradually develops a hectic spiking fever curve, rising to 39° to 40°C. The WBC count also rises only gradually but may reach alarming levels in an untreated patient. Early evaluation with pelvic ultrasonography may reveal a fluid collection, leading to a presumptive diagnosis of an infected pelvic hematoma or abscess.

Whenever pelvic cellulitis or an abscess is suspected, broad-spectrum antibiotics capable of covering both anaerobic and aerobic bacteria should be initiated through a parenteral route. If there is any suggestion of an infected pelvic hematoma or abscess of the vaginal vault, attempts should be made to open the vaginal cuff to achieve drainage. Should the patient continue a septic course that does not respond to antibiotics, it may be necessary to undertake surgical drainage of the abscess, irrigation, and placement of pelvic suction drains.

The respiratory tract may be the source of postoperative fever; and aside from the microatelectasis, which resolves spontaneously with increased pulmonary expansion, aspiration pneumonia or a bacterial pneumonia must be considered in patients with fever and pulmonary findings. Aspiration pneumonia in particular may occur in the operating room with induction of anesthesia or upon extubation yet remain unrecognized for hours after surgery. The chest radiograph is usually diagnostic in these more serious pulmonary

complications. Aggressive management with appropriate broad-spectrum antibiotics, pulmonary toilet, and even ventilatory support may be necessary.

Infections of the urinary tract may also cause a postoperative fever. Usually these infections are recognized several days after surgery and may vary between causing a low grade fever to the high spiking fever curve of pyelonephritis. Prolonged use of an indwelling urinary catheter and preexisting urinary tract infections are the most common etiologies of urinary tract infections following surgery. Ureteral injury or obstruction may lead to urinary stasis and pyelonephritis. On the other hand, ureteral obstruction following pelvic surgery may be entirely asymptomatic and go unrecognized until years later, when it is found that the patient has lost kidney function. Lower urinary tract infection may be reasonably asymptomatic or may be associated with suprapubic tenderness, urinary frequency, and dysuria. Costovertebral angle pain on percussion is usually pathognomonic for pyelonephritis. Urinalysis should demonstrate an increased number of white blood cells and bacteria. A urine specimen should be obtained for urine culture and antibiotic sensitivity at the first suggestion of a urinary tract infection. Because of the high probability of urinary tract infection acquired in hospital being caused by resistant organisms, initial empiric antibiotic coverage should be either with a second-generation cephalosporin or an aminoglycoside antibiotic, with the antibiotic coverage being adjusted appropriately once sensitivity is known.

Thrombophlebitis in the lower extremities or pelvic veins may be the etiology of a fever with little or no other symptoms. Evaluation and management of deep vein thrombosis and pulmonary embolism are discussed later in this chapter. Finally, in some patients an antibiotic initiated for presumed infection may actually be the source of a continuing fever. If the patient's clinical course is not septic and the fever continues (usually below 38.5°C), consideration should be given to a drug fever, which is managed by discontinuation of the antibiotics and observing the patient's course.

The workup of a postoperative fever is many times broadly based, as the source of the fever is not initially obvious. A complete physical examination, including auscultation and percussion of the chest, auscultation of the heart, searching for a cardiac murmur, inspection of the abdominal incision, percussion of the costovertebral angle, and inspection and palpation of the legs are important. A history of previous infection, pelvic inflammatory disease, or chronic bronchitis should be reviewed. Pelvic examination early in the postoperative course, as previously noted, is usually of little value, as the patient is usually tender and the pelvic tissues are indurated.

Laboratory tests should include a complete blood count and urinalysis. Cultures should be obtained from the urine, sputum, and blood, as well as from the wound drain sites or vaginal cuff if these sites appear to be clinically infected. A chest radiograph is indicated as part of the evaluation for a fever source, although usually there are auscultatory findings on physical examination. In patients with an unremitting fever, an abscess should be suspected and may be diagnosed by ultrasound, computed tomography, or an indium 111 leukocyte scan. Clearly, the early diagnosis of the source of postoperative fever and the appropriate management should minimize the seriousness of the infection and avoid prolonged morbidity.

POSTOPERATIVE HEMORRHAGE

Hemorrhage following gynecologic surgery is a serious, life-threatening complication. Because of the extensive blood supply to the pelvic viscera and the vascular pedicles that are created in the routine procedures such as hysterectomy, this risk is always present. Intraoperative hemorrhage and its management is discussed in Chapter 4. Clearly, patients who have suffered intraoperative hemorrhage are at high risk to have postoperative hemorrhage, especially during the immediate recovery phase. Most postoperative hemorrhage occurs within the first 48 hours of surgery and is usually the result of a vascular pedicle becoming freed from its ligature. Common sites of hemorrhage after hysterectomy are the ovarian pedicles, uterine vessels, and vaginal cuff.

The bleeding may be clinically obvious as vaginal bleeding, although in many instances it is intraperitoneal or retroperitoneal and is suspected only because of signs and symptoms of contracting vascular

volume. Tachycardia, hypotension, diminished urinary output, and increasing urinary specific gravity are all signs suggesting the possibility of intraabdominal hemorrhage.

In the patient in whom postoperative hemorrhage is suspected, a hematocrit and vital signs should be checked serially. Immediate transfusion of the anemic patient and correction of any coagulopathy should be instituted. Patients who have had significant intraoperative bleeding and large volumes of blood replacement may have depleted their coagulation factors and may be bleeding from an unrecognized coagulopathy. Therefore it is always appropriate to check a platelet count, prothrombin time, partial thromboplastin time, and bleeding time. In patients with an iatrogenic coagulopathy or with disseminated intravascular coagulation (DIC), correction of the coagulopathy may control the bleeding without further surgery. In most instances of severe postoperative hemorrhage, immediate surgical reexploration to control the bleeding point(s) is advised. Finally, obvious bleeding from the vaginal cuff can usually be managed by resuturing the vaginal cuff, achieving control of the vaginal artery. This bleeding usually arises in the lateral fornices of the cuff where the blood supply originates.

It is clear that many patients with limited postoperative bleeding go unrecognized except for the fact that their postoperative hematocrit falls more than would have been expected. Occasionally a retroperitoneal hematoma or a hematoma at the vaginal cuff becomes infected and thereby manifests as an infected hematoma, evolving into an abscess. Depending on the longevity of the suture material used, delayed bleeding from the vaginal cuff or vascular pedicles may occur one to two weeks postoperatively. This complication is rare. Patients should be advised that some vaginal spotting after hysterectomy is expected for a week or two, but that any heavier bleeding should be brought to the attention of her surgeon. The patient should be immediately reexamined for the possibility of a vaginal cuff bleeder.

Vascular embolization by way of a percutaneous catheter may be able to control postoperative pelvic bleeding. Arteriographic study of the pelvic vasculature and ovarian blood supply should be performed in an attempt to identify a vascular "blush" of the bleeding point. Selective embolization may then be performed, directed at the specific artery. Because the blood supply to the pelvis arises from the hypogastric artery, the inferior mesenteric artery, or the ovarian artery, arteriographic evaluation may be complicated. Control of difficult pelvic bleeding may require ligation of the anterior division of the hypogastric artery (Chap. 4).

URINARY TRACT COMPLICATIONS

The lower urinary tract (ureters, bladder, urethra) are always at potential risk of incurring injury and other complications following gynecologic surgery. Depending on the extent of the operation, which may even involve the urinary tract, the degree of potential complications may be anticipated. A thorough knowledge of the lower urinary tract anatomy, blood supply, and physiology aids in the reduction of these complications. Complications may be minor, such as transient urinary retention or an uncomplicated urinary tract infection, or they may be major life-threatening problems, such as gram-negative sepsis or vesicovaginal fistula.

To minimize trauma to the bladder, catheterization and drainage of the bladder is usually performed prior to pelvic surgical procedures. An indwelling Foley catheter is placed for major operations, whereas the bladder may be drained with a straight catheter on a one-time basis at the institution of minor procedures such as dilatation and curettage (D&C) or cold-knife conization. A Foley catheter placed at the time of surgery may be removed the evening of surgery or the morning after surgery, and thereafter the patient usually resumes a normal voiding pattern. After extended dissection (such as for radical hysterectomy or posterior exenteration) or after extensive surgery to the bladder (such as anterior colporrhaphy or retropubic cystourethropexy) it is wise to leave the catheter in for a longer period to allow resolution of bladder wall edema and pain prior to expecting the patient to be able to void. Patients who are critically ill and who require urinary output monitoring on an hour-by-hour

basis should also have the urinary catheter left in place.

For patients in whom prolonged bladder drainage is required, placement of a suprapubic catheter is often advised. The suprapubic catheter, by virtue of its location, is less contaminated and therefore associated with decreased risk of urinary tract infection. In addition, a trial of voiding is often necessary before complete bladder function recovery. With the suprapubic catheter, the catheter may be clamped, allowing the bladder to fill, and the patient may then void through the urethra as she is able. If the patient is unable to void, the suprapubic catheter may be unclamped and the bladder drained. This method of bladder "training" avoids a need for repeated removal and replacement of a transurethral Foley catheter, minimizing the use of expensive equipment as well as the potential for a urinary tract infection. Many surgeons give patients prophylactic (suppressive) antibiotics if the catheter is left in for more than a few days, but the benefit of this practice remains controversial.

Urinary Retention

After pelvic surgery a small proportion of patients are unable to void when the catheter is removed. Usually this problem can be resolved by a single straight catheterization of the bladder and allowing the patient to attempt to void a second time, or by replacement of the Foley catheter for 24 hours. The physiologic mechanism of this urinary retention is not clear, but it is likely related to abdominal wall pain, bladder wall edema, and psychological mechanisms. The patient may fear discomfort when attempting to void or may be unable to relax in the unfamiliar hospital environment. The psychological component is the most likely cause of urinary retention and usually resolves when the patient is able to relax and attempts to void in an unpressured, unsupervised fashion.

For patients who have repeated episodes of urinary retention, initial management is prolonged bladder drainage. Repeated attempts at voiding and then replacing the catheter only leads to further psychological trauma and frustration for the patient, the nursing staff, and the physician. Allowing the catheter to drain for several days after initial attempts to void have failed is the usual recommendation. If on repeated attempts the patient is unable to void, she should be evaluated further. Cystoscopy with urodynamic studies can further elucidate the etiology of the urinary retention. In most instances the prolonged urinary retention is due to psychological abnormalities, although on occasion it may be the first sign of preexisting neurologic disease, e.g., multiple sclerosis or a neurogenic bladder secondary to diabetes.

Certain surgical procedures are likely to be associated with postoperative urinary retention. Radical pelvic surgery for cancer with wide resection of the paracervical tissues, uterosacral ligaments, and extensive dissection along the base of the bladder interrupts some of the innervation of the bladder, thereby leading to a hypertonic bladder during the initial postoperative phase. In most patients, routine bladder drainage should be considered for at least one week and up to six weeks after a radical hysterectomy or posterior exenteration before attempting voiding trials. When the spontaneous voiding trial is allowed, care should be taken not to overdistend the bladder, as it may lead to further difficulties with voiding.

Occasional patients after radical surgery have prolonged urinary retention or incomplete emptying with a large postvoid residual volume. These patients should be taught intermittent self-catheterization to reduce the risk of repeated urinary tract infections secondary to a large postvoid residual urine volume carried in the bladder.

Surgical procedures aimed at the correction of stress urinary incontinence (e.g., anterior colporrhaphy, retropubic cystourethropexy) cause significant acute alteration in the preexisting anatomy of the base of the bladder and urethrovesicle junction. The surgical trauma with resultant edema further contributes to difficulties in voiding initially after surgery. An overly enthusiastic attempt to resuspend the urethrovesicle angle may actually kink or obstruct the proximal urethra, thereby creating outflow obstruction. This obstruction, easily recognized by urethroscopy and cystoscopy, should be managed conservatively initially in the hope that it will resolve spontaneously once edema has resolved and the tissues have relaxed as the suture material absorbs. On rare occasions surgical reexploration and removal of the offending suture may be necessary.

Urinary Tract Injury

Even though the urinary tract is intimately associated with most gynecologic surgical procedures, surgical injury of the urinary tract is relatively infrequent. Avoidance of these complications depends on a thorough knowledge of the anatomy of the lower urinary tract and careful dissection to identify the anatomy before proceeding with surgical resection of an adjacent organ. Complications are more likely to arise in situations where anatomy is significantly distorted by disease, as with surgery for acute pelvic inflammatory disease, endometriosis, or cancer.

The most frequent urinary tract injury is cystotomy. This accident may occur at the time of abdominal wall incision or as the bladder is being advanced from the uterus, cervix, and upper vagina when performing an abdominal or vaginal hysterectomy. Most often cystotomy is recognized immediately and may be repaired without long-term complications.

Because most cystotomies are in the dome of the bladder (away from the trigone) the risk of fistula is small. Management of a cystotomy in the dome of the bladder requires repair with absorbable suture material and continuous bladder drainage for five to six days postoperatively. Cystotomy at the bladder base, near the trigone, is more likely to result in a subsequent fistula.

Careful repair of these cystotomies requires that the surgeon identify the location of the ureters and ureteral orifices and be certain that they are not obstructed or incorporated in the closing sutures. If any doubt is present, ureteral catheters should be placed for better identification of the ureters and ensured patency as the cystotomy heals. To avoid overdistention of the bladder or any tension on the suture line while it heals, prolonged urinary bladder drainage (for up to six weeks) is advised: In this setting prophylactic antibiotics should be given to minimize the risk of bladder wall infection or pelvic cellulitis. Drainage of the retroperitoneal space in the pelvis may prevent hematoma or abscess formation, which might further compromise blood supply to the injured bladder.

The cystotomy that goes unrecognized intraoperatively may provide a diagnostic dilemma postoperatively, thereby increasing the significance of the complication. The most frequent symptoms of an unrepaired cystotomy relate to the spill of urine into the peritoneal cavity. This problem may initially present as increasing abdominal pain postoperatively, abdominal distention, and ileus. Suspicion of this problem should be evaluated promptly with a cystogram; and if cystotomy is identified, immediate repair and prolonged bladder drainage are recommended. An unrecognized cystotomy at the base of the bladder may be recognized only by profuse and continued vaginal drainage of serosanguineous fluid (urine mixed with blood) and be identified as a vesicovaginal fistula. Alternatively, vesicovaginal fistula may result from devitalization of the base of the bladder or the ureter following extensive pelvic dissection. Although the bladder wall may not be injured in the operating room, it may take several days before the bladder wall or ureter completes the course of ischemia, necrosis, and slough, with the ultimate appearance of clinical signs of a fistula. Pelvic cellulitis following surgery further contributes to the possibility of fistulization.

Most fistulas are initially suspected by the patient's complaint of watery, prolonged vaginal drainage. Pain may be minimal, although abdominal, back, and flank pain may be apparent, especially if there is an infectious component or pyelonephritis.

When a fistula is suspected, immediate evaluation should be undertaken to prove or disprove the possibility and institute appropriate corrective measures, if needed. A simple bedside technique to detect fistulas utilizes a dye such as indigo carmine or methylene blue. First, the bladder is distended to 200 to 300 ml volume using saline dyed with indigo carmine and the vagina examined for any leaking of the dye. The vaginal apex is inspected carefully. Alternatively, a tampon may be placed in the vagina and left in for 30 minutes with the bladder distended. The tampon is then removed and inspected for any dye stain. If there is stain on the tampon or dye is noted on vaginal examination, it is strong presumptive evidence of a vesicovaginal fistula (Fig. 5-1). If no dye leaks from the

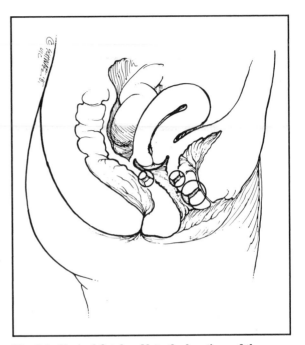

Fig. 5-1. Vaginal fistulas. Note the locations of the fistula arising between the bladder and vagina (vesicovaginal fistula), ureterovaginal fistula, urethrovaginal fistula, and rectovaginal fistula. They may result from complications of surgery or radiation therapy.

bladder, the possibility of a ureterovaginal fistula still must be excluded: Indigo carmine is then injected intravenously and a tampon placed in the vagina. Indigo carmine is cleared by the kidneys and appears in the urine within a few minutes. The tampon is left in place for 30 to 40 minutes until the dye appears in the bladder. The tampon is then removed and inspected for any blue staining. Staining of the tampon following intravenous injection of methylene blue strongly suggests the possibility of a ureterovaginal fistula. Further radiographic evaluation, including intravenous pyelogram, cystoscopy, and retrograde pyelograms, should then be undertaken to delineate the exact location of the fistula.

Management of a vesicovaginal fistula is discussed in more detail in Chapter 19. It may be the surgeon's initial tendency to wish to repair the fistula immediately, but past experience has clearly demonstrated that the safest and most successful outcome is achieved by allowing complete healing of all adjacent pelvic tissues and complete evolution of the fistula. Over the ensuing weeks, further necrosis and sloughing of the base of the bladder may occur, and therefore it is important to allow demarcation of the fistula tract before attempting to close tissue that may be inadequate for repair. This process may take anywhere from three to six months. It is clearly a difficult time for the patient because in most cases urinary leakage is constant; and depending on the size of the fistula, it may also be nearly complete. Patients with a small vesicovaginal fistula may benefit from placement of a urethral or suprapubic catheter to drain most of the urine before bladder wall distention and pressure are increased. Ultimately, the fistula can usually be closed with careful attention to surgical technique, a layered closure, and careful postoperative management. For patients in whom the blood supply was compromised (especially after radical surgery or radiation therapy), a new blood supply should be brought into the area of the fistula repair to improve the possibility of healing. This blood supply may come from the omentum or the bulbocavernosus muscle of the vulva (Martius flap).

Ureterovaginal fistula is managed by placement of ureteral catheters. Ureteral catheters divert most of the urine across the fistula and thereby minimize drainage from the fistula tract. Furthermore, as healing progresses, it is not infrequently noted that the fistula closes spontaneously (due to scarring around the ureteral catheter). Therefore if the fistula is closed and urinary tract patency is maintained, a major surgical procedure can be avoided. Immediate repair of a ureterovaginal fistula low in the pelvis should be considered. This choice is in contradistinction to repair of a vesicovaginal fistula because the injured tissue in the ureterovaginal fistula is not used for part of the closure. In most instances, ureteral injury low in the pelvis is managed by ureteral reimplantation (ureteroneocystotomy), which is usually easily accomplished, implanting a healthy ureter into an area of the bladder that is also healthy. Injuries of the ureter closer to the pelvic brim cannot be managed by ureteroneocystotomy and require some other method to reestablish continuity of the urinary tract, such as ureteroureter reanastomosis.

Obstruction of the ureter postoperatively may go completely unrecognized, as it may be asymptomatic. On the other hand, ureteral obstruction with pyelonephritis should be considered in any patient with a postoperative fever, especially when associated with abdominal or flank pain. In the course of a hysterectomy, there are three anatomic locations where the ureter is particularly close to the operative site and in jeopardy of injury. (1) At the pelvic brim the ovarian vessels (infundibulopelvic ligament) cross the ureter and may be injured or ligated at the time of salpingooophorectomy. (2) When performing an abdominal or vaginal hysterectomy, the clamping, dividing, and ligating of the uterine vessels and cardinal ligament bring the surgeon and ligatures within 1 to 2 cm of the pelvic ureter. Because the ureter crosses under the uterine artery approximately 1.5 cm from the cervix, care must be taken when placing sutures in this area. The most frequent cause of ureteral injury is bleeding from the vascular pedicles that requires additional sutures, which may be placed too deep in the tissues and incorporate the ureter. (3) Finally, as the ureter passes through the distal few centimeters before the bladder trigone, it is only 1 cm away from the vaginal canal. This proximity makes the ureter vulnerable during the incision or closure of the vaginal cuff. Sutures in the vaginal cuff, especially those placed wide of the cuff to control bleeding from the vaginal artery, may incorporate the ureter.

Whereas the ureter should be easily identified in its location at the pelvic brim and recognized separately from the ovarian vessels, the course of the ureter in the lower pelvis is not so easily seen. Some surgeons routinely palpate the ureter through the paracervical tissues; but to completely visualize the ureter, an extended dissection such as that performed for radical hysterectomy must be performed. Recognition of ureteral ligature or injury in the operating room allows immediate repair and optimal chance for full recovery. A crushing injury to the ureter by hysterectomy clamps is managed by reimplantation of the ureter (ureteroneocystotomy).

Ureteral obstruction postoperatively must be evaluated by intravenous pyelography or retrograde pyelography. In many cases a ureteral stent may be passed either antegrade or retrograde across the area of stenosis. If there is no concomitant ureteral fistula, the injury may be allowed to heal over the stent. As the absorbable suture material adjacent to or around the ureter absorbs, ureteral patency may be reestablished and the stent ultimately removed with no long-term sequelae. If ureteral obstruction cannot be relieved by passage of a stent or if the obstruction persists after a reasonable period of conservative management, surgical correction is required.

PERITONEAL ADHESIONS

Any surgical procedure is associated with a potential for scarring and adhesion formation. Most peritoneal adhesions remain clinically occult and never bother the patient. Probably the most obvious result of postoperative peritoneal adhesive disease is acute intestinal obstruction requiring lysis of adhesions (enterolysis) or even small bowel resection or bypass. These infrequent serious complications are shared by general surgeons and gynecologists alike. Adhesions induced by surgery may also contribute significantly to a patient's subsequent difficulty achieving pregnancy. It is therefore reasonable to consider the prevention and treatment of pelvic adhesive disease, especially as it relates to the fallopian tubes.

As any experienced surgeon can attest, it is difficult to predict which patient will develop postoperative adhesions. It is always interesting to observe the intraperitoneal findings in a patient who has previously undergone an abdominal operation. In many cases there are minimal or few adhesions, whereas in some cases most of the intestine is densely adherent to other intestinal serosa, mesentery, and parietal peritoneum. Clearly, there are genetic factors we do not yet understand that predispose some patients to develop adhesions.

There are also obvious etiologic factors that contribute to adhesion formation, the most common of which is infection. Peritonitis, whether diffuse throughout the peritoneal cavity or confined to the pelvis (e.g., pelvic inflammatory disease), is a key etiologic factor of adhesions. Any other trauma or inflammation of peritoneal surfaces caused by surgical manipulation, packing the intestines with gauze packs, or trauma to tissues at the edges of the surgical resection or where suture material is applied may lead to a nidus of inflammation and subsequent adhesion formation. Talcum powder or starch on the surgeon's gloves that falls into the operative field could be the nidus for adhesion formation and granuloma.

Because of the devastating outcome of adhesive disease in the pelvis and the difficulties with correction of adhesive disease when it contributes to infertility, every attempt should be made to minimize adhesions during gynecologic surgery or other surgery in the abdomen and pelvis. Key principles of adhesion prevention include careful surgical technique, atraumatic (gentle) manipulation of tissues, minimal necrotic tissue remaining in the surgical field, and use of nonreactive suture material. Other maneuvers such as the use of prophylactic antibiotics, corticosteroids, antihistamines, and intraperitoneal dextran or heparin are part of the armamentarium of many surgeons, although none has undergone definitive clinical trials.

Tubal adhesions and obstruction are not diagnosed during the immediate postoperative period and may not become apparent until a patient attempts and is unsuccessful at achieving pregnancy. The diagnosis of tubal occlusion secondary to adhesions is strongly suggested by a hysterosalpingogram (Chap. 13) that shows clubbing and an obstruction or free spill of contrast into the pelvic peritoneal cavity. Diagnostic laparoscopy with insufflation of the uterus and fallopian tubes with dye (chromotubation) (Chap. 13) can confirm tubal occlusion. Management of infertility associated with tubal occlusive disease is detailed in Chapter 13. The patient with pelvic adhesions may also complain of chronic pelvic pain developing months to years after her surgical procedure. This problem is often difficult to identify and even more frustrating to treat successfully. The management of chronic pelvic pain and its other etiologies is discussed in Chapter 21.

Chronic pelvic pain may be aggravated by dyspareunia and decreased sexual function. The pain may be entirely due to adhesions, scarring, and fixation of the vaginal cuff. In addition, the ovary(s) may be adherent to the posterior cul-de-sac, leading to additional pain during sexual intercourse. If this *retained ovary syndrome* is suspected, the appropriate management is surgical removal of the adherent ovary.

In summary, the conscientious surgeon operating in

the female pelvis should be aware of the devastating complications of adhesive disease occluding fallopian tubes in women who wish to remain fertile. Whereas adhesions in the upper abdomen may be of little consequence, adhesions in the pelvis may lead to extended evaluation and subsequent surgical procedures in hopes of reestablishing tubal patency. Attention to careful surgical technique and appropriate selection of suture material are paramount.

GASTROINTESTINAL COMPLICATIONS

Any surgical procedure that enters the peritoneal cavity, whether transabdominally or through the vagina, may predispose to a number of gastrointestinal complications. Most patients who undergo major abdominal surgery have a transient decrease in coordinated bowel function. Auscultation of the abdomen on the day after surgery usually reveals minimal or hypoactive bowel sounds. This relative ileus, which may best be characterized by decreased intestinal motility, although not uniform throughout all segments of intestine, usually resolves within two to three days. During these first days the patient may display some abdominal distention, belching, and some cramping abdominal pain secondary to uncoordinated intestinal motility. If this problem continues past the first several days after surgery, diagnosis of postoperative ileus is usually made. The diagnosis of ileus is further supported by abdominal radiographs showing distended gas-filled loops of small *and* large bowel, with gas apparent in the rectosigmoid colon. It is important to attempt to distinguish between an ileus (which may easily resolve with conservative measures) and an acute small bowel obstruction, which may require more urgent surgery for correction. Plain radiographs usually suggest ileus.

As previously noted, conservative management can usually successfully resolve an ileus and return the patient to normal gastrointestinal function. The patient should remain NPO; and in cases of significant abdominal distention, a nasogastric tube is placed for gastrointestinal decompression. A gastric sump tube is the preference of most surgeons, although some surgeons prefer placing a long intestinal tube that ulti-

mately migrates into the proximal small bowel. Suction on these tubes decompresses the stomach of liquid contents and removes swallowed air, thereby preventing further distention of the small bowel. It does not necessarily, however, decompress the gas and fluid that is already in the distal small intestine or colon. During nasogastric decompression, the patient should receive appropriate intravenous fluids and electrolyte replacement. Fluid replacement requirements should consider not only the usual maintenance fluids but also the volume of fluid removed via the nasogastric tube and the estimated amount of fluid being "third-spaced" into the peritoneal cavity and the bowel lumen. This conservative approach of medical management usually promotes resolution of an ileus within a few days.

If the patient does not show improvement clinically or on plain abdominal radiographs, further investigation is warranted to exclude the possibility of small bowel obstruction. A barium enema followed by an upper gastrointestinal (GI) series is usually advised. On occasion the barium enema or the upper GI series appears to initiate the resolution of an ileus, and the patient returns to reasonably normal GI function within a day or so. If patency of the large and small bowel is confirmed, one must always consider the possibility of other sources for an ileus. In particular, electrolyte disturbances and ureteral injury should be considered.

Small bowel obstruction following gynecologic surgery is reasonably rare, occurring in approximately 1 percent of major gynecologic surgical procedures. Small bowel obstruction is usually due to the acute formation of adhesions, with the intestines rotated and adherent in a configuration that causes obstruction. Delayed small bowel obstruction (up to several years after surgery) may also be caused by adhesions. These adhesions are often bands ("banjo string") around which loops of intestines may coil, become edematous, and thereafter obstruct. Small bowel obstruction occurring weeks or years after surgery necessitates immediate surgical management with lysis of adhesions, bowel resection, or both. However, in a patient developing a small bowel obstruction a few days after a surgical procedure, a more conservative approach is warranted in hopes of resolving the obstruction spontaneously and without further surgery. The general measures outlined for the management of ileus with nasogastric tube decompression, intravenous fluid hydration, and close observation for a fever or rising white blood cell count (which might suggest intestinal infarction or perforation) should be given a trial of several days prior to considering surgical re-exploration. Total parenteral nutrition in this setting might also be considered for nutritional support while conservative measures are employed. Clearly, any evidence of intestinal infarction or perforation mandates immediate emergency surgical exploration.

Many patients undergoing gynecologic surgery develop adhesions between loops of small bowel (especially a terminal ileum) and the pelvic floor, which has been denuded at the time of surgery, but most patients suffer no sequelae. The patient who undergoes postoperative radiation therapy, however, is at increased risk to develop radiation-induced terminal ileitis, obstruction, or fistula. The pathophysiology is directly related to the fact that the small bowel segment is fixed in the pelvis by adhesions and therefore receives the entire dose of pelvic radiation therapy. This situation is in contrast to the patient who has freely mobile intestines that receive a less than full dose of pelvic radiation because different segments of the small bowel may be in the radiation port during the daily treatments.

Colonic complications following gynecologic surgery are rare. Most are related to injury at the time of surgery and may be corrected during surgery with no untoward sequelae. The most common surgical complication to the colon is injury to the rectosigmoid colon during a difficult dissection to free the uterus and cervix from adhesions in the posterior cul-de-sac. During the course of this dissection, the colon may be entered. If the patient has had an adequate mechanical bowel preparation, this injury can usually be repaired and the pelvis irrigated and drained without need for a colostomy. On the other hand, in an infected field or with an extended injury to the rectosigmoid, a temporary colostomy is advised to eliminate the fecal stream across the segment of rectosigmoid that is badly injured. Once healing has been achieved, the colostomy may be taken down six to twelve weeks postoperatively.

Colonic perforation and spill of fecal contents into the pelvis and peritoneal cavity postoperatively is a serious, life-threatening problem. Sigmoid injury and perforation should be considered in any patient with signs and symptoms of postoperative pelvic peritonitis or abscess formation. In most instances the colonic perforation is located in the rectosigmoid segment or the cecum and results from an unrecognized colonic injury, a necrotic appendiceal stump, or diverticulitis. Identification of the site of perforation and then reexploration with a diverting colostomy, irrigation, drainage, and broad-spectrum antibiotics are necessary.

Acute colonic obstruction following gynecologic surgery is rare. In nearly all instances it is related to an unresectable pelvic mass (e.g., ovarian carcinoma) or a large sarcomatous uterus. Progressive dilatation of the colon is noted on abdominal radiographs. Dilatation of the cecum beyond 10 cm warrants immediate Gastrografin enema to confirm the obstruction and then a diverting colostomy prior to perforation of the cecum.

COMPLICATIONS OF THE ABDOMINAL INCISION

Many gynecologic surgical procedures require an abdominal incision. Selection of the type of incision depends on the specific needs of the surgeon and his or her ability to satisfactorily perform the surgical procedure through the selected incision. Patient habitus, the need for an extended exposure or access to the upper abdomen, and cosmetic considerations are important factors when selecting the most satisfactory incision.

Among the complications of the abdominal wound, the most serious and potentially life-threatening is *dehiscence* (disruption of *all* layers of the wound) and evisceration. Prevention of this major complication begins with selection of the appropriate incision and then the appropriate wound closure technique. Key to preventing dehiscence is an adequate reapproximation of the rectus fascia. Important considerations in fascial closure include the suture material used and the type of closure performed. Statistically, the mass closure incorporating the fascia, muscle, and peritoneum with reapproximation of the fascia as a second portion of the closure (Smead-Jones closure) is associated with the lowest dehiscence rate. This type of closure for a midline incision should be seriously considered in patients at risk for poor wound healing. Such patients include those with cancer, those who are immunosuppressed or on corticosteroid therapy, those who have had abdominal or pelvic radiation therapy, diabetics, the obese, and those who have contaminated wounds from intraabdominal infection or bowel surgery.

Suture material that retains adequate tensile strength through the important portion of the healing phase includes permanent suture (e.g., monofilament nylon or wire) and the long-lasting absorbable materials (e.g., polyglycolic acid and polydioxanone). In addition, these particular suture materials induce minimal tissue reaction, thereby promoting healing. In contrast to these general principles of optimal wound closure is the technique of closing the wound with a running closure using a reactive absorbable material such as chromic catgut. Although many gynecologic abdominal wounds have been closed in this manner, the method is not associated with the best outcomes.

Wound dehiscence usually occurs several days after surgery and is often preceded by ileus and increasing incisional drainage. The drainage from the wound is usually clear (and in fact is peritoneal fluid). When the superficial layers of the wound open, the fascia should be inspected and carefully probed with a sterile Q-tip or sterile gauze. The recognition of a fascial defect requires immediate return to the operating room, where the wound is reclosed after excision of necrotic fascia muscle and subcutaneous tissue. In most instances of wound dehiscence, it is found that the suture material did not break in the fascial layer; rather, the suture pulled through the fascia, which was weakened and possibly under increased tension because of ileus or other postoperative problems. The wound dehiscence should be closed using the Smead-Jones mass closure, with the subcutaneous tissue being left open to heal by secondary intention or delayed closure.

In the past wound dehiscence was associated with up to 50 percent mortality, but with modern medical care the mortality is closer to 10 percent. Nonetheless, wound dehiscence is a serious complication requiring early identification, excellent surgical repair, and careful postoperative management.

Superficial separation of the abdominal wound, through the skin and subcutaneous tissue, is also a distressing problem, although not nearly so life-threatening. The superficial wound infection and separation is a nuisance that prolongs the patient's hospitalization and requires management after hospital discharge while the subcutaneous tissue granulates and closes by secondary intention. Most superficial wound separations are associated with a wound infection. Increasing erythema in the wound, drainage from the wound (although not always purulent), and possibly a low-grade fever portend a wound infection. Recognition of this problem should prompt immediate opening of the wound to allow drainage and débridement. Usually antibiotics are not required to control a fever.

Other causes for wound separation include incisional hematoma or seroma secondary to poor hemostasis prior to wound closure, or a hematoma that may have been induced by anticoagulent therapy or low-dose heparin venous thrombosis prophylaxis. The opened wound should be cleaned and packed with sterile gauze several times a day in order to débride necrotic subcutaneous tissue and to promote granulation. Over a period of four to six weeks, even a deep wound granulates and reepithelializes satisfactorily.

During long-term follow-up, an *incisional hernia* (ventral hernia) may become apparent. It is especially obvious when the patient is in the upright position and performs a Valsalva maneuver. This hernia results from inadequate fascial approximation and healing; and although the patient did not have dehiscence postoperatively, the intestines now protrude through the fascial defect. The risk of an incisional hernia is increased in obese patients, those with poor nutrition, those with chronic pulmonary disease, and diabetics. Postoperative distention of the abdomen and wound infection are also associated with the development of a postoperative incisional hernia. The hernia may cause pain, intermittent nausea and vomiting, or an obvious small bowel obstruction with potential for incarceration and strangulation of the small bowel protruding into the hernia. As mentioned previously, the diagnosis can usually be made on examination, and the patient may be aware of a bulging in the incision itself. Repair of the hernia requires tension-free reapproximation of fresh fascial edges. If the fascia cannot be reapproximated, substitution of a permanent mesh can be used satisfactorily to achieve integrity of the abdominal wall.

VAGINAL VAULT COMPLICATIONS

Following hysterectomy, be it vaginal or abdominal, extrafascial or radical, problems can occur with healing of the vaginal vault. It may seem that there are about as many ways to close the vaginal vault at the time of hysterectomy as there are surgeons performing the operation. In general, the surgeon may choose to close the vaginal vault or leave it open. When leaving the vaginal vault open, the goal is to allow drainage of pelvic and retroperitoneal serum and blood, thereby minimizing the chance of infection. In most uninfected cases, however, there is no clear-cut advantage to leaving the vaginal vault open. In fact, within a few days the vault is ultimately sealed and heals closed within a few weeks.

A frequent but minor problem is the formation of *granulation tissue* in the vaginal vault. This friable tissue usually causes a blood-tinged vaginal discharge. Granulation tissue in the vaginal vault can be removed by excision or cauterization, thus promoting complete epithelialization.

Prolapse of the fallopian tube through the vaginal vault is a rare complication following hysterectomy where the fallopian tubes are not removed. Tubal prolapse may cause a watery vaginal discharge or mild pelvic or abdominal pain. On pelvic examination, the pink to red fimbriated end of the fallopian tube is noted in the vaginal vault. On occasion, this tissue is mistaken for granulation tissue. The appropriate management of fallopian tube prolapse is excision of the prolapsed portion of the fallopian tube and reclosure of the vaginal vault.

Complete *dehiscence* (separation) of the vaginal vault with evisceration of small bowel through the vault is a rare complication that requires immediate abdominal exploration and resection of injured small intestine and closure of the vaginal vault.

Loss of support of the vaginal vault following hys-

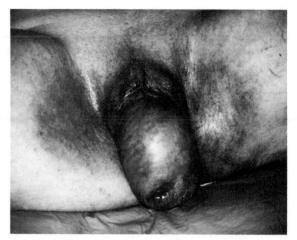

Fig. 5-2. Complete vaginal vault prolapse.

terectomy is a frequent problem that may not fully develop for several years or decades after surgery. When performing hysterectomy, supporting structures of the vaginal vault (cardinal and uterosacral ligaments) are severed. To reduce the occurrence of *vaginal vault prolapse* (Fig. 5-2), attempts should be made at the time of hysterectomy to resupport the vaginal vault by incorporating it into the transected uterosacral and cardinal ligaments. Obliteration of a large posterior cul-de-sac is also important to minimize the chances of enterocele formation. Vaginal vault prolapse occurs slowly over a period of years. The patient may note increased pelvic pressure or a bulging sensation in the pelvis or perineum. Complete prolapse is easily recognized by the patient, especially when she is in the upright position. Surgical correction of the vault prolapse offers several technical challenges but is usually successful; it is discussed further in Chapter 19.

DEEP VEIN THROMBOSIS AND PULMONARY EMBOLISM

Pulmonary embolism accounts for approximately 40 percent of deaths following gynecologic surgery and is one of the leading causes of death following radical surgery for pelvic cancer. To prevent this catastrophic event, prophylactic methods must be employed that prevent deep vein thrombosis in the lower extremities and pelvis. The recognition of risk factors associated with postoperative deep vein thrombosis and appropriate strategies for the prevention of this complication are discussed in Chapter 4.

Despite the aggressive use of prophylactic measures to prevent deep vein thrombosis, the clinician must remain vigilant for signs and symptoms of deep vein thrombosis or pulmonary embolism so that they may be recognized and treated properly. The signs and symptoms of *deep vein thrombosis* are often vague and inconclusive. Leg edema and pain, palpable venous thrombi in superficial veins ("venous cords"), and pain on dorsiflexion of the foot (Homan's sign) are suggestive of deep vein thrombosis. On the other hand, these signs and symptoms are due to other causes in approximately 50 percent of cases. Conversely, deep vein thrombosis is often a clinically silent disease that is suspected only after the patient has developed a pulmonary embolus. In fact, only 20 percent of patients with pulmonary emboli have prior signs or symptoms of deep vein thrombosis. In patients who are suspected of having deep vein thrombosis, immediate confirmation is necessary with the use of an accurate diagnostic technique. Today there are several noninvasive methods that may be used to accurately diagnose deep vein thrombosis: Doppler ultrasound, flow studies, venous imaging, impedance plethysmography, and iodine 125 fibrinogen leg scanning. The gold standard for diagnosis of deep vein thrombosis is ascending contrast venography, which should be used in any case where the less invasive tests are inconclusive or unavailable.

Pulmonary embolism may be suspected by subtle changes in vital signs, e.g., tachycardia or fever. Chest pain (usually pleuritic), hemoptysis, tachypnea, heart failure, or respiratory collapse suggest pulmonary embolism. With any of these events, a perfusion/ventilation lung scan or pulmonary arteriography should be performed for prompt diagnosis.

Although anticoagulant therapy carries some risk for hemorrhage in the postoperative patient, it is clear that the risks of fatal outcome from deep vein thrombosis or repeat pulmonary embolism are high, and immediate therapy is required. The goal of therapy is to achieve anticoagulation such that the patient does not develop further venous thrombi and does not have a pulmonary embolism. Heparin is usually instituted by continuous intravenous infusion (although some clinicians prefer a subcutaneous or intermittent intravenous route) for initial anticoagulant therapy. Intravenous heparin anticoagulation should have as its goal a prolongation of the activated partial thromboplastin time (APTT) to approximately 1½ times control value. Heparin anticoagulation is continued for 7–10 days. In the interim, oral anticoagulant therapy (warfarin) should be instituted. This oral anticoagulant therapy should be continued for 3–6 months postoperatively or longer if the patient's predisposing factors (e.g., advanced cancer) keep her at high risk for repeat deep vein thrombosis. Although anticoagulation therapy does not lyse the embolus or thrombus, the patient's own fibrinolytic system usually recannalizes a deep vein thrombosis or embolus. Plasminogen activators such as streptokinase or urokinase can cause immediate fibrinolysis, but they should not be used in postoperative patients because of the excessively high risk of hemorrhage and wound breakdown.

Septic pelvic thrombophlebitis is a variant of deep vein thrombosis associated with gynecologic and other pelvic surgery. Septic pelvic thrombophlebitis is associated with pelvic infection, usually after the delivery of a full-term pregnancy or a spontaneous or therapeutic abortion. Other postoperative pelvic infections or pelvic inflammatory disease may also lead to septic pelvic thrombophlebitis. The pathophysiology of this condition appears to be a mixed anaerobic infection in the pelvis that progresses to the plexus of hypogastric and ovarian veins, leading to venous thrombosis. Deep vein thrombosis not associated with infection may also occur in the pelvic veins postoperatively.

Pelvic vein thrombophlebitis is difficult to diagnose because of its lack of specific signs and symptoms and because there are no standard diagnostic methods to confirm the clinical suspicion of pelvic venous thrombosis. There are a few reports on the use of magnetic resonance imaging (MRI) or indium 111-labeled platelet scanning to identify pelvic and ovarian vein thrombosis. The diagnosis of septic pelvic vein thrombophlebitis is usually a presumptive one that follows either the acute onset of a pulmonary embolism or a septic postoperative course that does not resolve with broad-spectrum antibiotic coverage. The fever associated with septic pelvic thrombophlebitis is described as hectic with high temperature spikes, yet the patient appears relatively well. Tachycardia may be present, but the patient many times does not have an elevated white blood cell count. Usually the patient has been undergoing treatment for pelvic cellulitis, a pelvic abscess, or myometritis with broad-spectrum antibiotics. Despite adequate coverage for the infection, the temperature remains elevated.

In this setting, septic pelvic thrombophlebitis may be strongly suspected, and a diagnostic and therapeutic trial of intravenous heparin is recommended. If the fever resolves within 48 to 72 hours of institution of intravenous heparin therapy, a presumptive diagnosis of septic pelvic thrombophlebitis is made. Prior to anticoagulant therapy, the only treatment for septic pelvic thrombophlebitis was ligation of the ovarian veins and inferior vena cava.

COMPLICATIONS ASSOCIATED WITH SPECIFIC GYNECOLOGIC SURGICAL PROCEDURES

The risks of most gynecologic surgical procedures are similar to risks of any major abdominal operation and should be included in the preoperative discussion with the patient when obtaining informed consent. The most common and serious of these complications were outlined earlier in this chapter. Several gynecologic operations have additional unique complications associated with them that are discussed in this section.

D&C and Cold-Knife Conization of the Cervix

Dilatation of the cervix and curettage of the endocervix and endometrium (D&C) and cold-knife conization of the cervix are frequently performed minor surgical procedures. In general, they are associated with a low risk of complications and are most often performed on an outpatient basis. Nonetheless, serious complications can occur.

Perforation of the uterus at the time of D&C is a not infrequent complication. In most cases it is of no consequence because the uterus is perforated in its muscular fundus, which after the instrument is removed contracts to achieve hemostasis. Uterine perforation laterally in the broad ligament, however, does carry increased risk of hemorrhage and broad ligament hematoma. Additionally, perforation with a curet or suction curet may injure the bladder or intestines. Depending on the circumstances, it may be necessary to perform diagnostic laparoscopy or laparotomy to assess and repair potential injury of adjacent viscera. In most instances, patients are satisfactorily managed with close observation to ensure that hemorrhage is not developing and that injury to a viscus is not a problem.

The D&C procedure may also cause intrauterine *synechiae* or *adhesions* that may partially or completely occlude the endometrial cavity. The synechiae formed in the uterine cavity are most often associated with D&C performed under infected conditions or with a vigorous D&C required to control postpartum hemorrhage. The pathophysiology of uterine synechiae is probably due to complete denuding of the endometrium down to the basalis layer with concomitant infection and subsequent intrauterine adhesion formation. The management of Asherman's syndrome is discussed in Chapter 13.

Cold-knife conization is usually performed for the diagnosis and treatment of cervical intraepithelial neoplasia. With outpatient diagnostic modalities such as colposcopy (Chap. 25), the frequency of cold-knife conization has diminished significantly. When performing cold-knife conization, a cone-shaped portion of the cervix is removed for histologic study. This specimen usually contains a greater or lesser portion of the exocervix and the endocervical canal. Removed along with the epithelium of concern is a modest amount of cervical stroma.

Immediate or delayed postoperative *bleeding* may be a serious complication that requires resuturing the surgical site; on rare occasion, hysterectomy is needed to control the bleeding.

As the cervix heals, it may develop *stenosis,* which may subsequently lead to problems with dysmenorrhea, oligomenorrhea, and infertility. Furthermore, the scarred stenotic cervix may not dilate properly during subsequent labor and delivery, or it may dilate only by tearing, leading to a rapid second stage of labor. The removal of cervical stroma may also leave the patient with an *incompetent cervix* that dilates prematurely (during the second trimester of pregnancy) leading to premature delivery of a previable fetus. Management of this complication requires early recognition and placement of a cervical cerclage to prevent the cervix from premature dilation.

Complications of cervical stenosis are frequent; and depending on the particular definition, cervical stenosis may occur in up to 50 to 60 percent of patients after conization. Actual dysfunction due to cervical stenosis may occur in approximately 10 percent of patients. Incompetent cervix, on the other hand, although a serious complication, occurs in only 2 percent of patients undergoing cold-knife conization.

Laparoscopy

The laparoscope is being used with increasing frequency for the diagnosis and treatment of many gynecologic diseases. Its initial introduction in the United States was primarily for diagnosis of pelvic disease and to accomplish tubal sterilization. To a layman, the procedure was considered outpatient "Band-Aid surgery" because of the small puncture holes, which could be covered with a Band-Aid. Clearly, the minimal incisions required to insert the instruments offered major advantages over procedures that previously required laparotomy incisions.

The simplicity of the small abdominal incisions is deceptive, however, as serious complications can result from laparoscopy. Initial entry into the peritoneal cavity is a "blind" insertion of an insufflating needle, through which carbon dioxide is introduced to elevate the abdominal wall away from the abdominal and pelvic viscera. Insertion of this needle or the subsequent trochar may *injure viscera or blood vessels*. The potential for this injury is increased in patients who have had previous abdominal operations or adhesions from infection or endometriosis that may cause the intestines to be fixed to the anterior abdominal wall in the region where the trochar is being inserted. The slender patient is at increased risk for a *vascular injury* because the anterior abdominal wall is only a few

centimeters away from major abdominal and pelvic vessels. When major injury to viscera or vessels occurs, immediate laparotomy is necessary to repair the defect.

Insufflation of carbon dioxide creates space in the abdomen and pelvis for the laparoscope and other instruments to be inserted and manipulated safely. However, the insufflation of approximately 3 liters of carbon dioxide elevates the diaphragms, decreasing respiratory excursion, which may lead to *anesthetic complications*. Furthermore, carbon dioxide is absorbed and may cause *hypercapnia* with subsequent cardiac arrhythmias or arrest. Again, although laparoscopy appears to be a relatively minor surgical procedure, careful anesthetic management and observation throughout the surgical case for compromise in respiratory or cardiac function is absolutely mandatory.

Many laparoscopic procedures, such as tubal cautery and lysis of adhesions, are performed with electrocautery. Electrocautery does carry the potential for *thermal injury* to viscera; especially when the intestine is injured, potential perforation and serious complications may ensue. Reducing these complications by visualization of the intestine and areas to be cauterized is mandatory. In addition, the surgeon must have complete control over the activating device for the cautery so that it is not accidentally activated. Bipolar cautery has somewhat minimized the complications of tubal cautery. Many surgeons have completely eliminated the use of cautery for tubal sterilization, replacing it with the use of Silastic bands or clips. The early recognition of thermal injury is probably the most important key to preventing serious postoperative outcome. Recognition of burn to the bowel requires immediate laparotomy with resection of the injured segment. Because thermal injury extends beyond the area of obvious cautery injury, an adequate margin of resection must be achieved to have adequate healing without stenosis or perforation.

The *laser* is also applied through the laparoscope for treatment of pelvic disease, and it carries the hazards of injury to adjacent organs. Bleeding from small vessels that occurs during laparoscopic surgery is often controlled with electrocautery but sometimes requires laparotomy.

Complications of Abdominal and Vaginal Hysterectomy

In general, abdominal and vaginal hysterectomies, commonly performed major gynecologic procedures, are accomplished with great safety in the hands of a skilled pelvic surgeon. Most of the complications associated with hysterectomy are similar to those seen with any other major abdominal operation.

Because of the myriad pelvic blood vessels, *hemorrhage* may occur more frequently than one might initially expect; and because of the close approximation of bladder, rectosigmoid, and ureters, *injury to adjacent organs* is always a hazard. Establishment of anatomic planes and identification of adjacent important anatomy are critical steps of the surgical procedure in order to avoid serious complications. Injuries to adjacent organs are increased in patients who have severe anatomic distortions such as those caused by endometriosis, pelvic inflammatory disease, benign pelvic masses obstructing visualization of the pelvis, advanced cancer, and obesity. Complications following hysterectomy also may include *vault prolapse* due to transection of the support ligaments of the vagina, which are not appropriately reconstituted into the vaginal cuff closure.

Finally, *psychological problems* following hysterectomy are not infrequent and often relate to many issues of female sexuality and loss of reproductive function. Although this change in the patient's sexual function may cause transient depression or psychological disturbance, stable patients who are otherwise psychologically healthy can usually cope with these changes. The surgeon must be aware of the potential problems of more severe depression, grieving, and perception of loss. Support of the patient both pre- and postoperatively and appropriate psychological counseling when necessary are all part of a successful surgical outcome.

Radical Hysterectomy with Pelvic Lymphadenectomy

Radical hysterectomy and pelvic lymphadenectomy may be performed as definitive therapy for a Stage IB or IIA carcinoma of the cervix. This extended operation (outlined in Chapter 4) requires resection of the paracervical tissues and paravaginal tissues, which contain lymphatics and lymph nodes draining from the cervix and which may harbor cervical cancer. This extensive dissection also requires dissection of the base of the bladder and terminal ureter, which may lead to complications unique to this operation.

Denervation of the bladder is frequent, with incomplete ability to void, lasting several weeks for most patients. Many surgeons leave a catheter in the bladder to allow it to drain completely for up to six weeks following surgery. Others attempt to remove the catheter at an earlier point, as soon as the patient has established an ability to void with minimal postvoid residual.

Because of the extensive dissection in the pelvis, vesicovaginal and ureterovaginal *fistulas* are more common with radical hysterectomy than with total abdominal hysterectomy. The overall incidence of these major urologic complications is approximately 1 to 2 percent. Injury to the rectum with subsequent fistula formation occurs less frequently.

The extensive dissection of the pelvis may lead to intraoperative or delayed postoperative hemorrhage or infection. The three leading causes of death following radical hysterectomy in order of frequency are *pulmonary embolism, infection*, and *hemorrhage*. The surgical procedure is clearly an extended operation that requires a patient who is medically fit to tolerate several hours of anesthesia and large volumes of blood loss. The pelvic lymphadenectomy performed in conjunction with radical hysterectomy increases the risk of bleeding and infection.

Additionally, collection of lymph fluid draining from interrupted lymphatics may lead to a *lymphocyst*. Many lymphocysts are totally asymptomatic and resolve over a period of months with conservative management. On the other hand, they can lead to obstruction of adjacent ureter or venous blood supply, or they may become infected. All of these complications require surgical drainage.

Radical Vulvectomy and Inguinofemoral Lymphadenectomy

The standard therapy for vulvar carcinoma is radical vulvectomy with inguinofemoral lymphadenectomy.

Because of the location of this operation, the wound is always contaminated with vaginal and anal bacteria, leading to a high incidence of *wound infection* and *breakdown*. Furthermore, the reconstruction and wound closure following radical resection brings together tissues that are somewhat devitalized (due to subcutaneous undermining) and under tension. This tight closure of the vulvar and inguinal incisions further contributes to wound infection, necrosis, and breakdown. Inguinofemoral lymphadenectomy completely exposes the femoral artery and vein, which if wound breakdown occurs might be exposed with a risk of subsequent major blood vessel necrosis and hemorrhage. Surgical techniques to minimize this complication employ mobilization of the sartorius muscle to overlie the femoral vessels at the completion of the operation, bringing a new blood supply and protection over the vessels should superficial wound breakdown occur.

Lymphedema is a chronic problem following inguinal lymphadenectomy and is heightened by the addition of pelvic or inguinal radiation therapy postoperatively. Some degree of lymphedema is noted by up to 60 percent of patients following radical vulvectomy and inguinal lymphadenectomy and may be a major cause of disability. Today there is no satisfactory means for managing lower extremity lymphedema. Conservative management with leg elevation, gradient compression stockings, and diuretics offers some symptomatic relief, yet is incomplete. Sequential compression pumps placed around the leg seem to be of more benefit to the patient in reducing the leg swelling, although these measures must be used on a chronic basis. Operations to reestablish lymph channels or provide collateral lymphatic circulation have not been developed to the satisfaction of most patients or surgeons.

Resection of the medial levator muscle plate and external genitalia as part of the radical vulvectomy contributes to a high incidence of postoperative *stress urinary incontinence* and *pelvic floor relaxation*. Moreover, many patients undergoing radical vulvectomy are elderly and already have a component of pelvic floor relaxation or stress urinary incontinence. If pelvic floor relaxation is recognized preoperatively, a combination of a surgical method for resuspension of the urethrovesicle junction should be considered at the time of radical vulvectomy.

Finally, the radical nature of this operation, with subsequent scarring of the vulva and introitus leads to considerable *sexual dysfunction* for many patients. Obviously, psychological support and counseling should be given to all patients. Less radical surgery has been advocated for early stages of vulvar carcinoma (Chap. 29), and reconstructive methods to recreate a new vulva have been employed successfully by skin grafting and myocutaneous flaps.

Pelvic Exenteration

Pelvic exenteration is most frequently performed for recurrent carcinoma of the cervix following radiation therapy. This ultraradical pelvic operation is designed to achieve adequate clearance of a centrally recurrent malignancy, thereby affording the patient cure by secondary therapy. In order to achieve adequate surgical margins, vital organs must be removed.

The unique complications of pelvic exenteration include acute problems with *fluid loss and replacement* during the surgery and for the first several days postoperatively. Central venous monitoring and intensive care management are usually necessary during the acute perioperative period. Massive blood loss and requirements for fluid replacement are the ultimate strain on the cardiovascular and renal systems.

As the patient recovers further from surgery, *reduced wound healing* and *infection* become important potential complications. Usually, the surgery is performed following radiation therapy, and therefore pelvic tissues are considerably injured and devitalized, contributing to reducing wound healing.

In addition, tissue perfusion is diminished and the extensive dissection with tissue necrosis and devitalization puts the patient in a position to develop serious pelvic *cellulitis*. In fact, infectious complications occur in up to 70 percent of patients following pelvic exenteration. The most common infection is cellulitis of the pelvic floor, although pneumonia and urinary tract infections occur frequently.

The denuded, often infected pelvic floor predisposes to intestinal adhesions, leading to *bowel obstruction* and *fistulas*. Initial management with gastrointestinal decompression by suction tube is routinely employed until bowel function is established. Bowel function is further compromised by the intestinal surgery required during the reconstruction phase of the operation to create a urinary conduit and colostomy. Healing of the bowel anastomosis may be delayed because the bowel in the pelvis was previously irradiated. Likewise, the ureteral anastomoses in the urinary conduit may have problems with healing, leading to *dehiscence* of the anastomosis or subsequent *stricture* and *stenosis*.

In summary, pelvic exenteration from a surgical and medical management point of view is the most extended gynecologic procedure, requiring the most skill surgically and for postoperative management of any gynecologic operation. The psychological adjustment, sexual disfigurement, and identity alterations of the patient are also great. In most instances, the patient is left with a permanent urinary conduit and colostomy, and may not have a functional vagina. Gynecologic oncologists have now developed techniques to create a neovagina and thereby allow sexual function postoperatively for many patients. In selected cases, a colostomy may be avoided by use of a low rectal reanastomosis facilitated by circular stapling devices. Finally, a continent urinary conduit may be considered, although it is not routine at this time because of the complexity of its construction and additional significant operating time.

COMPLICATIONS OF RADIATION THERAPY

Radiation therapy is frequently used for treatment of gynecologic cancer. The combination of external radiation therapy (teletherapy) and intracavitary therapy (brachytherapy) provides optimal treatment for most patients with cervical and vaginal cancer, as well as selected patients with endometrial, vulvar, and ovarian cancer. Because radiation is widely used to treat gynecologic cancers, complications that may be encountered should be considered.

Factors Associated with Radiation Injury

Although radiation therapy may be used successfully to treat several gynecologic malignancies, it may also lead to devastating complications. Discussions of radiosensitivity of tumors are important, yet nearly any tumor may be eradicated with a high enough dose of radiotherapy. The limitation to successful radiation therapy for all patients is that prior to achieving a tumoricidal dose to some tumors serious injury and complications of normal tissues may lead to fatal outcomes.

Key factors associated with radiation injury include the total radiation dose and the volume of tissue irradiated. In addition, the period of time over which the radiation therapy dose is given is inversely proportional to the complication rate.

Normal organs and tissues are more or less sensitive to radiation therapy. Fortunately, in the pelvis most tissues are reasonably radioresistant. The most radiosensitive tissues in the pelvis are the ovaries followed by the small intestine. The ovary can withstand approximately 1000 rads before loss of ovulatory function, and the small bowel can absorb approximately 4500 rads before intervening complications develop. In the upper abdomen, the liver and kidneys tolerate only approximately 3000 rads before developing radiation hepatitis and nephritis, respectively. The dose of radiation therapy delivered to a particular area therefore must consider the sensitivity of organs in the radiation field.

Most radiation complications follow cell injury and subsequent obliterative endarteritis. This endarteritis leads to hypoxia, fibrosis, and further obliteration of the tissue's blood supply. Fibrosis, ischemia, and necrosis of normal tissues contribute to the major complications associated with radiation therapy. Other vascular diseases compound this problem of endarteritis and poor tissue profusion. Therefore patients with artherosclerotic cardiovascular disease and diabetes are at high risk to develop radiation therapy complications. Fixation of the small intestine in the pelvis due to prior pelvic surgery, pelvic inflammatory disease, or endometriosis increases the risk of small bowel complications because the segment of small bowel fixed in the pelvis cannot move out of the radiation field during part of the therapy. Most frequently it is the terminal ileum.

Surgery following radiation therapy may also contribute to increased radiation therapy complications because of further devitalization of tissues. In addition, because of the poor tissue healing caused by radiation therapy, surgery must be undertaken with care in the radiation field and strategies employed to bring in a new blood supply from tissues not previously irradiated, if possible.

Intracavitary radiation therapy plays a key role in the successful treatment of cervical and vaginal carcinoma. Factors associated with complications of intracavitary radiotherapy include uterine perforation by the uterine tandem, protruding radiation sources extending distal to the cervical os, or systems that shift from their proper position in the upper vagina adjacent to the cervix to the mid or lower vagina.

Radiation complications may be classified into two groups. (1) Those that occur during and immediately after radiation therapy are usually self-limited and may be managed by conservative measures. (2) Other complications may occur months to years after completion of radiation therapy and are a more serious group of complications. Often surgical intervention is necessary to correct them.

Acute Radiation Complications. Complications that occur during radiation therapy are usually self-limited and may be managed conservatively. During the course of fractionated whole-pelvis radiotherapy (extending over four to six weeks) the first two weeks are usually symptom-free. During the latter half of external beam radiation therapy, reaction from the ileum, rectum, and bladder may lead to symptoms of *diarrhea,* dysuria, urinary frequency, and intolerance to selected foods. Conservative management with alteration of the diet to a low fat, low residue diet and the use of antidiarrheal medications usually suffices to make the symptoms tolerable. Patients who have bladder symptoms should be evaluated for the possibility of a urinary tract infection and treated with appropriate antibiotics. Pyridium may be used to relieve dysuria.

Radiation of the pelvic bone marrow, especially in older patients, may lead to *pancytopenia.* Therefore blood counts should be checked on a weekly basis; and if significant pancytopenia is noted, radiation therapy must be interrupted until the bone marrow recovers.

Radiation sickness is usually minimal and self-limited but may present as malaise and nausea and vomiting. Conservative management with antiemetics and adjustment of the diet is usually satisfactory, although an occasional patient must be admitted to the hospital for intravenous hydration or total parenteral nutrition.

Most patients have some or all of these side effects during radiation therapy. Fortunately, the effects are self-limited, and the patient should be reassured that they resolve within a few weeks of the completion of radiation therapy.

Delayed and Chronic Radiation Complications. The most severe complications of radiation therapy are those that occur months to years after completion of radiation therapy. They are secondary to the obliterative endarteritis initiated by cell injury during radiation therapy. Because of the poor tissue perfusion caused by the endarteritis, fibrosis, ischemia, and necrosis may ultimately occur. Any organ in the radiation field is at risk to develop these complications.

Injury to the skin and subcutaneous tissue was more often a problem in the past when orthovoltage radiation equipment was used. With the higher energy therapy currently used, the skin and subcutaneous tissue is relatively spared, whereas a higher dose is delivered to the central pelvis. Nonetheless, occasional patients are still seen today with fibrotic leather-like skin and firm, hardened subcutaneous tissue. Subcutaneous tissue injury is rarely a complication that causes significant symptoms.

The small intestine may develop *intermittent diarrhea, intolerance to selected foods,* or *malabsorption.* A low fat diet and avoidance of green leafy vegetables and fried foods may be adequate management to prevent continuing gastrointestinal upset. Many patients find by trial and error that there are some foods they are unable to eat after radiation therapy. Chronic diarrhea due to radiation enteritis can be a life-long problem but may be managed with antidiarrheal medications. The fibrosis induced by radiation therapy contributes to the signs and symptoms of small bowel obstruction, fibrosis, and possible perforation or fistulization. Initial management of intermittent small bowel obstruction following radiation therapy should be conservative with nasogastric tube suction and intravenous fluids. Total parenteral nutrition during this time may be required. Because surgery on the small bowel that has been radiated is fraught with significant complications and poor healing, surgical resection or bypass should be considered only as a last resort. If small bowel obstruction or chronic intermittent obstruction does not resolve with conservative measures, surgery may be necessary.

Optimal preparation of the patient to aid in wound healing is mandatory. Rarely is this surgery performed under emergency circumstances; therefore the bowel should be prepared as best as possible and nutritional parameters optimized with total parenteral nutrition. The surgical approach to radiation-induced small bowel obstruction is somewhat controversial, although most surgeons prefer bowel bypass rather attempting resection of the injured and obstructed bowel. Resection in many reports is associated with numerous postoperative complications and high mortality, probably because of the devitalization of the bowel mesentery, leading to further ischemia, especially at the site of small bowel anastomoses. By leaving the mesentery intact and performing a side-to-side enterostomy (bypass), minimal blood supply is interrupted.

Small bowel fistulas may result from bowel wall necrosis. The direction of the fistulas may be out the top of the vagina (enterovaginal fistula), into another loop of bowel, into the bladder (enterovesicofistula), or out through the anterior abdominal wall skin (enterocutaneous fistula). Rarely do conservative measures with gastrointestinal decompression and total parenteral nutrition lead to spontaneous closure of the fistula, but it is reasonable to attempt for two to four weeks in hopes of avoiding major surgery, which is fraught with significant complications. This short course of total parenteral nutrition is probably necessary to optimize a patient's nutritional status prior to surgery anyway. Surgical correction of the fistula is usually managed by isolating the fistula, bringing up a mucous fistula on either side, and performing a small bowel reanastomosis of nonfistulized bowel. If the fistula can be easily resected, this course may be considered also.

Complications of the rectosigmoid colon are usually evidenced by *proctitis* with diarrhea, rectal bleeding, ulceration, and ultimately fistula into the vagina. Patients with rectal bleeding should be evaluated with proctoscopy, flexible colonoscopy, and barium enema to exclude other colonic lesions (e.g., carcinoma). The findings on proctosigmoidoscopy of an inflamed, friable, edematous rectal mucosa in the radiation field are usually pathognomonic for radiation proctitis. Conservative measures, including the use of stool softeners and avoiding constipation, and corticosteroid enemas relieve the patient's symptoms in many instances. If bleeding persists and multiple transfusions are required, the best management is a diverting colostomy.

Radiation-induced *stricture* of the rectosigmoid may lead to partial colonic obstruction with abdominal distention, tenesmus, and abdominal pain. Worsening of this lesion may lead to rectovaginal fistula (Fig. 5-3). In the setting of stricture or fistula, recur-

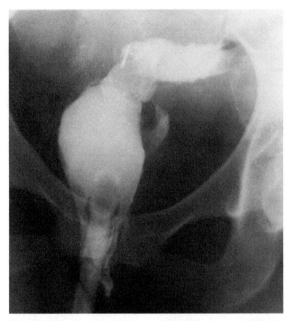

Fig. 5-3. Barium enema demonstrating a rectovaginal fistula. This fistula developed after rectosigmoid resection and reanastomosis, which was performed to alleviate radiation-induced proctitis and stenosis.

rent carcinoma must be considered and excluded by careful examination under anesthesia and carefully performed biopsy. Biopsy itself may lead to fistula formation and therefore should be performed with the utmost care by a surgeon familiar with radiation-induced complications. Repair of a rectovaginal fistula or resection of a rectal stricture in a radiated field is difficult and meets with failure in most instances. A diverting colostomy is the definitive therapy for these rectosigmoid complications. In selected patients, consideration might be given to resection of the stricture or fistula with end-to-end reanastomosis using a circular stapling device. The diverting colostomy should remain in place until the anastomosis is completely healed.

Complications of radiation therapy in the bladder may be noted as a change in voiding pattern, with frequency (secondary to fibrotic bladder with decreased compliance and decreased capacity) or dysuria secondary to chronic radiation *cystitis*. Episodes of urinary tract infection exacerbate the symptoms and are often associated with hematuria. Frankly bloody urine (hemorrhagic cystitis) should be initially managed by irrigation of the bladder through a three-way catheter. Fulguration of bleeding points that do not respond to irrigation should be performed carefully so as not to induce a vesicovaginal fistula. On rare occasions, hemorrhagic cystitis is so severe that cystectomy with a urinary conduit is the only remaining option.

Vesicovaginal and urethrovaginal fistulas are difficult problems to manage because of the poor blood supply in the irradiated tissues. Any attempt to close a vesicovaginal fistula in an irradiated field should include a plan for bringing in a new blood supply. The most frequently used sources are the omentum or bulbocavernosus (Martius) flap. A careful layered closure that is not under stress is the basic closure for a vesicovaginal fistula. Should fistula closure be unsuccessful, a diverting urinary conduit may be the best option to achieve patient comfort and hygiene. As with rectovaginal fistula, vesicovaginal fistula should be carefully evaluated and biopsied to exclude the possibility of recurrent carcinoma. Distal ureteral fibrosis, stenosis, and ultimate obstruction can be induced by radiation therapy, although it is much more

frequently associated with recurrent cervical carcinoma in the parametrium. Diversion or reimplantation of the ureters in the face of radiation fibrosis and stricture offers a permanent solution. Temporizing measures to preserve renal function include placement of a percutaneous nephrostomy or ureteral stinting across the stricture.

Although the vagina is one of the most radioresistant areas of the pelvis, the upper vagina receives some of the highest doses of radiation therapy, especially when it is combined with intracavitary cesium or radium application. Therefore *fibrosis and stenosis of the upper vagina* is a frequent complication of radiation therapy. Some of this problem may be reduced by the use of intravaginal estrogen cream and continued vaginal dilatation via sexual intercourse or the consistent use of a vaginal obturator. If nothing is done to preserve vaginal caliber and depth, it becomes stenotic and agglutinates; and ultimately the vaginal tube becomes a dimple only a few centimeters in length.

Less frequent and more severe complications in the vagina include radiation necrosis, which many times progresses to vesicovaginal and rectovaginal fistula. Pain and uncontrolled vaginal drainage with intermittent pelvic infections are difficult to manage conservatively. Attempts may be made to débride the area using half-strength hydrogen peroxide douches and daily application of intravaginal estrogen cream. On rare occasions in patients with intractable pain and multiple fistulas, a palliative pelvic exenteration offers the best outcome in terms of a reduction in symptoms.

SELECTED READINGS

Batres, F., and Barclay, D. L. Sciatic nerve injury during gynecologic procedures using the lithotomy position. *Obstet. Gynecol.* 62:925, 1983.

Berek, J. S., and Stubblefield, P. G. Anatomic and clinical correlates of uterine perforation. *Am. J. Obstet. Gynecol.* 135:181, 1979.

Buchsbaum, H. J., and Walton, L. A. *Strategies in Gynecologic Surgery.* New York: Springer-Verlag, 1986.

Clarke-Pearson, D. L., and Creasman, W. T. Diagnosis of deep venous thrombosis in obstetrics and gynecology by impedance phlebography. *Obstet. Gynecol.* 58:52, 1981.

Clarke-Pearson, D. L., Synan, I. S., Coleman, R. E., et al. The natural history of venous thromboemboli in gynecologic oncology: a prospective study of 382 patients. *Am. J. Obstet. Gynecol.* 148:1051, 1984.

Cuthbertson, A. M. The treatment of fistulas following irradiation damage. *Aust. N.Z. J. Surg.* 50:124, 1980.

DeStefano, F. Complications of interval laparoscopic tubal sterilization. *Obstet. Gynecol.* 61:153, 1983.

Dicker, R. C. Complications of abdominal and vaginal hysterectomy among women of reproductive age in the United States. *Am. J. Obstet. Gynecol.* 144:841, 1982.

Dudrick, S. J., Bane, A. E., Eiseman, B., et al. *Manual of Preoperative and Postoperative Care* (3rd ed.). Philadelphia: Saunders, 1983.

Gallup, D. G. Modification of celiotomy techniques to decrease morbidity in obese gynecologic patients. *Am. J. Obstet. Gynecol.* 150:171, 1984.

Krebs, H. B. Intestinal injury in gynecologic surgery: a ten-year experience. *Am. J. Obstet. Gynecol.* 155:509, 1986.

Loffer, F., and Pent, D. Indications, contraindications and complications of laparoscopy. *Obstet. Gynecol. Surv.* 30:403, 1975.

Muram, D. Postradiation ureteral obstruction: a reappraisal. *Am. J. Obstet. Gynecol.* 139:289, 1981.

Nichols, D. H. *Clinical Problems, Injuries and Complications of Gynecologic Surgery.* Baltimore: Williams & Wilkins, 1988.

Peterson, H. B. Deaths associated with laparoscopic sterilization in the United States, 1977–1979. *J. Reprod. Med.* 27:345, 1982.

Ratliff, J. B., Kapernick, P., Brooks, C. G., et al. Small bowel obstruction and previous gynecologic surgery. *South. Med. J.* 6:1349, 1983.

Ridley, J. H. Gynecologic surgery. In: *Gynecologic Surgery: Errors, Safeguards, Salvage.* Baltimore: Williams & Wilkins, 1981.

Rosenthal, D. M., and Colapinto, R. Angiographic arterial embolization in the management of postoperative vaginal hemorrhage. *Am. J. Obstet. Gynecol.* 151:227, 1985.

Rothenberger, D. A., and Goldberg, S. M. The management of rectovaginal fistulae. *Surg. Clin. North Am.* 63:61, 1983.

Wallace, D., Hernandez, W., Schlaerth, J. B., et al. Prevention of abdominal wound disruption utilizing the Smead-Jones closure technique. *Obstet. Gynecol.* 56:226, 1980.

Wingo, P. A., Huezo, C. M., Rubin, G. L., et al. The mortality risk associated with hysterectomy. *Am. J. Obstet. Gynecol.* 152:803, 1985.

6

Medical-Legal Issues in Gynecology

H. Alexander Easley III

Medical malpractice claims and settlements have increased dramatically. Parallel to this phenomenon has been an ever-increasing rise in malpractice insurance premiums paid by physicians. Of the medical specialties, obstetrics and gynecology has been one of the hardest hit by this "crisis." The cost of insurance (not always available) has changed the practice of some obstetricians and gynecologists, who have moved to less risky specialties or have left medical practice altogether. This chapter discusses the principles of medical malpractice, legal principles, informed consent, and areas of highest risk for the gynecologist.

MALPRACTICE LAW

As part of the tort system, which covers civil (not criminal) wrongs in American jurisprudence, medical malpractice law allows compensation of victims for injuries for which society dictates they are not responsible; it also promotes quality care by deterring substandard medical practice.

The quality of medical care today is high, and the possibility of a serious mistake occurs in only 1 in 100,000 events. However, the consumer of medical services, unlike the consumer of other services, is subject to a wide information gap. The ideal, fully informed patient could choose an efficient level of care suitable to her own desires. However, the medical consumer has limited ability to make informed choices and thus may not be able to protect herself. Therefore the medical provider is subject to a special malpractice system not applicable to providers of other services. Physicians are allowed considerable discretion, and their own desires for economic reward, satisfaction, and leisure may conflict with optimal patient care. Unfortunately, because of the patient's subordi-

nate position, market forces do not come to bear to eliminate physicians whose quality of care falls short.

More than 4000 years ago under the code of Hammurabi, a physician who injured a patient through negligence was tortured. Medical malpractice laws did not exist until the end of the fourteenth century, and the first malpractice case under English common law occurred in 1374. The surgeon won that case on a technicality. The first malpractice case in the United States, won by the plaintiff, was in 1794. However, before World War II, malpractice suits were virtually unheard of. Since then, malpractice litigation has exerted an increasing influence on physicians, patients, and society. Largely a consequence of the failure of physicians to meet the high expectations of society, the consequence of malpractice litigation may threaten the physician supply and the viability of the practice of certain high risk medical specialties in America.

LEGAL PRINCIPLES

Malpractice is a type of *negligence*. Negligence occurs when one owing a duty to another causes injury to the latter by failing to act as a reasonable person under similar circumstances. *Medical negligence* then is the failure of a physician to uphold the reasonable standard of care when treating a patient.

This *reasonable standard of care* is the crucial factor in most malpractice cases. Reasonable care does not require flawless care but does mandate that the physician possess the skill and knowledge of reasonably trained members of the specialty or subspecialty he or she was attempting to practice at the time the malpractice was allegedly committed and that this skill be exercised with diligence. Alternative methods of diagnosis and treatment may all be reasonable. So long as the method used is accepted by at least a respectable minority of similar practitioners, the standard is met. For many years only the standard practice in the community where the alleged malpractice occurred established the standard of reasonableness. However, this "locality rule" has been modified in recent years, and many states now apply national standards, particularly in regard to specialists.

Before the duty to exercise reasonable care arises, a

physician-patient relationship must exist. This relationship is usually implied by the conduct between the parties and does not arise out of a written or expressed verbal agreement. In fact, patients can refuse to enter the relationship and thus refuse treatment if they are mentally competent. There are several problem areas with this concept of refusal. For example, a Jehovah's Witness may be able to refuse a blood transfusion even if such a refusal may result in death. However, almost all jurisdictions would allow forced transfusion without the consent of such an individual if she were pregnant, had minor-age children, or were unconscious. Children cannot consent to treatment unless they are emancipated or are being treated for a venereal disease. A child is emancipated in most states if he or she is married, in the military, or in college. In most states a "mature" minor's consent to an abortion without the parent's consent may be sufficient. However, several states have attempted to legislate a requirement for parental consent for a minor's abortion. A parent's refusal to give such consent may be overcome in a special proceeding before a judge.

Proof of two other elements is required for an injured patient to maintain a malpractice case successfully. First, the plaintiff must show that the defendant physician's actions *caused* the injury sustained. Second, the plaintiff must present evidence of quantifiable damages resulting from the injury.

PROOF OF NEGLIGENCE

Proof of negligence, with the one exception described below, must be established by the plaintiff with *expert testimony*. This testimony is given by another physician, usually of the same specialty, who explains to the jury the standard of care that should have been practiced and if that standard was met. Then the jury, considering all expert testimony from both sides, determines if there was malpractice. The judge does not make this determination.

Some negligent events are so obvious to laymen that courts have decided that no expert testimony is necessary. These events are subject to the doctrine *res ipsa loquitur,* which means "the thing speaks for itself." More specifically, if the injury is one that usually occurs only with negligence, the cause was exclu-

sively under the physician's control, and the patient did not contribute to the cause, the doctrine is applied to establish negligence. *Res ipsa loquitur* is generally applied only in cases in which foreign objects were left in a wound or certain severe injuries occurred during surgery.

DAMAGES

The issue of damages recoverable in a malpractice case is a complex area embodying many social policy and economic considerations. Generally a patient can recover the following: actual costs and expenses incurred, lost earnings or profits, and the value of the pain and suffering occasioned by the injury. The direct out-of-pocket expenses, such as medical expenses and loss of earnings, are commonly called "economic damages." Intangible losses such as pain and suffering, loss of consortium, and loss of companionship are "noneconomic damages." The tremendous cost of caring for debilitating injuries such as infant brain damage over a lifetime, as well as the uncertainties of pain and suffering, have figured heavily in the large awards juries have given in contemporary malpractice cases.

SPECIFIC INCIDENTS OF MALPRACTICE IN GYNECOLOGIC PRACTICE

What constitutes gynecologic malpractice is usually determined by a jury. Such determination is based on facts revealed by the facts of the case and the opinions of the experts. The facts that give rise to the malpractice incident may not be completely recorded in the court documents after the case is decided. Cases decided at the trial level are not reported in published form but remain in court files. Only the records of cases appealed to higher courts are readily available as examples of malpractice incidents. Thus any compilation of incidents of malpractice is necessarily incomplete, and determining what incidents constitute malpractice in gynecology must derive from a thorough understanding of the appropriate standards of care.

Several areas of gynecologic practice are potentially hotbeds of malpractice activity. Such areas include contraception, dilatation and curettage, hysterectomy, and failure to diagnose gynecologic cancer.

Most of the malpractice cases involving contraception have involved the use of combination oral contraceptive and intrauterine devices. The medical-legal implications surrounding the prescription of *oral contraceptives* mandate that the physician discuss with the patient the possible adverse effects of the particular drug as well as its benefits. The manufacturer of the oral contraceptive has a duty to warn the physician of adverse consequences of its product. The manufacturer's duty generally is not to warn the patient, although the U.S. Food and Drug Administration (FDA) has ruled that the manufacturer of birth control pills must warn the consumer of the risks associated with the product in the informational insert that comes with the oral contraceptive pills.

In a 1980 case in which a 19-year-old woman with amenorrhea was placed on an oral contraceptive and subsequently suffered a stroke, the patient was awarded $1.1 million in a jury verdict. She alleged the physician failed to inform her of the indications and risks of the oral contraceptive. In that case expert testimony revealed that oral contraceptives are not a proper treatment for primary amenorrhea, that the standard of care required the physician to make a diagnosis of the amenorrhea prior to instituting contraceptive therapy, and that the physician should have informed her of the material risks associated with the medication. Other cases dealing with oral contraceptives have involved (1) a patient with a migraine disorder who had a stroke while taking the drug (Colorado, 1976) and (2) a physician's failure to diagnose lower extremity thrombophlebitis in a patient taking oral contraceptives (Illinois, 1979).

Any physician who prescribes an oral contraceptive must be familiar with the absolute contraindications listed by the FDA and monitor patients carefully for the onset of side effects. Although most of the serious side effects are related to estrogen dosage, and there is less use now of preparations with more than 50 μg of synthetic estrogen, patients should still be informed of the serious risks of thrombophlebitis, stroke, and hypertension prior to receiving the medication. Patients should receive and be encouraged to read the package inserts included with the medication.

Discussion of the medical-legal aspects of *intrauterine devices* (IUDs) centers around the Dalkon Shield marketed by the A. H. Robins Company. The initial cases against A. H. Robins disclosed that in 1971 a physician employed by Robins discovered that the multifilamented string at the tail of the IUD possessed wicking qualities that might lead to serious pelvic infection. This question was not researched by corporate microbiologists, but soon thereafter physicians prescribing the Dalkon Shield inquired if infections they were beginning to see in their patients may have been caused by the wicking effect. Over the next two years frequent reports of infections were publicized. Soon thereafter A. H. Robins published warnings about the product but stated that patients presently using the device and not having problems were safe. The massive litigation that followed alleged that the Dalkon Shield was both negligently designed and marketed, and that the company disregarded evidence of the lack of safety of the product.

In the wake of the Dalkon Shield litigation, Ortho Pharmaceuticals, producer of the Lippes Loop, and G. D. Searle and Company, producer of the Copper 7 Device, withdrew these devices from the market. There are still two devices available in the United States, the Progestasert (Alza Corporation) and the ParaGard (GynoPharma). The latter device was introduced during the summer of 1988. The prescription and insertion of the ParaGard involves a voluminous informed consent transaction.

Generally, for a parous woman in a stable relationship without a history of prior pelvic inflammatory disease, and who is not a good candidate for oral contraceptives or who strongly desires effective barrier contraception, the IUD is a reasonable contraceptive. A potential IUD user should understand the risks of infection, ectopic pregnancy, menorrhagia, and dysmenorrhea; furthermore, she should be encouraged to read the patient package information in detail.

The patient with an IUD should be monitored for excessive cramping and bleeding, suggestion of spontaneous expulsion or migration of the IUD into the pelvic cavity, pregnancy, and infection. Reasonable steps suggested with such monitoring included monitoring of hematologic indices if heavy bleeding is alleged. If the IUD string cannot be visualized, ultrasonography or pelvic radiography should be conducted for localization. The device should be removed if infection is diagnosed or suspected.

Sterilization procedures may give rise to malpractice litigation from complications arising out of the performance of the procedure and from failure of the procedure. Some authorities list previous abdominal or pelvic surgery as a relative contraindication to laparoscopic sterilization. Adhesions in these cases may increase the likelihood of bowel or vascular injury. An open laparoscopic technique is often suggested in such circumstances, but no overwhelming consensus exists as to this approach. Other significant risks during laparoscopic procedures include anesthetic complications, thermal injury to bowel, gas embolism, or subcutaneous emphysema (Chap. 5). Probably all of these risks should be disclosed to a patient contemplating this surgical procedure.

One of the most controversial medical-legal areas pertaining to sterilization deals with failed sterilization. Such failure has given rise to suits for "wrongful birth," "wrongful life," and "wrongful pregnancy." The courts have tended to use the terms interchangeably, creating confusion and inconsistency. There are important differences among the three definitions.

In most *wrongful pregnancy* cases the parents complain that the physician's negligence resulted in the birth of an unplanned but healthy and normal child. The crux of the action is that no child was supposed to have been born. In *wrongful birth* and *wrongful life* actions, generally the alleged negligence involves a physician's failure to advise the parents of available means for determining a fetal defect and thereby depriving the parents of the choice to terminate the pregnancy. As a further specific distinction, a *wrongful life* action is actually brought on behalf of the child for the harm of being born in a deformed condition. These cases are complex and involve highly charged public policy issues. For example, in *Turpin v. Sortini,* a 1982 California case, the court allowed a defective child to recover damages for deafness that could have been prevented had she not been conceived. The parents claimed she would not have been conceived if they had known of her potential for deaf-

ness. The court allowed the child to be compensated for the expenses necessary to treat her hearing loss. Other courts have rejected wrongful life as a viable cause of action. Those courts have held that there is no fundamental right to be born normal and whole. Other courts have stated that the measure of the value between life with and without handicap is too difficult to assess.

Some courts have allowed recovery of damaged for *wrongful pregnancy* if the negligence of the physician resulted in the delivery of a normal, healthy baby. In a 1982 case in Alabama, the court allowed the parents to recover for emotional distress as a result of the pregnancy, loss of consortium (sexual function), and medical expenses incurred as a result of the pregnancy. Damages for the care of a normal child are usually not recoverable.

Dilatation and curettage (D&C) is a frequently performed minor surgical procedure rarely accompanied by complications. Frequent causes of a malpractice suit resulting from D&C include laceration of the cervix, hemorrhage, perforation of the uterus, infection, incomplete removal of products of conception, damage to sacroiliac joints or the lumbosacral spine, Asherman's syndrome, and cervical incompetence. So long as the procedure is performed systematically and carefully and due diligence is exercised in recognizing immediate complications and in responding to a patient's complaints consistent with late complications, there is no negligence.

Hysterectomy is the most common major surgical procedure performed in the United States. The complications that may be associated with hysterectomy are legion (Chap. 5). Although a physician may be liable to a patient for injury that occurs during hysterectomy or inadequate postoperative care, most litigation involves claims that the physician performed an unnecessary hysterectomy. Diagnosis of the conditions warranting hysterectomy and alternative treatments must be carefully and systematically documented. For a complication of hysterectomy to constitute malpractice, the hysterectomy must have been performed with negligent technique. Identification of vital structures surrounding the organs to be extirpated, including the ureter, bladder, and rectum, should be mentioned in the operative note. Most malpractice cases for intraoperative injury involve the failure to recognize the injury or to repair it properly.

Misdiagnosis is a major area of malpractice litigation in gynecology; and failure to properly diagnose and treat breast cancer is the leading issue. Approximately one in every ten patients seen by gynecologists develop breast cancer during a lifetime. Delay in diagnosis results in poorer prognosis. Consequently, adequate breast examination, mammography, and timely biopsy of suspicious breast lesions are required.

One of the most important decisions confronting a physician is whether to biopsy the breast mass. Characteristics associated with malignancy include the absence of changes of shape during the menstrual cycle, persistence of a mass or area of abnormality through the menstrual cycle, lack of mobility, movement of surrounding breast tissue with the mass, skin dimpling, nipple retraction, and fixation to the chest wall. Generally, biopsy is indicated when the mass is persistent, dominant, and palpable. Mammography, although not supplanting the need for physician examination, is a critical, sensitive screening tool. Present recommendations for mammogram screening are listed in Chapter 24.

Failure to diagnose carcinoma of the cervix is one of the most confusing areas in gynecologic practice. The failure to obtain a Papanicolaou (Pap) smear in a timely fashion does not seem to be a major problem. Confusion arises, however, out of two shortcomings of the Pap smear. First, a significant percentage of Pap smears are falsely negative. The alleged false-negative rate ranges between 10 and 40 percent. Second, a significant percentage of Pap smears show "inflammation," "inflammatory atypia," and "koilocytotic (condylomatous) atypia." Although these Pap smear reports do not suggest malignancy or dysplasia, they are not "normal." Furthermore, the presence of the human papilloma virus suggests a high risk patient. Consequently, in view of the previously cited false-negative rate for Pap smears, many gynecologists feel compelled to perform colposcopy and biopsies in all cases of koilocytotic atypia. The significance of inflammation or inflammatory atypia is not clear. Inflammation alone on a Pap smear does not require special follow-up or evaluation. However, inflammatory *atypia* is probably an indication for treat-

ment of presumed infection and repeat cytology within three to six months.

In *Piel v. Gabol,* a 1977 Missouri case, the plaintiff's routine Pap smear was reported as "Class II, slightly active, but benign, no tumor cells." She was reexamined, but no lesion was found. Later that year, however, she was diagnosed as having cervical cancer. Although she was treated and cured, she sued the physician for malpractice in failing to diagnose a cervical cancer. The defendant won the case. However, the appellate court did not exclude the possibility that had expert testimony substantiated that the diagnosis should have been made despite the Pap smear in that case perhaps the physician would have been liable. This case, although won by the physician, does suggest that in certain cases one cannot rely totally on the Pap smear. If there are other suspicious symptoms, such as postcoital bleeding, bloody discharge, or a raised, friable lesion on the cervix, colposcopy and biopsy should be performed anyway.

INFORMED CONSENT

The root premise is the concept, fundamental in American jurisprudence, that every human being of adult years and sound mind has the right to determine what shall be done with his body. [*Canterbury v. Spence,* 464 F.2d 772 (DC Cir.) 1972]

True informed consent requires that a patient have an opportunity to knowledgeably evaluate the options available regarding her care and the risks associated with each option. The average patient must look to her physician for enlightenment to reach an intelligent decision. Consequently, the physician must make a reasonable divulgence to facilitate the decision. A well-informed patient who plays a major role in choosing her treatment plan accepts a major part of the responsibility for the risks and outcome associated with the plan.

A malpractice claim based on lack of informed consent arises when a patient formally consents to treatment but claims that she was not properly advised of the risks and options with regard to it. A claim based on lack of informed consent can succeed if the patient proves that the physician's performance in obtaining the consent fell short of the applicable standard of care. The standard of care for informed consent requires a reasonable disclosure of the *choices* with respect of the proposed therapy and the *danger* potentially involved. The *scope* of disclosure required is a crucial issue.

The scope of the disclosure required for adequate informed consent is defined by one of three rules depending on the jurisdiction involved. A minority of states require full disclosure of all risks and benefits without regard to their significance. Most states require disclosure of the risks and benefits that would be disclosed by a reasonable physician under similar circumstances. The remainder of the states follow a rule requiring disclosure of all risks and benefits that are *material* to the patient's decision about whether to undergo the proposed treatment. In jurisdictions adhering to this "reasonable patient" (in contrast to "reasonable physician") rule, the topics demanding a communication by the physician are the following.

1. Inherent and potential hazards of the proposed treatment
2. Acceptable alternatives to that treatment
3. Results likely if the patient remains untreated

The *likelihood of injury* and *the degree of harm* determine what is significant. Even a small chance of death or serious disability is significant. Yet there is no obligation to communicate dangers of which persons of average sophistication are aware or hazards the patient has already discovered. Patients must be educated to dispel the myths of medical perfection and of the infallibility of sophisticated equipment.

Exceptions to Informed Consent

In cases where the patient is unconscious or otherwise incapable of consenting and harm from failure to treat outweighs the possible harm from the proposed treatment, the physician may treat without obtaining consent. There is clear authority in emergency situations to treat incompetent patients even against their wishes. In these situations, the physician should attempt to secure a relative's consent.

A physician may withhold certain information for therapeutic reasons. If communication of the informa-

tion about risk would present a threat to the patient's well-being by preventing a rational decision or complicating the treatment, limited disclosure may be adequate. Again in this situation disclosure should be made to a relative.

Written Consent Form

Most consent forms presently in use in medical practice do not adequately demonstrate informed consent. The courts have recognized that a patient's signature on the consent form is no assurance that the patient had received sufficient information or has understood the information offered. Traditional consent forms are so full of medical and legal jargon and so fraught with compound, complex sentences that most patients cannot comprehend them. Even a comprehensible consent form, however, is not a guarantee that the physician and the patient communicated sufficiently. Figure 6-1 is an example of a consent form designed to comply with all of the informed consent requirements.

Always discuss with the patient and her family all information about the proposed therapy that is material to her decision, including the following.

1. Describing the procedure
2. Using the likelihood of occurrence of a particular risk in combination with the degree of harm foreseeable from that risk as a guide to which risks be disclosed
3. Divulging the alternative treatments
4. Answering questions
5. Using a comprehensive form for each procedure with all of the elements embodied in the same form such as in Figure 6-1

Remote, rare risks are not material unless catastrophic. More risks should be mentioned for purely elective surgery than for nonelective surgery. Before elective surgery, more items are likely to influence the patient's decision. The informed consent discussion should be documented. A letter to the patient or a note in the chart or section in the admission history and

Fig. 6-1. Example of a consent form.

CONSENT FOR VAGINAL HYSTERECTOMY

TO: Dr. _____ and _____ Hospital
                     (attending physician)

DATE: _____ TIME: _____

I have a condition known as: _____
                                   (use medical term with description)

1. *What my doctor has explained to me:*
   My doctor has explained:
   a. the operation to be performed
   b. the reasons why I need this operation
   c. the discomforts that I might experience
   d. the risks of the operation
   e. that a perfect result is not guaranteed
2. *What I consent to have done:*
   I agree to allow my physician and his assistants to remove my uterus (womb) and cervix through my vagina.
   My vagina will remain approximately the same size it is now.
   I know that medical students and other medical personnel in training are present at operations in this hospital and may be present at mine.
   I know that my physician may photograph the surgical area. My name will never be used to identify those photographs. They will be used for professional purposes only.
3. *Why I am having this operation.*
   I am having this operation because _____
                                            (patient to write here)

   _____
   _____
   _____

4. *Risks explained to me:*
   • hemorrhage
   • infection
   • making a hole in my bladder
   • making a hole in my rectum
   • injuring my ovary
   • developing a tract (fistula) between my bladder or rectum and vagina
   I know these problems are not likely to occur. I know that other complications that are even less likely could occur, such as death. Knowing all these risks, I have decided to have this operation.
5. *How I could treat my condition without surgery:*
   I could continue to take the medications already prescribed for me. I could have a D&C if my problem is too much bleeding. I could do nothing to treat my condition. I think my operation is the best treatment for my condition.
6. *Other surgery that may be necessary.*
   If one or more of the complications listed above should occur during my operation, other surgery may be necessary: I will allow my physician to decide what is necessary. My physician may discover during my operation such conditions as an abnormality of my ovary, fallopian tubes, or a protrusion of bowel or bladder into my vagina. I will allow my physician to correct these conditions and others to improve the results of my operation or prevent my having to have another operation to correct them in the future.
7. *Complications of anesthesia:*
   The anesthesia department of the hospital is responsible for explaining to me the risks of anesthesia.

SIGNED: _____
                           (patient or person authorized to consent for patient)

WITNESS: _____
                                     (title)

physical or a section in the operative note detailing the information given to the patient provides a permanent record. This documentation is perhaps more important than the consent form itself.

RISK MANAGEMENT

The systematic process of identifying, evaluating, and addressing potential and actual malpractice risks is termed *risk management*. Risk management employs both *mechanical* and *communicative methods* to reduce malpractice risks. Improved professional continuing education, staff education, documentation, incident reporting, use of informed consent, and contractual agreements are examples of mechanical methods of risk management. These methods are discussed below.

Nurses commonly complain about confusion over physicians' orders, the plan of therapy, physician unavailability, and unresponsiveness to their questions and calls. Resolving communication gaps with staff, responding to and educating them to promote cooperation and instilling confidence by a clear plan of care is paramount. Education and training of office personnel and nurses can significantly reduce malpractice claims. Emphasizing policies about telephone etiquette, greeting patients, scheduling, and referring calls about substantive medical questions recognizes that medicine has become a consumer service. It is therefore subject to many of the same market and public opinion forces as other commodities.

No area for improvement has received more effort and emphasis than documentation in record keeping. Rendering quality service without manifesting such service in the record is not sufficient in our litigious society. A weakness in documentation can severely hamper the defense of a malpractice suit. The patient's attorney scrutinizes every piece of the medical record to infer negligence. Such shortcomings as omissions, contradictions, delays, time gaps, illegible entries, extraneous remarks, and of course alterations and obliterations are serious pitfalls. The medical record is a major piece of evidence for a jury because jurors tend to believe what is recorded more than the testimony of a witness. Specific "dos" and "don'ts" include using a ballpoint pen; writing only in appro-

priate columns; dating, timing, and signing everything; making sure the patient's name is on the page; using the physician's first initial, last name, and title; making corrections by placing a single line through the material with the date and initial adjacent to it; documenting discharge instructions; and avoiding words reflecting judgments such as "inadvertently," "somehow," and "unexplainable."

The discharge summary should not be a repetition of the admission workup. It simply should state when the patient was admitted to the hospital and what happened. Likewise, the formal operative note should not be a narrative of how to do an operation. It should explain the indications for the surgery, what procedures were done, any variations from the standard technique, any unusual findings, and difficulties experienced.

COMMUNICATION WITH PATIENTS

In most cases it takes more than a poor outcome to produce a malpractice claim. Perhaps fewer than 5 percent of malpractice incidents actually result in malpractice claims. Anthropologist Irwin Press has analyzed the social and emotional predispositions and perceptions of patients that may result in filing a malpractice claim. A lawsuit expresses intense hostility by the injured patient. An act as hostile as a lawsuit is impossible to contemplate without anger. Suing the physician may be the only acceptable way a patient can satisfactorily express the anger she acquires during contact with the physician.

An important factor contributing to the increased malpractice activity of today may be that patients are *perceiving* more of their treatment experience negatively. When evaluating outcomes, patients must consider not only medical outcome but also their interactions with physicians and other members of the health care team. Patients often need medical care when they are least able to cope with anything less than the most tender and caring attention possible. They are anxious, afraid, and often in pain. Their "illness" is more than a physiologic disease process. It includes many societal, familial, and religiously derived symptoms, explanations, and treatment presumptions. Their understanding may differ markedly from standard medical teaching. Furthermore, the myth of medical perfection creates unrealistic expectations about outcome. All of these factors may *predispose* patients to form a negative *perception* of their care.

If a patient is *predisposed* to become litigious, the physician must carefully control her *perceptions* about her care. She must receive caring attention. Events such as receiving cold late meals, waking for 4 AM vital signs that may be unnecessary, wearing short robes with indwelling urethral catheters showing, failing to receive help when ambulating after surgery, and waiting long periods before receiving analgesics and other medications are examples of events that often exacerbate patients' already significant anxieties and lower their self-image.

Physicians must exert better efforts at educating patients, manifesting compassion, talking with their families, and training office personnel and office employees to be responsive and courteous. These activities should undermine the predisposition of many patients to perceive any error or poor outcome with animosity. By preventing the development of hostility, malpractice claims may be averted.

MALPRACTICE REFORM

Malpractice indemnity has increased geometrically during the 1980s. Consequently, the cost of malpractice insurance has risen sharply in most states and has become prohibitively expensive in some. Some critics allege that malpractice premiums have risen because of poor business practices by insurance companies or the general rise in inflation. The dynamics involved in creating the present high cost of the malpractice climate, however, are complex.

Claims made against obstetricians and gynecologists result in payment in almost two-thirds of cases— twice the rate for claims paid by other specialists. Statistics from malpractice insurance carriers show that the major burden of malpractice costs arise in obstetrics and gynecology claims.

The increased frequency and severity of malpractice claims have many reverberations. Well trained physicians, particularly in high risk areas such as obstetrics, have either ceased their high risk practice or ceased specialty practice altogether. It is alarming that nearly 25 percent of all obstetricians ceasing obstetric practice are under age 45. In addition, surveys show that more than two-thirds of obstetricians and gynecologists order more tests, obtain more consultations, and spend more time with patients because of the fear of malpractice.

Clearly, some physicians are committing negligent acts by failing to uphold the standard of care when treating patients. Physicians now are as well trained as ever, and medical schools are teaching students to maintain a caring attitude. Seemingly, the conditions necessary for physicians to avoid committing negligence are present.

There are no easy solutions. Although many proposals to alter the judicial system's method of dealing with malpractice claims have been proposed and many changes have become law in certain states, the frequency and severity of malpractice claims have not significantly lessened. For example, imposing changes in attorneys' contingency fee arrangements, the statute of limitations, and offsetting recoveries with amounts received from other sources (such as patients' personal insurance policies) have not affected the economics of the malpractice system. Caps—dollar limits placed on verdicts—do have some effect. However, state courts have not consistently upheld the constitutionality of this practice and other attempts to change patients' traditional rights under the tort system. Furthermore, the political realities of changing the traditional system for dealing with personal injury in the United States render proposed changes unpopular and difficult to achieve. Legislation to attain this type of "tort reform" has been passed usually when virtual crisis conditions exist.

More promising solutions are being explored. A concept of catastrophic reinsurance envisioned by Dr. William Curran of the Harvard School of Public Health would eliminate the physician's responsibility for malpractice insurance after the first $50,000, with the excess being carried by a social funding device. Alternative dispute resolution would remove malpractice cases from the traditional judicial arena to a more efficient system free of the high transaction costs and emotional reactions of juries. Binding contracts between physicians and patients providing for arbitration of claims of malpractice may be enforceable.

Individual casualty insurance purchased by patients upon their election to receive medical care could cover items of ordinary unintentional negligence by physicians. More thoughtful ways of handling specific injuries, e.g., catastrophic neurologic impairment in infants allegedly injured during delivery, have already been adopted in Virginia and Florida. Other states are considering proposals to provide reasonable compensation for babies born with cerebral palsy without lawsuits. The impetus for considering such proposals arises from a recognition of the catastrophic nature of neurologic impairment and the increasing evidence that the cause of the damage probably arises from obstetric management during delivery in perhaps only 1 percent of cases.

The tort system has always fairly considered the foreseeability of the injury, the culpability attributable to the alleged negligent activity, and the ability of society to continue to pay the high price demanded by the damages sought. In medical malpractice situations, the foreseeability of the resultant injury is often minuscule. The culpability of the physician's negligence often seems to exceed the magnitude of the exact error. The high cost of malpractice indemnity is passed on to all consumers for the benefit of a few injured patients. Discussion of malpractice reform must incorporate these factors. On the other hand, substan-dard practice of medicine cannot be tolerated. No discussion of malpractice reform can fail to incorporate meaningful peer review with sanctions requiring practice alterations and continuing medical education.

SELECTED READINGS

American College of Obstetrics and Gynecologists. Professional Liability Insurance and its Effects: Report of a Survey of ACOG's Membership. Washington, D.C.: ACOG, 1982.

Canterbury v. Spence, 464 F.2d 772 (DC cir 1972).

Danzon, P. M. The frequency and severity of medical malpractice claims: new evidence. *Law Contemp. Probl.* 49(2):57, 1986.

Easley, H. A., and Hammond, C. B. Informed consent in obstetrics and gynecology. *Postgrad. Obstet. Gynecol.* 7(4), 1986.

Easley, H. A., and Hammond, C. B. Management of malpractice risk. *Postgrad. Obstet. Gynecol.* 6(10), 1986.

Holder, A. R. *Medical Malpractice Law.* New York: Wiley, 1978.

Lewis, S. M. *Ob/Gyn Malpractice.* New York: Wiley, 1986.

Press, I. The predisposition to file claims: the patient's perspective. *Law Med. Health Care* 12:53, 1984.

Prosser, W. *Handbook of the Law of Torts.* St. Paul, MN: West Publishing, 1971.

II

Reproductive Endocrinology and Infertility

7

Endocrinologic Disorders of Childhood and Adolescence

Jay J. Gold and Erica Gold Sinsheimer

Normal differentiation of the female reproductive tract from its initial bisexual status to its final, normal, differentiated, and functional form is the culmination of a coordinated series of embryologic events. The gonads begin their development during the fifth to sixth week of embryonic life, initiating development of the genital ducts, urogenital sinus, and external genitalia.

Aging is a phenomenon that is initiated at the moment of fertilization. Once fertilization has occurred, the true sex of the individual is determined. All changes are in preparation for the mature role for which that individual is programmed after pubescence is completed. The timing of this role varies with the mores of the society into which that individual is born.

NORMAL PUBERTY

Puberty primarily represents the series of events culminating in sexual maturation and, secondarily, growth and psychic maturity. Usually during the earliest phases of puberty there is a preceding increase in adrenal activity, called *adrenarche,* that results in the development of pubic and axillary hair. With the onset of initial gonadal stimulation, more definitive changes of puberty occur, a phase described as *gonadarche.* Adrenarche usually begins several years before the gonadarche, but physiologic levels of adrenal androgens do not necessarily exert a major influence on timing of the onset of puberty. Furthermore, although adrenarche and gonadarche are sequentially linked, one may occur without the other.

Breast budding begins with the appearance of early puberty in the female. Figure 7-1 illustrates the five Tanner stages of breast development. Breast budding occurs as the earliest stage of change, i.e., Stage 2.

At that time there are early estrogen changes in the vaginal mucosa that reflect ovarian enlargement in response to gonadotropin stimulation. The labia majora begin to become more prominent and exhibit wrinkling, increased vascularity, and early hair follicles. The uterus also begins to grow, so that the cervix is no longer the dominant portion of the combined cervix and uterus; they are now of approximately equal size. The endometrium is still immature and shows no specific changes, but there are changes in the distribution of body fat. In addition, the episodic pattern of gonadotropin secretion and responsive sex steroids, with augmentation during sleep, continues to occur, but the typical feedback mechanism characteristic of the adult female is not yet present. Growth hormone is still secreted in increased amounts during sleep throughout this period.

When the girl reaches midpuberty, the ovaries continue to increase in size, from an ovarian weight of about 3 gm up to about 6 gm at menarche. Tubes increase in diameter and develop a ciliated epithelial lining. The internal reproductive viscera, including the ovaries, uterus, and tubes, appear lower in the pelvis as the entire pelvic cavity increases in size and breadth. The breasts increase in size to Tanner Stage 3 to early Stage 4, with the appearance of areolar tissue, glandular tissue, and ductile structure. Labia minora become prominent, and the vaginal mucosa, with an increase in hormonal stimulation and vascularity, changes from a reddish to a pinkish color. With the appearance of Bartholin glands and hormonal stimulation, vaginal secretions begin, and the vagina increases in depth from an initial length of about 4.0 cm up to 8.5 cm. In addition, vaginal pH becomes acidic, and the uterus is now the dominant portion of the uterus-cervix structure.

The initial hair follicles on the labia majora progress to the changes characteristic of pubic hair, with gradual increases in amount; and the early changes of hair development on the mons pubis now occur as noted in Figure 7-2. Pubic hair begins to take on a coarse appearance, and there may be axillary hair development at about this time as well as sweat gland activity and body odor.

In this stage, well before the onset of menarche, peak height velocity occurs much earlier in the female

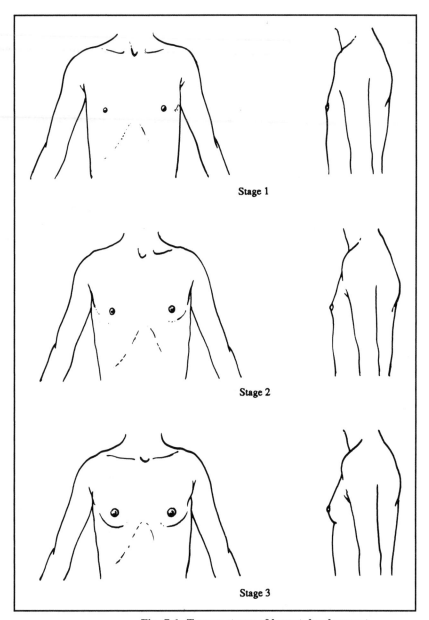

Stage 1

Stage 2

Stage 3

Fig. 7-1. Tanner stages of breast development.

than in the male. Moreover, the characteristic female changes in body fat distribution now progress, and acne changes may appear as well.

Although sleep augmentation of gonadotropin secretion is still prominent, there may be increases in quantities of gonadotropin noted during the waking periods as well. However, in the female, estradiol secretion is dissociated from gonadotropin peaks. It is also in this stage that some thyromegaly may be noted.

By late puberty, the breasts enlarge to Tanner Stage

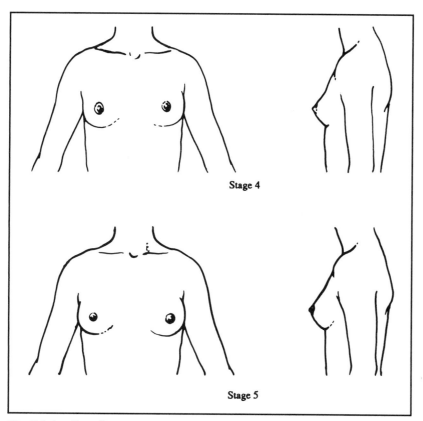

Stage 4

Stage 5

Fig. 7-1 (continued).

4 and in some cases to Stage 5 (Fig. 7-1). Ovarian enlargement continues up to adult size, and the vagina elongates to its adult length of about 15 cm with thickened mucosa and almost fully stimulated hormonal changes. The labia minora continue to elongate, and the pubic hair is now adult in form and well spread over the labia majora and mons pubis. Axillary hair is present in larger amounts, and the characteristic body fat changes of the female are now fully apparent, with greater prominence of the buttocks, hips, narrowing of the waist, and fullness in the breast area. The uterus is now at least two-thirds larger than the cervix, and adequate secretions by the cervical epithelium mirror the full estrogen stimulation.

The initiation of menarche occurs during this stage, although sometimes earlier, and by this time the average developing female has shown most of her growth, although there may be 2 to 3 inches of further growth over the ensuing two years. Females still manifest gonadotropin secretion of an augmented nature during sleep, but with menarche positive feedback occurs that ultimately leads to ovulation, evidenced by a fully mature hypothalamic-pituitary-ovarian relation. However, this ovulatory stage may take as long as two years until which time 55 to 90 percent of the cycles are anovulatory. It is not until five years postmenarche that 80 percent of the cycles are ovulatory.

With full adult status, the sleep augmentation of gonadotropins disappears, and growth in girls is complete. With menarche and adult status manifesting pulsatile secretion of gonadotropic hormone and releasing hormone (GnRH), cyclic fluctuations of plasma luteinizing hormone (LH) and follicle-stimulating hormone (FSH) lead to ovarian stimulation, allowing the

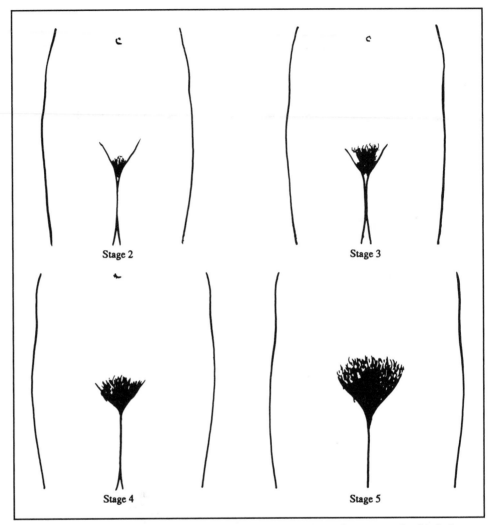

Fig. 7-2. Tanner stages and patterns of pubic hair growth.

typical menstrual cycle changes and hormonal responses associated with ovulation. The responses of estrogen and progesterone to such stimulation help to control the hypothalamic-pituitary cyclic activity, and estrogen acts in positive feedback to aid in this normal ovulation process.

A statistical study of American female children covering the period 1969 to 1974 showed that puberty may begin from ages 8.0 to 14.9 years with completion of their pubescence by ages 12.4 to 16.8 years. Breast development was completed at 11.3 to 17.7 years, and pubic hair reached adult status at 12.4 to

16.8 years. A peak height velocity preceded breast development in some instances by as much as 1 year. However, the peak height velocity occurred within six months of the appearance of pubic hair, and menarche occurred 1.2 to 2.8 years after breast development was apparent.

Sexual Precocity

The etiologies of sexual precocity are protean (Table 7-1), and it is best to categorize them into true or cen-

Table 7-1. Etiology of Isosexual Precocity

True and complete isosexual precocity	Pseudoprecocious puberty
Idiopathic (familial)	hCG-secreting tumors
Congenital anomalies	Hepatoma
Septooptic dysplasia	Chorioepithelioma (gonadal, extragonadal)
Hydrocephalus	Teratoma
Tumors of the central nervous system	Gonadal (ovarian)
Glioma of optic nerve of hypothalamus	Granulosa or theca cell tumor
(neurofibromatosis)	Follicular luteal cysts
Astrocytoma	Adrenal
Ependymoma	Congenital adrenal hyperplasia
Germinoma/pinealoma	Adrenal neoplasm, feminizing
Teratoma	Iatrogenic, surreptitious, or drug-contaminated sex
Hamartoma	hormone or hCG administration
Craniopharyngioma	Gonadotropin-independent
Cysts	Sporadic
Sarcoid granuloma	McCune-Albright
Postinflammatory: meningitis, encephalitis, brain	Tumorous sclerosis
abscess	Incomplete isosexual precocity
Posttraumatic	Premature thelarche
Other	Premature adrenarche
Following late treatment of congenital adrenal	Premature menarche
hyperplasia, or feminizing adrenal or gonadal	Other
tumor	Vaginitis, foreign body
Chronic renal failure	Vaginal or uterine neoplasm
After cranial irradiation	
Primary hypothyroidism (?)	
Isolated LH secretion (?)	

Adapted from Root, A. W., and Shulman, D. I. Isosexual precocity. *Fertil. Steril.* 45:749, 1986.

tral precocious puberty that is initiated by the early triggering of the hypothalamic-pituitary-gonadal axis caused by removal of normal inhibitory signals. Probably the most common is the idiopathic form, but other causes include any localized lesion that would permit hypothalamic secretions to initiate the normal hormonal interrelations. Pulsatile stimulatory changes are required to allow this change to occur, but it seems to be more critical in girls than in boys. A classic example was polyostotic fibrous dysplasia, as described by McCune and Albright many years ago, but the hypothalamic relation is no longer as tenable as it used to be. The patients present with indices of early sexual development in its entirety, and the problem is considered precocious puberty if it appears before the age of 8 years in girls. These indices are early breast budding (Fig. 7-1), rapid linear growth with in-

creased velocity of growth, appearance of pubic and axillary hair, body odor, and finally menarche. These children have full fertility potential and so must be watched carefully. Their fertility potential differentiates them from the group with pseudoprecocious puberty (*vide infra*), where the precocious sexual development is not central and occurs apart from the hypothalamic-pituitary-gonadal stimulation that is characteristic of true precocity.

With the development of synthetic GnRH and with the knowledge that puberty and menses require pulsatile secretion of hypothalamic and pituitary hormones, long-acting GnRH analogs have been developed that provide constant rather than pulsatile stimulation. They have been utilized therapeutically to produce regression of precocious puberty.

Incomplete sexual precocity along isosexual lines

includes *precocious adrenarche,* which precedes pubarche in normal female development and occurs well before the age of 8 in girls. Precocious adrenarche is adrenal in origin and usually initiates development of axillary hair, some pubic hair, and body odor. However, there is no gonadal stimulation, and so fertility potential does not exist. In fact, these children usually stay at that level until they go through a normal puberty. It may be associated with elevations in dehydroepiandrosterone sulfate (DHEAS), which is of adrenal origin.

Precocious pubarche usually refers to premature pubic hair and little else. Prior to age 8 in girls this situation is less common and is often confused with adrenarche, which is more common, especially in girls. There is no specific therapy for either of these events, as they are not associated with other indices of puberty and may become, in effect, nonentities once puberty starts.

Precocious thelarche is the development of breast tissue in girls less than 8 years of age, with no other indices of precocity. Most of these children have precocious breast development during the first year of life, but precocious puberty rarely follows. Breast tissue is often present during the neonatal period. This breast tissue usually regresses; and if precocious or premature thelarche then occurs, there is a secondary increase in this tissue. There are minimal or no indices of precocious puberty associated with it, and the child eventually goes on to a normal pubescent sequence. One may note that precocious thelarche usually appears during the first year of life, whereas true isosexual precocity occurs sometime after the fourth year.

Pseudosexual precocity may be due to a large variety of causes, including ovarian tumors secreting estrogen, adrenal hyperplasia, human chorionic gonadotropin (hCG)-secreting tumors such as chorioepitheliomas or hepatomas, or it may be iatrogenic, due to exogenous hormone administration. Such individuals may well manifest many of the indices of true precocity, but they do not have fertility potential. In fact, normal ovarian follicular function is often suppressed. Treatment here requires removal of the offending lesion or discontinuation of the exogenous

hormonal therapy. The flowchart in Figure 7-3 relates to the workup of the patient with various forms of puberty, outlining the multitude of causes.

DELAYED PUBERTY

When the onset of puberty is delayed beyond what is considered to be the upper range of normal for the female, i.e., age 16 years, and in the absence of any apparent cause of a disease or anomaly, delayed puberty is considered to exist. In fact, it is probably the most common cause of primary amenorrhea. It is usually hereditary and indicates an inherited failure to release GnRH. In these circumstances the pituitary and gonads have the capacity to respond normally but are unable to do so because the hypothalamic stimulus is not present.

It is important to distinguish between idiopathic delayed puberty, which is the most common variety, and delayed puberty secondary to specific structural or functional disorders that may occur at any level from the hypothalamus to the gonads. The reader may refer to the flow sheet for the workup of delayed puberty in Figure 7-4.

It is important to include the GnRH test as a means of distinguishing delayed puberty from hypothalamic, pituitary, or gonadal disease. The test requires administration of 100 μg of GnRH as an intravenous bolus, after a blood sample is obtained for a control serum LH level. Further samples are obtained for serum LH levels at 15, 30, 45, 60, and 120 minutes after the GnRH bolus. Normal control LH levels are 5 to 25 mIU per milliliter, and peak LH responses should be 20 to 120 mIU per milliliter. If there is an exaggerated peak response above these levels, one should consider primary hypogonadism. Responses markedly decreased below the normal ranges imply pituitary disease.

NORMAL MENSTRUAL CYCLE

The normal cyclicity of the menstrual cycle depends on specific pulsatile secretions of GnRH and pituitary gonadotropins affecting the growth of responding ovarian follicles. The ideal cycle duration, 28 days, is

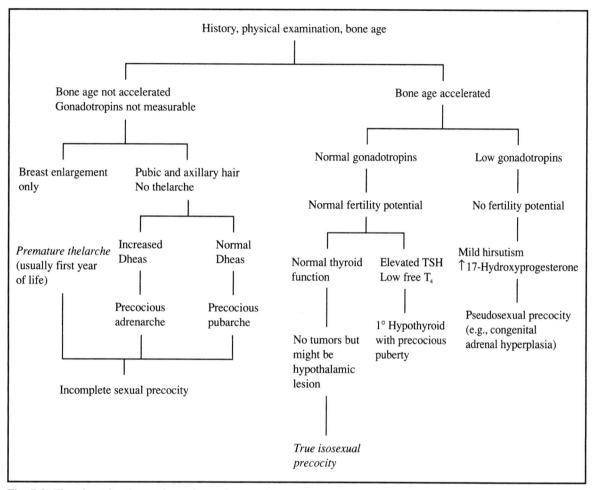

Fig. 7-3. Flowchart for the workup of sexual precocity.

counted from the first day of menstrual flow to the onset of the next menstrual flow. There may be normal variations in the duration of this cycle. Toward the end of the normal menstrual cycle, late in the luteal phase, there is a secondary rise in FSH that is a consequence of decreasing luteal function; the result is a fall in serum estrogen. This fall decreases the negative feedback that estrogen has on serum FSH, resulting in the FSH increase. The elevated FSH now initiates the growth of a new crop of ovarian follicles in preparation for the subsequent cycle. Although menstruation ensues during this phase, there is continuing stimulation of the follicles.

As the follicles grow, estrogen secretion slowly increases, starting to become detectable on or about the seventh day after the initiation of the period. The estrogen rise continues to a point where on or about the thirteenth day there is a marked increase in estrogen (in positive feedback to LH) and then a fall that leads to the LH surge, or release of LH itself. FSH at this point is decreasing (with negative feedback) and then begins to rise again after the estrogen fall. At midcycle, FSH peaks with LH coincident with the estrogen fall, but at a far lower level than the LH itself. Furthermore, as FSH stimulation of the responding graafian follicles selected for ovulation continues,

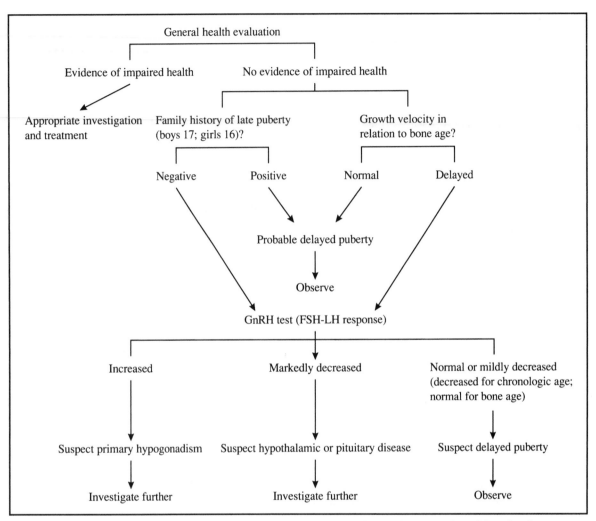

Fig. 7-4. Diagnostic approach to delayed puberty. (From R. Metz and E. B. Carson. *Blue Book of Endocrinology*. Philadelphia: Saunders, 1985.)

the receptors for FSH are increased, presumably by the FSH itself and by estrogen sensitization of the follicle, which also enhances LH receptor activity in this area. One may note low levels of progesterone rising at this point as well just prior to ovulation.

All of these hormonal events associated with full maturation of the selected graafian follicle result in eventual rupture of the prepared follicle and release of the ovum. The rising estrogen levels are also reflected in the vaginal mucosa by its increased number of superficial cells as well as a marked increase in proliferation of the endometrium.

Subsequent to ovulation there is a rapid fall in FSH and LH, with secondary rises in estradiol and progesterone. 17-Hydroxyprogesterone levels also rise at ovulation, then fall and secondarily rise to relatively low levels. At about the same time, progesterone peaks during the secretory phase of the menstrual cycle. The increase in progesterone secretion by the corpus luteum after ovulation may be seen in smears of the vaginal mucosa, which show a marked increase in exfoliation of intermediate cells and a decrease in the number of superficial cells. The endometrium reflects these changes as well in a specific sequential fashion that can be timed histologically with an increase in glandular activity and eventual secretion within the lumen. This sequence is all in preparation for the eventual implantation of a fertilized egg. In the absence of fertilization, hormone levels begin to fall; and a secondary rise in FSH with falling estrogen and progesterone levels initiates follicular growth for the subsequent cycle.

The basal body temperature reflects the hormonal events, as progesterone and its metabolites are thermogenic. Therefore with ovulation and secretion of progesterone by the corpus luteum, a temperature increase is initiated, is reflected in the basal body temperature, that is sustained so long as progesterone is produced. In the absence of pregnancy, progesterone levels fall, resulting in a fall in the basal temperature to its control level. If a pregnancy does occur, corpus luteum function persists for awhile, and the basal body temperature elevation is sustained. In fact, this rise may be an early indication of pregnancy.

PRIMARY AMENORRHEA

Primary amenorrhea may be defined as the absence of menses in an individual who has never had a menstrual period usually by the age of 18. Pubescent development may or may not be present. It occurs in fewer than 1 percent of patients with gynecologic disorders, although there are a multitude of disorders that may be associated with primary amenorrhea (Table 7-2).

An accepted technique for classification utilizes the gonadotropin level as the defining factor. Individuals with normal gonadotropins fall into one category, whereas patients with an elevated gonadotropin level and those with a low gonadotropin level fit into the other categories. However, it must be appreciated that the largest number of patients with primary amenorrhea are probably adolescents with delayed pubescence.

Normal Gonadotropins

Patients with normal gonadotropins represent about 20 percent of individuals with primary amenorrhea.

Table 7-2. Classification of Primary Amenorrhea

Physiologic causes	Other causes
Prepubescence	Gonadal dysgenesis and variants
Pregnancy	Primary hypogonadism: surgical, developmental, destruction by disease
	Panhypopituitarism: craniopharyngioma
	Hypothalamic hypogonadism: Kallman syndrome
	Anatomic: absence of uterus, imperforate hymen, altresia of vagina
	Chronic diseases and/or malnutrition
	Ovarian or adrenal tumors
	Adrenogenital syndrome
	Hypothyroidism
	Delayed puberty

Included in this group are patients with the Rokitansky syndrome. These individuals usually have a hypoplastic uterus associated with failure of fusion of the müllerian anlagen as well as associated vaginal agenesis. They have a normal 46,XX karyotype and normal pubescence but without menarche. The absence of a canalized vagina and of a clearly defined uterus on rectal bimanual examination should make one strongly suspicious of this syndrome. The gonadotropins are normal because ovarian function is normal, and the patient's general development is otherwise normal.

Cryptic menstruation occurs in individuals with an imperforate hymen or a transverse vaginal septum that prevents egress of the menstruum from a normal uterus. The individual with an imperforate hymen has primary amenorrhea but menstrual molimina; and, ultimately, bulging can be noted on the perineum with squeezing. In the presence of a transverse vaginal septum, there is a defect in the distal third of the vagina that does not canalize and can lead to backup of menstruum proximally. This disorder may be suspected not only by the absence of menses but also with menstrual molimina, palpation of a mass rectally, and inability to find an appropriate vagina at the introital area. The rectal mass is caused by a collection of menstruum deposited by retrograde flow through the fallopian tubes.

Elevated Gonadotropins

About 50 percent of patients with primary amenorrhea have elevated gonadotropins. The classic patient in this group has gonadal dysgenesis associated with a chromosomal abnormality. Most of these patients have an XO pattern with 45 chromosomes. Such individuals have the classic congenital anomalies: a webbed neck with cutis laxa, hypertelorism, shield chest, wide carrying angle, and short stature. Their lack of secondary sex characteristics associated with the primary amenorrhea is termed *Turner's syndrome*. There are mosaics associated with this grouping that may show XO/XY or XX/XO. In general, mosaics do not manifest all of the classic features of Turner's syndrome, but the patients usually do have short stature.

Another variant of the gonadal dysgenesis syndrome occurs in girls who have an apparent normal XX pattern but the karyotype shows a translocation of one of the arms of the X chromosome. Such patients may demonstrate initial pubarche and menarche, but they then develop what evolves as premature ovarian failure. In this subset, elevated gonadotropins are seen routinely. With chromosomal translocation, gonadotropin levels may be initially normal but become elevated as the characteristic premature ovarian failure and amenorrhea develop.

There are rare patients with primary amenorrhea who have a 46,XY pattern but develop as phenotypic females because they lack the HY antigen. The gonadal streaks in these individuals are liable to tumor formation, and so the gonads are prudently removed prophylactically.

Another disorder in this grouping is the *feminizing testis syndrome* (androgen resistance). Affected individuals have an XY chromosomal pattern but exhibit a female phenotype. Thus they are genotypically male but phenotypically female. The intraabdominal or inguinal gonads in these patients are testes that secrete testosterone. The mechanism of the abnormality is an end-organ and pituitary insensitivity to testosterone. This combination leads to an absence of feedback suppression and elevated gonadotropins. The mül-lerian inhibitory factor appears to function normally during embryologic development in these patients, indicated by an absence of müllerian structures. The patients lack a uterus and adnexae, in contrast to patients with XY gonadal dysgenesis, and they have no HY antigen. The latter group of patients, as noted above, require prophylactic surgical removal of the gonads because of the risk of tumor development. Some cases of amenorrhea in the high gonadotropin group result from a genetic deficiency of 17α-hydroxylase enzyme, which leads to an inability to form androgens and estrogens, with consequent primary amenorrhea, sexual infantilism, and hypertension.

Another abnormality in this category is the *ovarian resistance syndrome*. Here the ovaries fail to react to gonadotropins, presumably secondary to receptor deficiencies.

Low Gonadotropins

Patients with primary amenorrhea associated with low gonadotropins account for about 30 percent of all individuals with primary amenorrhea. Girls with *delayed puberty* may be seen among these patients, but they are also seen in the group with normal gonadotropins. The combination of low gonadotropins and delayed puberty indicates hypothalamic disturbances with loss of pulsatile secretion and hence an absence of stimulation of gonadotropin formation that is presumably of a temporary nature. These girls are normal individuals who are just slow to develop for varying reasons. Most commonly a hereditary factor is the cause. Such children may show evidence of adrenarche without evidence of gonadarche.

There may also be selective deficiency of gonadotropin, as in the *Kallman syndrome*. This syndrome is usually associated with midline craniofacial defects such as cleft palate, hare lip, and hyposmia to anosmia. Characteristically, these individuals have primary amenorrhea, are eunuchoid, and have no secondary sex characteristics. Their development of müllerian derivatives is intact, and they have a normal chromosomal pattern. Gonadotropins are low, but the other pituitary tropic hormones are intact.

Craniopharyngioma, which is the most common pituitary tumor of childhood, may result in panhypopituitarism, which manifests as short stature, lack of secondary sex characteristics, and primary amenorrhea. Primary hypothyroidism may also be associated with primary amenorrhea, as may congenital adrenal hyperplasia. Severe nutritional deficiencies, including anorexia nervosa and starvation, may be associated with primary amenorrhea as well. Occasionally, severe psychic trauma delays the onset or progression of normal pubescence. In addition, some patients with polycystic ovary syndrome manifest primary amenor-

rhea rather than secondary amenorrhea, as is more common.

Primary amenorrhea has also been noted to be associated with diabetes mellitus, insulin resistance, hirsutism, and acanthosis nigricans. It may also be associated with multiple endocrine neoplasia, and a hypothalamic form of hypogonadism has been described.

Diagnostic evaluation of primary amenorrhea is directed to the identification of the point of defect in the brain centers linking the hypothalamus, pituitary, gonads, and endometrium (Fig. 7-5). Initially, unstimulated plasma gonadotropin concentrations are measured to exclude primary ovarian failure or "ovarian

Fig. 7-5. Diagnostic workup for primary amenorrhea. (From R. Metz and E. B. Carson. *Blue Book of Endocrinology*. Philadelphia: Saunders, 1985.)

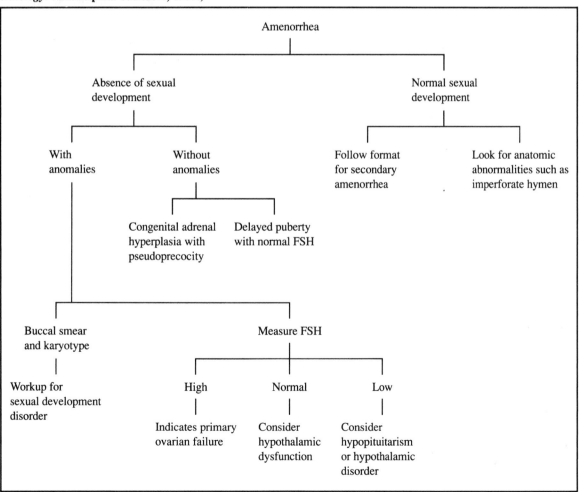

resistance." Depending on these results, the next step is usually determining the response of LH and FSH to GnRH to evaluate the capacity of the pituitary to respond to hypothalamic stimulation. Finally, the response of FSH and LH to clomiphene administration is determined to evaluate both hypothalamic and pituitary responsiveness. Analysis of the results usually pinpoints the locus of the defect, which is necessary to assess the prognosis and alternative forms of therapy.

There is also a clinical approach to the classification of primary amenorrhea, based on the presence or absence of breast and uterine development. Patients with no breast development but an intact uterus generally have hypogonadotropic hypogonadism. Patients with breast development but no uterus usually fall into the category of either testicular feminization syndrome or congenital absence of the uterus. Those who lack breast development as well as a uterus usually have congenital failure of gonadal development or a deficiency of a 17,20-desmolase enzyme. Finally, those patients with normal breast development and a normal uterus are usually found to have hyperprolactinemia, polycystic ovaries, or hypothalamic dysfunction.

SELECTED READINGS

Maschak, C. A., Kletsky, O. A., Davajan, V. E., and Mishell, D. R., Jr. Clinical and laboratory evaluation of patients with primary amenorrhea. *Obstet. Gynecol.* 58:715, 1981.

Pelliniemi, L. J., and Dym, M. The fetal gonad and sexual differentiation. In Tulchinsky, D., and Ryan, K. J. (eds.), *Maternal-Fetal Endocrinology.* Philadelphia: Saunders, 1980.

Prader, A. Delayed adolescence. *Clin. Endocrinol. Metab.* 4:143, 1975.

Root, A. W., and Shulman, D. I. Isosexual precocity: current concepts and recent advances. *Fertil. Steril.* 45:749, 1986.

Tanner, J. M. Growth and endocrinology of the adolescent. In Gardner, L. I. (ed.), *Endocrine and Genetic Diseases of Childhood* (2nd ed.). Philadelphia: Saunders, 1975.

8

Congenital Anomalies of the Reproductive Tract

Developmental anomalies of the female genital tract are often not discovered until the early adult period. Failure to recognize such anomalies at birth could be avoided by more careful routine examinations of the newborn or young child.

Many of the common congenital anatomic abnormalities do not involve either the external genitalia or the ovaries and hence do not manifest in any way until the menarche or perhaps even until marriage and unsuccessful attempts at conception or child-bearing prompt an infertility investigation that reveals their presence. Furthermore, only rarely does a delay in the detection of the more common simple anatomic anomalies have any unfortunate effects on the outcome of their treatment, which is often best postponed until adolescence or even maturity.

The situation is different, however, for the more profound disturbances of fetal genital tract development that originate in fundamental hormonal or chromosomal abnormalities and include the various forms of intersex or pseudohermaphroditism. Here the anomalies of the external genitalia invariably accompanying these disorders draw immediate attention to their presence at or shortly after birth. It is fortunate because in most such cases treatment is most successful if planned and carried out during infancy or early childhood.

ETIOLOGY AND CLASSIFICATION

A complete and accurate classification of the various anomalies that may be encountered according to anatomic type and etiology is certainly not possible because the basic causes of developmental errors are not yet always understood. Furthermore, similar genital anomalies may have entirely different fundamental etiologies. Finally, a theoretical classification devised

on purely embryologic grounds does not suffice, as it cannot take into account etiologic differences that may result in various combinations of reproductive tract abnormalities; nor would it allow for the genital tract anomalies that undoubtedly occur in conjunction with lethal anomalies elsewhere in the embryo and hence are never actually seen in the living female. Therefore for this chapter a clinical classification is adopted to present the common anomalies of various segments of the reproductive tract as they are encountered clinically, discussing the probable etiology of each separately on the basis of presently available information.

A few general concepts concerning etiology serve to orient and integrate the later discussion of individual anomalies. Broadly speaking, there appear to be three fundamental types of developmental error that give rise to congenital anomalies of the female reproductive tract.

1. *Simple retardation, arrest, or partial or complete failure of occurrence of normal embryologic events involving reproductive tract formation in an otherwise normal female embryo* (i.e., a genetically normal female with normally developing female gonads). The commonest anomalies of the female genital organs are of this type and involve varying degrees of failure of the normal union of the originally separate müllerian ducts, as is discussed later. Persistence of a double müllerian system in adult life is normal for some of the lower vertebrates (e.g., rabbits and other rodents), and its occurrence in the human female may in this sense be looked on as a reversion to a more primitive type of embryologic development. Nevertheless it remains a serious anomaly, often with unfortunate effects on the reproductive capacity of the woman. This phylogenetic relation emphasizes, however, that the group of anomalies does represent the result of retardation or arrest of an otherwise normally proceeding embryologic process.

There are many and varied causes of this retardation or arrest. Fetal environmental factors, primarily maternal or placental in locus or origin, are undoubtedly the most likely causes and include such diverse maternal conditions as poor nutrition, metabolic disorders (e.g., diabetes), and certain vital or inclusion-body diseases (e.g., German measles and, less frequently, measles, mumps, chickenpox, toxoplasmosis, cytomegalic inclusion disease, herpes simplex, varicella, and poliomyelitis). Because most of the significant events in the embryologic formation of the reproductive tract commence around the fifth or sixth week and are essentially complete by the end of ten to twelve weeks of fetal life, it is clear that the disturbances in fetal environment, whatever they may be, must have occurred during this crucial interval. Although hereditary factors and germ plasm defects may conceivably also be implicated, most women with this type of anomaly are otherwise normal except for associated urinary tract anomalies, which are found in 35 to 50 percent of women suffering from müllerian duct anomalies. This association is readily explained by the anatomic juxtaposition of the urinary and reproductive tracts in the fetus and the occurrence of crucial events in the embryologic development of both systems almost simultaneously. Other less common, though more obvious, causes might include exposure to toxic drugs or ionizing radiation.

2. *Genetic abnormalities involving the sex chromosomes.* The theory of sex determination that has been accepted for more than half a century holds that sex is determined at the moment of conception and depends on whether the fertilizing spermatazoon contains either the X or the Y sex chromosome of the original primary spermatocyte (which contained both) at the time of union with the ovum. The latter, of course, can contain only an X chromosome, derived as it is from the primary oocyte, which in turn always carries two identical X sex chromosomes. However, advances in genetics have revealed that the situation with regard to the sex chromosome pattern is not always this simple. The ability to count and identify human chromosomes using the banding technique and quinacrine or fluorescence labeling of the Y chromosome has revealed that some individuals have more than two or fewer than two sex chromosomes within the nuclei of most if not all of their cells; or they have two, but one or both are abnormal. Furthermore, many of these individuals characteristically present a typical pattern of anomalous development of the reproductive tract, the particular anomaly tending

to be correlated with a specific abnormality of the sex chromosome pattern. One of the two most frequently encountered examples of this type of sex chromosome-related anomaly is gonadal dysgenesis (Turner's syndrome). Although such individuals appear to be female, 80 percent are genetically neither female nor male, with their chromosome karyotype showing only one X sex chromosome and a total chromosome number of only 45 (i.e., 45,XO). The second is Klinefelter's syndrome, in which there are typically 47 chromosomes with an XXY sex chromosome pattern. Both of these disorders are discussed in more detail later. Because of the increased interest in this obviously important aspect of sexual differentiation, the basic information concerning the study of sex chromosomes and their abnormalities are also briefly summarized later in a separate section.

The mechanisms by which these chromosomal abnormalities can arise are varied. They usually involve either failure of the members of a chromosome pair to separate properly during the cell divisions necessary to form the ovum or spermatozoon (maternal or paternal origin), or there is a similar failure or nondisjunction after fertilization during the cell divisions of the early embryonic stages (perhaps the result of an adverse condition in the fetal environment). The underlying factors that might predispose to disruption of the normal pattern of chromosomal separation during cell division are even less clear. Parental age has been incriminated, as chromosomal abnormalities in general tend to occur more frequently in children born to older parents. The high incidence of Down syndrome in pregnancies in women in their late reproductive years is a case in point, although an autosomal rather than a sex chromosomal abnormality is involved. Maternal viral infections (measles, rubella) also seem to be followed by a high incidence of chromosomal aberrations, and anoxia and irradiation have been shown experimentally to produce them.

3. *Fetal endocrine disorders interfering with the normal embryologic development of the reproductive tract* in an otherwise normal female or male embryo (normal female or male sex chromosome pattern and normal female or male gonads). The most common reproductive tract anomaly arising through such a

mechanism is female pseudohermaphroditism (congenital adrenogenital syndrome), which occurs as a result of fetal adrenal hyperplasia. This syndrome accounts for well over 50 percent of all so-called intersex problems. This problem is discussed later in more detail. The testicular feminization syndrome is now known to be an anomaly of male embryos developing in response to a fetal endocrine-metabolic disturbance. Embryonic pituitary and thyroid disturbances have long been recognized as precursors of more generalized congenital disorders of growth and development, and it is possible that as yet unknown, more subtle, perhaps even transient fetal endocrine abnormalities play a role in the production of other anomalies involving the reproductive tract as well as other organ systems. As for the basic causes of these fetal endocrinologic errors, reference can be made again to potential hereditary constitutional deficiencies and the many possible maternal-fetal environmental factors already mentioned.

IMPORTANT EMBRYOLOGIC EVENTS IN FEMALE REPRODUCTIVE TRACT FORMATION

An outline of the normal sequence of principal events in the embryologic development of the female reproductive tract is helpful for understanding how the more common anatomic anomalies come about.

The genital system first makes its appearance during the fifth and sixth weeks of embryonic life. At this point it is indifferent, or neuter, in appearance, although the prospective sex of the individual is theoretically predictable on the basis of the sex chromosomal pattern irrevocably established at the moment of conception. Four key developmental processes occurring in the primitive genital tract and a fifth related, though less important, transition taking place in the adjacent embryonic urinary tract should be kept in mind. The following sections discuss these processes.

Gonadal Differentiation

The initially indifferent paired gonads, which make their appearance about the sixth week as medial thickenings in the urogenital ridges, have differentiated sufficiently within 1 to 2 weeks to assume the characteristics of ovaries and have begun to receive the migrating primordial germ or egg cells. These primordial germ cells appear to arise in the caudal end of the primitive streak in all mammalian embryos, and their migration may well be initiated by a chemical attractant secreted by the genital ridge epithelial cells. In the absence of the Y chromosome, this differentiation must proceed in the direction of the formation of an ovary. Conversely, the presence of a normal Y chromosome is absolutely essential to the development of a normal testis from the indifferent gonad. The primitive gonad originally contains both a cortical component (potentially ovarian) and a medullary component (potentially testicular). The presence of two normal X chromosomes is essential for proper development of the gonadal cortex to form a normal ovary. A normal Y chromosome plus an X chromosome is needed for normal growth and maturation of the gonadal medulla and formation of a normal testis.

Thus Turner's syndrome is primarily an instance of cortical gonadal dysgenesis, and Klinefelter's syndrome is principally an example of medullary gonadal dysgenesis. The few true hermaphrodites (individuals in whom both ovarian and testicular tissues are present) in whom complete chromosome studies have been done have mosaic chromosome patterns (e.g., XX/XY, XO/XY). Alternatively, some of the embryos with pure XX patterns are believed to have had elements of the Y chromosome transferred to an X (one X frequently abnormally large) through "translocation" during nuclear division and are thus the result of a combined corticomedullary gonadal dysgenesis. Hence sex chromosomal abnormalities may give rise to the persistence of completely indifferent gonads (gonadal dysgenesis), rarely to the formation of gonadal tissues of both male and female type in the same individual (true hermaphroditism), or to various intermediate gonadal aberrations; although rare, arrested or failed embryologic development at this stage may result in complete absence of gonadal tissue on one or both sides.

Finally, it should be noted that the primitive gonads arise fairly cephalad in the urogenital ridges but undergo a relative descent during growth of the embryo. In females they normally come to assume a more caudal position within the pelvis, and an abnormal ovarian descent is unusual. However, failure to complete the descent to the normal scrotal site is not uncommon in the male. Therefore having arisen from the same urogenital ridge area from which the kidney and adrenal form, the ovary may carry with it, during its descent, embryonic rests of kidneys or adrenals that may manifest later in life as either functioning or nonfunctioning, benign or malignant tissue of renal or adrenal origin.

Müllerian Duct Transformations

During the so-called indifferent stage, and regardless of the genetically predetermined sex, the paired müllerian ducts appear in the lateral portion of each urogenital ridge. Atresia or regression of the müllerian ducts depends on the appearance of müllerian-inhibiting factor, a protein produced in the male fetal testis and controlled by the Y chromosome. Thus in a female fetus and in the absence of the Y chromosome (and therefore of müllerian-inhibiting factor), the müllerian ducts undergo further development once gonadal differentiation is well under way. The müllerian ducts ultimately unite caudally to form a single uterine cavity and cervix and a provisional single upper vagina. Only the cephalic portion remains unfused as separate fallopian tubes. In the male embryo, both the development of the testis and the secretion of both androgen and müllerian-inhibiting factor cause regression of the müllerian duct system, only vestiges of which remain in the adult male genitourinary tract. However, if normal male gonadal development and embryonic androgen and müllerian-inhibiting factor secretion do not take place, the müllerian ducts continue to evolve as if the individual were a chromosomal female. This point is important for understanding the anomalous anatomy present in cases of gonadal dysgenesis or agenesis (Turner's syndrome), where only one X chromosome is present and there is no Y chromosome (XO chromosome pattern).

The most common anomalies of the human female reproductive tract involve failures of varying degrees in the process of normal müllerian duct fusion. Rarely, one or both of the müllerian ducts simply do not appear. Because the factors producing these apparently simple embryologic arrests of normal müllerian duct development might be expected to have an effect on simultaneously occurring events in the adjacent fetal urinary tract, the frequent coexistence of anomalies of the kidneys and ureters in patients with genital anomalies of müllerian duct origin is not surprising.

Formation of the External Genitalia

After the appearance of the genital tubercle during the sixth week of embryonic life, early modifications during the next two weeks result in the development of an "indifferent" external genital area that includes the phallus, a urogenital sinus from which ultimately arise both the urethra and the lower end of the vagina, and the paired labioscrotal swelling. Once gonadal differentiation occurs at about the eighth week, further modifications in this primitive external genital region result in the formation during the next six to eight weeks of either male or female external genitalia in accordance with the gonadal and hormonal (and normally the chromosomal) status of the embryo.

Obviously, incomplete or imperfect occurrence of this sequence of events due to unknown and nonspecific causes can produce a variety of simple anatomic abnormalities in both the genital and lower urinary tracts in either females or males who are otherwise sexually normal, but these abnormalities are uncommon.

Most important, however, are the more specific anomalies resulting from embryologic errors in the further evolution of the primitive, indifferent set of external genitalia caused by imperfect gonadal differentiation. In this regard, the crux of the matter lies in the organizing potential of the embryonic male gonad, or primitive testis, and its early secretion of androgen. Only in the presence of actively functioning testicular tissue or androgen from some other source do the embryonic modifications necessary to form a male set of external genitalia occur. Thus even in a genetically indifferent embryo—so long as normal male gonadal differentiation and androgen production fail to take place—a female type of external genitalia appears (Turner's syndrome and gonadal dysgenesis or agenesis are examples). In the presence of intermediate androgenic effects that are insufficient to produce the completely masculine type of external genitalia, varying degrees of partial virilization, often with hypospadias, result.

Equally significant for the genetically female embryo is the abnormal presence of androgens during this crucial phase of the development of the external genitalia. If androgens are present in large enough amounts in the developing female embryo at this time, a tendency toward male external genitalia and a masculine type of lower urinary tract anatomy are evident to a greater or lesser degree at birth, even though normal female gonads with a potentially normal functional capacity and a normal müllerian duct system (normal fallopian tubes, uterus, cervix, and upper vagina) are present. The two common examples of this phenomenon are (1) congenital adrenogenital syndrome (congenital adrenal hyperplasia or female pseudohermaphroditism), in which the fetal adrenal of a genetically and gonadally normal female secretes large amounts of androgenic steroids, and (2) the more recently encountered iatrogenic syndrome of virilization of the otherwise normal female fetus by the administration of androgens or, more commonly, progestational compounds with androgenic activity to the mother during the early months of pregnancy.

Union of the Fused Lower Segment of the Müllerian Duct System with the External Genital Tract

At the caudal end (Müller's tubercle) of the fused müllerian duct systems, a lumen normally develops below the cervix and between the rectum and urethra. When contact is made with the deepening external urogenital sinus, union ordinarily occurs, and the thin membrane so formed becomes the hymen. Usually the hymen assumes its normal perforate form during the latter months of embryonic life or shortly after birth. Thus the upper two-thirds of the vagina are of müllerian duct origin, whereas the lower one-third is of urogenital sinus origin.

Knowledge of these embryologic facts serves to explain the various congenital anomalies of the vagina and vestibule, most of which result either from failure of fusion or partial or complete failure of normal development of one or the other of the two initially independent forerunners of the completely formed, final vaginal tract. The simple abnormalities of imperforate hymen or imperforate vagina are easily understood, and complete absence of the upper vagina in the presence of normal external genitalia and a short, apparently normal lower vaginal canal are equally comprehensible. The mechanisms by which less common anomalies such as congenital rectovaginal and urethrovaginal fistulas might arise are also obvious.

Disposition of the Mesonephric (Wolffian) Duct System in the Female Fetus

Although the male embryo appropriates the mesonephric ducts and tubules and converts them to the male genital canals, the mesonephric duct system undergoes atrophy in the normally developing female fetus and largely disappears. However, portions do remain as normal vestigial remnants even in adults (the so-called rete ovarii, or complex of epoophoron and paroophoron and their ducts, which lie in the broad ligaments and the mesosalpinx and mesovarium). Other mesonephric duct remnants are often found retroperitoneally, in the ovaries or tubes, or in the walls of the uterus, cervix, vagina, and even the vulva. Although not strictly anomalies, numerous cysts (e.g., the common Gartner's duct cysts of the vagina, the hydatid cysts of Morgagni near the fimbriated ends of the tubes, and the frequently large parovarian cysts) and, more rarely, neoplasms arising from these residual mesonephric duct structures are often of considerable clinical interest and significance and are in a sense congenital in origin.

CHROMOSOME STUDIES OF SEX CHROMOSOME DISORDERS

A brief outline of the methods available for studying chromosomes and for interpreting the results can assist in the understanding and management of sex chromosomal disorders. Chromosome karyotyping can be readily carried out by culturing leukocytes obtained from blood in a culture medium to which colchicine is later added to arrest mitosis during metaphase. The individual chromosomes are scattered widely if the cultured cells are exposed to hypotonic

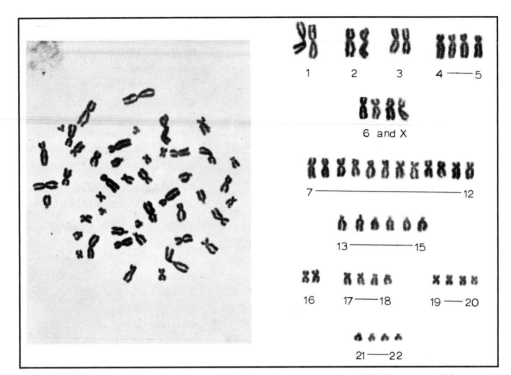

Fig. 8-1. Chromosomal analysis by means of the "squash preparation." On the left is the "squash smear" of a normal human female cell grown in tissue culture, with cell division arrested at the metaphase. On the right is the normal human female idiogram or karyotype constructed from these individual chromosomes.

saline solution to cause cellular swelling and disruption ("squash preparation"). By photomicrography, the various chromosome types can then be separately and accurately identified, paired off, and counted (Fig. 8-1). In this way the total number of chromosomes and their composition, normal or abnormal, can be precisely determined. It is through the use of this and similar complicated techniques that the exact chromosomal patterns of the various known anomalous clinical entities have been established. The chromosomes can be individually recognized easily by employing the "banding" technique in the karyotype preparation. The Y chromosome can also be specifically identified or tracked with a fluorescence method using quinacrine hydrochloride.

A much simpler, quicker, and clinically readily available test for sex chromosome complement is the determination of the nuclear sex chromatin pattern of an individual's cells. As described in Chapter 2, the buccal smear is ordinarily used because the surface epithelial cells of the oral mucosa are ideal for the purpose and are readily available. The determination

depends on the fact that in most cells of normal females a sex chromatin body—the Barr body—can be regularly seen and identified in the cell nucleus at or close to the nuclear membrane (Fig. 2-4). This chromatin, or Barr, body represents a coiled, temporarily inactivated X chromosome in the nucleus of female cells, according to the Lyon hypothesis. Thus the Barr body count of female cells is never 100 percent and actually fluctuates, particularly in adult women during the monthly menstrual cycle, possibly in response to varying estrogen levels. When most of the cell nuclei display the sex chromatin body, the individual is termed chromatin-positive, and an XX sex chromosome pattern can generally be assumed. If three X chromosomes are present, as is the case with certain genetic abnormalities, two sex chromatin bodies are usually visible (i.e., the number of Barr bodies is equal to one less than the number of X chromosomes). However, the presence of a sex chromatin body does not necessarily connote absence of the Y chromosome but, rather, indicates only that two X chromosomes exist. In Klinefelter's syndrome, for example, the individuals are chromatin-positive, and the sex chromosomal pattern is XXY.

On the other hand, absence or virtual absence of sex chromatin bodies in an individual's cells implies that no more than one X chromosome is present, and the individual is termed chromatin-negative. This situation exists in a genetically normal male with the normal XY chromosome pattern. However, a chromatin-negative status by no means establishes the presence of a Y chromosome, as was originally assumed. Again, for example, in Turner's syndrome or gonadal dysgenesis the individuals are chromatin-negative, a fact that at one time was believed to indicate they were genetic males, whereas the usual sex chromosomal pattern is now known to be XO.

Within these limitations, however, the sex chromatin determination can be a helpful clinical test. Because there are only three major sex chromosomal abnormalities of clinical significance, correlation of the clinical picture with the sex chromatin pattern nearly always suffices to establish a definite clinical diagnosis.

The normal number of chromosomes within human cell nuclei is 46, and the chromosomes are made up of 22 paired autosomes and one pair of sex chromosomes. The autosomes are responsible for some specific aspects of growth and maturation of body structures or organ systems, and the presence and nature of the sex chromosome determines the genetic sex and subsequent sexual and reproductive tract development. One-half of each pair of chromosomes (a total of 23) is of male parental origin, the other half being of female parental origin (the male and female gametes contain only 23 chromosomes each as a result of the meiotic division necessary for the formation of either the ovum or the spermatozoon). At the time of fertilization the two sets of 23 chromosomes differ. Normal female cells contain two identical X chromosomes, whereas normal male cells contain an X chromosome and a smaller Y chromosome. Herein

lies the basis for the genetic determination of sex. All normal female gametes (ova) contain one X chromosome, whereas half the normal male gametes (spermatozoa) contain an X chromosome and half a Y chromosome. Thus there is ordinarily a 50 percent chance at the time of fertilization that the resulting zygote will be gentically female (XX) and an equal chance that it could be male (XY).

The normal nuclear divisions and unions involving these chromosomal transfers during gametogenesis and conception (Fig. 8-2) fortunately take place in an orderly fashion with the greatest regularity. However, abnormal chromosomal transfers occasionally occur through a number of mechanisms and may result in a

Fig. 8-2. Normal germ cell divisions involved in gametogenesis and conception.

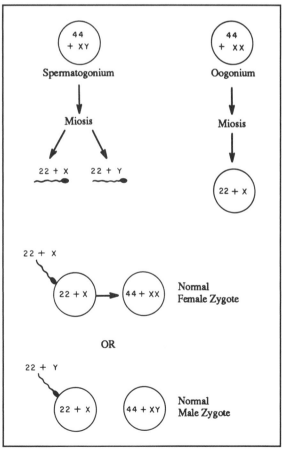

sex chromosome pattern (in either the male or female gamete or the fertilized ovum and developing zygote) that is neither male nor female. The various mechanisms by which these chromosomal abnormalities may arise are as follows.

1. *Nondisjunction,* or failure of the two members of a chromosome pair to separate during the meiotic divisions that occur during the formation of ova or spermatozoa
2. *Reciprocal translocation,* or exchange of portions of chromatin material by members of two chromosome pairs during either meiosis of the embryonic mitotic divisions
3. *Deletion,* or loss of part or all of a chromosome
4. *Reduplication,* or nondisjunction of only a part of a chromosome
5. *Mosaicism,* in which nondisjunction occurs during the mitotic divisions of the early embryonic stages, with persistence of more than one type of nuclear chromosomal pattern, the various cell types having different total chromosome numbers

About 0.56 percent of all newborn babies have major chromosomal abnormalities, giving an incidence of 1 in 200 live births. Sex chromosome abnormalities occur in 0.2 percent, or 1 in every 400 newborn males and 1 in every 680 newborn females. Abnormalities of autosomal chromosome number (e.g., trisomies) occur in 0.12 percent, and structural abnormalities of autosomal chromosomes (e.g., translocations) occur in 0.24 percent. A major and clinically significant abnormality involving the autosomal chromosomes is the consistent finding of 47 chromosomes in mongoloid infants, where an extra autosomal chromosome (derived from number 21) is present—hence the descriptive phrase "trisomy 21 syndrome" (Down syndrome). Several other trisomies involving autosomes have also been discovered, i.e., trisomy 13 (Patau syndrome) and trisomy 16–18 (Edwards syndrome), but they are less frequent than Down syndrome. This paucity of known autosomal abnormalities may well exist because loss or any other major abnormality of an autosome is more often lethal.

In contrast, abnormalities of the sex chromosomes are not only frequently compatible with life but also are recognized to be the basic cause of some of the more common reproductive tract anomalies. Currently, the three most common abnormal sex chromosomal patterns that have been encountered are the following.

1. XO sex chromosomal constitution in phenotypic females with 45 chromosomes, which is the usual

Fig. 8-3. Types of abnormal germ cell division that may lead to disorders. A. Turner's syndrome. B. Klinefelter's syndrome. C. Poly-X syndrome.

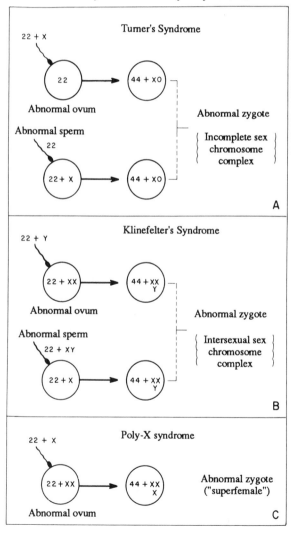

situation in the anomaly of gonadal dysgenesis with Turner's syndrome. (A buccal smear is chromatin-negative.)

2. XXY sex chromosomal constitution in phenotypic males with 47 chromosomes, or Klinefelter's syndrome. (A buccal smear is chromatin-positive.)

3. XXX sex chromosomal constitution in phenotypic but mentally retarded females, the so-called superfemale, or poly-X syndrome. (A buccal smear reveals that most of the cells contain two sex chromatin bodies.)

Numerous variants of these three basic abnormal sex chromosome patterns have been identified in individuals presenting any one of the three typical clinical pictures. These variants involve the presence of abnormal or additional X or Y chromosomes as well as sex chromosomal mosaics (several sex chromosome patterns in various cells of the same individual). (For example, in Klinefelter's syndrome, although the 47,XXY chromosomal pattern is the most frequent, various other patterns have also been encountered and reported, including 48,XXXY, 48,XXYY, 49,XXXXY, and a variety of mosaic patterns. Similarly, a 48,XXXX "superfemale" type has been observed, and mosaics of various types as well as some individuals who are chromatin-positive have been encountered in 20 percent of patients with Turner's syndrome.)

Although considerably simplified, the diagrams in Figure 8-3 indicate the gross mechanisms by which these three principal types of sex chromosomal aber-

rations might arise. An outline of the essential features of these disorders is presented in Table 8-1.

Finally, with the intense interest in precise study of sex chromosomal abnormalities and the application of the findings to clinical problems, basic information about specific chromosomal functions and variations and their correlation with particular features of the resulting gross anatomic and functional disturbances has been accumulating. The information that is valuable for a better understanding of the various clinical entities as well as useful in their differential diagnosis is summarized in the next sections.

X Chromosomes

1. Two normal X chromosomes are definitely necessary for differentiation of the primitive, indifferent gonads into normal functioning ovaries.

2. The genes responsible for the well-known sex-linked conditions of hemophilia and color blindness are known to be carried by the X chromosome.

3. The gene or genes that determine a person's ultimate height appear to be located on one or both short arms of the X chromosome. Evidence for this statement rests in the observation that stature in most patients with Turner's syndrome is markedly shorter than normal, and the chromosome pattern is either XO or the second X is abnormal and small, with one or both of the short arms of the second X partially or completely absent. In a small number of patients with otherwise typical gonadal dysgenesis, the sex chro-

Table 8-1. Nuclear Sex Chromatin and Sex Chromosome Patterns in the Principal Genetic Disorders Associated with Reproductive Tract Anomalies

Condition	Nuclear sex chromatin pattern (buccal smear)	Sex chromosome karyotype	Total no. of chromosomes
Normal female	Positive	XX	46
Normal male	Negative	XY	46
Turner's syndrome[a]	Negative	XO	45
Klinefelter's syndrome[a]	Positive	XXY	47
Superfemale[b]	Positive	XXX	47

[a]Only the most common chromosomal patterns are indicated.
[b]Two chromatin bodies.

mosome pattern is an apparently normal XX, and these individuals are normal in height.

4. When too many X chromosomes are present, as in the "superfemales" or poly-X syndrome (XXX, XXXX), or as in Klinefelter's syndrome (XXY), the individuals are always mentally deficient.

5. Early in embryonic life one of the two X chromosomes may be rendered physiologically inactive in the somatic cells of normal females (Lyon hypotheses), although it is not yet clear if this situation is also true for cells of the germ line. Similarly, it appears that even when too many X chromosomes are present only one tends to remain active.

6. The incidence of X chromosome abnormalities varies from 1 in every 200 to 400 live-born infants to an estimated 1 in 1800 in a general population of adults. Klinefelter's syndrome, the triple-X syndrome, and Turner's syndrome are by far the most common anomalies, in that order.

Y Chromosomes

1. The Y chromosome unquestionably contains genetic material strongly determinant for the male phenotype, or masculine appearance and developmental tendencies. Thus even in Klinefelter's syndrome the presence of two X chromosomes along with the Y chromosome still results in a masculine-appearing individual.

2. The Y chromosome, especially the short arm, is in general absolutely essential for differentiation of the primitive gonad into a functioning testis. There may be infrequent exceptions to this rule, for the rare, true hermaphrodites so far studied have always shown an XX or, more rarely, an XO sex chromosome pattern. Furthermore, a few cases of an even rarer "male XX syndrome" have been recorded. However, it is also possible that a small, abnormal Y chromosome is actually present but has not yet been identified (it may even be located on an X chromosome or an autosome), or that a Y chromosome had been present during an early period of fetal life but was subsequently lost. Even more rarely, a female phenotype has been observed in the presence of a 46,XY karyotype and

bilateral streak gonads; this syndrome appears to be a familial genetic disorder.

3. The fetus with a chromosomal opposite of Turner's syndrome, a YO sex chromosome pattern, is probably not viable, as no living individuals with this pattern have ever been encountered. Whether such a chromosomal disorder does in fact occur occasionally remains to be established by examining early abortion material. However, the Y chromosome carries loci, either in its short pairing segment or on its long arm, that are homologous with the loci on the short arm of the X chromosome, the absence of which is responsible for the short stature and congenital anomalies seen in Turner's syndrome. Thus these homologous loci on the Y chromosome guarantee normal height and absence of congenital anomalies in normal 46,XY males. Therefore, as might be predicted, a few individuals have been encountered with probable Y chromosome aberrations (X–abnormal Y) who have short stature and other stigmata of Turner's syndrome as well as defective testicular development.

4. The occurrence of an XYY sex chromosome complement in some individuals has been recorded and is discussed in more detail later in the chapter.

SIMPLE EMBRYOLOGIC DEVELOPMENTAL ANOMALIES: CLINICAL ASPECTS

Having considered the basic underlying genetic and embryologic mechanisms responsible for their development, the common genital anomalies are now presented from the clinical standpoint. In the case of the simpler specific developmental abnormalities, it seems most convenient to consider them according to their anatomic location. Some of the more complex, generalized congenital reproductive disorders of genetic or fetal endocrine origin, particularly those associated with either true or pseudointersexuality, are discussed separately.

Vulvar Anomalies

Invariably, true congenital vulvar anomalies are encountered only in connection with pseudohermaphroditism. Labial adhesion or agglutination, sometimes simulating absence of the vagina, is a simple condition not uncommon in young girls. The labia minora become adherent to each other usually from behind forward, bearing only a tiny opening through which urine passes. The adhesed area is usually translucent but becomes thicker with time. Some believe this abnormality to be a congenital condition, but adhesions may develop after the neonatal period. Estrogen cream applied to the area of adhesion is the recommended treatment.

Vaginal Anomalies

Vaginal anomalies may be of urogenital sinus origin (imperforate hymen, female hypospadias, persistent urogenital sinus membrane) or müllerian duct origin (congenital absence or atresia of the vagina, double or septate vagina).

Imperforate Hymen. Imperforate hymen is the simplest and perhaps most frequent genital anomaly. It may not be recognized until the menarche, when cyclic monthly distress is experienced but no overt menses occur. At this point, the vagina behind the intact and bulging hymeneal membrane may be distended with old menstrual secretions (hematocolpos). In the late stages, with further backing up of secretions, secondary distention of the uterus (hematometrium) or even of the tubes (hematosalpinx) may occur, with palpable abdominal and adnexal cystic "masses." The diagnosis is usually now readily apparent, and the treatment is simple hymenotomy or hymenectomy.

Rarely, distention of the vagina by simple mucoid vaginal secretions produced by maternal hormone stimulation occurs in a newborn infant or young child (hydrocolpos); and because of pressure or secondary infection the vagina may require drainage at this time. In this situation, differentiation from congenital absence of the vagina as well as the safety of hymenotomy are afforded by the vaginal distention. It is important to note that the hydrocolpos occurring in a newborn infant may be of considerable size and not only may interfere with bladder emptying but, more significantly, may present as an abdominal mass. The possibility of hydrocolpos must therefore always be

kept in mind in this situation lest an ill-advised, unnecessary laparotomy be undertaken for an "abdominal tumor." Once catheterization has eliminated bladder retention as the sole source of the mass, abdominal roentgenograms following injection of a small amount of iodized oil (Lipiodol) into the distended vaginal portion of the mass nearly always reveals the true nature of the abdominal component, and simple incision of the hymenal membrane can effectively deal with the problem. Ultrasonography may be helpful for identifying the mass.

If discovered early in infancy or childhood, and if it is asymptomatic, an imperforate hymen is best treated expectantly until the anatomic structures are sufficiently developed and large enough to distinguish it definitely from congenital vaginal absence and to permit a safe hymenectomy. If it becomes necessary to perform hymenotomy in the absence of distention in a child, the presence of an intact vaginal canal above the imperforate hymen should be ensured by rectal examination and by roentgenograms after injection of radiopaque dye through the hymen. At operation, a finger in the rectum and a sound in the urethra and bladder should be used to guide and control the incision.

A variant of imperforate hymen is the "microperforate hymen." In infants and young children, this condition may be a cause of both recurring vulvovaginitis and recurring urinary tract infections due to retention of a pool of infected urine behind the hymenal membrane. The condition is promptly relieved by hymenoplasty.

Occasionally, variation in aperture size or in the thickness and rigidity of the hymen requires dilatation or formal hymenectomy under anesthesia before maturity, but these problems are not considered true anomalies.

Congenital Absence of the Vagina. Congenital absence of the vagina most frequently involves only the upper two-thirds of the vagina, the lower one-third usually being normal. It is one of the commoner anomalies and is usually associated with an absent or rudimentary uterus and tubes; the ovaries, however, are invariably present and normal. Less often (in about 10 percent of these patients), a normal uterus and tubes are present, and with the onset of menstrual function a situation analogous to that of the hematocolpos behind an imperforate hymen may develop, except that only hematometrium and hematosalpinx result. At this point, if the diagnosis is made and treatment carried out early, fertility may be preserved by avoiding irreparable damage to the tubes and uterus. When the uterus and tubes are normal, this anomaly is usually not accompanied by anomalies of the urinary tract. If it is discovered during infancy or early childhood, further diagnostic maneuvers and treatment should be delayed because of possible damage to adjacent structures by ill-advised probing or exploration in the tiny patient.

If cyclic menstrual phenomena suggesting the presence of a normally functioning uterus appear at the menarche, prompt laparoscopy and, when necessary, laparotomy followed by plastic reconstruction of the vagina are indicated to prevent the development of a significant hematometrium or hematosalpinges that might interfere with attempts to preserve normal reproductive function. If the anomaly is discovered either before or after the menarche but in the absence of any signs of a normally functioning uterus, creation of an artificial vagina should be delayed until maturity has been reached and preferably until sexual activity is imminent or likely. The surgeon can then count on the normal functional use of the artificially created vagina postoperatively to maintain its integrity and functional capacity.

TYPES OF REPAIR

1. Surgical dissection of the perineum and rectovaginal septal area (space between the bladder and rectum) with placement of a full-thickness skin graft temporarily held in position by a suitable plastic mold is often employed.

2. Williams vaginoplasty, which consists in a vulvovaginal plastic procedure creating a new vaginal pouch lined by vulvar skin. This operation is easily performed and is notably free of complications. The results in terms of coital function have been satisfactory. Although equally useful in patients with congenital absence of the vagina, this procedure appears to be especially applicable to the problem of vaginal reconstruction after any radical pelvic cancer operation that of necessity includes a total vaginectomy.

3. Use of an isolated loop of small or large bowel in place of a skin graft. After the preliminary perineal and rectovaginal septal dissection, the mobilized segment of gastrointestinal tract is brought down to the introitus with its mesenteric blood supply intact; the upper end is closed, and the lower end is sutured to the perineal skin edges.

4. Various sliding and pedicled skin flaps transported from the perineum and thighs and then sutured in place in the previously dissected space between bladder and rectum.

5. Method of Frank, in which simple pressure at the proper perineal site is used to form a skin pit slowly. By means of a bluntly rounded, solid tube of plastic or metal, the patient gradually produces progressively deeper indentation of the skin by daily pressure for several months until a reasonably satisfactory, functioning vaginal canal is created. Progressively larger vaginal molds are used and could be left in the indented neovagina or pit each night in addition to manual pressure dilatation several times a day. Although successful in a few, this method has not proved feasible for most patients. However, it is worth trying before embarking on surgery, especially if the patient is not ready or has no need for sexual activity as yet.

Congenital Vaginal Atresia. Although seen rather infrequently, membranous or partial fibrous obliteration (congenital vaginal atresia) may occur at various levels of the vaginal canal. The manifestations and physical findings may be indistinguishable from those of either imperforate hymen or congenital absence of the vagina, and the final differential diagnosis may depend entirely on the findings at the time of surgical exposure.

Double or Septate Vagina. Double or septate vagina rarely if ever occurs in the absence of one of the uterine duplications (usually uterus didelphys) and is discussed later.

Hypospadias. Female hypospadias due simply to faulty urogenital sinus development is rare, as are congenital urethrovaginal and rectovaginal fistulas, which presumably arise through similar mechanisms. However, a characteristic type of hypospadias is encountered in association with congenital adrenal hyperplasia and is discussed with that entity.

Uterotubal Anomalies (Müllerian Duct Origin)

Uterotubal anomalies of müllerian duct origin are frequently accompanied by congenital anomalies of the urinary tract (e.g., double ureters, absent kidney), but the gonads are usually normal.

Failure of Formation

UNILATERAL ABSENCE. With unilateral absence (uterus unicornis), the vagina and cervix are invariably normal, but the uterus possesses only one cornu and one tube; and usually only one ovary is present.

BILATERAL ABSENCE. Bilateral absence may be complete or partial [congenital absence of the uterus and vagina (except the lower third), with or without rudimentary tubes, and usually with normal ovaries]. Although the presence of normal ovaries ensures normal female secondary sex characteristics, obviously these patients suffer from primary amenorrhea. Before the menarche, it may be impossible to distinguish such patients from those with simple congenital vaginal absence, and laparoscopy and or laparotomy may be necessary to establish the diagnosis. In the absence of a utuerus, it is usually prudent to delay construction of an artificial vagina until sexual activity is contemplated.

Congenital absence of the cervix, with an otherwise normal uterus and a normal vagina, is a rare anomaly. It actually represents cervical atresia due to failure of the normal process of canalization. The clinical picture is one of pseudoprimary amenorrhea, with the appearance of cyclic, monthly bouts of abdominal pain and the eventual development of a hematometrium behind the obstruction produced by the absence of a normal cervix. As the retained menstrual secretions accumulate, a palpable suprapubic mass becomes evident. Hematosalpinges may also develop,

and associated pelvic endometriosis has been reported, presumable secondary to tubal reflux and intraperitoneal spillage of viable endometrial cells (Chap. 12). This developmental disorder was formerly treated by hysterectomy, but successful operative correction has been reported in a few cases by creating a fistula between the endometrial cavity and the vagina below it and then allowing the fistulous tract to epithelialize and heal over a rubber or polyethylene plastic tube.

Failure of Fusion, or Imperfect Fusion. Failure of fusion, or imperfect fusion, constitutes the largest group of müllerian duct anomalies, the so-called duplications, or double uterus. Although a number of nomenclatures and systems of classification have been devised, the following seems simple, accurate, descriptive, and most helpful, particularly with reference to selection of proper surgical treatment.

DOUBLE UTERUS (SYMMETRICAL DUPLICATIONS)

1. Externally unified, with two internal chambers formed by an intracavity septum
   a. Uterus subseptus (subseptate uterus) (Fig. 8-4)
   b. Uterus septus (septate uterus with or without a double or septate vagina) (Fig. 8-4)
2. Externally divided, with two cavities formed by two hemiuteri
   a. Uterus arcuatus (arcuate uterus or heart-shaped uterus often of no significance) (Fig. 8-4)
   b. Uterus bicornis unicollis (bicornuate uterus with a single cervix) (Fig. 8-4)
   c. Uterus bicornis bicollis (didelphys); double uterus and double cervix with a double or septate vagina frequently present (Fig. 8-4)

ASYMMETRIC DUPLICATIONS. With an asymmetric duplication, the embryologic development of one müllerian duct proceeds along normal lines, but on the opposite side there is arrested or imperfect development at some phase in the evolution of the upper portion as well as a variable degree of failure of fusion at the level of the uterus. It results in the development of a rudimentary hemiuterus or horn; the vagina

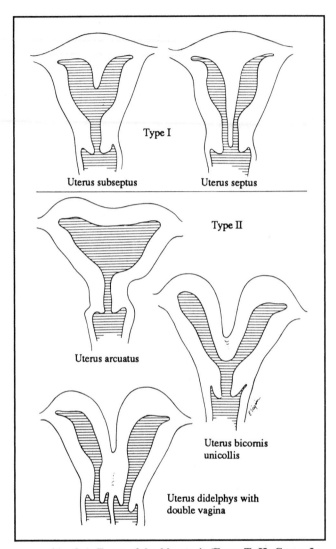

Fig. 8-4. Types of double uteri. (From T. H. Green Jr. Gynecology. In G. L. Nardi and G. D. Zuidema [eds.], *Surgery: A Concise Guide to Clinical Practice* [4th ed.]. Boston: Little, Brown, 1982.)

and cervix are usually normal. These rudimentary horns may vary considerably in size as well as the nature of their communication with the normal horn, or definitive uterus and cervix. In some instances the connecting lumen is tiny; in others it is totally absent (no communicating rudimentary horn). If the rudimentary horn is small and communicates by a wide opening with the uterus, it may remain totally asymptomatic and unsuspected throughout the life of the individual. If it is large enough to permit the implanta-

tion and growth of an early pregnancy, a surgical emergency may arise during the childbearing age owing to progressive distention and the inevitable rupture and hemorrhage that often follows—in a sense, a form of ectopic pregnancy. A similar acute abdominal emergency may arise in connection with a rudimentary horn that lacks an adequate communication with the main uterus, cervix, and vagina. Distention and ultimate rupture secondary to the accumulation of menstrual secretions in the postmenarchal female may occur. This mechanism may also be responsible for patients having progressively increasing dysmenorrhea and the gradual development of a "lateral pelvic mass" or "uterine tumor." This condition must be borne in mind in the differential diagnosis of either of these clinical pictures in young women.

SYMPTOMS OF DUPLICATIONS. Approximately 25 percent of women with the various uterine duplications have no symptoms whatsoever, exhibiting a normal menstrual pattern, normal fertility, and no complicated pregnancies or deliveries. Far more often, however, symptoms appear after the menarche and tend to increase in severity. The more commonly encountered manifestations include dysmenorrhea, menorrhagia, irregular bleeding, dyspareunia, infertility, the occasional surgical emergency mentioned earlier, and repeated bouts of pelvic inflammation secondary to hematometrium and hematosalpinx in a rudimentary horn. Perhaps the most common complications that immediately suggest the possible existence of a uterine duplication are repeated abortions, miscarriages or premature deliveries, and difficult labors with malpositions, dystocia, and postpartum hemorrhage. Such a history strongly indicates the need for appropriate studies to confirm or rule out the presence of a uterotubal anomaly.

DIAGNOSIS OF DUPLICATIONS. A history of repeated abortions and menstrual disorders and discomfort may be the initial clue. Physical examination, if carefully done, should certainly reveal the presence of uterus didelphys and a bicornuate uterus. The presence of a rudimentary horn is sometimes detected on bimanual pelvic examination, particularly if the index of suspicion is high. The externally unified, septate uterus obviously cannot be recognized in this way.

In most cases, however, definite and anatomically precise diagnosis depends entirely on the findings by hysterosalpingography and, more recently, vaginal sonography. Actual radiographic visualization of the anatomic configuration of the uterus and tubes can invariably establish the presence and nature of the anomaly, except in the case of a rudimentary horn that does not communicate with the main uterine cavity. Here, in the face of symptoms, exploratory laparotomy may be necessary before a definite diagnosis can be made.

It is essential to include intravenous pyelography in the total diagnostic evaluation to discover any of the frequently associated urinary tract anomalies. Often no treatment for the urologic abnormality is indicated or necessary, but it is nevertheless important to be aware of its presence.

TREATMENT OF DUPLICATIONS. Symmetric duplications of all types can nearly always be corrected by metroplasty using the unification operation of Strassman or modifications of this procedure, including the Tompkins procedure or the Jones variations. As depicted in Figure 8-5, the separate horns are united by a plastic surgical procedure, and any septum present in the fundus, cervix, or vagina is divided or resected. It should be emphasized that no corrective surgery should ever be undertaken until endocrine or metabolic causes for menstrual disorders, infertility, and repeated abortions have been completely ruled out. The results with regard to relief of symptoms, improvement in fertility, and reduction in fetal mortality have been highly satisfactory. In Strassman's series of 128 operated patients, only 4 percent had carried a pregnancy to term prior to corrective surgery, the abortion or miscarriage rate having been 70 percent and the incidence of premature deliveries 15 percent. After the plastic unification operation, however, 85 percent carried pregnancies to term, and the incidence of abortion was only 12 percent. Most of these patients can be delivered vaginally safely and easily, despite the previous rather extensive uterine surgery, provided there are no other contraindications to vaginal delivery. In Strassman's own patients, 85 percent were subsequently delivered vaginally, and there were no cases of uterine rupture and no maternal deaths.

In the case of asymmetric duplications, the symptomatic rudimentary horn should be totally excised; unification procedures are usually difficult or impossible and unnecessary, as the larger hemiuterus is nearly always functioning normally and capable of carrying a normal pregnancy to term.

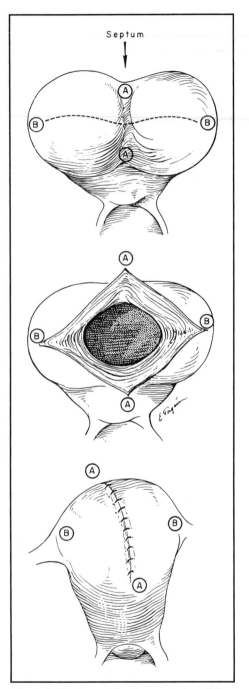

Fig. 8-5. Uterine unification operation of Strassman. (From T. H. Green Jr. Gynecology. In G. L. Nardi and G. D. Zuidema [eds.], *Surgery: A Concise Guide to Clinical Practice* [4th ed.]. Boston: Little, Brown, 1982.)

Obviously, simple resection is all that is required in the case of vaginal or cervical septa unaccompanied by any uterine abnormality. In asymptomatic patients having uterus bicornis bicollis (double uterus and double cervix) and who do not have recurrent abortions or are able to carry their pregnancy satisfactorily, metroplasty is not indicated; the vaginal septum, however, if present, requires simple resection.

Hypoplasia of the Uterus (Infantile or Juvenile Uterus)

Hypoplasia of the uterus is often more apparent than real and is probably not a true anomaly. It is sometimes, but by no means always, associated with relative infertility and various menstrual disorders. Such a diagnosis has customarily been made in the past when a tiny uterus with a cervical-fundal length ratio of 2:1 or 1:1 was encountered, instead of the normal 1:2 ratio in the mature adult female. Its significance, if any, is debatable. Most often, it is simply a reflection of ovarian inadequacy. Uterine hypoplasia can be corrected with estrogen replacement or supplementation if the patient has inadequate ovarian function.

Congenital Absence or Hypoplasia of the Ovary

Bilateral absence of the ovaries is rare. Occasionally women are encountered in whom there is unilateral absence of the ovary, and it is nearly always associated with absence of the fallopian tube on the same side, with a normal uterus and normal adnexa on the opposite side. Presumably, an embryonic vascular accident of some type during gonadal descent best explains this abnormality, which is usually of no clinical significance.

Exstrophy of the Bladder

Although the genital tract in females is usually entirely normal, exstrophy of the bladder, which is primarily a musculoskeletal and urologic anomaly, results in a shift of the vaginal canal anteriorly into the suprapubic area. There is also poor support due to absence of the musculature of the lower abdominal wall and pelvic floor. The uterine and vaginal prolapse that develops may require surgical correction.

ANOMALIES DUE TO GENETIC OR FETAL ENDOCRINE DISORDERS: INTERSEX PROBLEMS

With rapid advances in genetics, endocrinology, and molecular biology, many of our concepts concerning intersex problems need to be reexamined. The old terms true hermaphroditism and female and male pseudohermaphroditism have lost much of their significance and nearly all their meaning with respect to clinical management of these conditions. The qualifying adjectives male and female could be eliminated, because it is apparent that these individuals are often genetically and gonadally neither basically male nor basically female but are in fact something in between, having too many or too few sex chromosomes to be called more one than the other with accuracy.

Therefore the common intersex problems of genetic origin are presented as a group of separate syndromes, in most instances now eponyms, followed by the known fetal endocrine-metabolic disorders, testicular feminization syndrome, and congenital adrenal hyperplasia. Where applicable, the old hermaphroditically oriented nomenclature formerly used is indicated in parentheses after the name of the syndrome or disorder, primarily to serve as a point of reference for correlation with the older literature as well as with current and future communications in which the old terminology may continue to be employed.

Genetic Disorders Due to Sex Chromosome Abnormalities

Gonadal Dysgenesis (The Broad Spectrum). With normal gonadal genesis, the XX sex chromosome constitution is accompanied by the development of normal ovaries and a normal female genital tract and phenotype; the XY sex chromosome constitution is accompanied by the development of normal testes and a normal male genital tract and phenotype. A variety of abnormal sex chromosomal patterns lead to different degrees of abnormal gonadal develop-

ment, or gonadal dysgenesis, the spectrum of which ranges from mere vestigial streaks of primitive stroma (usually accompanied by an XO sex chromosomal complement) to structures that may be thought of as hypoplastic ovaries (in association with abnormal "female" types of sex chromosome constitution, e.g., X–abnormal X and various mosaics such as XO/XX or XO/XX/XXX) or that may more appropriately be viewed as dysgenetic testes (in association with abnormal "male" types of sex chromosome patterns, e.g., X–abnormal Y and various mosaics such as XO/XY or XO/XYY). Thus individuals with gonadal dysgenesis may have been potentially either female or male from a sex chromosomal-genetic standpoint. However, a normally functioning testis is essential for repression of müllerian activity and development of the male genital tract and phenotype; and in its absence—and regardless of whether normal ovarian tissue is present—the development of the genital tract and the body configuration or phenotype proceeds along feminine lines. Thus with rare exceptions (some patients with mixed gonadal dysgenesis and some with dysgenetic male pseudohermaphroditism), patients with the various forms of gonadal dysgenesis are generally phenotypic females, which is of obvious importance to the gynecologist. Only the more frequently encountered major forms of gonadal dysgenesis are discussed, as the more obscure variants are rare.

Turner's Syndrome (Gonadal Dysgenesis). Turner's syndrome, formerly termed ovarian agenesis, is the most common clinical form of gonadal dysgenesis, occurring about once in every 10,000 normal female births. In this disorder there is complete aplasia, with all germ cells absent and no development of either the cortical or the medullary components of the gonads; the latter are represented only by thin streaks of fibrous connective tissue in the broad ligaments, the *streak gonads.* The presence of streak gonads is the characteristic feature of all forms of gonadal dysgenesis. In the case of Turner's syndrome, the accompanying short stature and frequently associated spectrum of congenital anomalies outside the pelvis set it apart as a distinct, readily recognizable clinical entity.

The genetic abnormality in Turner's syndrome involves either complete absence or partial deletion of one X chromosome. It is now known that loss of the short arm of one X chromosome is the specific cause of the short stature and possibly a contributing factor to the other congenital malformations.

Turner's syndrome (and, much less often, some of the other variants of the abnormality of gonadal dysgenesis) and testicular feminization (see below) are responsible for approximately 50 percent of all cases of primary amenorrhea in apparent females. The importance of performing a buccal smear for the determination of somatic nuclear sex chromatin type in any patient whose chief complaint is primary amenorrhea is therefore obvious: As previously noted, the most common chromosomal pattern (in 60 to 80 percent) associated with Turner's syndrome is 45,XO, yielding a negative sex chromatin pattern. In the other 20 to 40 percent, the pattern is either 46,X–abnormal X or a variety of mosaic types (e.g., XO/XX, XO/X–abnormal X), and the nuclear sex chromatin pattern is positive. However, the nuclear sex chromatin smear may yield clues to the presence of an abnormal X: Barr bodies that are either smaller or larger than normal or a chromatin count that is intermediate between normal male (less than 2 percent) and normal female (more than 20 percent). The chromosomal pattern for the testicular feminization syndrome is always a normal 46,XY; therefore it too is accompanied by a negative sex chromatin pattern. The two syndromes are usually readily distinguished from one another on more or less obvious clinical points but can be precisely differentiated in doubtful cases by chromosome karyotyping and fluorescence labeling of the Y chromosome if necessary. Genetically normal females with primary amenorrhea on some other basis are invariably of normal height, and the positive sex chromatin pattern of the normal female is present on buccal smear.

In addition to showing primary amenorrhea and other evidence of hypoestrogenism (e.g., lack of breast development), patients with Turner's syndrome are characteristically of short stature (most being less than 4 feet 8 inches in height). As might be predicted, the müllerian duct system is usually normally developed, with uterus, tubes, and vagina present, though small owing to lack of estrogen. However, only rudimentary fibrous tissue is present in the anatomic location normally occupied by the gonads (ovaries). In general, these individuals continue to maintain a feminine appearance, although the lack of estrogen prevents the development of adult secondary sex characteristics. Rarely, although no true gonadal tissues or germinal cells are ever present, there may be functioning hilus cells in the rudimentary fibrous tissue. In this case, hilus cell activity is occasionally sufficient to produce hirsutism and even true virilization, with clitoral enlargement and a masculine habitus. Although this situation may result in a confusing clinical picture, the basic features of the syndrome remain the same, and diagnosis is still not difficult if these basic features are integrated with the results of a chromosome karyotype and if laparoscopy (or laparotomy) reveals the typical internal genital appearance.

These patients also show a high incidence of other congenital anomalies elsewhere in the body, including webbing of the neck, *high-arched* palate, deformed ears, low posterior hairline, cubitus valgus, shield chest, coarctation of the aorta, other cardiovascular defects, and kidney malformations. With the exception of the typical short stature, these other anomalies probably arise on some basis other than the sex chromosomal aberration per se, as they are also seen in both males and females with normal sex chromosome patterns. Patients with Turner's syndrome are usually of normal intelligence.

A few cases of "unilateral gonadal dysgenesis" (female patients with many of the features of Turner's syndrome but with a streak gonad on one side and a normal or hypoplastic ovary on the other) have been reported. In all these patients there was essentially normal secondary sexual development at puberty, including the appearance of regular, ovulatory menstrual cycles. Ultimately, however, oligomenorrhea that progresses into complete, secondary amenorrhea or precocious menopause develops in most of these patients. It is also of interest that although in Turner's syndrome with the XO chromosome pattern the patients have primary amenorrhea and are sterile, a few patients with the clinical features of Turner's syndrome but with mosaic chromosome pattern XO/XX have exhibited menstrual activity and occasionally have been fertile. In an even less common variant of this disorder associated with either an XX or an XY chromosome pattern (Noonan's syndrome), the patient is relatively fertile, is often taller (e.g., 5 feet), and may have minor or no somatic abnormalities.

DIAGNOSIS. The association of short stature with primary amenorrhea and poorly developed breasts, when accompanied by webbed neck, cubitus valgus, low-set ears, and the other somatic congenital abnormalities, frequently renders the diagnosis of gonadal dysgenesis obvious on clinical grounds alone. During infancy and early childhood, the condition may also be suspected by virtue of the multiple, characteristic anomalies present and the retarded growth rate; and in newborn infants it is identified by a characteristic, diffuse lymphedema involving both upper and lower extremities. The nuclear sex chromatin pattern (usually negative) confirms it absolutely. In rare instances the sex chromatin pattern is positive owing to mosaicism such as XO/XX. Pituitary gonadatropin levels are also frequently elevated after puberty. Except for the doubtful cases, laparoscopy or laparotomy (to establish the nature of the pelvic organs and confirm the presence of gonadal agenesis) is usually not necessary.

TREATMENT. These individuals are invariably of feminine psychological orientation and have a feminine appearance and functioning vagina. Because they invariably have been or will be easily raised as females, no problem arises as to assignment of sex. Treatment by cyclic hormone therapy with estrogen and progesterone not only produces the further development of normal female secondary sexual characteristics but also results in fairly normal, although artificially induced, cyclic menstrual function. Even in the face of absolute infertility, monthly menstrual flow may be of tremendous psychological import to the young woman. The estrogen-progesterone regimen to be employed is as described in the chapter on menopause. The dose of estrogen employed may have to be increased or adjusted to a higher dose at the beginning if necessary to induce or assist with development of secondary sexual characteristics. The hormone treatment additionally protects against premature development of osteoporosis or increased risk of cardiovascular disease. However, it is essential to postpone cyclic therapy until after epiphyseal closure and maximum growth have been obtained. The use of estrogens except in small doses prior to this event leads to premature epiphyseal closure and further depression of growth in a person already tending toward short stature.

Because the risk of malignancy developing in the dysgenetic gonads associated with Turner's syndrome (streak gonads in patients with a sex chromatic complement of 45,XO/46,X–abnormal X or any form of mosaicism not involving the presence of a Y chromosome) is apparently remote, surgical removal is not necessary or indicated. However, the contrary is true for all forms of gonadal dysgenesis in which the sex chromosome constitution is XY or any form of mosaicism involving the presence of a Y chromosome (see next section).

Pure Gonadal Dysgenesis. Far less common than Turner's syndrome is the syndrome of pure gonadal dysgenesis, in which streak gonads are present in phenotypic females who are of normal height and who lack the associated congenital anomalies and other stigmata of Turner's syndrome. These patients are also of normal intelligence and have good general health. Almost all of them prove to have a 46,XY (normal male) karotype and are correspondingly chromatin-negative. Rarely, a 46,XX complement or XO/XX and other more complex types of mosaicism have been seen, so that occasional individuals with the syndrome are chromatin-positive. The multiple occurrence of the XY form of pure gonadal dysgenesis in one or more sibships in the same family has frequently been recorded. This strong familial tendency (entirely similar in nature to that noted for the testicular feminization syndrome) suggests that it is a genetic disorder transmitted by ostensibly normal female carriers, with the abnormality in either an X-linked gene or an autosomal dominant gene (abnormal autosomes have been noted in some of these patients) capable of expression only in chromosomal males. It is not known whether the abnormal genes directly suppress testis-determining loci on the Y chromosome or block some early stage of testicular development. In view of these features, the most common example of this syndrome has sometimes been termed familial XY pure gonadal dysgenesis.

DIAGNOSIS. As with Turner's syndrome, these

patients possess uteri and fallopian tubes (underdeveloped though they may be). They neither menstruate nor spontaneously undergo any pubertal changes. They completely lack any normal secondary sexual development. Pituitary gonadotropin levels are usually elevated. Their normal height and the absence of any of the other features of Turner's syndrome, together with the results of chromosomal analysis, make the distinction between the two syndromes an easy one.

At first glance, pure gonadal dysgenesis is apt to be confused with the testicular feminization syndrome. In both instances the disorders show a strong familial tendency, the general appearance is feminine, the patients are normal in height, there is failure of spontaneous menstrual function (usual reason for seeking medical attention), and the karyotype is XY, with a negative nuclear sex chromatin pattern (always with testicular feminization, almost always with pure gonadal dysgenesis). However, here again the differential diagnosis is usually made readily on the basis of several fundamental and obvious differences, as follows.

1. In patients with the testicular feminization syndrome, there has been complete suppression of müllerian development in the embryo, and examination discloses absence of the uterus and the fallopian tubes. Furthermore, although imperfectly developed and cryptorchid in location, functioning male gonads are present, not dysgenetic streak gonads. These imperfect testes are nevertheless capable of the normal secretion of both androgen and estrogen. However, because of the androgen insensitivity of the normal target tissues, the fetal external genital tract development is forced to proceed along feminine lines, and only the effect of estrogen is manifested clinically later, when with the onset of puberty gonadal stimulation and secretion of both androgen and estrogen ensue. Thus these patients undergo pubertal changes with normal female secondary sexual transformation, including excellent breast development, and the pituitary gonadotropin levels are normal. Furthermore, examination reveals normal vulvar and clitoral development and a normal lower vaginal tract, the result of estrogen acting on the normal female type of external genitalia formed during fetal life.

2. In contrast, in patients with pure gonadal dysgenesis, the uterus and fallopian tubes, though hypoplastic and infantile in type, can always be found on examination, and artificial menstrual flow can be induced by cyclic hormone administration. Obviously, the fundamental and most distinguishing feature is the presence of the dysgenetic or streak gonads, which consist of undifferentiated embryonic stroma totally lacking in normal germ cells or ovarian or testicular elements. Therefore such gonads are incapable of the estrogen (or androgen) secretion required to initiate normal pubertal events. These patients never undergo spontaneous puberty, and they exhibit minimal or complete lack of breast development. The basically female external genitalia remain infantile, but many of these patients tend toward a eunuchoid body build and frequently show mild degrees of virilization, with clitoral hypertrophy and a masculine type of hirsutism. The latter features are believed due to activity of the hilar Leydig cells usually present in dysgenetic gonads, as these virilizing manifestations tend to regress following removal of the streak gonads and institution of cyclic estrogen-progesterone therapy. Laparotomy is usually necessary for confirmation of the presence of streak gonads as well as for proper treatment of the patient.

TREATMENT. Once the diagnosis has been tentatively established, the first step in treatment involves laparotomy to confirm the diagnosis definitely and to remove the abnormal streak gonads completely, usually with the accompanying fallopian tubes. Removal is strongly indicated because of the frequent presence, or subsequent development, of malignancy in dysgenetic gonads, especially in patients with an XY chromosomal complement of any form of mosaicism involving the presence of a Y chromosome. Estimates of the incidence of malignant change have varied between 30 to 50 percent or higher. Gonadoblastomas and dysgerminomas, the tumors most often encountered, are frequently bilateral. Bilateral gonadectomy and salpingectomy, preserving the uterus, are also helpful in that they remove the source of hilar Leydig cell activity and therefore usually cause at least partial regression of any tendency to hirsutism or virilization present. Preservation of the uterus may provide an opportunity for applying the new developing technology of artificial reproduction, i.e., ovum or embryo donation and transfer to the remaining uterus with exogenous hormone support. This procedure has been successfully carried out in a few patients with premature ovarian failure. After the gonadectomy, cyclic estrogen-progesterone therapy (see details in Chapter 23) is instituted to promote normal female secondary sexual development. With the uterus still present and intact, the resulting artificial menstrual cycles may offer important psychological benefits to these young patients. Because they have invariably been reared as females, there is no problem in gender assignment and gender identity. Except for the infertility, they are able psychologically, physiologically, and anatomically to function as normal adult females. Any abnormal uterine bleeding in these patients should be promptly investigated.

Mixed Gonadal Dysgenesis and Dysgenetic Male Pseudohermaphroditism. Mixed gonadal dysgenesis and dysgenetic male pseudohermaphroditism are the two remaining, somewhat similar and obviously closely related forms within the broad spectrum of gonadal dysgenesis so far identified. Each is rare. With mixed gonadal dysgenesis, a streak gonad is found on one side and a poorly developed dysgenetic testis on the other. With dysgenetic male pseudohermaphroditism, bilateral dysgenetic testes are present. Thus from the gonadal standpoint, these abnormalities are intermediate between gonadal dysgenesis, with bilateral streak gonads on the one hand and true hermaphroditism with normal testicular and ovarian tissue on the other. As has been found true for all dysgenetic testicular tissue, gonadal tumors frequently develop in these patients.

Testicular development is abnormal with both disorders; and although the dysgenetic testes are capable of secreting androgen, the testicular inducer (müllerian-inhibiting factor) is deficient, either in amount or embryonic timing. Hence müllerian duct suppression is minimal or absent, and wolffian duct stimulation as well as masculinization of the external genital tract are incomplete. Almost all these patients have a uterus and at least one fallopian tube, although occasionally a vas deferens is present on one side. At birth, the par-

tially masculinized external genitalia vary from an essentially female type, with clitoral hypertrophy, to an essentially male type, with or without hypospadias and cryptorchidism. At puberty, almost all these patients undergo further virilization, with a masculine type of hirsutism, deep voice, and phallic enlargement. Clinically, these patients are thus either first recognized as newborns with ambiguous sexual development or are seen later in adolescence because of primary amenorrhea, virilism, or both.

Both disorders are usually associated with XY/XO mosaicism. Hence the patients are invariably chromatin-negative, a valuable diagnostic point when evaluating any patient, especially a newborn infant, who presents with ambiguous external genitalia and sexual development. When considering the two other most likely causes of sexual ambiguity, particularly in the newborn, it is helpful to remember that all patients with female pseudohermaphroditism (congenital adrenal hyperplasia in the female) and 80 percent of all true hermaphrodites are chromatin-positive. Chromosome karyotyping can confirm the true karyotype for each patient.

True Hermaphroditism. The occurrence of true hermaphroditism, or the presence of both ovarian and testicular tissue in the same individual, is rare. Such patients may be either chromatin-positive or chromatin-negative and present a chromosome pattern of either XX or XY, although the occurrence of mosaicism (e.g., XY/XO, XY/XX) has been reported in some true hermaphrodites. Only 80 percent are chromatin-positive with an apparent 46,XX karyotype. There is now good evidence that the second X chromosome in these individuals probably contains the portion of a Y chromosome carrying loci normally determining testicular differentiation and that this transfer could have taken place during the meiotic divisions of gametogenesis, when the pairing of X and Y chromosome occurs. Thus during spermatogenesis an X spermatozoon containing a testis-determining factor could result, and the resulting 46,XX zygote would have genetic material capable of inducing both ovarian and testicular development. In the case of the less common mosaic forms, it is postulated that double fertilization occurred (two spermatozoa fertilizing two ova, or one ovum and its polar body), the resulting double zygote fusing to evolve into a true hermaphrodite instead of separating to form fraternal twins of opposite sex. As a result, in these individuals either a testis or an ovotestis develops on one side and an ovary or an ovotestis on the other. Usually the gonads remain in an intraabdominal position, but occasionally a testis migrates to an inguinal or labioscrotal location. The parental choice of sex of rearing varies considerably, depending on the development of the internal and external genitalia, body type, and endocrine status. Usually a uterus is found, and at least one fallopian tube is present on the ovarian side. On the side of the testis there may be just a vas deferens, occasionally with an epididymis, or there may also be a second tube. Because the presence of functioning testicular tissue usually produces some degree of external genital tract masculinization, most of the true hermaphrodites have been reared as males. However, the external masculinization is rarely complete, and hypospadias and cryptorchidism are frequently present and serve as potential clues to the actual situation. Gynecomastia and ovulatory menstrual function usually appear at puberty in most of these patients. However, there is often nothing particularly characteristic about the obvious clinical manifestation in cases of true hermaphrodites that absolutely distinguishes them from those with more common types of ambiguous sexual differentiation due to specific sex chromosomal abnormalities or congenital fetal endocrine disorders. Hence a definite diagnosis can be made only by laparotomy (or inguinal and labioscrotal exploration in some cases), with biopsy and histologic study of gonadal tissue from any and all apparent gonads present, including careful bisection to ensure that an ovotestis is not overlooked as a result of inadequate sampling.

It is important that the disorder be recognized as soon after birth as possible, so that the optimal choice of gender can be made and appropriate therapy begun early. Further discussion of the definitive treatment of the true hermaphrodites is covered in the concluding section in this chapter, in which the general principles of management of all the conditions associated with sexual ambiguity are discussed.

Klinefelter's Syndrome. Patients with Klinefelter's syndrome are phenotypic males, and the abnormality is therefore of no immediate clinical significance to most gynecologists other than for infertility problems. It is the commonest major chromosomal anomaly in masculine-appearing individuals (about 1 in every 1000 normal male births).

The syndrome was originally thought to be due to acquired testicular atrophy, with resulting palpable small testes, sparse pubic hair, sterility, azoospermia, gynecomastia, and even eunuchoidism. The associated increased urinary excretion or elevated levels of serum pituitary gonadotropins and decreased urinary excretion of 17-ketosteroids was thought to complete the diagnostic picture. When chromosome analysis became available, all these apparent males were found to be chromatin-positive, with most having 47 chromosomes and an XXY sex chromosome pattern. In some of the others, 48,XXXY, 48,XXYY, 49,XXXXY, and various mosaic chromosome patterns have been reported. Histologically, the gonads are male in type but show atrophy and hyalinization of the seminiferous tubules with no spermatogenesis despite normal interstitial or Leydig cells, which are sometimes increased in number. Mental deficiency is frequently an associated feature, which has been demonstrated consistently for the sex chromosomal disorders that involve the presence of "too many" X chromosomes. Both external and internal genitalia are of the male type, and it is only after puberty that a tendency to eunuchoidism or even slight feminization (absent beard, high-pitched voice, gynecomastia, feminine fat distribution) occurs. Androgen therapy frequently corrects this problem and allows the individual to function normally as a male with the exception of the usually associated infertility. However, an occasional patient with an otherwise typical Klinefelter's syndrome has been fertile, possibly owing to unrecognized mosaicism, with an XY as well as an XXY cell line.

"Superfemale" Syndrome (Triple-X and Poly-X Syndromes). The apparent females in which triple-X chromosome patterns have been discovered, far from being superior examples of femininity, have tended to be sexually infantile, with amenorrhea or infertility

and underdeveloped external genitalia and breasts; they are also severely retarded mentally. In fact, most such patients have been discovered in mental institutions. The condition occurs about once in every 1000 normal female births, making it a common genetic abnormality, not accompanied by a recognizable clinical syndrome. Aside from a tendency to infantilism, the presence of the extra X chromosome does not appear to result in any major anatomic anomalies of the genital tract, presumably because of the capacity for functional suppression of X chromosomes when they are present in excess (Lyon hypothesis). This finding is in marked contrast to the severe adverse effects on embryonic development produced by autosomal trisomy.

Many of these women menstruate, though often abnormally, and some have been fertile. The extra X chromosome is apparently responsible for the subnormal intelligence. The chromosome pattern is 47,XXX (a few examples of 48,XXXX have also been reported in patients with similar clinical characteristics), and the nuclear sex chromatin pattern is positive but with two (or three) Barr bodies visible in the cells of a buccal smear.

XYY and Related YY Syndromes. Sex chromosomal surveys carried out on male populations in prisons and mental institutions have uncovered another male sex chromosomal disorder, the YY syndrome. Most have been XYY, though a few XXYY or XXXYY have been found. This chromosomal abnormality was originally linked with violent criminal and antisocial behavior, high-grade mental retardation, and excessive height (two-thirds or more of those affected were over 6 feet tall). Aside from tallness, no other distinguishing physical characteristics are usually present, though a tendency to persistent acne and a slightly increased frequency of genitourinary anomalies have been noted.

As more routine population studies are made, it becomes apparent that the YY syndrome may represent one of the more common sex chromosome disorders. The observed incidence is estimated to be 1 per 1000 live-born male infants. Although they are impulsive and overreact to both internal and external environmental stimuli (poor impulse control or decreased ability to restrain themselves), most in fact do not actually exhibit criminal or out-and-out antisocial behavior. Many are apparently of normal intelligence, and only a small percentage are confined in penal or mental institutions.

Genetic Disorders Due to Fetal Endocrine-Metabolic Abnormalities

End-Organ Resistance: Testicular Feminization Syndrome (Male Pseudohermaphroditism). Testicular feminization (androgen insensitivity) syndrome is another form of male pseudohermaphroditism, also familial in type. It is a fetal endocrine-metabolic disorder in which there is usually complete (occasionally partial) androgen insensitivity on the part of target tissues and organs that should be responding to testosterone secreted by the fetal testes. Despite a genetically normal male XY karyotype, these patients are characterized by a female phenotype, complete absence of female internal genitalia, and cryptorchid testes as gonads. The differentiation of this syndrome from XY pure gonadal dysgenesis and dysgenetic male pseudohermaphroditism has already been presented.

It is unusual for *complete testicular feminization syndrome* to be diagnosed in the neonate on routine examination, as the baby appears completely female in external appearance; the exception is if a 46,XY karyotype has been obtained through prenatal genetic amniocentesis. Sometimes an inguinal hernia with a testis in an apparent female infant suggests the diagnosis. In cases presenting later, the adult is feminine in appearance, of normal height, has normal fat deposits and breast tissue, has sparse or absent pubic and axillary hair, and exhibits normal female external genitalia but a shorter than normal vagina ending in a blind pouch. The uterus and tubes are absent, and bilateral testes may be found in the inguinal canals or intraabdominally in the ovarian fossa. These testes show tubules lined with immature germ cells and Sertoli cells, but there are disproportionately more Leydig cells. The chromosome karyotype is 46,XY. There is a strong familial tendency, and therefore several "sisters" may have the condition. The disorder is probably genetic in origin, though a definite sex chromosomal disorder has not been identified. A negative nuclear sex chromatin pattern plus the clinical picture suggest the diagnosis, but confirmation by laparotomy is usually necessary.

Both androgens and estrogens are secreted by the gonads of these patients, and adrogen levels are as high as those of normal male controls. Müllerian inhibition is complete owing to end-organ resistance to testosterone. The end-organ resistance is due to *absence of the androgen receptors* (receptors for dihydrotestosterone) in the target tissues (wolffian duct structures—vas deferens, seminal vesicles, epididymis—as well as prostate, penis, breast, hair follicles, larynx, and so on). In the face of androgen insensitivity in the target tissues, the effect of estrogen secretion dominates the picture and feminization results.

A more rare defect is *postreceptor resistance* to dihydrotestosterone in the target tissues, where the clinical picture may be identical with that of the complete testicular feminization syndrome or varying degrees of it. Both types, with an absence of androgen receptors and postreceptor resistance, have normal levels of the enzyme 5α-reductase in the genital tissues. Morphologically and psychologically, these individuals are oriented as females. Except for absolute infertility, they can function satisfactorily as females and are usually anxious to do so. Because of the significant incidence (4 to 10 percent or more) of malignant change in these "imperfect testes," the abnormal gonads should be removed surgically after puberty, following which these patients require cyclic estrogen therapy. The vaginal pouch is usually of adequate length for satisfactory function and elongates further with regular intercourse, so vaginal reconstruction is rarely necessary.

Incomplete testicular feminization syndrome (Reifenstein's syndrome) is a variant of the testicular feminization syndrome. Patients with incomplete testicular feminization syndrome commonly present as a male neonate with perineoscrotal hypospadias. Cryptorchidism is common; and although they contain normal Leydig cells, the testes are usually small. The clinical picture is varied, ranging from gynecomastia and azoospermia to the presence of a pseudovagina.

After puberty, these patients have elevated levels of testosterone, LH, and estradiol, findings similar to those seen with the complete form of testicular feminization syndrome. The end-organ primary abnormality appears to be a quantitative defect in androgen receptors. Interestingly, a relative deficiency of androgen receptors may also be responsible for some types of simple hypospadias. Most patients with Reifenstein's syndrome are psychosexually male and should be accordingly assigned to this gender for management. Treatment may therefore involve repair of hypospadias, orchiopexy, gonadectomy, androgen therapy, and occasionally mastectomy. Often sexual function can be restored, although sterility remains irreversible.

In the past, *5α-reductase deficiency* was thought to be responsible for the classic complete testicular feminization syndrome, but it is now clear that at birth subjects with this enzyme deficiency have a markedly bifid scrotum that appears labia-like, a clitoris-like phallus, and a urogenital sinus with a blind vaginal pouch. Again the testes may be in the abdomen, inguinal canal, or scrotum. Whereas müllerian structures are inhibited, wolffian ducts develop normally. After puberty, testosterone levels increase normally as for males, the phallus elongates, the scrotum becomes rugose and pigmented, and in most patients the testis descends into the scrotum. Penile erections are attained, and ejaculation occurs through the perineoscrotal urethral orifice. Sizable numbers of such patients have been found in Santo Domingo. Although reared as females originally, they undergo behavioral changes to become males after puberty, thus underscoring the powerful effects of male androgen levels and the culturally acceptable psychosexual transformation from female to male concomitant with a phenotypic transformation. With the familial types, the 5α-reductase deficiency is thought to be due to the homozygous state of an autosomal recessive gene manifested only in males. It is important to recognize this entity, infrequent as the condition may be, because of the noninvasive nature of the management pending the eventual normal transformation to a male and the need not to assign female gender with removal of the phallus. The hypospadias may need surgical repair, later if necessary.

Congenital Adrenal Hyperplasia, or Congenital Adrenogenital Syndrome (Female Pseudohermaphroditism). Although congenital adrenal hyperplasia may affect males (in whom it produces a precocious and overvirilizing type of masculine puberty), it is most commonly seen and recognized in newborn females. When it is mild in degree, the gross anatomic genital abnormalities may be so minimal that the condition is not recognized until later in childhood or at puberty. An acquired form that develops later in life exists but is more often due to tumor than to hyperplasia. The disorder is important because it is responsible for about 50 percent of all cases of apparently ambiguous sexual differentiation and because it is nearly always correctable.

There is a strong familial tendency, and the condition is genetic in origin. The sex chromosome and nuclear sex chromatin patterns are always normal female 46,XX and chromatin-positive; when encountered in males, the 46,XY and chromatin-negative patterns are just as uniformly present.

At birth, the characteristic anatomic abnormality consists in clitoral enlargement, sometimes to the point of simulating the penis of a newborn male, with a varying amount of apparent hypospadias, so that the urethra opens directly into the vaginal canal at a level somewhat higher than the usual site of the normal female urethral meatus, creating the effect of a partial urogenital sinus (Fig. 8-6). It is often accompanied by varying degrees of vulvar ("labioscrotal") fusion. Rarely, the urethra is actually phallic in type, and the infant or child may be mistakenly assumed to be a bilaterally cryptorchid male unless a nuclear sex chromatin study is done. The uterus, tubes, ovaries, and upper vagina are invariably normal, so it is obvious that an abnormal androgenic hormone stimulus during the critical phase of the development of the external urogenital tract has been at work in an otherwise normally developing female embryo. If untreated, the newborn child subsequently exhibits manifestations of continuing excessive androgenic stimulation: increased growth rate, increasing signs of virilization including progressively enlarging phallus formation or clitoral hypertrophy, and markedly increased urinary 17-ketosteroid excretion.

Because the gonads are normal ovaries histologically and functionally, the source of the androgens in the spontaneous form of the disease is known to be the fetal adrenals, which lack one of the hydroxylating enzymes necessary to complete glucocorticoid biosynthesis. The more common enzyme deficiencies include 21-hydroxylase deficiency (commonest form) and 11β-hydroxylase deficiency, but enzyme deficiencies at each step of the biosynthetic pathway for corticosteroid have been described (Fig. 8-7). Because of the low levels of glucocorticoids, the fetal pituitary compensates by secreting increasingly larger amounts of adrenocorticotropic hormone (ACTH). Because the adrenals are unable to produce corticosteroids, hyperplasia ensues, with increased production of other adrenal steroids, particularly precursors or compounds with androgenic activity (Fig. 8-8). Apparently this sequence usually occurs or has its maximum effect during the maturation of the external urogenital tract but after the normal gonadal and müllerian duct development has taken place. After birth, the abnormal androgen production continues to increase, with progressively more pronounced virilization of the infant.

Dangerous electrolyte disturbances of a salt-losing type may also develop in these infants having the 21-hydroxylase enzyme deficiency, an enzyme required for the production of desoxycorticosterone and aldosterone, which are important to electrolyte metabolism. An addisonian type of crisis is occasionally encountered, with vomiting, diarrhea, dehydration, and circulatory collapse in acute adrenal insufficiency with the typical low sodium, high potassium serum electrolyte disturbance. Because such a course of events is often fatal, it is important to bear this possibility in mind in newborns with this genital anomaly so as to anticipate and prevent it if possible and to treat it early, correctly, and vigorously should it appear.

DIAGNOSIS. The diagnosis is based on the presence of the typical anatomic configuration in a female infant showing a normal positive nuclear sex chromatin pattern on buccal smear and with increased urinary excretion of 17-ketosteroids, which, however, are not consistently increased until after two to three weeks of life. Alternatively, elevated levels of serum 17α-hydroxyprogesterone are detected. The chromosome

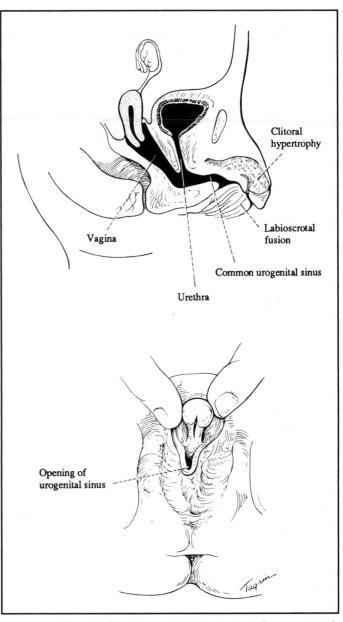

Fig. 8-6. Typical urogenital tract anomaly encountered in congenital adrenal hyperplasia of the female (female pseudohermaphroditism).

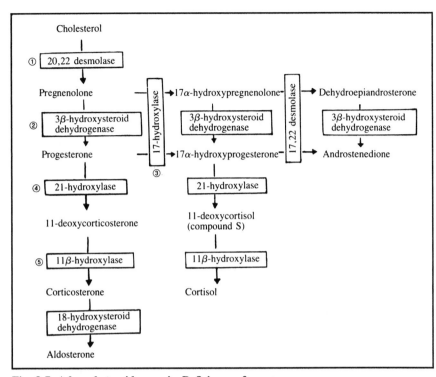

Fig. 8-7. Adrenal steroidogenesis. Deficiency of an enzyme (1–5) results in congenital adrenal hyperplasia. The most common deficiencies are 21-hydroxylase (4) and 11 β-hydroxylase (5).

karyotype is normal (46,XX). Cystoscopic examination of both urethra and vagina and the vaginal introduction of radiopaque dye for the purpose of radiographic visualization for definite confirmation of the presence of a vagina are frequently helpful maneuvers for identifying the characteristic external urogenital anomaly in newborn infants and young children. In the older child, pelvic or rectal examination can confirm the presence of an essentially normal vagina, cervix, and uterus; or if a small vaginal transducer is available, vaginal sonography may confirm the presence of a uterus. In the face of this clinical picture, laparotomy to determine the status of the gonads or internal genital tract is rarely necessary.

TREATMENT. Treatment with cortisone or any of the related corticosteroid preparations now available is usually dramatically successful. The administered corticoids substitute for what is normally produced by the adrenals. The excessive ACTH formation and adrenal stimulation are suppressed, and the production of androgens promptly falls to normal levels (Fig. 8-8). If the 17-ketosteroid excretion level or appropriate plasma androgen level does not fall rapidly, the possibility that an adrenocortical tumor is present should be considered, although this occurrence is rare. Under such circumstances, a computed tomography scan or magnetic resonance imaging of the adrenal may reveal the tumor. If an associated electrolyte disturbance is also present, it must be corrected by administration of desoxycorticosterone; and careful attention must be paid to the sodium, potassium, and fluid balance in these young, particularly vulnerable patients. Continued lifelong maintenance on cortisone results in subsequent normal growth and development, normal puberty and adolescence, and continued normal ovarian function in adult life. Ovulation, normal estrogen and progesterone production, fertility, normal pregnancy, and delivery can be anticipated in most instances, though the menarche is somewhat delayed in some patients.

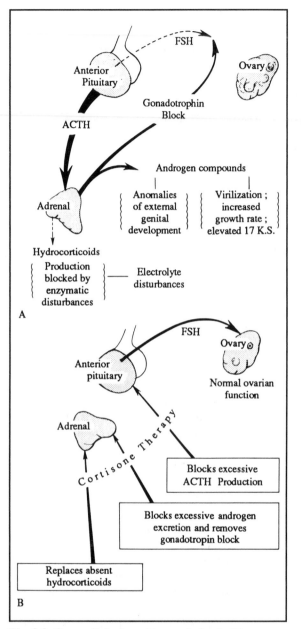

A

B

Fig. 8-8. Congenital adrenal hyperplasia. A. Biochemical mechanisms involved in pathogenesis. B. Biochemical mechanisms involved in successful therapy.

The external genital anomaly itself can of course be corrected only by an appropriate operative procedure. The procedure ordinarily consists in relatively minor local surgery and usually includes total resection of the phallus and a simple vulvovaginal plastic operation to restore the normal female relation between the urethra and the vaginal canal. The best psychological results for both the patient and her family are achieved when the operation is performed early, usually at around 18 months of age, before the child develops an awareness of the genitalia and gender role and after she has grown sufficiently to permit easy identification of the vaginal canal, so that it can be properly exteriorized at the time of surgery. In cases of clitoromegaly sufficiently large to require reduction but with no involvement of the urethral opening or introitus, recession of the clitoris without resecting it can be readily undertaken by surgery. This technique has an apparent advantage of leaving clitoral sensation intact.

Iatrogenic Masculinization of the Female Fetus. An iatrogenic type of "female pseudohermaphroditism" is being increasingly recognized. The condition is characterized by the presence of the identical external genital anomalies seen with the true congenital form of adrenal hyperplasia but with a different etiologic mechanism. Adrenal function is entirely normal. The abnormal androgens exposed to during early fetal life are certain steroid hormones with androgenic activity given to the mother during the early months of the pregnancy. Testosterone and certain progestational agents employed in the management of women for threatened or habitual abortion given during the first two to three months after conception have been incriminated. These progestational and androgenic agents include compounds such as members of the 17-ethinyl testosterone groups, nortestosterone derivatives such as norethindrone acetate, and compounds such as danazol used for treatment of endometriosis. Rarely, a maternal arrhenoblastoma or other androgen-producing ovarian tumor, luteoma, theca lutein cyst, or virilizing adrenal tumor results in masculinization of the female fetus through the same mechanisms.

These iatrogenically masculinized infants do not show any further tendencies to virilization or abnormalities of growth and development, nor is there any disturbance of electrolyte balance after they are born and the source of the androgenic substance is removed. The diagnosis rests primarily on finding normal urinary 17-ketosteroid excretion or plasma androgen levels, a normal female sex chromatin pattern, and of course a history of prenatal administration of any of the compounds mentioned. Because adrenal function is normal, no hormonal therapy of any kind is necessary. Normal subsequent growth and development are ensured. Again, minor vaginal plastic surgery is indicated to correct the external urogenital anomalies.

It should be emphasized that only a few women receiving prenatal steroid therapy give birth to infants with masculinized external genitalia. It is not clear whether this finding simply reflects the critical role of dosage and timing or there is some abnormality of maternal metabolism or placental permeability to these steroid compounds. At any rate, the possibility should by no means be construed as a contraindication to the **proper use** of supportive steroid hormone therapy during pregnancy in diabetic women or other women with true progestational deficiencies who might otherwise not carry successfully to term. If indicated, it is more prudent to give progesterone rather than a synthetic progestin.

Management of Intersex Problems

It is apparent that several disorders may result in ambiguous sexual development. They include true hermaphrodites, most patients with mixed gonadal dysgenesis, most patients with dysgenetic male pseudohermaphroditism, most patients with congenital adrenal hyperplasia (female pseudohermaphroditism), and some patients with the testicular feminization syndrome (familial male pseudohermaphroditism). Once a definite diagnosis has been established, a decision regarding optimal management must be made for each patient. Except in the case of congenital adrenal hyperplasia, fertility cannot be readily restored. Thus the chief goal of treatment is to create the endocrine and anatomic foundation for as satisfactory function as possible later on as either a male or a female. The success of treatment in turn depends primarily on an

intelligent decision as to which gender should be assigned. In those with a uterus present, embryo transfer combined with hormonal support (which is still at an early stage of development) can probably offer the last hope of carrying a pregnancy.

When making sex assignment in the infant, the sex chromatin pattern (or genetic or chromosomal sex) is of little significance. Far more important is the anatomic configuration and potential functional capacity of the external genitalia.

If the anatomy is essentially male in type with an adequate phallus, regardless of the chromosomal sex the child should be reared as a male. Having reached this decision, further treatment involves removal of all ovarian tissue and any other undesirable female internal structures (it may require complete removal of all gonads in the case of ovotestis formation, though at times the testicular and ovarian components can be separately dissected and one or the other preserved). Surgical repair must also be undertaken for any external genital defects such as hypospadias or bifid scrotum that might interfere with the normal male outward appearance and function. It is important to remove all nonconforming gonadal tissue, lest it function at puberty and produce undesirable feminization or masculinization.

On the other hand, if the external genitalia are essentially female in type, with a vagina present, surgery is performed to make the internal gonadal picture conform, if possible (otherwise, gonadal removal is appropriate). A phallus, if present, should be excised and the infant raised as a female.

In either case, appropriate substitution hormone therapy (androgenic or estrogenic) is indicated at puberty to ensure the development of as nearly normal secondary sex characteristics and sexual function as possible. Ideally, the decision and necessary surgical transformations should be completed before the age of one and a half to two years. After that time, an attempt at reversal of the already parentally assigned sex of rearing, if it differs from the optimal gender role dictated by the external genital tract configuration, usually creates serious psychological problems.

In the older child or young adult, the sex of rearing or psychologically assumed gender role plays the dominant role in decisions about therapy, and attempts to reverse it should rarely if ever be made. Both surgical and hormone therapy should consist of procedures and medication that might help the patient function more effectively sexually, physically, and psychologically in the gender role already assumed.

Summary

There are basically six aspects to sex determination in the broad, total sense: the chromosomal pattern (genetic); the three morphologic factors (the status of the gonads and the anatomic configurations of the internal and external genital tracts); the endocrine pattern (hormonal status); and finally the psychological orientation (the sex of rearing or spontaneously assumed gender role). In the normal female or male, all conform with each other. In the person with an intersex problem or ambiguous sexual differentiation, one or more of these six aspects fail to conform with the others to a greater or lesser extent.

In the case of congenital adrenal hyperplasia of the female (female pseudohermaphroditism), the disharmony is often minimal: the genetic sex, internal genitalia, and gonads are normally female. Because the endocrine disorder is reversible, the hormonal status and reproductive capacity can also be brought into line with proper therapy. The external genitalia are basically female, except for the phallic enlargement, which can be corrected by simple plastic surgery. Finally, if the phallic enlargement is pronounced, medical advice and treatment are sought early. If it is not, most of these children are raised as females, and hence rarely if ever is there any psychological conflict in the matter of gender role, regardless of the age at which therapy is undertaken.

At the other extreme are the true hermaphrodites and the various other intersex disorders in which there may be profound disharmony among the six basic aspects of sex determination, with no possibility of bringing more than two or three of them into conformity and usually little hope of restoring fertility. In these situations, as already emphasized, the functional potential of the external genitalia and, if the patient is beyond 2 years of age, the psychological orientation are the two key factors to be considered when deciding on the most satisfactory permanent gender role for the patient to assume. Once this decision has been made, additional treatment is undertaken to bring as many of the other modifiable factors into conformity as possible—whether it is surgery on the gonads or internal genital tract, plastic reconstructions of the external genitalia, or hormone substitution therapy. In any case, in the older patient who has already assumed a gender role, the psychological orientation almost without exception is the sole determining factor in gender assignment, regardless of the status of the external genitalia. These basic principles apply equally to the problems of management of either "true" hermaphrodites or "pseudohermaphrodites."

These fundamental genetic disorders of ambiguous sexual development are entirely unrelated to the purely psychological disorders of sexual ambiguity such as transsexualism, transvestism, homosexuality, and neurotic or psychotic problems accompanied by confusion or anxiety regarding sexual identity. The latter occur in persons whose chromosomal, anatomic, and endocrinologic status are completely in accord and entirely consistent with one or the other sex. A detailed consideration of these purely psychological ambiguities in sexual development and role fulfillment are beyond the scope of this text but can be found in excellent monographs elsewhere.

SELECTED READINGS

Dewhurst, C. J., and Gordon, R. R. *The Intersexual Disorders.* London: Balliere, Tindall and Cassell, 1969.

Jones, H. W., and Rock, J. A. *Reparative and Constructive Surgery of the Female Genital Tract.* Baltimore: Williams and Wilkins, 1983.

Patton, G. W. The Uterus in Infertility Evaluations. In S. J. Behrman, R. W. Kistner, and G. W. Patton (Eds.), *Progress in Infertility* (3rd ed.). Boston: Little, Brown, 1988. Chap. 13, p. 197.

Simpson, J. L. Ovarian Failure (Gonadal Dysgenesis). In S. J. Behrman, R. W. Kistner, and G. W. Patton (Eds.), *Progress in Infertility* (3rd ed.). Boston: Little, Brown, 1988. Chap. 14, p. 239.

White, P. C., New, M. I., and DuPont, B. Congenital adrenal hyperplasia. *New. Engl. J. Med.* 316:1519, 1987.

Wilson, J. D., George, F. W., and Griffin, J. E. The hormonal control of sexual development. *Science* 211:1278, 1981.

9
Normal Menstrual Cycle

From menarche to menopause, disturbances in the normal physiology of the reproductive tract and its endocrine control give rise to symptoms that constitute the single most common type of problem presenting to the gynecologist. These disorders may be transient and are not necessarily life-threatening, but when they are persistent they frequently lead to excessive blood loss and secondary anemia. They also may cause serious disability and may be accompanied by infertility. It is important to establish the definitive diagnosis of menstrual disturbances as well as avoid overlooking the presence of more life-threatening organic disease arising in the genital tract or endocrine disorders of the ovaries, thyroid, adrenal, or pituitary gland.

This chapter reviews the basic physiology of the normal menstrual cycle as it relates to a fundamental understanding of the mechanism or mechanisms involved in bringing about deranged menstrual cycles and the accompanying symptoms. The next two chapters cover the main types of menstrual disorders in some detail with special emphasis on the endocrine basis of the disorder and how to employ such an understanding for diagnosis and management of the specific conditions.

A brief and somewhat oversimplified outline of the endocrine control of the reproductive system is provided primarily for a conceptual grasp of deviations from such an integrated normal physiology when attempting to understand, diagnose, and manage menstrual disturbances. For a completely integrated and harmoniously functional menstrual cycle and rhythmicity, it is necessary that the hypothalamic-pituitary-ovarian-uterine axis functions in a coordinated manner with input from other regions of the brain, the thyroid, and the adrenals.

HYPOTHALAMIC-PITUITARY-OVARIAN AXIS

The initiation of cyclic menstrual function at puberty was briefly summarized in Chapter 7. As soon as regular periodic flow has become established in a completely mature, adult pattern, the regulation of the normal cycle is under the control of neurohormonal mechanisms with its feedback systems present in the hypothalamic-pituitary-ovarian axis. The fundamental features of this regulatory system and the endometrial response patterns are illustrated in Figure 9-1.

Hypothalamus and Anterior Pituitary Gland

The anterior pituitary gland is under the control of the hypothalamus, which secretes regulatory peptides that are carried to the anterior pituitary gland via the rich vascular arcade of the hypothalamic-pituitary portal system. The median eminence in the hypothalamus consists of neural, vascular, and epithelial components. The neural component is made up of densely packed nerve endings from which all cell bodies arise in the ventral hypothalamus. These neurons may be (1) peptidergic, producing small peptides (i.e., the releasing or inhibiting factors or hormones); or (2) bioaminergic, producing amines such as dopamine and norepinephrine. The peptidergic neurons secrete the gonadotropin-releasing hormone (GnRH), which is sometimes referred to as luteinizing hormone-releasing hormone (LHRH). This peptide reaches the anterior pituitary gland to stimulate release of mainly luteinizing hormone (LH) and to a lesser extent follicle-stimulating hormone (FSH) from specialized cells referred to as gonadotropes. Thus GnRH, a decapeptide, is a chemical messenger between the cerebral cortex and the anterior pituitary gland via the hypothalamus. Similarly, the releasing factor for thyroid-stimulating hormone (TSH) known as thyrotropin-releasing factor (TRF), a tripeptide, and corticotropin-releasing factor (CRF) for andrenocorticotropin (ACTH) are secreted by the hypothalamus into the hypothalamic-hypophyseal portal system to stimulate release of their respective hormones by the anterior pituitary gland.

The release of GnRH by the hypothalamus is pulsa-

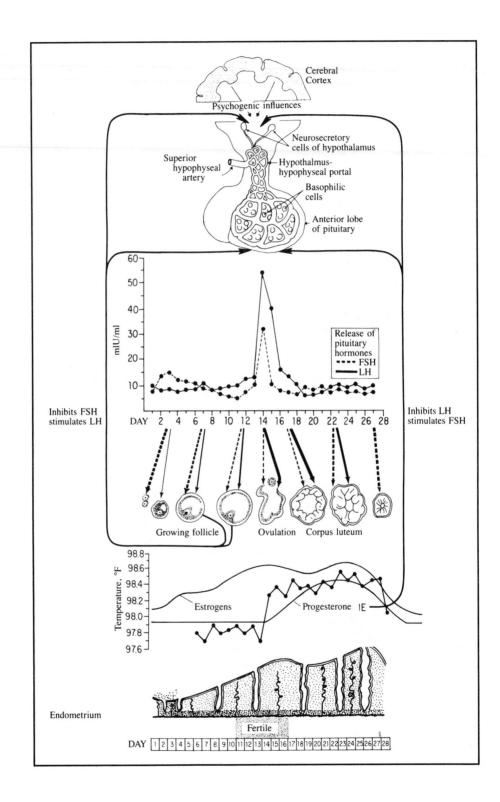

Cerebral Cortex

Psychogenic influences

Neurosecretory cells of hypothalamus

Superior hypophyseal artery

Hypothalmus-hypophyseal portal

Basophilic cells

Anterior lobe of pituitary

Inhibits FSH stimulates LH

Inhibits LH stimulates FSH

Release of pituitary hormones
---- FSH
—— LH

mIU/ml

DAY

Growing follicle

Ovulation

Corpus luteum

Temperature, °F

Estrogens

Progesterone

Endometrium

Fertile

DAY

tile, with pulses occurring every 90 minutes. This pattern leads to pulsatile release of FSH and LH. The rhythmic pulsatile release of GnRH and consequently of FSH and LH is critical to the recruitment and rate of growth of the ovarian follicles, which are essential to the normal ovulatory cycle as reflected by normal regular menstrual cycles. Loss of this synchronized rate of pulsatile stimulation leads to aberrations of the normal cycle and therefore clinical manifestations. Both normal physiology and pathophysiology of the menstrual cycle, at least in terms of central control, can be explained by mechanisms that affect the pulsatile secretion of GnRH.

The pulses of GnRH and its secretion into the tubes in the tuberoinfundibular tract and portal system appear to be directly under the influence of a dual catecholaminergic system: norepinephrine, which is facilitatory, and dopamine and serotonin, which are inhibitory. Most of the norepinephrine in the brain is synthesized in cell bodies in the mesencephalon and lower brainstem. The same cells also synthesize serotonin. Axons from these sites then transport the norepinephrine and serotonin into the medical forebrain to terminate in various brain structures including the hypothalamus.

Dopamine synthesis takes place in the cell bodies of the arcuate and periventricular nuclei. Dopamine is then transported via the tuberoinfundibular tract to the median eminence. Dopamine exerts its effect on GnRH release by suppressing GnRH activity in the arcuate nucleus but has no direct effect on pituitary secretion of LH. However, dopamine also is transported via the portal system to directly suppress pituitary secretion of prolactin.

Emotional influence, stress, light, and other cerebral factors affect the hypothalamus through the catecholaminergic system and therefore the control of the cycling center and GnRH pulses. Feedback effects of steroids such as estrogens and progesterone, produced by the ovaries as the follicles develop, affect the hypothalamus and the anterior pituitary gland on go-

nadotropin secretion. These feedback effects may be mediated also through the catecholamine system and opioid activity in the hypothalamus to effect GnRH pulsatility.

A large variety of brain peptides may function as neurotransmitters, including neurotensin, substance P, cholecystokinin, vasoactive intestinal peptide, somatostatin, and the endogenous opiates (the endorphins). Somatostatin inhibits release of growth hormone, prolactin, and thyrotropin from the pituitary gland. Endorphins are derived from the ACTH-lipotropin family of polypeptides. β-Lipotropin is a 91-amino-acid molecule that shares with ACTH a high-molecular-weight common precursor called proopiomelanocortin. Proopiomelanocortin is split into two fragments, an ACTH intermediate fragment and β-lipotropin, the latter having no opioid activity. β-Lipotropin is, however, broken down into α-melanocyte-stimulating hormone, enkephalin, and α-, γ-, and β-endorphins. Enkephalin and the α- and γ-endorphins are equipotent to morphine, and β-endorphin is five to ten times more potent. In the hypothalamus the major product is β-endorphin, located mainly in the region of the arcuate and the ventromedial nuclei.

The endogenous opioids stimulate growth hormone, prolactin, and ACTH and inhibit FSH, LH, and TSH. Opioid receptors are present on dopamine neurons. Through these receptors endogenous opioids in the hypothalamus exert their effect on dopamine and, in turn, on the pulsatility of GnRH secreted. Endogenous opioids also can directly inhibit GnRH neurons in the arcuate area. Estrogens and progesterone, through their feedback mechanisms, modulate the opioid tone and the effects of endogenous opioids on GnRH pulsatility. Thus high estrogens increase opioid tone, and progesterone stimulates release of β-endorphins, which further increase opioid tone, inhibition of the GnRH pulse, and LH secretion. Exercise and stress may exert effects on the menstrual cycle through increased secretion of endogenous opioids and their action on gonadotropins and prolactin. Endogenous opioids increase prolactin secretion through inhibition of the dopamine neurons.

Prolactin, an anterior pituitary hormone, with structural similarities to growth hormone, is now shown to be distinct and different from it. Both prolactin and

Fig. 9-1. Normal menstrual cycle. Note the suprahypothalamic (cerebral, pineal), hypothalamic, pituitary, ovarian, and endometrial interrelations.

growth hormone are produced by acidophils in the anterior pituitary gland but from separate cells. The lactotropes (acidophils secreting prolactin) constitute at least one-third of the pituitary cell population, and therefore most pituitary tumors are prolactinomas. The secretion of prolactin by the pituitary is under the inhibitory control of a prolactin-inhibiting factor (PIF), which in women is dopamine from the hypothalamus as no distinct peptide that acts as PIF has been found. Dopamine administration inhibits release of prolactin and dopamine, but no norepinephrine is present in the hypophyseal-portal blood. Dopamine agonist also suppresses prolactin secretion, whereas a dopamine receptor antagonist such as metoclopramide stimulates prolactin release. Prolactin secretion is also influenced by other neurotransmitters such as γ-aminobutyric acid, which stimulates prolactin release in humans. Serotonin receptor stimulation also leads to prolactin release, as does 5-hydroxytryptophan, a precursor of serotonin. A prolactin-releasing factor from the hypothalamus has been implicated in the release of prolactin and has been suggested to be present, but this proposal awaits confirmation.

Thyrotropin-releasing factor (TRF) from the hypothalamus not only stimulates pituitary TSH release but also prolactin secretion. The prolactin response to TRF is greater in women than men, and circulating thyroxine and triiodothyronine modulate TRF-induced prolactin release. Hypothyroidism with low thyroxine and triiodothyronine increases TRF-induced prolactin release. Thus the feedback mechanism in pituitary prolactin secretion is through a short feedback loop between dopamine and TRF in the hypothalamus and prolactin in the anterior pituitary gland.

Prolactin has a diurnal variation, with highest levels during the early morning hours and lowest between 10 AM and noon. Prolactin is released episodically, like the gonadotropins. During sleep, episodic prolactin release reaches a nadir during rapid eye movement (REM) sleep, which is dependent on catecholaminergic activity with peaks during non-REM sleep that are serotonergic-dependent.

Other physiologic factors regulating pituitary prolactin release include exercise, stress (e.g., surgery), pregnancy, puerpuerium, suckling, and parturition, all of which stimulate and increase prolactin secretion. Estrogen in sustained high levels stimulates prolactin release by both a direct effect on the growth and number of lactotropes as well as on the hypothalamus and the dopaminergic system. The hypothalamic opioids (see above) also stimulate prolactin release.

Throughout the menstrual cycle, serum prolactin levels do not show consistent differences between the follicular and luteal phases, although high luteal phase prolactin levels have been implicated as being responsible for some forms of luteal phase defect. However, prolactin response to TRF is greater during the normal luteal phase than the follicular phase. The role of prolactin on human ovarian function is not well defined, but it probably regulates ovarian steroidogenesis and modulates the action of pituitary gonadotropins on the ovary. Prolactin in high concentrations inhibits progesterone secretion in early follicular growth but in low doses enhances progesterone secretion during the luteal phase. Prolactin appears to modulate the number of LH receptors in the ovary, with suppressed prolactin levels markedly decreasing LH receptors.

Ovary

After the onset of menstruation, during the first few days of each cycle, the basophilic, or "beta," cells of the anterior pituitary gland are stimulated by GnRH to secrete increasing amounts of FSH. Primordial follicles in the ovaries are recruited in response to the FSH and develop. FSH induces growth of the follicular cells as well as LH receptors in these cells. During the spontaneous cycle of a woman, although several primordial follicles may be recruited, usually a single follicle becomes the dominant one. This dominant follicle continues to respond and progress in maturation and function. Occasionally two follicles or more are stimulated to the point of ovulation in spontaneous cycles and account for biovular twinning.

During the earliest phases of ovarian follicle response, while some growth is occurring in a number of follicles, the pituitary gonadotropes begin also to elaborate LH. Under the combined stimulation of a small amount of LH and by now the large amounts of FSH, the granulosa and theca cells begin to secrete estrogens. At first there are low levels of both estrone and estradiol, but by midcycle the levels are increasing rapidly and the estradiol/estrone ratio is markedly increased. As circulating estrogen levels rise, a reciprocal inhibition or negative feedback effect on the pituitary output of FSH comes into play. Although FSH secretion begins to decline, the pituitary continues to produce more LH because of the positive feedback effect of estrogen on pituitary secretion of LH alone. At a crucial point, approximately at or shortly before midcycle, with both estrogen and LH levels on the rise and already approaching a maximum, and with FSH well on the decline but still present in a small but critical amount, the one dominant follicle undergoes characteristic vascular, cellular, and secretory changes and moves to a position near the surface of the ovary. Thereafter ovulation is stimulated, probably by a sudden surge in pituitary LH production (and possibly FSH as well) initiated by the outpouring of LH-releasing factor elaborated by the hypothalamus.

The mechanism by which a single follicle is selected to be the dominant follicle is unknown. The remaining partially stimulated follicles simply persist in a resting state or ultimately become atretic, although they continue to secrete variable amounts of estrogen throughout the rest of the cycle.

Midcycle Gonadal Steroid Feedback

The classic concept about ovulation was that the steroid feedback centers were in the hypothalamus and that rising estrogen and progesterone levels around the midcycle exerted the positive and negative feedback effects on the hypothalamus with release of GnRH followed by gonadotropins. Findings in primates indicate that, in women, GnRH in the hypothalamus plays only a permissive role and that the center for midcycle surge of gonadotropins is in the pituitary. Therefore in women the feedback responses regulating gonadotropin levels are controlled by ovarian follicle steroid feedback on the gonadotropes of the anterior pituitary gland.

Cycle with Conception

If ovulation should be followed by conception and implantation of the fertilized ovum, placental formation proceeds. The early chorionic villi attain a functional capacity adequate for the elaboration of sufficient chorionic gonadotropin to reserve and maintain the corpus luteum in optimum secretory activity, even in the face of falling pituitary gonadotropins. This situation, in turn, prevents the onset of the expected menstruation and preserves and rapidly further modifies the endometrium into decidua favorable to the maintenance and subsequent normal development of the pregnancy. Placental gonadotropin secretion is adequate to this end within the first week of implantation. The levels of chorionic gonadotropin are thus high enough to be detectable as a positive index of pregnancy by current radioimmunoassay pregnancy tests employing specific antiserum sometimes as early as two to three days before the expected menstrual cycle, usually at the time of the missed period, and certainly a few days after missing a period.

CEREBRAL, PINEAL, THYROID, AND ADRENAL FACTORS

What has been presented thus far concerns only the basic regulatory physiology of the normal menstrual cycle and the modification introduced when pregnancy intervenes. Three other influences on the hypothalamic-pituitary-ovarian-uterine axis should be considered: cerebral, thyroid, and adrenal factors.

Cerebral Cortical Centers

The anatomic proximity and functional connections between the higher cortical centers and the hypothalamus are shown in Figure 9-1. Although the exact nature of whatever may be the neural equilibrium between cortex and hypothalamus essential for normal cycle regulations is unknown, disturbances in this equilibrium are common causes of functional menstrual disorders. Thus psychogenic influences of a great variety and apparently mediated via this cortical-hypothalamic pathway often can profoundly affect a previously (and subsequently) perfectly normal, regular menstrual pattern. The frequent, often prolonged, so-called hypothalamic amenorrhea of college women away from home for the first time is a familiar example, as is the delayed period in the young single woman who fears she may have recently conceived though her fear ultimately proves to be without foundation. Grief reactions, acute or chronic anxiety states, too frantic a pace of living, periods of high excitement, and a multitude of mental problems or emotional difficulties are often wholly or partly responsible for the alterations in normal cyclic menstrual function that are so commonly encountered. (The potential role of the pineal gland in regulating the hypothalamic control of pituitary gonadotropin secretion is discussed later in this chapter.)

The availability of synthetically prepared GnRH offers the possibility for testing and differentiating whether the derangement is at the hypothalamic or the pituitary level. Thus the diagnosis is rendered more accurate and specific, and management and treatment are more appropriate and successful.

Likewise, variations in steroid hormone levels and balance may affect various areas of the central nervous system, including cortical function. This situation may account for the various emotional changes and disturbances sometimes encountered in relation to the menstrual cycle, pregnancy and parturition, and oral contraceptive programs. Because the so-called mood changes often parallel a weight increase and fluid retention, it is possible that they are caused by activation of the reninangiotensin-aldosterone system as the levels of ovarian hormones fluctuate. Migraine headaches that occur regularly in association with the menstrual cycle are probably related to the sharp premenstrual drop in estradiol.

Pineal Gland

The hypothalamus is probably also under the inhibitory control of the brain through the pineal gland. The parenchymal cells of the pineal, which develop as an outgrowth of the roof of the third ventricle, also receive sympathetic innervation. Thus the pineal serves as a neuroendocrine gland, responding to photic and hormonal stimuli. The pineal makes melatonin from tryptophan. Norepinephrine stimulates tryptophan entry into the pineal cell as well as adenyl cyclase activity in the membrane, which leads to increased cyclic adenosine monophosphate (AMP). *N*-Acetyltransferase activity, the rate-limiting step in melatonin synthesis, is increased by the increased cyclic AMP. Norepinephrine is liberated by sympathetic stimulation of darkness (absence of light) leading to stimulation of adenylate cyclase and melatonin. Melatonin in turn is antigonadal, with increased melatonin causing decreased ovarian weight. In women the pineal gland probably exerts a permissive type of inhibitory control of the brain on the hypothalamus, as pinealectomy or blindness does not necessarily affect long-term ovarian function and fertility.

Thyroid Function

Normal thyroid function is an essential feature for normal cyclic female reproductive tract activity because the adenohypophysis also elaborates TSH. Gonadotropins and TSH secretion may well regulate the menstrual cycle and thyroid function together through the hypothalamic-pituitary level. The tripeptide TRH not only stimulates TSH from the thyrotropes but also prolactin from the lactotropes in the anterior pituitary gland. Thus elevated levels of TRH, as occurs with hypothyroidism, can induce hyperprolactinemia, which can induce menstrual irregularity or amenorrhea-galactorrhea. Furthermore, the general effect of thyroid hormone on tissue metabolism is obviously important to proper functioning of the entire neurohormonal regulatory mechanism, as well as to the cellular metabolic and cytochemical events that must take place in the ovary and subsequently in the rest of the target organs in the reproductive tract for the estrogen and progesterone produced by the properly maturing follicle.

In view of these facts, it is obvious that thyroid disorders, either hyper- or hypothyroidism, characteristically are accompanied by functional menstrual disorders. In fact, in the case of mild degrees of hypothyroidism, menstrual dysfunction may be the sole or principal clinical manifestation prompting the patient to seek medical advice.

Adrenal Function

The relation of adrenal function to hypothalamic-pituitary-ovarian activity is even more complex and intimate. The ACTH elaborated by the pituitary, though normally stimulating primarily the adrenal production of corticosteroids, may, particularly in excess amounts, elicit the production of androgens and estrogens by the adrenal. Rising levels of these hormones, though of adrenal rather than ovarian origin, inhibit pituitary secretion of FSH and LH and drastically interfere with normal gonadal function, as in congenital adrenal hyperplasia. Furthermore, both LH and prolactin (PRL) stimulate the adrenals to produce androgens. Obviously, deficient or excessive adrenal stimulation or adrenal hypofunction or hyperactivity is accompanied by fundamental disturbances of cyclic menstrual function, as seen clinically with the menstrual disorders commonly associated with Cushing's disease, Addison's disease, and the adrenogenital syndrome, whether due to adrenocortical hyperplasia or tumor.

Finally, there are inherent biochemical similarities between adrenocortical cells and ovarian cortical and stromal cells in terms of the potential ability of each to synthesize a wide variety of steroids of both androgenic and estrogenic activity. Such abilities are sometimes reflected in the apparent production of androgens and even adrenal-like steroids by the ovary itself in certain pathologic states.

ENDOMETRIUM AND MYOMETRIUM

During the first half of the cycle, when the uterus and the other target organs that are responsive to hormones of ovarian origin are primarily under the influence of estrogen, growth or proliferation is the keynote of their response. This preovulatory phase is hence often referred to as the proliferative, follicular, or estrogenic phase of the cycle.

Estrogen activity is initiated in the target organs by the binding of estradiol to specific estrogen receptor (proteins) in the cells. Estrogen receptors are present not only in the endometrium but also in the hypothalamus, vagina, and breast, all of which are target tissues for estrogens. Similar specific progesterone receptors are also present in the uterus. The endometrium proliferates rapidly, causing complete reepithelialization of the functioning layer and a threefold increase in its thickness by midcycle. An endometrial biopsy specimen obtained during this portion of the cycle exhibits the typical histologic changes characterized by the pathologists' term *proliferative endometrium* (Fig. 9-2A). The myometrial cells also enlarge and elongate, and the spiral arteriolar capillary bed of the functioning endometrial layer proliferates to afford an adequate blood supply for the growing endometrial lining.

On the other hand, during the second half of the cycle, following ovulation, the ovarian production of progesterone dominates and the response of the target organs is essentially one of functional change or activity rather than significant further growth. Because it involves secretory activity and is primarily dependent on adequate amounts of progesterone, the postovulatory phase of the cycle is usually called the secretory, luteal, or progestational phase. An endometrial biopsy taken well along in the second half of the cycle shows the typical histologic features of a normal response, which the pathologist designates *secretory endometrium* (Fig. 9-2B). The endometrial glands have assumed their familiar, coiled, elongated, tortuous, sawtooth appearance; the cells show secretory vacuoles, and the tubular lumens are bulging with secretion. The endometrial stroma becomes edematous, and the stromal cells begin to show predecidual changes. The spiral arteriolar network also becomes increasingly prominent and tortuous.

With the cycle nearing completion, one of two things must happen. If pregnancy has occurred, the corpus luteum continues to be supported by the chorionic gonadotropin of the early placenta; and with the continued production of estrogen and progesterone in increasing amounts, the endometrium and myometrium undergo further anatomic and functional changes, resulting in the decidual transformation that favors maintenance and further development of the pregnancy. If pregnancy does not occur, a rapidly increasing rate of decline in estrogen and progesterone levels accompanying normal corpus luteum degeneration produces the typical sequence of events in the uterus leading to menstruation. The endometrium itself shrinks during the days immediately preceding menstruation, and the arterioles begin to collapse and ooze underneath the outer, functional layer, forming blood "lakes" that cause further endometrial ischemic and pressure necrosis.

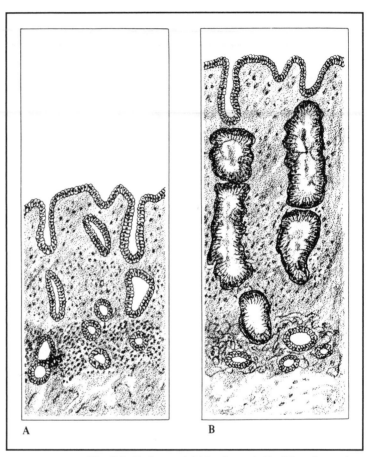

Fig. 9-2. Endometrial histology. A. Proliferative endometrium. B. Secretory endometrium.

With the rapid decrease in progesterone due to regression of the corpus luteum, there is labilization of the intracellular lysosomes and release of lysosomal enzymes. It is this lysosomal labilization that constitutes the initial endometrial cellular disruption and forms the basis of our current understanding for the onset of menstruation. It is the release of lysosomal enzymes, one of which is phospholipase A_2, that hydrolyzes the phospholipids of endometrial cell membranes to generate arachidonic acid. The availability of arachidonic acid, combined with the cellular trauma taking place, provides the right stimuli and favorable conditions for the biosynthesis of prostaglandins through the arachidonic acid cascade (Chap. 10).

Prostaglandin (PG) $F_{2\alpha}$ is a potent vasoconstrictor and stimulates uterine contraction. It has been shown that in the normal ovulatory cycle endometrial $PGF_{2\alpha}$ increases two- to threefold during the luteal phase and sixfold during the menstrual phase with maximum active uterine pressure seen at this time. This vasoconstrictive effect plus the increased myometrial tone in the normal cycle causes the myometrial layer to have an additional tourniquet-like constrictive effect on the more proximal portion of the spiral arterioles, thereby avoiding excessive blood loss during the menstrual period. These same two hemostatic mechanisms are also largely responsible for the premenstrual and early menstrual uterine cramps so characteristic of the normal ovulatory menstrual flow. By the end of four to seven days, the old functioning endometrial layer has been completely shed, and a new growth cycle is already under way.

OTHER PARTS OF THE REPRODUCTIVE TRACT

Fallopian Tubes

Increases in the number and activity of the ciliated cells of the tubal epithelium, tubal peristaltic activity, and tubal secretions are clearly evident just before and for some days after ovulation. In addition, slow contraction of the tubal musculature and shortening of the ovarian ligament at ovulation time tend to draw the fimbriated end of the tube into closer apposition with the ovary. These mechanisms facilitate retrieval of the ovum by the fimbriated end and its further passage and nourishment in transit through the length of the fallopian tube. Each mechanism in turn is brought into play as a result of the stimulus of estrogen and progesterone applied to the cellular activity of the tissues involved in the proper sequence and in the correct total and relative amounts.

Changes in the volume and composition of tubal secretions are equally important during this critical time of ovum transport for facilitating the passage of sperm in the opposite direction, as normally they are favorable to sperm motility and survival. It has also been established that an appropriate biochemical environment within the tube is necessary to prepare both ovum and sperm for the fertilization process and to provide a life-support system for the morula (fertilized egg) during the early days prior to the implantation.

Cervix

Alterations in the amount and chemical constitution of the cervical secretions occur during the critical few days around ovulation and are dependent on the increasing levels of estrogens during the five to seven days just before ovulation. As a result of change in volume and in protein and electrolyte composition, the normally thick, gelatinous, opaque cervical secretions become thin, abundant, stringy, clear, and rich in nutrient materials; moreover, the pH shifts from an acidic range of about 4.0 to a decidedly alkaline range of 7.0 to 8.0. Thus the cervical mucous plug, ordinarily a complete barrier to both bacteria and spermatozoa, is converted to a liquid medium of entry entirely favorable to sperm penetration, motility, and survival by virtue of its altered physical characteristics, its alkalinity, and its glucose, electrolyte, and protein composition.

These important physiologic changes are reflected in the various measurable items utilized clinically as tests of the adequacy of cervical response and as indirect evidence of the status of ovarian function (estrogen output) and the presence or absence of ovulation. The *fern test,* measurement of cervical *pH,* quantitative determination of *spinnbarkeit* (the ability of normal cervical mucus to be drawn out into long threads only at ovulation time), and the postcoital test of actual *sperm penetration* of the cervical mucus at ovulation time are valuable clinical indexes of the normality of the ovarian cycle and cervical response. After ovulation, under the influence of luteal phase progesterone secretion by the corpus luteum, the mucus thickens, it becomes less stretchable, and its ability to fern disappears. The quantity of mucus is also markedly reduced. Obviously, inadequate cervical response may also be seen in the presence of significant local disease such as severe chronic endocervicitis, even though ovarian function is normal.

Breasts

Mammary tissue, an integral part of the female reproductive tract, is responsive to the monthly stimulus of estrogen and progesterone elaborated by the ovary during the normal cycle. During the estrogenic phase of the ovarian cycle, there appears to be some ductal and glandular proliferation; during the progestational phase, this epithelial activity may be enhanced and may be accompanied by edema and vascular congestion of the supporting stroma. Clinically, these changes are manifested by typical breast symptoms (discomfort, tenderness, and swelling) experienced by most women during the premenstrual phase of the cycle. As might be expected, as the hormonal stimulus is removed at the onset of menstruation, the breast symptoms usually promptly subside.

Examination of the breast during the ovulatory cycle reveals a smooth, soft texture during the proliferative phase and a more "granular," or "coarse," texture during the luteal phase. Therefore, for both self-examination and adequate reliable examination by a physician, it is best to examine the breasts at the end of the menstrual flow, during the proliferative phase of the cycle.

GENERAL BODY CHANGES DURING THE NORMAL CYCLE

Basal Body Temperature Changes

The most obvious and most readily verified and quantitated of all the systemic changes in the reproductive cycle is the abrupt shift in the level of the basal body temperature that occurs at or shortly before ovulation as a result of the thermogenic effect of progesterone. Its purpose, if any, is unknown, but this thermal shift is of course the basis for the use of the basal body temperature chart as an indicator of ovulation and adequate progesterone production by the corpus luteum.

Changes in Electrolyte and Fluid Balance

There are numerous other cyclic fluctuations in general body physiology, with the majority most pronounced during the premenstrual or early menstrual phase. However, many of these fluctuations are as yet neither well defined nor clearly understood. One deserving of mention because of its frequent clinical significance when exaggerated is the tendency toward salt and fluid retention that manifests during the late progestational and premenstrual phase. This change in electrolyte and fluid balance is apparently a reflection of the steroid hormone pattern characteristic of the last week or so of the normal cycle. It becomes more pronounced when estrogens (aldosterone or similar compounds of ovarian or adrenal origin may also be involved, at least under certain circumstances) are in relative excess, as they may be when corpus luteum function is not entirely adequate and progesterone deficiency of varying degree is present. At any rate, many of the systemic premenstrual molimina of the normal cycle are probably the result of this change in fluid and electrolyte metabolism. At least some of the somatic symptoms of one of the menstruation-related disorders not accompanied by failure of ovulation, i.e., the premenstrual syndrome, may be explained on the basis of an exaggeration of this normal physiologic phenomenon.

SELECTED READINGS

Andersen, A. N., Hagen, C., Lange, P., et al. Dopaminergic regulation of gonadotropin levels and pulsatility in normal women. *Fertil. Steril.* 47:319, 1987.

Filicori, M., Santoro, N., Merriam, G. R., and Crowley, W. F. Characterization of the physiological pattern of episodic gonadotropin secretion throughout the human menstrual cycle. *J. Clin. Endocrinol. Metab.* 62:1136, 1986.

Fritz, M. A., and Speroff, L. Current concepts of the endocrine characteristics of normal menstrual function: The key to diagnosis and management. *Clin. Obstet. Gynecol.* 26:647, 1983.

Knobil, E. The neuroendocrine control of the menstrual cycle. *Recent Prog. Horm. Res.* 36:53, 1980.

Lenton, E. A., and Landgren B-M. The Normal Menstrual Cycle. In R. P. Shearman (Ed.), *Clinical Reproductive Endocrinology.* Edinburgh: Churchill Livingstone, 1985. Pp. 81–108.

10

Menstrual Cycle-Related Disorders of Ovulatory Cycles

The events and physiology of the normal menstrual cycle were outlined in Chapter 9. This chapter reviews those menstrual cycle-related disorders that occur only during ovulatory cycles. These disorders can be classified as related to (1) bleeding, (2) pain, and (3) the premenstruation period.

BLEEDING-RELATED DISORDERS

Bleeding may occur in nonreproductive tract tissues at the time of menstrual flow during ovulatory cycles. Vicarious menstruation or bleeding and recurrent catamenial pneumothorax are such bleeding-related disorders of ovulatory cycles.

Recurring catamenial pneumothorax is an episodic phenomenon that occurs occasionally but only in women who have regular ovulatory cycles. Although an occasional case associated with pleural or diaphragmatic endometriosis has been reported, the syndrome almost invariably occurs as a result of the spontaneous rupture of pulmonary alveoli. Actual pulmonary blebs are usually absent, and only rarely is there demonstrable underlying pulmonary pathology produced by exaggeration of the normal physiologic changes during ovulatory cycles just before or just after the onset of menstruation. Perhaps the increased levels of prostaglandin F at this time are responsible. $PGF_{2\alpha}$ is known to cause bronchospasm as well as pulmonary arteriolar vasoconstriction. Invariably, the pneumothorax occurs on the right side, never occurs at any other time in the cycle, and can be prevented by ovulation-inhibiting drugs. Immediate treatment consists in prompt reexpansion of the lung by appropriate intercostal needle aspiration or tube drainage. If the pneumothorax persists despite drainage or if it con-

tinues to recur, thoracotomy and operative pleurodesis may be necessary.

PAIN-RELATED CONDITIONS

Pain is a common presenting complaint in ovulatory cycles. In addition to its location, the relation of the pain to the particular phase of the menstrual cycle is often a clue to its origin and diagnosis. Pain due to ovulation (mittelschmerz), pain from a ruptured corpus luteum or ruptured corpus luteum cyst, pain from menstruation (dysmenorrhea), pain from pelvic congestion, and pelvic pain occur during ovulatory cycles.

Mittelschmerz: Ovulation and Postovulation Pain

Mittelschmerz, or ovulation discomfort, is common and is probably due to ovarian capsular distention, the result of the final peak of intrafollicular pressure just prior to ovulation, as well as to the slight intraperitoneal leakage of fluid during the event itself. It is ordinarily transient and dull and aching in character; it occurs almost exactly at midcycle and is more frequently felt in the right lower quadrant than on the left side. Many women experience it each month to a mild degree, some only when they ovulate from one ovary more than the other, some never.

Physical examination ordinarily reveals only minimal lower quadrant abdominal tenderness and a slightly tender, perhaps slightly enlarged ovary on the affected side. There should never be any real difficulty distinguishing this normal physiologic event from truly significant intraperitoneal disorders. If there is still difficulty distinguishing or diagnosing this condition based on history and clinical findings, vaginal ultrasound at the time the patient has the symptoms can reveal either a preovulatory follicle (on the same side as the pain) that is about to rupture or one that has already ruptured, in which case follicular fluid is also seen in the cul-de-sac.

Ruptured Corpus Hemorrhagicum

Many of the clinical features of ruptured corpus hemorrhagicum are somewhat similar to those of simple follicle rupture. However, ruptured corpus hemorrhagicum may occur at any time during the luteal phase of the cycle, typically about one week before the menstrual period. The pain is more severe, more generalized, and of longer duration. Considerable bleeding from the site of rupture of the ripening corpus luteum results in peritoneal irritation of varying extent and degree. Depending on the amount of blood accumulating, generalized abdominal pain and tenderness, radiation of pain to the back, shoulder, or leg, and rectal or bladder discomfort may ensue. If bleeding is massive, as it occasionally is, actual hemorrhagic shock develops and requires emergency laparotomy to control hemorrhage by suture of the bleeding site. When bleeding is moderate, the findings may suggest the possibility of any of a number of other acute intraabdominal disorders, such as appendicitis, mesenteric adenitis, acute salpingitis, ureteral colic, pyelonephritis, or ectopic pregnancy. In most cases, however, a carefully elicited history of the sudden nature of the onset of the acute episode and its chronologic relation to the menstrual cycle, the usual absence of associated symptoms suggestive of gastrointestinal or urinary tract disease (although there may be nausea and vomiting), and clinical and laboratory findings pointing to simple, chemical peritoneal irritation rather than infection or inflammation (relatively little if there is any elevation of temperature, pulse, or white blood cell count), and a negative serum beta human chorionic gonadotropin (β-hCG) level to rule out an ectopic pregnancy should permit a correct diagnosis. In doubtful cases or if bleeding continues, laparoscopy can easily resolve the problem of differential diagnosis. Exploratory laparotomy is rarely necessary, except to control massive hemorrhage. The symptoms usually subside spontaneously within a day or two, and no specific treatment is required once the diagnosis is established.

Ruptured Corpus Luteum Cyst

An entity related to ruptured corpus hemorrhagicum, with somewhat similar manifestations, is ruptured corpus luteum cyst. This cyst may develop during the current cycle or in some instances may have originated in a previous cycle. Development of a corpus luteum cyst is initiated by excessive hemorrhage into the center of a corpus luteum, with resulting hematoma formation and ultimately a cystic cavity lined by luteinized granulosa and theca cells. Actual rupture may be preceded by an interval of several days of increasing adnexal discomfort caused by slow bleeding within the cyst capsule and steadily rising intracystic pressure. Because about two-thirds of these luteal cysts have some functional activity, the preceding menstrual period may have been scanty, the present expected period may be delayed, sometimes for three to four weeks (rarely for as long as four to six months), and the endometrium may show a pseudodecidual change histologically. Rupture usually occurs either late in the cycle or during or after the delayed period, and bleeding is often extensive.

Because of the sudden, often massive hemoperitoneum, and in the face of the described menstrual irregularities and endometrial abnormalities, this entity may closely simulate ruptured ectopic pregnancy. In its milder forms, the ruptured corpus luteum cyst may suggest a ruptured endometrioma, acute salpingitis, twisted ovarian cyst, or any of the other previously mentioned acute abdominal disorders. In fact, the corpus luteum cyst is the greatest masquerader of all and is a frequent cause of either acute or chronic pelvic pain and menstrual irregularities. Diagnosis is frequently facilitated by laparoscopy.

When massive bleeding has occurred, laparotomy with resection of the cyst is necessary. It can nearly always be accomplished with preservation of the ovary.

Although many corpus luteum cysts undoubtedly are spontaneously resorbed, either with or without rupture, a significant number persist and manifest as tender ovarian enlargements, producing chronic intermittent pelvic pain and menstrual irregularities. Such irregularities are most commonly menorrhagia or metrorrhagia due to excessive secretion by the cyst of both estrogen and progesterone, although occasionally there is oligomenorrhea or secondary amenorrhea if the cyst persists for more than a few months. These cysts too usually ultimately require surgical removal for relief of symptoms, even when rupture does not occur.

Dysmenorrhea

Dysmenorrhea refers to painful menstrual cramps. It is classified or divided into primary or secondary dysmenorrhea. Descriptive classifications such as idiopathic, spasmodic, congestive, and membranous dysmenorrhea have been previously employed, but they add little to the diagnosis and management of painful menstrual cramps. *Primary dysmenorrhea* is painful menstrual cramps or menstruation without visible pathology in the pelvis to account for it. With *secondary dysmenorrhea,* visible pelvic pathology responsible for the menstrual cramps is present. The causes of secondary dysmenorrhea are listed in Table 10-1. With the exception of intrauterine device induced secondary dysmenorrhea, the treatment of secondary dysmenorrhea is elimination or treatment of the specific underlying lesion, which then provides relief of the dysmenorrhea. In most instances the treatment is surgery; specific management of the various lesions is outlined in the chapter dealing with the particular condition.

Incidence. Dysmenorrhea is one of the most frequently encountered gynecologic disorders and is recognized as an extensive personal and public health problem for women. However, with the advent of oral contraceptive and nonsteroidal antiinflammatory drug therapy, primary dysmenorrhea can be relieved significantly and readily. About 50 percent or more of menstruating women are affected by dysmenorrhea,

Table 10-1. Causes of Secondary Dysmenorrhea

Endometriosis
Intrauterine device
Pelvic inflammation and infections
Adenomyosis
Uterine myomas, uterine polyps, uterine adhesions
Congenital malformations of the müllerian system (bicornuate and septate uterus, transverse vaginal septum, blind uterine horn)
Cervical strictures or stenosis
Ovarian cysts
Pelvic congestion syndrome

and 10 percent of them have severe dysmenorrhea that renders them incapacitated for one to three days each month. Because women constitute 42 to 45 percent of the adult work force in the United States, it is estimated that about 600 million work hours are lost annually in the country because of untreated, incapacitating dysmenorrhea. Dysmenorrhea causes considerable personal and family disruption as well.

Primary dysmenorrhea occurs most commonly between the ages of 20 and 24. Women in this age group are also disabled by it most severely. For those over 25, the incidence of primary dysmenorrhea, particularly of the disabling type, is reduced. Marital status has some influence, with primary dysmenorrhea occurring more frequently in unmarried women (61 percent) than in married ones (51 percent). The incidence of primary dysmenorrhea tends to decrease with age more rapidly in married women than in unmarried ones, possibly in relation to childbearing. However, pregnancy and vaginal delivery do not necessarily cure primary dysmenorrhea.

The frequency of disabling dysmenorrhea does not appear to be related to the type of occupation or physical condition. Many women do not go to work when they experience severe dysmenorrhea, and when they do work they have a reduced work capacity, resulting in a lower work output. Dysmenorrheic women have lower marks and more school adjustment problems than do nondysmenorrheic ones. Exercise does not appear to have a significant effect on the incidence of dysmenorrhea, as the frequency of the disorder among gymnastics and nongymnastics students is similar.

Clinical Features. Primary dysmenorrhea occurs almost invariably during ovulatory cycles and usually appears within 6 to 12 months after menarche, when ovulatory cycles are established. The pain usually begins several hours before or just after the onset of menstruation. The discomfort is most severe and may be incapacitating on the first or second day of menstruation. The pain is described as characteristically spasmodic and is strongest in the lower abdomen, although it may also radiate to the back and along the inner aspects of the thighs. The uterine cramps are accompanied by one or more systemic symptoms in more than 50 percent of dysmenorrheic patients. These symptoms include nausea and vomiting (89 percent), fatigue (85 percent), diarrhea (60 percent), lower backache (60 percent), and headache (45 percent). Nervousness, dizziness, and in some severe cases even syncope and collapse are associated with dysmenorrhea. The symptoms may last a few hours to one day but seldom persist for more than two to three days. In some patients, primary dysmenorrhea disappears after the first childbirth, but the relief may be temporary. The symptoms often decrease with age.

Diagnosis. All too often primary dysmenorrhea is diagnosed on the basis of the exclusion of other causes of dysmenorrhea and serves as a wastebasket in which many forms of dysmenorrhea and even pelvic pain are dumped. Primary dysmenorrhea should be diagnosed by its clinical features. The following are its important hallmarks.

1. The initial onset of primary dysmenorrhea is at or shortly after menarche. A history of dysmenorrhea starting two years or more after menarche should arouse suspicion of secondary dysmenorrhea. Endometriosis can be difficult to exclude, as the dysmenorrhea of endometriosis remarkably resembles primary dysmenorrhea.
2. The duration of the dysmenorrhea is usually 48 to 72 hours, with the pain starting a few hours before or, more often, just after the onset of the menstrual flow. Therefore dysmenorrhea beginning more than just a few hours and as long as several days before the onset of the menstrual flow is less likely to be primary dysmenorrhea. The duration of the pain with primary dysmenorrhea closely reflects the period of maximum prostaglandin release in the menstrual fluid.
3. The character of the pain is cramping, or labor-like.
4. The pelvic examination, including rectovaginal inspection, is normal.

The differential diagnosis of primary dysmenorrhea includes all the causes of secondary dysmenorrhea: endometriosis; intrauterine device; pelvic inflammatory disease and infections; adenomyosis; uterine myomas,

polyps, and adhesions; congenital malformations of the müllerian system (bicornuate and septate uterus, transverse vaginal septum); cervical strictures or stenosis; ovarian cysts; pelvic congestion syndrome; and Allen-Masters syndrome. Endometriosis must be a particular consideration, as it can closely mimic primary dysmenorrhea, can begin with the onset of menarche or shortly thereafter, and occurs as frequently in teenagers and blacks as in whites. Therefore in patients who have a strong index of suspicion for endometriosis, such as those whose sisters or mothers have a history of endometriosis, laparoscopy should be undertaken fairly early in treatment after medical therapy has failed.

Etiology. For simplicity, the etiologies implicated in primary dysmenorrhea can be categorized as: (1) psychological factors; (2) endocrine factors; (3) cervical factors; (4) increased, abnormal uterine activity; and (5) increased production and release of prostaglandins by the endometrium. Currently, the objective scientific data indicate that most women with primary dysmenorrhea have abnormal uterine activity brought about to a large extent by excess prostaglandin release.

Psychological factors have been shown to be no more unique to the pain of primary dysmenorrhea than to any other type of acute or chronic pain. Therefore, although not necessarily the initiating factor for primary dysmenorrhea, psychological factors should, however, be considered and skillfully incorporated into the pharmacologic treatment plan as in the overall management of any type of pain, particularly in women who have not responded to medical therapy. With respect to endocrine factors, primary dysmenorrhea occurs only in ovulatory cycles. Investigations have suggested that circulating vasopressin levels are increased during the menstrual phase of these women, giving rise to dysrhythmic uterine contractions, and a small preliminary trial reported that primary dysmenorrhea was relieved with a vasopressin antagonist. There is no evidence suggesting that cervical stenosis is responsible for primary dysmenorrhea. Cervical stenosis secondary to a cervical lesion or trauma can, of course, produce secondary dysmenorrhea.

Current evidence suggests that with primary dysmenorrhea there is increased abnormal uterine activity, usually due to elevated uterine prostaglandin production coupled with declining ovarian steroid hormone levels at the time of menstruation. During the menstrual phase of the normal menstrual cycle, the uterine basal tone (resting pressure) is lowest (10 mm Hg), the active intrauterine pressure is highest (120 mm Hg), and the number of contractions is least (three or four per 10 minutes), compared with the other phases of the cycle. In women who have primary dysmenorrhea, abnormalities of uterine activity include (1) elevated uterine basal tone (10 mm Hg); (2) elevated intrauterine active pressure; (3) increased frequency of contractions (more than five per 10 minutes); and (4) incoordinate uterine activity. When more than one abnormality of uterine activity is present, they potentiate each other, and clinical symptoms are therefore produced with smaller deviations of these uterine activities from normal. Elevated basal tone of the uterus appears to be a common finding in many studies. With the increased and abnormal uterine activity, uterine blood flow has been demonstrated as being concurrently reduced in women who have primary dysmenorrhea, giving rise to uterine ischemia and pain. When the abnormal uterine activity is suppressed, there is enhancement of uterine blood flow, with simultaneous accompaniment of pain relief clinically. Thus uterine ischemia secondary to abnormal uterine activity contributes significantly to the genesis of pain in primary dysmenorrhea.

Evidence for the role of prostaglandins in the pathophysiology of primary dysmenorrhea can be summarized as follows.

1. The side effects of prostaglandin $F_{2\alpha}$ ($PGF_{2\alpha}$) administration for termination of midtrimester pregnancy and induction of term labor include nausea, diarrhea, headache, vomiting, and uterine cramps, which are similar to the symptoms of primary dysmenorrhea.
2. Measurements of endometrial and menstrual fluid prostaglandin levels in several studies have indicated significantly higher levels of prostaglandins in women who have primary dysmenorrhea than in those who do not have dysmenorrhea.
3. Measurement of the metabolite of $PGF_{2\alpha}$ (15-keto 13,14-dihydro-$PGF_{2\alpha}$) in plasma showed higher

levels in women who have primary dysmenorrhea than in normal women.
4. Certain prostaglandin synthetase inhibitors, e.g., fenamates, indoacetic acid derivatives, and arylpropionic acid derivatives, have been shown to be effective in the treatment of primary dysmenorrhea.

Prostaglandins are C20 hydrocarbon lipids with hydrophilic and hydrophobic properties. The biosynthesis of prostaglandin is shown in Figure 10-1. At the end of the luteal phase, if pregnancy does not occur, the corpus luteum regresses and progesterone levels fall, resulting in labilization of the lysosomes within the endometrial cells, leading to release of the lysosomal enzyme phospholipase A_2. Phospholipase A_2 hydrolyzes the phospholipids present in the bilipid cell membrane to generate free arachidonic acid, which is the main obligatory precursor for prostaglandin biosynthesis. Several enzymes—cyclooxygenase, isomerase, and reductase—often referred to as prostaglandin synthetase, are involved in the biosynthesis of $PGF_{2\alpha}$ and PGE_2. Trauma and the availability of arachidonic acid are two important factors that stimulate the generation of prostaglandins. The nonsteroidal antiinflammatory drugs are prostaglandin synthetase inhibitors, and corticosteroids block the production of prostaglandin through stabilization of the cell membrane by forming intercalating molecules between the phospholipids on the bilipid cell membrane.

The cause of the increased prostaglandin production and release in primary dysmenorrhea is currently unknown. Figure 10-2 outlines the pathophysiologic mechanism of pain originating in the pelvis in primary dysmenorrhea. The afferent limb of the pain originating in the pelvis in primary dysmenorrhea is thought to be due to three factors: (1) increased abnormal uterine activity; (2) uterine ischemia; and (3) sensitization of the nerve terminals to prostaglandins and their intermediates by lowering the threshold of these nerve terminals to the action of chemical and physical stimuli. The uterine cramps and pain of primary dysmenorrhea correlate closely with the quantity of menstrual fluid prostaglandin released over the same period and with the reduction in uterine blood flow that coincides with the increased abnormal uterine

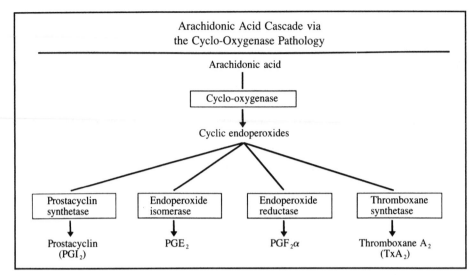

Fig. 10-1. Pathway for biosynthesis of prostaglandin $F_{2\alpha}$ and prostaglandin E_2.

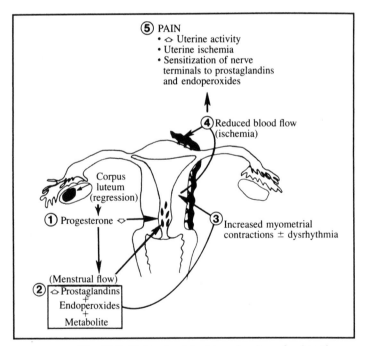

Fig. 10-2. Pathophysiologic mechanism of pain originating in the pelvis as it involves prostaglandins in primary dysmenorrhea. (From M. Y. Dawood. Hormones, Prostaglandins, and Dysmenorrhea. In M. Y. Dawood (ed.), *Dysmenorrhea*. Baltimore: Williams & Wilkins, 1981.)

activity. With primary dysmenorrhea, the greatest amount of prostaglandin is released during the first 48 hours of menstrual flow, which coincides with the duration of the clinical symptoms.

Treatment. For proper therapy it is essential to identify whether the dysmenorrhea the patient is suffering is primary or secondary. The overall approach to the treatment of both primary and secondary dysmenorrhea should include manipulation of both the psychological and behavioral factors in addition to the specific therapy, be it pharmacologic or surgical. The pain from both primary and secondary dysmenorrhea is the sum total of the organic factors that cause the pain and the psychological components, which comprise the inherent factors that influence the response to pain and the recurring pain itself, which in turn influence the response to subsequent cycles of dysmenorrhea. A careful assessment of the proportion that each of these various factors contributes to the final pain experienced by any given woman is necessary so that appropriate therapy can be given. Pain is difficult to quantify; the proportions that the various factors contribute to the total pain are even more difficult to identify. However, in day-to-day clinical practice an overall assessment can be made if the physician spends enough time taking a careful history. The efficacy of any kind of treatment for any type of dysmenorrhea can be enhanced greatly if simple psychotherapy in the form of a physician-patient dialogue, explanation, and reassurance is offered informally by the physician.

Various modalities of treatment that have been used for primary dysmenorrhea are summarized in Table 10-2. The two groups of drugs that are highly effective and specific are the oral contraceptives and the prostaglandin synthetase inhibitors.

ORAL CONTRACEPTIVES. If the patient wishes to use the oral contraceptive pill for conception control, it would be the agent of choice for the treatment of primary dysmenorrhea. Oral contraceptives can effectively treat primary dysmenorrhea and have been the main method of treatment since their introduction. Menstrual fluid prostaglandin is reduced below normal levels in women using oral contraceptives, probably the result of a reduction in the menstrual fluid

Table 10-2. Treatments That Have Been Used for Primary Dysmenorrhea

Type of therapy	Specific procedure or medication
General measures	Psychotherapy; reassurance
Surgery	Dilatation and curettage; presacral neurectomy
Endocrine therapy	Oral contraceptives; vasopressin antagonist
Tocolysis	Alcohol; terbutaline; nifedipine
Analgesics	Narcotics; nonnarcotics
Prostaglandin synthetase inhibitors	Ibuprofen; naproxen; mefenamic acid; flufenamic acid; indomethacin
Nonmedication	Transcutaneous electrical nerve stimulation

volume accompanying the use of birth control pills, which suppress endometrial tissue growth and development and thus reduce the accompanying menstrual fluid. Inhibition of ovulation, resulting in an endocrine milieu similar to that of the early proliferative phase of the menstrual cycle when prostaglandin levels are lowest could also contribute to the relief of dysmenorrhea.

About 90 percent or more of women can be relieved of their primary dysmenorrhea with an oral contraceptive, which can be tried for three or four months and continued if the patient responds to it. If the dysmenorrhea is not alleviated, an appropriate prostaglandin synthetase inhibitor can be added. The choice of the most suitable or optimal inhibitor should be based on clinical evidence of its efficacy, safety, and cost. It may be necessary to increase the dosage if relief is incomplete during the first cycle of treatment with the inhibitor concerned. If there is still no improvement, a change or a trial of a new prostaglandin synthetase inhibitor might become necessary.

PROSTAGLANDIN SYNTHETASE INHIBITORS. If birth control pills are not required for contraceptive purposes, the drug of choice for the treatment of primary dysmenorrhea is a prostaglandin synthetase inhibitor

(PGSI). Unlike oral contraceptives, PGSIs are taken only for two or three days of the menstrual cycle. Also, PGSIs do not suppress the pituitary ovarian axis, nor do they produce the metabolic side effects of the oral contraceptive. A trial of up to 6 months with a PGSI, with any necessary change in dosage or change from one inhibitor to another should the one originally chosen prove unsatisfactory, can demonstrate if relief can be obtained through this drug.

At present there are five groups of PGSI: (1) benzoic acid derivatives (aspirin); (2) butyrophenones (phenylbutazone); (3) indoleacetic acid derivatives (indomethacin); (4) fenamates (mefenamic acid, flufenamic acid); (5) arylpropionic acid derivatives (ibuprofen, naproxen, ketoprofen). Most of the agents shown to be effective provide relief for 70 to 80 percent of patients with primary dysmenorrhea. With ibuprofen, indomethacin, naproxen, and suprofen, there is a reduction in endometrial prostaglandin released during treatment of primary dysmenorrhea. Suppression of endometrial prostaglandin synthesis restores normal uterine activity and provides clinical relief because it eliminates all of the pain mechanism outlined in Figure 10-2. Clinical trials with PGSIs for treatment of primary dysmenorrhea indicate the following: Aspirin is no better than a placebo; butyrophenones are type II inhibitors; and indomethacin is effective, but the high incidence of gastrointestinal side effects caused high dropout rates in clinical trials. Thus the PGSI of choice for treatment of primary dysmenorrhea is either a fenamate or an arylpropionic acid derivative.

Pretreatment with a rapidly absorbed PGSI is not necessary. Treatment should be given during the first 48 hours of menstruation; but because the time of onset of menstrual flow is variable, it is more practical to prescribe medication for the first three days of menstruation. Dosages for the effective PGSIs are shown in Table 10-3. Contraindications to the use of PGSIs include the presence of gastrointestinal ulcers and hypersensitivity to these agents. Side effects of PGSIs as used for primary dysmenorrhea therapy are relatively mild and usually tolerable, but significant complications such as the known side effects of PGSIs (Table 10-4) can occur.

Table 10-3. Dose of Prostaglandin Synthetase Inhibitors Used for Treatment of Primary Dysmenorrhea

Prostaglandin inhibitor	Dose
Indomethacin	25 mg 3–6 times a day
Flufenamic acid	100–200 mg 3 times a day
Mefenamic acid	250–500 mg 3–4 times a day
Tolfenamic acid	133 mg 3 times a day
Ibuprofen	400 mg 4 times a day
Naproxen sodium	275 mg 4 times a day
Ketoprofen	50 mg 3 times a day

Table 10-4. Known Side Effects of Prostaglandin Synthetase Inhibitors

Gastrointestinal symptoms
    Indigestion, heartburn, nausea, abdominal pain, constipation, vomiting, diarrhea, melena
Central nervous system symptoms
    Headache, dizziness, vertigo, visual disturbances, irritability, depression, drowsiness, sleepiness
Other symptoms
    Allergic reactions, skin rash, edema, bronchospasm, hematologic abnormalities, eye effects, fluid retention, liver and kidney effects

OTHER TREATMENTS. If the patient does not respond to a PGSI, it is appropriate to reconsider the possibility of a pelvic pathologic condition. At this point, laparoscopy is probably indicated. If pelvic disease is discovered, appropriate treatment for the underlying pathologic condition should alleviate the dysmenorrhea. If no pelvic pathology is found, it is unclear if any pharmacologic agent could be helpful to these patients. Beta-mimetic agents have been generally disappointing and have many side effects, but they may be worth trying in such patients. Calcium antagonists, e.g., nifedipine, hold promise as an additional therapy. If no satisfactory response is obtained, referral for psychiatric help might be appropriate. If the diagnosis is correct, however, only a small group of patients with primary dysmenorrhea reach this point after the proper steps have been taken in management.

Secondary Dysmenorrhea

The more common causes of secondary dysmenorrhea are listed in Table 10-1. The age of onset of dysmenorrhea is often helpful for distinguishing primary from secondary dysmenorrhea, although endometriosis can occur soon after the onset of menarche. A history of recurrent pelvic inflammatory disease, irregular menstrual cycles (especially associated with anovulation), menorrhagia, the use of an intrauterine device, and infertility may point toward secondary dysmenorrhea or even to its underlying cause.

Useful investigations for identifying the cause of secondary dysmenorrhea include a complete blood count, erythrocyte sedimentation rate, pelvic sonograms, hysterosalpingography, and genital cultures for pathogens. The final diagnosis often can be made with the help of diagnostic laparoscopy, hysteroscopy, and dilatation and curettage (D&C). Hysteroscopy and D&C can usually be done together with laparoscopy when the latter is indicated. Hysteroscopy can provide valuable information on small intrauterine lesions that a D&C may miss.

Abdominal and pelvic examinations, including a rectovaginal examination, are likely to reveal positive findings for many causes of secondary dysmenorrhea, e.g., ovarian cysts, uterine malformations, uterine myomas, the presence of an intrauterine device, pelvic inflammatory disease, and some cases of endometriosis.

The differential diagnosis of secondary dysmenorrhea includes primary dysmenorrhea and chronic pelvic pain. With chronic pelvic pain there is no relation between the pain and the menstrual cycle, whereas with dysmenorrhea the pain is confined to the menstrual phase or the period of time shortly before.

Prostaglandins and Secondary Dysmenorrhea. The role of prostaglandins in the pathophysiology of secondary dysmenorrhea is less clearly defined than for primary dysmenorrhea. Endometrial prostaglandins were found to be high with uterine myomas, but prostaglandin synthetase inhibitors are not the definitive therapy except for possible temporary relief while waiting for myomectomy or hysterectomy. With endometriosis the endometriotic tissue has increased prostaglandin levels and could synthesize more prostaglandins than normal. Again, the mechanisms of pain for endometriosis are often multiple, and treatment with a PGSI is often not effective and does not take care of the endometriosis lesions. With the intrauterine device (IUD) in place inside the uterus, there is a mild inflammatory response around the IUD with an increase in endometrial $PGF_{2\alpha}$ levels. This increased endometrial prostaglandin level contributes to the basis for the secondary dysmenorrhea due to the IUD as well as contributing to the IUD-associated menorrhagia. Dysmenorrhea and menorrhagia are two common and frequent side effects of the IUD.

Treatment. As mentioned earlier, treatment of secondary dysmenorrhea is directed toward the specific cause or disease. However, for secondary dysmenorrhea due to the presence of an IUD, relief is readily and effectively obtained with the PGSIs. Medication is started in the same dosage as for primary dysmenorrhea, starting from the onset of menstrual flow and continued throughout the menstrual period. In addition to relieving the dysmenorrhea, such treatment also corrects the menorrhagia if it is due to the IUD. Ibuprofen, naproxen, and mefenamic acid have been shown to be particularly effective for treating IUD-related dysmenorrhea and menorrhagia.

Pelvic Congestion Syndrome

The pelvic congestion syndrome is a vague disorder characterized by chronic but often intermittent pelvic and lower abdominal pain, secondary dysmenorrhea, low backache, and dyspareunia. It invariably increases in severity during the premenstrual and menstrual phases of the cycle but is often symptomatic throughout the cycle. There is sometimes an associated menorrhagia that fails to respond to the usual conservative management. It appears to be a real entity, the associated symptoms and some of the etiologic mechanisms involved resembling in part those of the premenstrual syndrome but with the addition of a local pelvic vascular and autonomic nervous system disorder that produces grossly visible vascular congestion, tissue edema, hypersecretion, and muscle spasm throughout the pelvis and pelvic viscera. A frequent, almost pathognomonic sign is extreme tenderness and pain on motion of the boggy pelvic organs and supporting structures.

An even more specific variant of the pelvic congestion symptom complex, the Allen-Masters syndrome ("universal joint syndrome"), was described by Allen and Masters as a common cause of the pelvic congestion syndrome and as due to obstetric trauma. In some patients with the symptom complex, they were able to demonstrate a laceration of the broad ligament resulting in an unstable cervicofundal junction resembling a universal joint and a characteristically retroflexed, retroverted uterus with excessive and independent mobility of the fundus and cervix. Dilatation of the venous system with the appearance of huge pelvic varicosities results from poor support and torsion of the veins, and continued engorgement further softens the lower uterine segment and weakens its supports. The symptoms are definitely acquired ones and can usually be shown to have developed after a traumatic delivery. In the experience of Allen and Masters, operative repair of the broad ligament fascial defects with uterine suspension was highly successful in alleviating the condition in patients who wished to preserve their childbearing potential. In those not desiring further pregnancy, hysterectomy is probably the procedure of choice when the diagnosis is firmly established.

Great care should always be taken when arriving at the diagnosis of chronic pelvic congestion, with or without the associated Allen-Masters syndrome. In a small number of patients with well documented pelvic congestion, hysterectomy may be indicated, which completely relieves the problem. If the patient desires sterilization as well as relief from her disabling symptoms, abdominal hysterectomy is clearly the treatment of choice.

Chronic Pelvic Pain

There are basically two categories of chronic pelvic pain: chronic pelvic pain due to an organic cause (organic pelvic pain) or chronic pelvic pain without obvious pelvic pathology and sometimes referred to as functional chronic pelvic pain.

Organic Pelvic Pain

Diseases in the pelvis that could give rise to chronic pelvic pain include malignant or benign tumors; ovarian cysts with adhesions, torsion, slow leaks, or hemorrhage; severe uterine malpositions including the Allen-Masters syndrome (see above); chronic pelvic inflammatory disease; chronic or recurrent urinary tract infection or inflammation (e.g., cystitis); chronic bowel or gastrointestinal inflammation; endometriosis.

The diagnosis is dependent upon a good history and is strongly influenced by how chronic and variable the pain is, the timing of the pain, provoking or accentuating factors, and associated symptoms and features. An organic etiology should always be sought before making a final diagnosis of chronic pelvic pain without obvious pathology.

The differential diagnosis, characteristic features, and management of each of the causes of organic pelvic pain referred to above have been described in appropriate chapters. Laparoscopy and cystoscopy play important roles, especially the former procedure when the diagnosis is not readily and confidently made with the results of clinical and laboratory examinations.

Chronic Pelvic Pain
Without Obvious Pelvic Pathology

Chronic pelvic pain without obvious pathology has in the past been referred to as pelvic congestion syndrome, pelvic sympathetic syndrome, or pelvic neurodystonia. The prevalence of the syndrome is difficult to ascertain, as it varies according to the cultural background of the population concerned. Chronic pelvic pain without obvious pathology is found in 25 to 28 percent of women undergoing laparoscopy for pelvic pain. It should be remembered that this group represents only those patients who have enough pain to warrant laparoscopy; it does not include those seen in the outpatient clinic only. Most of the patients are married and are 20 to 40 years of age.

The precise etiology of chronic pelvic pain without

obvious pathology has not been worked out but may include the following.

1. Increased prostaglandin levels in the peritoneal fluid, although no such increase was found when measured
2. Traumatic laceration of uterine support (see below)
3. Circulatory disturbances in the uterus
4. "Sclerocystic oophoritis" or "painful ovarian dystrophy"
5. Morphologic or functional modification of the parametrium or reproductive tract
6. Psychogenic mechanisms

The symptoms usually start after a delivery. Clinically, the most important symptom is lower abdominal pain and, less frequently, low back pain. The abdominal pain may be felt over the whole lower abdomen, in one iliac fossa, or in both iliac fossae. The back pain is usually located over the sacrogluteal region or only one-half of this area. The pain usually is severe for several days before menstruation and improves on the first or second day of flow. However, continuous pain is not unusual. The pain is accentuated by prolonged upright standing, jumping, or sitting down suddenly; it is relieved by the horizontal position (lying down). Deep dyspareunia is common. Although not common and not essential, other associated symptoms may include leukorrhea, menstrual disturbances, constipation, cystalgia, asthenia, depression, and anxiety. Physical examination reveals tenderness of the uterus and adnexa, often with marked tenderness of the posterior parametrium.

The diagnosis of chronic pelvic pain without obvious pathology is usually made by fulfilling the following conditions.

1. The patient's pain is not due to a nongynecologic cause.
2. The pain has the characteristics of pain of gynecologic origin.
3. No definite lesions are found to account for it.
4. The pain is not due to one of the acknowledged causes of gynecologic pain.

Chronic pain of gynecologic origin has its own characteristics and is dealt with in greater detail under the specific conditions in other chapters. Details on pain due to nongynecologic causes can be readily found in standard textbooks of medicine or surgery.

Management of chronic pelvic pain without obvious pathology requires sensitive and tactful handling of the patient combined with medication. If analgesics have failed to provide relief, laparoscopy is indicated to rule out pathologic causes or lesions that may be responsible for the pain as well as to confirm the diagnosis of chronic pelvic pain without obvious pathology. Laparoscopy is at times therapeutic or can lessen the anxiety by having excluded organic diseases.

Once the diagnosis is firmly established, it is important that the clinician does not compound the situation with implications that it is all "just nerves." Because the condition is frequently associated with psychological problems or with a neurotic disorder, it is important to examine the relation between psychological factors and the pain complaints. Information should be obtained regarding family and personal history, marital life, and general behavior. Referral to a psychiatrist conversant and interested in this field is useful for some patients.

Cyclic estrogen and progestin or birth control pills have been helpful in some and should be tried. Progestins alone, e.g., 2.5 to 5.0 mg of norethindrone acetate for several months, have relieved the pain in some patients. The dyspareunia may also be lessened by changing coital position and avoiding vigorous, rapid, deep penetration during intercourse.

For pain due to tears or large defects in the broad ligament or extreme mobility of the uterus due to defects at the uterosacral ligament to the uterus, repair of the defects or suturing the uterosacral ligament may be attempted if nonsurgical management has been unsuccessful. Most recently, painful localized spots detected either on pelvic or abdominal examination have been employed as target points for injecting local anesthetic agents or alcohol to obtain relief of pain. These agents can also be injected into the uterosacral ligaments either transvaginally or abdominally through the laparoscope or at laparotomy.

Finally, short wave electrotherapy has been employed in the past, but more recently transcutaneous electrical nerve stimulation (TENS), which is simpler and easier to use, is available for relieving various types of pain. TENS employs small units that the patient can use but remain mobile and functional. It provides relief by stimulating the nerve terminal over the dermatome with the same segmental innervation as the structure from which the pain originates. Relief of pain by TENS is brought about through two main mechanisms: (1) gate blocking, which alludes to the dorsal spinal ganglion being saturated by the electrical stimulation and therefore blocking further stimuli brought about by the pain itself; and (2) release of endorphins by the nerves being stimulated, thereby providing sufficient endogenous opiates to the appropriate dermatomes.

Hysterectomy has been resorted to for chronic pelvic pain, but the results have not been uniformly good. The psychological component to the pelvic pain must be carefully and adequately assessed; if psychological disturbance is deemed to constitute a large basis for the pain, hysterectomy may not provide relief. In general, if other simpler measures discussed have been tried and were unsuccessful, hysterectomy may be considered if the patient is fully aware of the low percentage of good long-term results with hysterectomy.

PREMENSTRUAL DISORDERS

Many conditions are noted to worsen only during the premenstrual phase and sometimes during menstruation. Depressive illness or bipolar affective disorders may be accentuated premenstrually; the incidence of suicide is increased premenstrually, as are a number of somatic conditions. However, two specific conditions that present especially to the gynecologist are premenstrual syndrome, or premenstrual tension syndrome, and cyclic breast disorders.

Premenstrual Syndrome

Although premenstrual syndrome and dysmenorrhea are both related to the menstrual phase, current evidence suggests that they are probably not directly interrelated disorders. Premenstrual syndrome is present in some women with dysmenorrhea, and the reverse is equally true. The two disorders tend to occur in different age groups, however, with primary dysmenorrhea more common in young women and improving with age, whereas premenstrual tension is more frequent in the 30- to 40-year age group. Moreover, the etiology and therapy of primary dysmenorrhea is well established, whereas premenstrual tension syndrome is still a disorder shrouded with controversy.

A striking aspect of premenstrual syndrome is the lack of a widely accepted definition of what it is, which leads to difficulty when interpreting the results of studies, proliferation of the theories responsible for the disorder, and lack of sensitive and accurate methods for assessing it. The definitions that have been used include the following.

1. Changes in certain mental and physical symptoms in women relative to the menstrual cycle with increasing intensity and frequency of these symptoms premenstrually
2. A condition with cyclic mood changes whose symptom development is closely related to the luteal phase
3. The collective name given to the problems that occur during the two-week period before menstruation
4. A cluster of symptoms, both psychological and physical, that appear episodically in relation to the phases of the menstrual cycle

Premenstrual syndrome was first recognized by Frank as a clinical disorder. He defined it as a specific and severe syndrome of "indescribable tension and irritability" with a "desire to find relief by foolish and ill-considered acts" and relieved by the onset of menses. A reasonable working definition of premenstrual syndrome is "a clinical condition comprising distressing behavioral, psychoemotional (e.g., anxiety, irritability, tension, depression, emotional lability), and physical signs and symptoms (e.g., headache, backache, abdominal pain, bloating, painful and swelling breasts, leg swelling and craving for sweets) that present episodically and predictably during the two-week period premenstrually with the patient becoming spontaneously and completely symptom-free for at least one week postmenstrually."

Incidence. Premenstrual syndrome has been reported in a number of ethnic groups throughout the world. The incidence is reported as 20 to 90 percent, the wide variability being a function of the definition and criteria for diagnosis of premenstrual syndrome employed by different authors. Careful analysis of most reports indicates that premenstrual syndrome is present in about 30 percent of otherwise healthy females in the reproductive age group. It is important to note that most of the reports on the incidence of premenstrual syndrome were retrospective analyses and involved self-reporting, both of which conditions are well known to result in overreporting. One critical assessment suggested that, based on data extrapolated from limited surveys, the incidence of premenstrual symptoms may be closer to 2 to 5 percent.

In a prospective evaluation and analysis of three groups of symptoms (breast symptoms, abdominal symptoms, mood), it was found that patients who believed they had premenstrual syndrome perceived that they had these symptoms whereas controls did not. However, the study found no difference in the frequency of the three groups of symptoms between those who thought they suffer from premenstrual syndrome and controls.

The widespread media attention given to premenstrual syndrome can readily influence the way women perceive these symptoms and their entrainment to the premenstrual phase. Because it can be socially more acceptable to have premenstrual syndrome than a psychiatric disorder, many patients with varying degrees of bipolar affective disorder not infrequently insist on having premenstrual syndrome and to be treated for their "hormonal imbalance."

Women who suffer from premenstrual syndrome may have serious repercussions in their interpersonal relationships premenstrually. Such effects of premenstrual syndrome include marital discord, baby battering, and criminal behavior. It is estimated that absenteeism caused by premenstrual syndrome in the United States generated a loss of $5 billion in 1969 alone.

Etiology. The etiology of premenstrual syndrome is not known. There is a plethora of theories about the pathogenesis of the syndrome, many of which have not been substantiated by acceptable scientific methodology but continue to be perpetuated as facts. The concepts may be summarized as follows.

1. *Psychological causes.* Premenstrual syndrome patients have been suggested to be more neurotic than normal women, but critical studies have found that the neuroticism scores in premenstrual syndrome patients were similar to those in normal women. There is little evidence to substantiate a psychosomatic origin of premenstrual syndrome. Although women with premenstrual syndrome had a higher score on the comprehensive psychiatric rating scale than normal women, it is unlikely that psychological factors alone could give rise to the premenstrual syndrome.

2. *Estrogen excess or progesterone deficiency.* According to this hypothesis, patients with premenstrual syndrome have progesterone insufficiency or deficit giving rise to a relative estrogen excess. The symptoms intensify as progesterone levels decline late in the luteal phase. Unopposed estrogen could cause fluid retention, hyperplasia of breast tissue, and abnormal carbohydrate metabolism. Estrogen accumulation within the limbic system could give rise to the central nervous system manifestations of premenstrual syndrome. Progesterone deficit results in a lack of its usual natriuretic effect and antiestrogenic effects, thereby compounding the estrogen effect. Careful review of many reports of women with premenstrual syndrome and normal women showed no significant difference in the circulating progesterone and estradiol levels of the two groups. Also, the former group of women had adequate corpus luteum function as judged by endometrial biopsies and serum estrogen and progesterone assays. The effectiveness of progesterone therapy is yet to be scientifically confirmed, with all controlled clinical trials showing only similarity between placebo and progesterone for relieving symptoms of premenstrual syndrome.

3. *Vitamins B_6 and A deficiency.* Vitamin B_6 acts as a coenzyme (pyridoxal phosphate) in the biosynthesis of dopamine and serotonin. Lack of this vitamin could therefore lead to decreased synthesis of these biogenic amines. It is speculated that estrogen could induce a "relative deficiency" of vitamin B_6 by

altering tissue distribution and producing hepatic enzymes, which compete for vitamin B_6. A deficiency in pyridoxine diminishes synthesis of serotonin from tryptophan and could produce depression in women with premenstrual syndrome. Treatment of premenstrual syndrome with pyridoxine, however, showed benefit in one study but no effect in another.

Uncontrolled studies of successful treatment of premenstrual syndrome with vitamin A have been reported. Vitamin A is believed to relieve premenstrual syndrome by opposing thyroid hyperfunction or by direct antiestrogenic or diuretic effect. These hypotheses remain to be substantiated.

4. *Prolactin.* Several early studies suggested elevated luteal phase prolactin levels in premenstrual syndrome patients, but subsequent studies failed to confirm the finding. It is postulated that prolactin is important in fluid balance, but no osmoregulatory role of pituitary prolactin has been established in humans. Suppression of prolactin secretion with bromoergocriptine in premenstrual syndrome patients relieved breast symptoms but had little or no significant beneficial effects on the other symptoms.

5. *Endogenous hormone allergy.* Because premenstrual urticaria and other skin eruptions could occur, it is suggested that hypersensitivity to endogenous hormones or their metabolites may be responsible for the symptoms of premenstrual syndrome. Allergy to progesterone or pregnanediol has been suggested. In inadequately controlled studies, up to 80 percent overall relief from premenstrual syndrome was obtained with small desensitizing doses of pregnanediol. Many aspects of the effects of gonadal steroids in human allergic response, however, remain unknown, and it is unlikely that endogenous hormone allergy plays a significant role in the etiology of premenstrual syndrome.

6. *Aldosterone and fluid retention.* Fluid retention as a factor responsible for the other symptoms of premenstrual syndrome is a widely held clinical concept that forms the basis for diuretic therapy. Careful studies, however, have been unable to document significant alterations in total exchangeable sodium or body water or any association between water retention and mental symptoms in women with premenstrual syndrome. Progesterone has a natriuretic effect, and the premenstrual decline in progesterone could contribute to the fluid retention. In addition, progesterone is responsible for the increase in renin concentration leading to an increase in plasma renin activity and plasma aldosterone levels. In premenstrual syndrome patients, elevated premenstrual urinary aldosterone excretion but not plasma aldosterone has been reported. The mechanism of this increased aldosterone excretion is unclear, but altered activity of dopamine may be involved, as aldosterone secretion is normally under maximal tonic dopaminergic inhibition.

7. *Hypoglycemia.* Although gonadal steroids induce changes in insulin action and may account for the flattened glucose tolerance curves with delayed hypoglycemia during the luteal phase, it is unlikely that hypoglycemia is a significant etiologic factor in premenstrual syndrome, as it occurs in normal women.

8. *Prostaglandins.* There are high prostaglandin concentrations in the central nervous system, and they influence the excitability of neurons. Together with other prostaglandins in local tissues, e.g., the breast, kidneys, and uterus, prostaglandins could account for the symptoms of premenstrual syndrome. There are, however, no data on prostaglandins in premenstrual syndrome other than a clinical trial with a prostaglandin synthetase inhibitor, which relieved a few somatic but not the major mental symptoms of the premenstrual syndrome.

9. *Endogenous opiate peptides.* It is hypothesized that excessive exposure to or abrupt withdrawal of the endogenous opiate peptide stimulus may trigger psychoneuroendocrine manifestations of premenstrual syndrome. During the luteal phase, progesterone acting alone or together with estrogen can increase central endogenous opiate peptide activity, giving rise to cyclic exposure to be followed by withdrawal from endogenous opiate peptides during the normal luteal phase. Acute withdrawal of the inhibition of endogenous opiate peptides at the approach of menstruation may lead to rebound hyperactivity of the dopaminergic pathways because of slowly acquired hypersensitivity to endogenous opiates. It may then manifest as irritability, tension, and aggression. High doses of the

opiate receptor antagonist naloxone given to normal volunteers apparently produced behavioral changes similar to those seen with premenstrual syndrome.

Clinical Features. Premenstrual syndrome generally occurs in mature women. Premenstrual anxiety and sadness are more frequent and severe with increasing age.

The common symptoms of premenstrual syndrome are summarized in Table 10-5. There are four patterns of premenstrual symptoms, as depicted in Figure 10-3. The symptoms may (1) last four to seven days before menstrual flow and abate with onset of menstruation; (2) last throughout the two weeks premenstrually and abate with the menstrual flow; (3) occur for a few days at midcycle, followed by relief for a few days and recurrence of symptoms again followed by relief after menstrual flow begins; or (4) last throughout the two weeks premenstrually and throughout the menstrual period.

Premenstrual syndrome usually begins with varying degrees of fatigue, emotional lability, and depression as early as 10 to 14 days before menses. Crying spells or emotional outbursts may occur for apparently little reason. With more severe forms, there could be complete withdrawal from the family and all social engagements. Somatic complaints such as painful breast swelling, abdominal bloating, constipation,

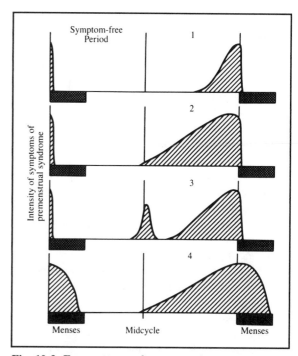

Fig. 10-3. Four patterns of symptoms in premenstrual syndrome in relation to the phase of the menstrual cycle and menstruation.

generalized swelling, weight gain, and edema may then set in. A noticeable increase in appetite or specific cravings for sweets (especially chocolates) or salty foods with episodes of binge eating appears in many women during the premenstrual week. During the five to seven days premenstrually, symptoms usually reach a peak, with many of the psychoemotional symptoms increasing in intensity such that the feelings of anxiety, inward tension, and anger often lead to physical unrest, insomnia, combativeness, and repeated angry confrontations for trivial matters. Under these conditions, child, spouse, and partner battering may occur, and murders have been committed.

The severity of premenstrual syndrome may be graded as follows.

Mild: only the woman is affected, with the change perceived by the family but not affecting social or working life

Table 10-5. Symptoms of Premenstrual Syndrome

Altered emotional state
  Tension, anxiety, depression, irritability, lethargy, aggression, loss of concentration
Behavioral changes
  Avoidance of social contact, change in work habits, crying spells, change in libido (increased or decreased), tendency to pick fights
Somatic symptoms
  Feeling bloated, feeling of weight increase, breast swelling, change in bowel habit, skin eruptions
Altered appetite
  Food craving or avoidance of certain foods
Motor effects
  Poor coordination, clumsiness, accidents

Moderate: disruption of intrafamily relations and social life, with work capacity affected but work can still be done

Severe: symptoms intense enough to disrupt family relations with no social life or ability to work; need for medication

Diagnosis. The following critera can be employed for the diagnosis of premenstrual syndrome.

1. There is a cyclicity of the patient's symptoms, with higher ratings during the premenstrual than the preovulatory weeks.
2. Mental symptoms comprise one of the more prominent manifestations, with moderate to severe mood changes present.
3. The symptoms must be relieved after menstrual flow, and there should be a symptom-free period postmenstrually, preferably for a week.
4. Premenstrual symptoms must recur every menstrual cycle for at least a year, although the severity may vary from cycle to cycle.

The patient should be assessed *prospectively,* which is the key to understanding the extent and severity of the problem. A careful history and interview should be carried out. Although a variety of psychometric and psychological tests have been employed, most of these tests assess mood or behavior rather than the relation of the symptoms to the menstrual cycle. A practical method is to have the patient keep a menstrual calendar on a single card with the months running horizontally and the dates vertically (Fig. 10-4). She then enters her specific symptoms with an abbreviation for each day they occur as well as when menstruation occurs. This record should be kept for at least three consecutive menstrual cycles and be reviewed by the physician. It allows assessment of the onset and duration of symptoms and the symptom-free period in relation to menstruation.

Premenstrual syndrome must be distinguished from exacerbation of chronic conditions, e.g., idiopathic edema, fibrocystic disease of the breast, aggression, depression, anxiety neurosis, and other intercurrent stressful events. Thus a thorough psychiatric history may be necessary, as psychiatric disorders may present with vague somatic complaints. In addition, stress life changes, such as divorce and family problems, should be identified and dealt with because they can either exacerbate or present as apparent premenstrual syndrome. Usually little or no laboratory investigation is necessary. Thyroid function may have to be checked if it is thought to be responsible for some of the psychoemotional symptoms. Premenstrual pelvic pain is seldom present with premenstrual syndrome. If present, suspicion of endometriosis or other forms of secondary dysmenorrhea should be entertained.

Management. Both general measures and specific pharmacotherapy are necessary in the management of patients with premenstrual syndrome.

GENERAL MEASURES. Education and reassurance are central and critical to the management of patients with premenstrual syndrome. The patient and family should be informed that the disorder is common in women of reproductive age and is probably caused by cyclic neuroendocrine derangement. Discussion about intercurrent stress or provoking environmental or social conditions may assist the patient to come to grips with these factors. Avoidance or reduction of caffeine intake and smoking often leads to improvement of many mild to moderate symptoms. It is unclear whether the observed improvement is due to a placebo or a physiologic effect. Small, frequent meals rather than large, predominantly carbohydrate-containing meals during the luteal phase can be helpful in reducing the postprandial rebound hyperglycemia.

SPECIFIC THERAPY. There is as yet no scientifically rational, validated, and proved effective drug therapy for premenstrual syndrome. A large placebo effect is ever present in the management and treatment of the syndrome, however. The following are some of the drug therapies that have been employed for premenstrual syndrome, but it is prudent to keep the number of medications prescribed to a minimum (preferably one).

1. *Psychotropic agents.* Tricyclic antidepressants and lithium carbonate are ineffective, although the latter is sometimes used for controlling recurrent psychotic or cyclothymic behavior. Alprazolam, an agent used for panic attacks, has been found to be signifi-

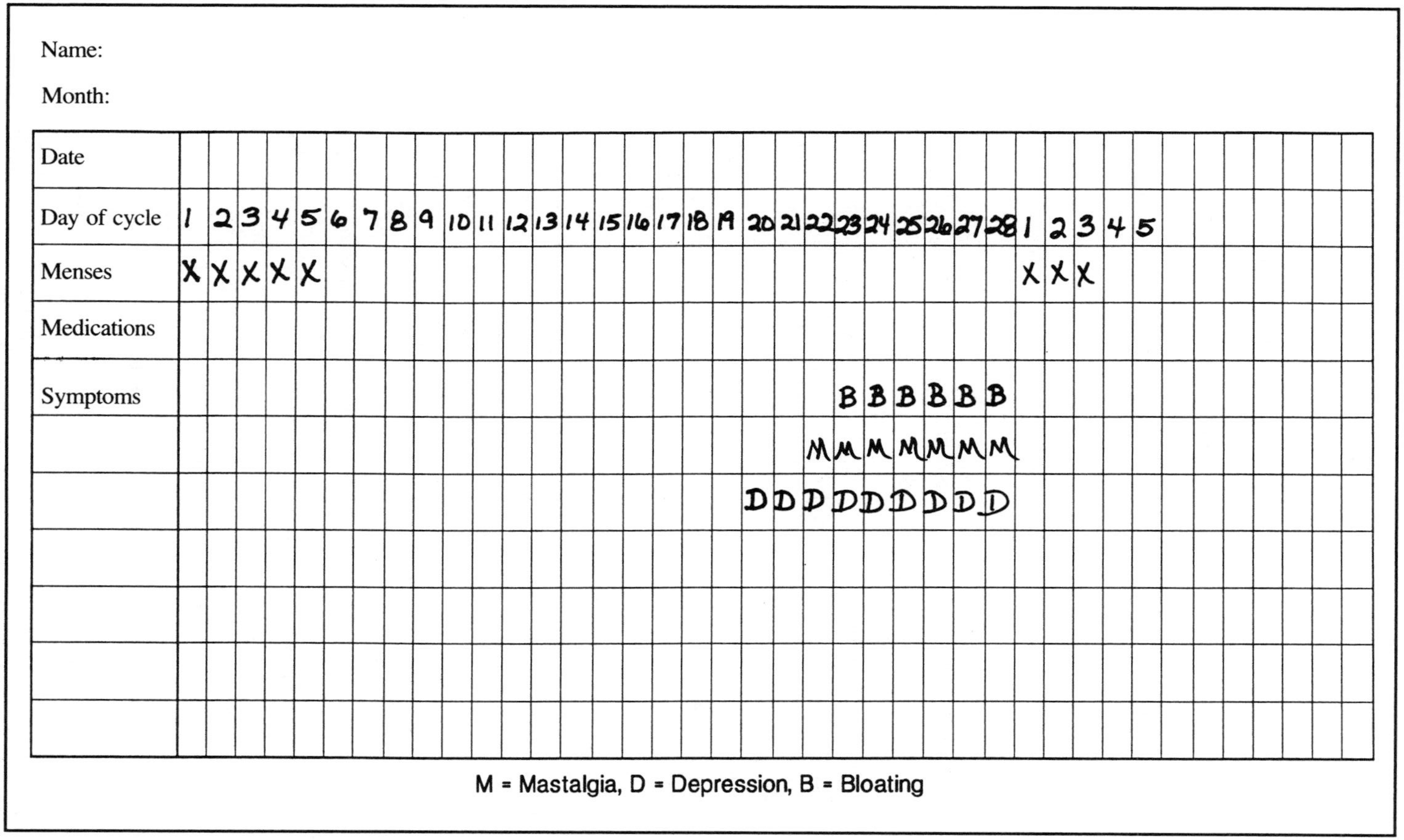

Fig. 10-4. Simple diary card for charting symptoms of premenstrual syndrome prospectively by the patient.

cantly better than placebo for relieving premenstrual syndrome.

2. *Diuretics*. Diuretic therapy has been widely abused for treatment of the premenstrual syndrome on the premise that the disorder is associated with salt and water retention. Uncontrolled studies with diuretics have shown efficacy and remarkable success. A history of diuretic abuse frequently found in women having severe cyclic edema is a good reason to be concerned about indiscriminate use of diuretics for the treatment of premenstrual syndrome. In double-blind studies of chlorthalidone the results were variable. In one double-blind placebo-controlled study, spironolactone 25 mg four times a day from days 18 to 26 of the menstrual cycle improved mood and weight significantly and reduced psychological symptoms in more than 80 percent of the patients. Therefore when there is evidence of water retention diuretics may be useful, but the risk of secondary hyperaldosteronism should be considered. Spironolactone is the preferred diuretic because it is an aldosterone antagonist and its steroid-like structure may allow it to act as a steroid agonist or antagonist at the central nervous system.

3. *Progesterone therapy*. Progesterone therapy has been widely used by Dalton, who recommended it on the basis that premenstrual syndrome patients have either progesterone insufficiency or a high estrogen/progesterone ratio premenstrually. This rationale is without basis in fact, as the balance of evidence indicates no such demonstrable endocrine derangement in premenstrual syndrome patients. Progesterone has usually been given as vaginal suppositories, each suppository containing 200 or 400 mg progesterone. The dose is 800 mg daily in two divided doses beginning just before the onset of premenstrual symptoms until menstruation starts. Double-blind controlled studies of progesterone therapy for premenstrual syndrome could not show progesterone to be better than placebo. Many questions about progesterone therapy remain unanswered. The dose of progesterone recommended is high even if only a portion of it is absorbed through the vagina, which has a good blood supply and clearly absorbs drugs and hormones. Although the production rate of progesterone is 25 mg per day during the luteal phase and 200 mg per day during the third trimester of pregnancy, the dose used for premenstrual syndrome therapy is 800 mg per day, which far exceeds the amount of any deficiency. Caution must be exercised, and patients must be accurately informed. Progesterone has also been used intramuscularly, rectally, and as an implant for therapy of premenstrual syndrome. The progestogens that have been used at one time or another for treatment of premenstrual syndrome include norethisterone, dimethisterone, ethisterone, medroxyprogesterone, and dydrogesterone.

4. *Oral contraceptives*. If cyclic ovarian activity is essential to the pathogenesis of the premenstrual syndrome, it should make sense to see a reduction or improvement of the premenstrual syndrome when cyclic ovarian activity is suppressed by the oral contraceptives. The general "clinical impression" is that premenstrual syndrome could worsen or improve with oral contraceptives. The incidence of premenstrual syndrome has been reported as being 29 percent less in oral contraceptive users than in nonusers. The more progestogenic oral contraceptives appear to be associated with fewer symptoms. However, in one double-blind study there was no difference between oral contraceptive and placebo therapy for premenstrual syndrome.

5. *Bromocriptine*. Clinical trials of bromocriptine for premenstrual syndrome have produced conflicting results. The balance of evidence indicates no significant improvement with bromocriptine. Improvements, if any, were mainly in breast symptoms, edema, and weight increase. Therefore bromocriptine, if considered for premenstrual syndrome therapy, is best reserved for the breast and water retention symptoms.

6. *Prostaglandin synthetase inhibitors*. There are no studies that have examined the levels of prostaglandins in premenstrual syndrome or induction of the syndrome with administration of prostaglandins. However, a preliminary double-blind placebo-controlled study of the PGSI mefenamic acid showed alleviation of some of the symptoms of premenstrual syndrome. The evidence, however, is too preliminary to warrant recommending PGSIs for treatment of premenstrual syndrome. In patients who also have dys-

menorrhea, however, these agents should be given during menstruation.

7. *Other therapies. Vitamins A* and *B₆* have been used for treating premenstrual syndrome. Vitamin B_6 (pyridoxine) has been used on the basis that it is a co-enzyme for dopa-decarboxylase and would therefore stimulate serotonin and dopamine metabolism from tryptophan and thus reduce prolactin levels. The studies were uncontrolled; and in view of the adverse effects of excessive amounts of vitamins A and B_6, caution should be exercised concerning the dose of these vitamins when used. In the few controlled trials on the efficacy of pyridoxine on premenstrual syndrome, the results have been conflicting. *Danazol* is effective for treatment of benign breast disease and significantly improves the breast symptoms but not most of the other symptoms of premenstrual syndrome. *Bilateral oophorectomy* with or without hysterectomy has been resorted to by some, but cyclic symptoms have been found to persist despite the surgery.

Cyclic Breast Disorders

The normal mild premenstrual breast discomfort (often attended by slight swelling and tenderness) that accompanies the physiologic interstitial edema and increased glandular activity produced by the hormonal stimuli present at this phase of the cycle has already been noted. The exaggerated form of this phenomenon invariably associated with the premenstrual syndrome has been discussed.

Not infrequently, repeated occurrence of these cyclic breast changes leads to palpable anatomic abnormalities that may be either transient (subsiding postmenstrually) or ultimately chronic. Sometimes these changes have been erroneously referred to as fibrocystic disease. A more appropriate term is fibrocystic changes of the breast. The lesions are usually bilateral and multiple. Pain and tenderness, which are accentuated premenstrually, are the cardinal symptoms.

Fibrocystic changes occur in three stages with overlapping of the symptoms at any stage. Early changes are seen in the late teens and early twenties with premenstrual painful, tender breasts, particularly in the axillary tail. Tenderness and fullness of the breast with a pseudolump in the axilla are present. This stage is followed by the stage of multinodular breast, sometimes referred to as "Schimmelbusch disease," characterized by multinodularities and occasionally a dominant mass. This stage is sometimes difficult to differentiate from carcinoma. The final stage is that of cystic changes, when the patient complains of pain or a burning sensation in conjunction with the appearance of a mass in the breast. The cyst may increase in size rapidly; is well circumscribed, tender, and mobile; and it transilluminates. A deep-seated cyst can be difficult to differentiate from breast carcinoma, but ultrasound of the breasts may show up the cystic areas. The fluid aspirated is usually yellow or clear if there are fibrocystic changes of the breast. The peak incidence of cystic changes occurs between 30 and 50 years of age.

This cyclic breast condition may start with a progesterone/estrogen imbalance, perhaps with excess estrogen playing a dominant role in the formation of the cyst, although the premenstrual progesterone must also play an etiologic role in the pain and discomfort. However, in many women the cause may not be a hormone imbalance but, rather, an abnormal breast tissue response.

These cyclic breast disorders present two major problems for the physician: diagnosis and relief of discomfort. For diagnosis, mammography is useful and can be diagnostic when used in conjunction with ultrasound, especially for identifying small or deep-seated cysts. Aspiration of the cyst may be necessary. Further details of the workup, diagnosis, and management of breast disorders are given in Chapter 24.

With regard to troublesome cyclic breast symptoms, whether in association with premenstrual syndrome or alone, judicious use of diuretics can provide adequate relief. Avoiding caffeine or caffeine-containing products or methylxanthine-containing foods during the luteal phase of the cycle can provide relief. Additionally, some studies suggest that danazol (Chap. 12) may be effective for treatment of cyclic breast tenderness or chronic cystic mastitis. Along the same principles, testosterone has been used with good response. The danazol and testosterone presumably bring about relief through an antiestrogenic effect.

SELECTED READINGS

Cunanan, R. G., Courey, N. G., and Lippes, J. Laparoscopic findings in patients with pelvic pain. *Am. J. Obstet. Gynecol.* 146:586, 1983.

Dawood, M. Y. *Dysmenorrhea.* Baltimore: William and Wilkins, 1981.

Dawood, M. Y. Dysmenorrhea and prostaglandins: Pharmacological and therapeutic considerations. *Drugs* 122:42, 1981.

Dawood, M. Y., McGuire, J. L., and Demers, L. M. *Premenstrual Syndrome and Dysmenorrhea.* Baltimore: Urban & Schwarzenber, 1985.

Dawood, M. Y. Premenstrual tension syndrome. *Obstet. Gynecol. Annu.* 14:328, 1985.

Dawood, M. Y. Nonsteroidal anti-inflammatory drugs and changing attitudes toward dysmenorrhea. *Am. J. Med.* 84:23 (Suppl. 5A), 1988.

Dawood, M. Y., and Ramos, J. Transcutaneous electrical nerve stimulation (TENS) for treatment of primary dysmenorrhea: A randomized cross-over comparison with placebo TENS and ibuprofen. *Obstet. Gynecol.* 75:656, 1990.

Reid, R. L., Yen, S. S. C. The premenstrual syndrome. *Clin. Obstet. Gynecol.* 26:710, 1983.

Rubinow, D. R., Hoban, M. C., Grover, G. N., et al. Changes in plasma hormones across the menstrual cycle in patients with menstrually related mood disorders and in control subjects. *Am. J. Obstet. Gynecol.* 158:5, 1988.

Smith, S., Rinehart, J. S., Ruddock, V. E., and Schiff, I. Treatment of premenstrual syndrome with alprazolam: Results of a double-blind, placebo-controlled, randomized crossover clinical trial. *Obstet. Gynecol.* 70:37, 1987.

Youngs, D. D., Reame, N. Psychosomatic aspects of menstrual dysfunction. *Clin. Obstet. Gynecol.* 26:777, 1983.

11

Disorders of Anovulatory Cycles

The events and physiology of the normal menstrual cycle described in Chapter 9 form the basis for understanding the deviation from such normal cyclic physiologic mechanisms that are common to menstrual disorders associated with anovulatory cycles. Disorders associated with anovulatory cycles almost always present with menstrual irregularities of one kind or another. Although there could be a functional hormonal basis for the menstrual irregularity and the anovulation, it is important to identify the specific pathology responsible for the clinical manifestation so that the underlying cause is specifically treated.

Disturbances of ovulation and, therefore of the ovulatory cycle, can present with infrequent ovulation or oligoovulation to complete anovulation. Although both forms of ovulatory disturbances can present with menstrual irregularities, amenorrhea is usually associated with anovulation. Whereas anovulation itself usually gives rise to amenorrhea, the associations with variable estrogen levels and their fluctuations can bring about irregular shedding of the endometrium and therefore irregular bleeding superimposed on the amenorrhea. These true endocrine disorders may be (1) of primary ovarian origin, (2) the result of a more generalized endocrine-metabolic disorder disturbance in one of the endocrine glands (pituitary, thyroid, or adrenal), or (3) disturbance in the hypothalamic regulatory centers.

This chapter discusses the menstrual and gynecologic disorders that occur during anovulatory cycles. To understand the common basis for all dysfunctional or acyclic menstrual disorders, the abnormal physiology of anovulation is discussed first. The next section then covers primary ovarian disorders, followed by generalized endocrine-metabolic disturbance. The last section of this chapter deals with two common presenting symptoms, amenorrhea and hirsutism.

ABNORMAL PHYSIOLOGY OF ANOVULATORY CYCLE

Unopposed by progesterone, estrogen stimulates the endometrium continuously in an unimpeded manner. However, an absolute or relative decline in estrogens below the critical level necessary for continued endometrial growth and hormonal support causes periodic uterine bleeding called withdrawal (anovulatory) bleeding. Such bleeding is typically irregular in amount and duration, the flow varying in accordance with the length of time and degree of prior estrogenic stimulation, as well as with the degree and duration of the estrogen withdrawal. The absence of progesterone results from failure of any of the active ovarian follicles to mature to the point of ovulation and subsequent corpus luteum formation. Such cycles are therefore termed anovulatory (Fig. 11-1). The fluctuating estrogen levels that lead to periodic bleeding episodes alternating with intervals of amenorrhea of varying duration are due to intermittent variations in the number and functional status of the active ovarian follicles present at any present time. If a number of follicles are present and active, and if new ones are recruited to develop as some degenerate, high or even increasing levels of estrogen are present. Simultaneously, the endometrium may continue to proliferate for weeks or months, even to the point of undergoing simple glandular hyperplasia (cystic, or "Swiss cheese," hyperplasia) and ultimately gross, polypoid change if the stimulus to growth is sufficiently protracted (Fig. 11-2). If proliferation continues, though estrogen levels remain constant, a relative estrogen inadequacy ultimately occurs and leads to bleeding. One or more follicles may simultaneously deteriorate; and if they are not replaced promptly by actively functioning new ones, absolute estrogen withdrawal results and endometrial bleeding ensues.

As already noted, in an anovulatory cycle the endometrium is stimulated to proliferate only, so that a specimen obtained by endometrial biopsy or curettage

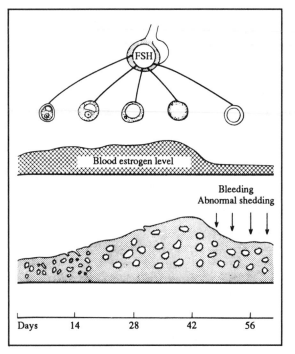

Fig. 11-1. Pathophysiology of the anovulatory cycle.

done at any time during such a cycle or during the bleeding phase reveals either simple proliferative endometrium or hyperplasia, with or without polypoid change, on histologic examination. Thus a biopsy performed at a time when a secretory endometrium would chronologically be expected if ovarian function was normal is usually diagnostic of the anovulatory nature of the cycle.

Anovulatory bleeding is usually not accompanied by cramps, is frequently excessively heavy, and may be prolonged because of reduced or absent vasoconstriction and myometrial contractions that are induced by progesterone in the normal ovulatory cycle. Excessive and prolonged flow is also due to the often much thicker superficial endometrial layer, the accompanying richer blood supply, and the irregular uncontrolled desquamation that occurs without the effect of progesterone.

The abnormal, continued, unopposed estrogen stimulation also exerts its effect on other ovarian hor-

mone-sensitive target tissues, bringing about symptoms. Prolonged, uninterrupted breast glandular activity induced by estrogen alone may lead to severe mastalgia and even to gross cystic changes. Similar unphysiologic responses are elicited in the fallopian tubes, cervix, and vagina. Such a pattern of reproductive tract function is an infertile one, not only absolutely and because of anovulation but also because of inadequacy of all the other mechanisms designed to promote ovum pickup and safe transfer, sperm penetration, survival, and transport, and a proper uterine environment prepared for and favorable to the implantation and further growth of the early embryo. Thus even if an ovum were to be supplied, conception would be most unlikely; implantation and further development of even a hypothetically fertilized ovum would be impossible.

This broad view on the overall fertility effect of the anovulatory cycle is relevant to the recognition, understanding, and treatment of infertility. Poor or defective ovulatory cycles may present with less obvious but more subtle menstrual disruptions such as temporary shifts in intermenstrual intervals, transient variation in menstrual flow, and premenstrual spotting, but the woman is infertile. Therefore infertility may be the only presentation with some forms of poor or defective ovulatory disturbance (as with an inadequate luteal phase) as well as with anovulation with gross menstrual irregularities or amenorrhea.

It is not the lack of ovulation per se that is responsible for the various types of menstrual dysfunction that may accompany the anovulatory cycle but the failure of normal follicle maturation and corpus luteum function (specifically progesterone production), of which failure of ovulation is just one manifestation, though an important one in its own right.

Anovulatory menstrual function is characteristic of the first year or two following the onset of puberty. Ordinarily, the resulting irregularities are of minor importance, and excessive bleeding does not occur. However, persistence of an anovulatory type of ovarian function further along during adolescence or its reappearance later in adult life is responsible for most of the clinically significant functional menstrual disorders encountered.

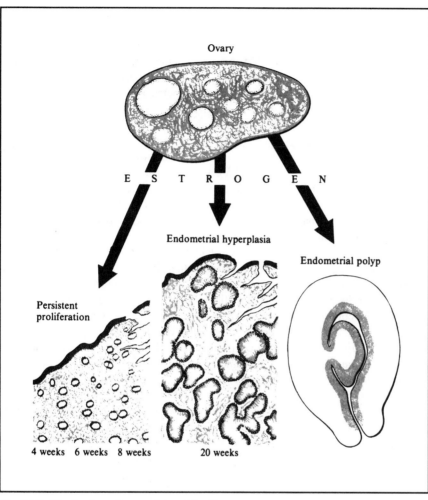

Fig. 11-2. Mechanism of anovulatory bleeding.

DYSFUNCTIONAL UTERINE BLEEDING

Although many acyclic menstrual disturbances are accompanied by short intervals of amenorrhea or involve oligomenorrhea, the most prominent clinical feature is the occurrence, sooner or later, of excessive bleeding: too frequent flow, too heavy flow, too prolonged flow. Hence this spectrum of functional menstrual irregularities is often considered under the term *dysfunctional uterine bleeding* or *anovulatory uterine bleeding*.

Dysfunctional uterine bleeding is responsible for the largest single group of clinical problems that confront the gynecologist. In its strict definition, dysfunctional uterine bleeding is irregular vaginal bleeding without underlying uterine pathology (e.g., myomas, polyps), bleeding diathesis, specific ovarian lesions, or a fundamental endocrine disorder.

In a small percentage of women, the anovulatory cycles and irregular bleeding are due to a more fundamental endocrine disorder.

1. Thyroid disease (hyperthyroidism, hypothyroidism)

2. Adrenal disease (hyperplasia, benign or malignant tumors)
3. Pituitary disease (failure or neoplasms)
4. Diabetes mellitus, with its generalized metabolic and steroid hormonal disturbances

The anovulatory cycles leading to irregular uterine bleeding may also be due to a specific primary ovarian lesion, of which the following are the principal ones encountered.

1. Stein-Leventhal syndrome; ovarian hyperthecosis (see below)
2. Functioning ovarian tumors; arrhenoblastoma, granulosa or theca cell tumors, hilus cell tumors (Chap. 18).
3. Chronic pelvic inflammatory disease (or, more rarely, extensive pelvic endometriosis), in which there are severe pathologic changes in the ovaries leading to disturbances of follicular function

Any of the conditions cited may lead to a disturbance in the normal pituitary-ovarian axis, anovulation, and resulting irregular cycles characterized by amenorrhea, oligomenorrhea, or dysfunctional uterine bleeding ("functional menometrorrhagia").

Certain other generalized metabolic disturbances also seem to predispose to the development of an anovulatory type of menstrual function:

1. Marked obesity (even in the absence of diabetes or thyroid disease)
2. Severe malnutrition, e.g., anorexia nervosa syndrome
3. Chronic, debilitating, systemic disease, e.g., tuberculosis

In obese patients, there is increased extraovarian production of estrogens from androgens in the adipose tissues, often giving rise to elevated tonic luteinizing hormone (LH) secretion and therefore anovulation. With severe malnutrition and in anorexia nervosa patients, pituitary gonadotropin function and secretion revert to a more infantile form and therefore anovulation. With these conditions the major therapeutic effort should be directed at the underlying systemic abnormality. Treatment aimed at restoring ovulatory cycles can be of considerable symptomatic value but should not be attempted by itself only.

In some patients the temporary development of an anovulatory type of ovarian function leads to a functional type of amenorrhea, in which there is no basic underlying impairment or abnormality of reproductive tract potential. Here the problem is invariably one of a temporary, reversible disturbance in the hypothalamic-pituitary-regulating mechanism; hence this type of functional amenorrhea is often referred to as *hypothalamic amenorrhea*. These patients have no organic lesion at any point in the reproductive tract or its regulatory apparatus, and their anovulatory state and associated oligomenorrhea or functional amenorrhea has usually been initiated by (1) emotional stress at some point in their life situation; (2) marked variations in weight—either an abrupt loss induced by crash dieting or a sudden gain (conversion of ovarian and adrenal C19 androgens to estrone in the peripheral adipose tissue compartment may account for the frequent occurrence of anovulatory cycles and functional amenorrhea in obese women); or, less often, (3) nonspecific metabolic and endocrine effects of a chronic systemic illness. The history, physical findings, and response to a test dose of progesterone are often sufficient to confirm the presence of a functional hypothalamic amenorrhea, without the need for a more elaborate endocrine workup; however, the latter is necessary in some cases and is discussed below in detail.

Treatment of simple functional amenorrhea is usually expectant, first explaining the situation to the patient and reassuring her that spontaneous recovery is the rule. Ordinarily, oral contraceptive treatment or cyclic estrogen-progesterone therapy to produce an artificial menstrual cycle in these patients should be avoided because it only perpetuates hypothalamic-pituitary inhibition and prevents spontaneous return of the normal regulatory mechanism. A cyclic program of an oral progesterone alone for five days can be given every month or two to produce withdrawal bleeding without interfering with spontaneous resumption of ovulatory function, but this measure is rarely necessary. In the case of women with hypothalamic amenorrhea who want to begin childbearing without further delay, ovulation induction with clomiphene can be employed (see below).

In most patients with dysfunctional bleeding, the problem is usually of short duration, is frequently prone to spontaneous correction, and is nearly always temporary if handled properly. Furthermore—and most important—no basic underlying endocrine or metabolic disorder is present. However, certain contributing or precipitating factors invariably lurk in the background, of which the following are the most common examples.

1. Transient, acute physical or psychic stress.
   a. The temporary emotional influences leading to the menstrual irregularities (occasionally even to hypothalamic amenorrhea) of college freshmen or first-year student nurses.
   b. Emotional upsets that may affect any woman in the prime of reproductive life, e.g., family illness or death, marital discord, problem children, pressure of outside activities, social or occupational personality clashes.
   c. A febrile illness that leads to a delayed or missed period followed by dysfunctional bleeding (the high fever interfering with normal follicular development and resulting in failure of ovulation, inadequate progesterone production, or both).
   d. Prolonged administration of substantial amounts of certain tranquilizers, which may produce anovulatory cycles with associated menstrual disturbances.
2. Moderate fluctuations in body weight; chronic physical, mental, or emotional fatigue.
3. Seasonal variations. For reasons that are not entirely clear, anovulatory cycles with short periods of amenorrhea or episodes of dysfunctional bleeding are more common during the summer months, particularly July and August.

Finally, as already noted, dysfunctional bleeding is definitely more common at the beginning and at the end of active menstrual life, i.e., during adolescence and the premenopausal and menopausal phases, because the ovarian cycle is apparently more unstable and more subject and vulnerable to disruptive influences early and late in life.

Diagnostic Approach

The probability that abnormal bleeding is dysfunctional in origin is nearly always suggested by a careful and accurate history. The various clinical manifestations of the anovulatory type of ovarian function include (1) a premature or delayed period that is then prolonged; (2) oligomenorrhea or polymenorrhea, with the episodes of bleeding irregular in duration and amount; and (3) amenorrhea of short duration followed by the onset of a continuous type of bleeding that may vary in amount from day to day. Although highly variable in amount, the bleeding is at some time or another profuse but invariably painless. Possible factors precipitating the change from a previously perfectly normal, regular menstrual pattern may be uncovered in the history. Finally, the general physical survey and pelvic examination usually reveal no evidence of an underlying endocrine or metabolic disorder and no sign of any local pelvic disease. (The presence of incidental but asymptomatic local pelvic disease must be carefully evaluated and integrated with the overall clinical picture when arriving at a correct explanation for the abnormal bleeding.)

In the differential diagnosis, it is particularly important to exclude disorders of early pregnancy, as the history accompanying an early tubal pregnancy or a threatened, incomplete, or missed abortion may be similar (Chap. 16). The presence of cancer of the cervix or corpus uteri, submucous fibroids, symptomatic uterine adenomyosis, or endometrial polyps must be excluded. An endometrial biopsy or a curettage that reveals a secretory rather than a proliferative or hyperplastic endometrium is often a clue to the presence of primary uterine disease as the source for the abnormal bleeding.

One other group of disorders that sometimes simulate dysfunctional uterine bleeding and actually represent a type of "functional bleeding" (because again no local uterine disease is present) are the hematologic diseases with prolonged bleeding or clotting times or increased capillary fragility, and the diagnostic screening program for assessing generalized hemorrhagic disorders in a patient with excessive uterine bleeding described in Chapter 2. For example, easy bruising, menorrhagia, and even significant midcycle hemorrhage are common first manifestations of von Willebrand's disease, a coagulopathy characterized by a prolonged bleeding time seen in association with a reduced plasma Factor VIII level, a capillary defect, and probably deficient platelet adhesiveness as well. A correct diagnosis can often be made on the basis of an accurate history (there is a strong familial tendency, as it is an autosomal dominant hereditary disorder) and a simple bleeding time determination, thereby avoiding the need for diagnostic curettage, which carries the risk of provoking even more excessive hemorrhage. The immediate arrest of any major bleeding episode can nearly always be achieved by intravenous infusions of plasma or Factor VIII preparations (cryoprecipitate) and platelet transfusions if indicated.

1. *Adolescents and young women (early twenties).* A detailed history, careful general physical examination, and pelvic or rectal examination (or both) in a patient with suspected dysfunctional bleeding are usually sufficient to exclude other conditions and establish the diagnosis of a functional menstrual disorder. Thyroid function studies are frequently indicated and may be helpful. A complete endocrinologic survey is required if there are symptoms or findings suggestive of some more basic underlying endocrine disturbance or if there is failure of response to adequate therapy. It is particularly important to rule out the presence of blood dyscrasias and abnormal bleeding tendencies in this age group. As discussed more fully below, the possible existence of polycystic ovary syndrome should also be carefully considered. *Curettage or endometrial biopsy is rarely necessary* as either a diagnostic or a therapeutic maneuver. However, for obese women, endometrial tissue sampling for histology is necessary to rule out endometrial hyperplasia or carcinoma due to the excess extraglandular estrogen production.

2. *Women in the prime of menstrual life (age 25 to 40).* Early pregnancy disorders are the most important conditions to be differentiated in this age group. Pregnancy tests and, in acute situations, laparoscopy to rule out an ectopic gestation may be indicated. Curettage is occasionally necessary, either to exclude the presence of submucous fibroids or endometrial polyps or to control excessive bleeding if the response to conservative management is unsatisfactory. Obviously, pelvic malignant disease must also be excluded by thorough examination, cytologic studies, and biopsies if indicated. Except for thyroid disturbances, endocrine disorders or blood dyscrasias seldom manifest for the first time in women of this age group, but thyroid function studies again are worth doing.

3. *Premenopausal and menopausal women.* Although the same general principle applies to these women, *curettage is almost always necessary* to be certain of ruling out endometrial or endocervical cancer.

Therapy

In patients in whom dysfunctional bleeding is merely a secondary symptom of some fundamental endocrine disorder, treatment should be directed at the primary cause. However, symptomatic control of the anovulatory bleeding may be temporarily achieved with the methods used for dysfunctional uterine bleeding. In most cases the dysfunctional bleeding is temporary, and the disturbed ovarian function is completely reversible by simple therapeutic measures.

Because the underlying feature is failure of normal follicular maturation and hence inadequate progesterone production, these patients bleed abnormally and irregularly from a proliferative or hyperplastic (occasionally atrophic) endometrium. It is the lack of progestational change in the endometrium that results in the irregularity of the onset of flow and in the frequently excessive and prolonged bleeding. The various therapeutic programs therefore aim to supply progesterone in some form to promote normal endometrial maturation artificially and ultimately to achieve complete shedding of the secretory type of endometrial lining so produced, in place of the prolonged and incomplete sloughing and accompanying abnormal bleeding of the proliferative and hyperplastic endometrium. In cases where there has been prolonged bleeding and therefore shedding of the endometrium or if there is definite evidence of atrophic endometrium, estrogen therapy is initially employed to stop the bleeding. Specific hormone regimes for dysfunctional uterine bleeding are now given.

SINGLE COURSE OF PROGESTERONE. A simple course of progesterone is useful if the bleeding is of short duration (one or two cycles) in women in the prime of menstrual life with little or no history of previous irregularities. A single intramuscular injection of progesterone in oil (short-acting) 25 to 50 mg or one of the more potent long-acting progestational preparations such as hydroxyprogesterone caproate (Delalutin) 250 mg can be conveniently given. The current bleeding usually ceases within a few days of the injection as the endometrium undergoes progestational change, but after a few days to as long as one or two weeks this phase is followed by the artificially produced "normal period" or withdrawal flow from the resulting secondary type of endometrium. This form of therapy is sometimes referred to as "medical curettage." The patient should be warned that during the first 48 hours of this "normal period" the flow may be excessive because of the varying degrees of endometrial overproliferation prior to the administration of progesterone. She should be reassured that the flow will thereafter be more normal and will ordinarily cease within the usual 5 to 7 days.

Similar beneficial effects can be obtained with a single, short course of oral progestins using norethindrone acetate (5 to 10 mg) or dydrogesterone (10 to 20 mg), each given daily for 10 to 14 days. Whether given by injection or by mouth, this single course of progesterone results in the return of normal ovulatory ovarian function in the following cycles in approximately 85 percent of patients in whom the functional disturbance has been an isolated event. Currently, progesterone itself cannot be given orally as it is poorly absorbed. Other progestins that could be used include (1) the 19-norsteroid compounds; (2) the 17-hydroxyprogesterone compounds, including medroxyprogesterone acetate, hydroxyprogesterone caproate, and dydrogesterone (6-dehydroretroprogesterone). Dydrogesterone is structurally related to natural progesterone but is more than 30 times as potent pharmacologically, does not inhibit ovulation, and has no thermogenic or androgenic effects.

It is important to note that improvement in the secretory pattern of the endometrium and other beneficial effects are obtained only when progestins are given during the latter half of the cycle. When therapy is begun during the first half of the cycle, normal proliferation is somewhat inhibited and final maturation is less complete.

CYCLIC PROGESTERONE THERAPY. Supplemental progesterone therapy more prolonged than single-course therapy invariably is required in patients (1) who fail to respond to a single course of therapy, (2) whose bleeding irregularities are of considerable duration, (3) whose "periods" remain fairly regular but who suffer from increasing menorrhagia (excessive and prolonged flow), and (4) who required curettage to control the original bleeding episode but the anovulatory cycles promptly recur. Supplemental progesterone therapy is most effectively given during the latter half of the cycle so that the normal progestational phase is simulated as closely as possible. Any of the current oral progestogens in the dosages previously indicated can be employed and are usually begun on the fourteenth or sixteenth day of the cycle and continued for 12 or 10 days, respectively (e.g., Provera 5 to 10 mg daily; Norlutate 5 to 10 mg daily). Cyclic therapy should usually be continued for three or four cycles and then stopped.

In most patients, return to spontaneous normal ovarian function and ovulatory cycles follows such a program. Presumably, the artificially created, relatively normal estrogen-progesterone balance aids in reestablishing the normal reciprocally related pituitary-ovarian regulatory mechanism; and normal follicle stimulation and subsequent maturation, ovulation, and corpus luteum function are restored. If a satisfactory response is not obtained, further investigation is definitely indicated to rule out a more fundamental endocrine disturbance or a local organic cause for irregular bleeding.

CYCLIC ESTROGEN-PROGESTERONE THERAPY. The addition of estrogen to the cyclic program of supplemental progesterone therapy may be required in adolescents and premenopausal women because in both age groups an estrogen as well as a progesterone deficiency is commonly present. Endometrial biopsies that show an atrophic type of proliferative endometrium is helpful for determining if the patient requires estrogen as well as progesterone for therapy.

Estrogen in the form of Premarin (1.25 mg) once or

twice daily is begun on day 1 and continued for 25 days, adding the progestational agent as usual on the fourteenth day and continuing until the twenty-fifth treatment day, when both drugs are discontinued. Bleeding usually ensues two to three days later. The treatment course is repeated for three or four cycles, beginning with estrogen again on the first day of each withdrawal flow. If withdrawal flow is substantially delayed beyond the usual two to three days, it usually indicates that the patient has ovulated spontaneously. Therapy can be discontinued then and a return of normal ovulatory cycles is frequently observed thereafter.

An alternative to cyclic estrogen-progesterone therapy is use of an oral contraceptive that contains both estrogen and progestin. It is started on day 1 and continued for 21 days. Initially, if there is still breakthrough bleeding, the dose could be increased to 1 tablet twice a day.

Management of Acute Bleeding Episodes. Dysfunctional uterine bleeding is sometimes heavy. An acute episode of profuse hemorrhage with a fall in hemoglobin and blood volume sufficient to require transfusions is not uncommon. In this situation, prompt arrest of the bleeding is obviously desirable, and curettage is often the most rapidly effective way of achieving control. Curettage is not helpful if bleeding has been profuse and prolonged, as the endometrium has already been shed.

In this case and in cases in which for any of a number of reasons it may not be safe or advisable to proceed with immediate curettage, short-term hormone therapy can quickly arrest excessive dysfunctional bleeding. Estrogens are usually more rapid than progestogens in this respect and can be given as a single intravenous injection (e.g., Premarin 20 mg) or orally (e.g., Premarin 2.5 mg) every 2 hours until bleeding ceases or abates considerably. A maintenance dose should be continued for 20 to 25 days and progesterone added during the last two weeks in an attempt to create a more normal secretory endometrium, withdrawal bleeding is allowed to occur at the end of that time. Cyclic estrogen-progesterone therapy is then advisable for another three or four months. Perhaps an even simpler alternative, when the oral medication route is feasible, is the use of one of the combination

oral contraceptive agents, administering 1 tablet two to four times daily to arrest the hemorrhage, then allowing a more normal withdrawal menstrual flow. Thereafter, cyclic oral contraceptive therapy may be wise for three or four months to minimize the chance of recurrent dysfunctional bleeding.

If curettage has become necessary, it may be followed in 40 to 60 percent of cases by return to a normal ovulatory pattern without further maneuvers or by a remission of months or years. This regimen is often sufficient to tide the premenopausal patient over completion of the menopause. At the same time, curettage has served to exclude any organic lesions. If abnormal bleeding should recur within a few months of the curettage, cyclic hormonal management can then be undertaken.

Additional Measures. Attention to more general factors may be indicated and prove helpful in the correction of the anovulatory pattern with its associated dysfunctional bleeding. Reassurance, a thorough explanation of the mechanism involved, and efforts to ferret out and modify, when possible, any underlying psychogenic or general health factors should be a routine part of the general management of all patients. Regulation of the body weight also may be important.

If repeated curettage and adequate attempts to control recurrent refractory dysfunctional uterine bleeding by supplemental hormone therapy fail and excessive bleeding persists, hysterectomy may ultimately prove necessary in some patients.

OVARIAN ENDOCRINE DISORDERS

Ovarian endocrine disorders are due to either hormone-producing tumors (sometimes referred to as functioning ovarian tumors) or nonneoplastic ovarian endocrinopathies. Hormone-producing ovarian tumors are described in greater detail in Chapter 18. Hormone-producing ovarian tumors include the granulosa cell tumor, theca cell tumors, arrhenoblastomas, sclerosing stromal tumor, gynandroblastoma, gonadoblastoma, hilus cell tumor, lipoid cell tumor, adrenal-like tumors, struma ovarii, stromal luteinization, and luteoma of pregnancy. Nonneoplastic ovarian endocrinopathies include a variety of ovarian disorders (discussed below). The most common cause is polycystic ovarian disease, which in its extreme form was originally referred to as the Stein-Leventhal syndrome.

ENDOCRINOPATHIES CAUSED BY OVARIAN NEOPLASMS

See Chapters 18 and 28.

NONNEOPLASTIC OVARIAN ENDOCRINOPATHIES

Polycystic Ovarian Disease (Stein-Leventhal Syndrome)

Stein and Leventhal first described the syndrome that now carries their names in a group of women with the classic form of the disease, all of whom had bilaterally pale, smooth, markedly (three to five times) enlarged polycystic ovaries and varying combinations of the typical symptom complex of amenorrhea, infertility, obesity, and hirsutism. Polycystic ovarian disease is now recognized to be a somewhat broader clinical entity than what Stein and Leventhal observed, which represented the more extreme examples of the condition. Thus polycystic ovarian disease occurs more frequently than the original classic syndrome but may have somewhat different clinical manifestations.

Clinical Features. The typical patient is a young woman in her late teens or twenties in whom, following a menarche at the normal age and after a few years of somewhat irregular and invariably anovulatory cycles, either oligomenorrhea (perhaps one to three, often scanty periods yearly) or secondary complete amenorrhea developed. However, approximately 10 to 15 percent of these patients complain of menometrorrhagia, with episodes of prolonged and somewhat profuse bleeding alternating with intervals of amenorrhea. There is a tendency to obesity in many patients. Hirsutism is present in 50 to 60 percent of the patients, but actual virilization is rare, although slight clitoral enlargement has occasionally been noted. The patients are otherwise normally female in appearance, although many have small breasts (50 percent) and a small, infantile type of uterus (75 percent).

The symptom complex mirrors the fact that, with few exceptions, there is complete failure of ovulation as a result of the basic disturbance in ovarian function. Hence infertility, the other chief feature of the syndrome, is often the presenting complaint. Pregnancy has been known to occur, and evidence of occasional ovulation is seen in a small percentage of patients at the time of laparoscopy or laparotomy. The disturbance in ovulation is often reversible with treatment.

Pathologic Features. There is always bilateral ovarian involvement. Both ovaries are often grossly and usually symmetrically enlarged, sometimes approaching three to five times the size of normal ovaries, but this degree of enlargement is not necessarily always present. The ovaries may be only slightly enlarged or essentially normal in size. The ovarian surface is usually smooth and pearly white with prominent surface vessels, in contrast to its normal, pale yellowish, wrinkled appearance. Although the ovarian capsule is characteristically thick and fibrous, often the more superficial follicle microcysts can be seen shining through. On sectioning the ovary, the increased capsular thickness is apparent, and the many small cysts, usually 5 to 10 mm in diameter, are seen lying within a dense, fibrous stroma.

On microscopic examination the markedly thickened capsule (tunica albuginea) is noted, the ovary being literally surrounded by a dense layer of collagenous tissue. Multiple subcapsular follicular cysts are seen in all stages of development or atresia, many with a normal granulosa cell layer and an active, at times hyperplastic, theca interna, the latter showing characteristic, often excessive luteinization. The degree to which luteinization of the theca cells of the cysts themselves is present varies considerably but appears to be most marked in patients with hirsutism and other evidence of an androgenic effect. Occasionally, there is some hyperplasia of the stroma in the central portion of the ovary as well. The final typical feature, as clinically suggested by anovulation or oligoovulation, is the virtual absence of any corpora lutea or corpora albicantia except occasionally.

Pathogenesis. Although the basic cause remains unknown, mechanical prevention of ovulation by the thickened ovarian capsule is no longer acceptable. Current biochemical and endocrine evidence indicates that patients with polycystic ovarian disease have an abnormal, constantly elevated *tonic secretion* of pituitary LH, which in turn continuously stimulates both ovaries. Ovarian stimulation by follicle-stimulating hormone (FSH) leads to folliculogenesis, but the constantly elevated *tonic* LH level leads to arrest of follicular development and premature luteinization, resulting in multiple subcapsular cysts arrested at various stages of development—hence the description and term applied, polycystic ovarian disease or syndrome. The constantly elevated *tonic* levels of LH are thought to be due to a positive estrogen feedback on LH surges.

Production rates of estrone (E_1) are markedly increased in women with polycystic ovarian disease (PCO), and this elevated estrone drives the pituitary in an estrogen positive feedback manner to sustained, elevated LH levels. Estrone is increased presumably because of the constant stimulation on the ovarian stroma to produce androgens such as androstenedione and testosterone. Androstenedione is then aromatized either in the ovary or in the peripheral adipose tissues to estrone or converted peripherally to testosterone. Hence androgen levels are elevated to varying degrees in women with PCO, and consequently the clinical manifestation of hirsutism is seen in these women. Estradiol levels are not increased.

Because of the increased estrone production rates in women with PCO, some have elevated prolactin secretion secondary to the hyperestronemia. Therefore galactorrhea is also present in some of them. The absence of a true midcycle LH surge further contributes to the absence of ovulation seen with PCO. The irregular secretion of estrogens but elevated production rates of estrone stimulate the endometrium to proliferate, and irregular uterine bleeding, menometrorrhagia, and endometrial hyperplasia are frequently encountered. Thus the incidence of endometrial hyperplasia and endometrial carcinoma in women with PCO, if left untreated, is higher than in ovulatory women.

Despite the above current understanding, it is still not clear whether the primary defect is originally (1) at the hypothalamic-pituitary level and compounded by the increased estrone and its positive LH feedback or (2) at the ovarian level and compounded by the sustained, elevated tonic LH secretion by the pituitary. Consensus suggests that the primary defect is at the hypothalamic-pituitary level and may involve the opiodergic control of pituitary gonadotropin secretion through a variety of factors including estrogen feedback. Alteration in light exposure and stress can produce PCO in rats. Certainly PCO is not infrequently seen in young women in urban societies with a high level of daily stress in their lives.

Enzymatic defects in the ovaries or adrenal glands have been implicated in the pathogenesis of PCO, but these mechanisms may be operating in only a small proportion of cases, if any. Deficiency of enzyme(s) in the ovarian steroidogenic pathway resulting in elevated androgen production, and therefore estrone, have been described. Similarly, deficiency in the adrenal steroidogenic enzyme pathway have been described, but these disorders are probably true variants of mild adrenal hyperplasia, which gives rise to interference of the hypothalamic-pituitary-ovarian axis and therefore secondary ovarian changes. Indeed patients with Cushing's disease or patients given corticosteroids for prolonged periods develop ovaries with thickened, glistening white capsules owing to the corticosteroid effects and resembling ovaries of women with Stein-Leventhal syndrome. It is important to identify these patients from the standpoint of differential diagnosis and management, but they do not have PCO as such. In addition, elevated levels of dehydroepiandrosterone sulfate (DHEAS), an adrenal steroid, are found in some patients with PCO, and rats given DHEAS produce ovarian and hormonal changes similar to those seen with PCO.

Diagnosis. The finding of bilaterally grossly enlarged ovaries on pelvic examination in a patient with a typical history is strongly suggestive of the disorder. However, pelvic examination findings are often inconclusive because the frequently associated obesity makes ovarian palpation and evaluation of its size difficult. Vaginal ultrasonography is useful, as the enlarged ovaries with subcapsular cysts can be demonstrated and measured. As the ovaries are not enlarged in some patients, the diagnosis can never be made or excluded on the basis of pelvic findings alone. Neither are all patients obese. The diagnosis is frequently and readily supported by hormonal levels. The diagnostic plan in all suspected cases of PCO is as follows.

1. Basal body temperature recordings, serum progesterone levels, and endometrial biopsy are done if necessary to determine if the patient is ovulating.

2. Serum FSH and LH levels are measured. In classic full-blown cases, LH is elevated and FSH is within normal limits. In other cases at various stages of derangement between the hypothalamic-pituitary axis and the ovary, the serum LH/FSH ratio is often 2:1 and sometimes 3:1 or more with or without an absolute increase in the LH level itself. Although patients with PCO show an exaggerated LH and diminished FSH response to gonadotropin-releasing hormone (GnRH) stimulation, this test is often not necessary in clinical practice but could be employed in biochemically questionable cases.

3. Serum DHEAS and cortisol assays in the morning are useful if an adrenal component, adrenal hyperplasia, or mild Cushing's disease is suspected. Serum levels of androgens such as androstenedione and testosterone are useful; they are usually elevated in the presence of hirsutism or virilization. If the serum DHEAS level is elevated and obvious adrenal hyperplasia or tumors have been ruled out, dexamethasone suppression can be employed overnight and continued for 6 months. A good response with respect to the hirsutism and reestablishment of ovulation is expected if the adrenal is largely responsible. To rule out adrenal tumors, a computed tomography (CT) scan of the adrenals is useful. Laparoscopic ovarian biopsies could confirm the ovarian histologic changes and can confirm PCO; in early or mild forms of PCO, however, the ovarian biopsy specimen may not be representative or may not show the classic changes (outlined in paragraphs 4, 5, and 6).

4. Thyroid studies [thyroid-stimulating hormone (TSH), triiodothyronine (T_3), throxine (T_4)] (Chap. 2) are indicated in some cases to rule out hypothyroidism.

5. Androgenic tumors of the ovary, ovarian hyperthecosis, and precocious menopause should be con-

sidered in the differential diagnosis. The ovarian tumors rarely present diagnostic problems because the history and physical findings are usually totally different; moreover, tumors are much less common than is PCO. Elevated serum FSH and LH and reduced serum estradiol levels identify patients with premature menopause; associated hirsutism is rare. The clinical picture and findings in patients with ovarian hyperthecosis may be almost identical and may represent a different phase of the same basic disorder as that causing PCO disease. Because treatment is often similar for these two conditions, the frequent inability to make an absolute distinction between them except on pathologic examination of resected ovarian tissue causes no serious difficulties in clinical management.

6. If the ovaries are palpably enlarged or infertility is a complaint, laparoscopy may be performed but is reserved as the final diagnostic procedure. Laparoscopy is often not necessary when the ovaries are not enlarged and infertility is not a complaint. The characteristic gross appearance of Stein-Leventhal ovaries is readily recognized, firmly establishing the diagnosis. Such diagnosis can be readily accepted if the serum gonadotropins and history are characteristic of PCO.

Surgical Treatment. Before ovulation-inducing agents became available, bilateral ovarian wedge resection, in which one-third to one-half or more of each ovary was frequently removed, to reduce the total mass to normal size and the ovaries were then resutured (Fig. 11-3). Wedge resection of the ovary is rarely necessary in current practice except for severe hyperandrogenism, hirsutism, or virilization that are not satisfactorily controlled with medication. Wedge resections are rarely needed to restore fertility alone if there is no severe hyperandrogenism. Wedge resections of the ovaries may give rise to postoperative periovarian and peritubal adhesions and therefore compromise fertility itself. If performed for the proper indications, wedge resection of the ovaries restores ovulatory cycles in 80 to 90 percent of patients, with a rapid decline in serum testosterone levels to normal as early as seven days; menstruation is restored as early as four weeks postoperatively, and hirsutism regresses

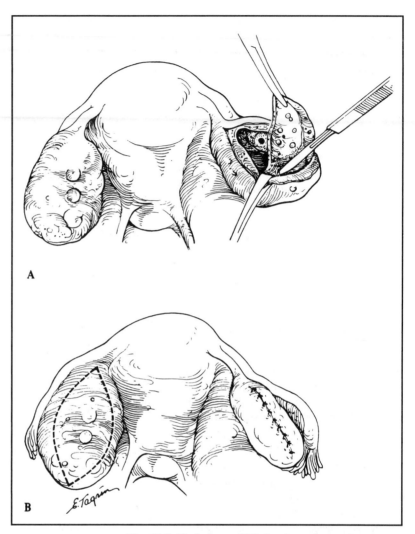

Fig. 11-3. Technique of bilateral ovarian wedge resections in polycystic ovarian disease. A. Wedge resection of the right ovary under way, exposing the thickened capsule and multiple microfollicular subcapsular cysts. B. Right ovary is resutured. Wedge-shaped area to be resected from left ovary is shown by dotted lines.

subsequently. However, ovarian wedge resections do not cure PCO permanently; and often in the absence of pregnancy occurring, the basic LH overdrive on the ovary slowly returns and menstrual irregularities recur. On an average, without pregnancy, wedge resection of the ovary probably produces a remission of 18 to 20 months.

Medical Treatment. Medical management of patients with PCO depends on the specific desires of the patient concerning her need for fertility. If she does not wish to become pregnant, the oral contraceptive pill can be administered cyclically, as for contraception (Chap. 22), to suppress pituitary gonadotropins and therefore ovarian stimulation. This treatment can be continued until she desires and is ready to conceive so long as there is no contraindication to the use of the oral contraceptive pill.

Oral contraceptive pills can also be given to manage hirsutism due to PCO. The estrogen-progesterone pill (1) suppresses pituitary LH secretion and therefore stimulation of ovarian stromal androgen; (2) increases sex hormone-binding globulin and therefore reduces free unbound testosterone; and (3) probably also inhibits 5α-reductase activity at target tissues to reduce the conversion of testosterone to 5α-dihydrotestosterone, which is more active at the androgen receptor site. Through these three mechanisms, oral contraceptive pills can reduce the hyperandrogenemia and hirsutism.

Other agents used for treatment of hirsutism associated with PCO include cyproterone acetate and GnRH agonist. Cyproterone acetate is an antiandrogen and is given orally in combination with an estrogen. Cyproterone acetate promotes urinary excretion of testosterone and binds to the androgen receptor in competition with 5α-dihydrotestosterone, and the estrogen increases the levels of circulating sex hormone-binding globulin. Several GnRH agonists, e.g., buserelin, leuprolide, and nafarelin, are available clinically or will soon become available at the time of this writing. They can be given as either an intranasal spray, subcuticular injection, or depot injection. GnRH agonists, after initially stimulating pituitary gonadotropin secretion, rapidly down-regulate pituitary GnRH receptors and reduce pituitary gonadotropin secretion to low or subnormal levels, resulting in "medical oophorectomy" or "medical castration." The final result is ovarian suppression of the PCO and therefore hyperandrogenism and hirsutism. To overcome any potential long-term osteopenia or bone depletion effect of the medical castration, estrogen can be given concurrently.

If the patient wishes to conceive, ovulation induction can be readily and successfully carried out with clomiphene citrate (see below). If hyperprolactinemia is present, bromoergocriptine is the agent of choice for the induction of ovulation. If clomiphene citrate is unsuccessful in producing a pregnancy and maximum doses of up to 200 mg daily have been tried, human menopausal gonadotropins (hMG) can be tried. However, when using hMG, much caution should be exercised in view of the sensitivity of patients with PCO to hMG with the accompanying risk of ovarian hyper-

stimulation. For this reason, pure human follicle-stimulating hormone (hFSH) may be preferable to hMG for ovulation induction in patients with PCO in view of already elevated endogenous LH secretion in these patients.

Although GnRH is successfully used for inducing ovulation in patients with hypothalamic amenorrhea, it appears to be less successful for PCO patients and may need further studies regarding the optimal dose regimen and route of administration. GnRH agonist could be used to down-regulate GnRH receptors in the pituitary and therefore reduce the elevated pituitary LH secretion followed by hMG induction of ovulation. This approach has been shown to work and has a rational endocrine basis.

Finally, various regimens could be employed, switching from one to the other if one is not successful and coming back to the original regimen. For example, clomiphene citrate could be switched to hMG after appropriately increasing the clomiphene citrate dose to a maximum followed by a treatment-free cycle during which pregnancy could ensue. Subsequently, if hMG is unsuccessful, one could switch back to clomiphene citrate; pregnancies have occurred with this regimen. Therefore bilateral wedge resection of the ovaries need be resorted to only rarely.

One other aspect of the medical treatment of patients with PCO concerns management of the recurring endometrial hyperplasia that may develop. In 15 percent of patients with Stein-Leventhal syndrome, recurring and prolonged dysfunctional bleeding is the chief problem. Adenomatous hyperplasia of the endometrium can develop in a significant number of these patients if prolonged anovulation and unopposed effects of estrogens persist. This potentially premalignant lesion of atypical endometrial hyperplasia is often reversible with cyclic progestin therapy. Such patients should be carefully followed because the atypical, adenomatous hyperplasia sometimes persists, recurs, or progresses to carcinoma in situ and ultimately to invasive carcinoma of the endometrium. If childbearing is completed, hysterectomy may be considered.

Relation Between Stein-Leventhal Syndrome and Endometrial Carcinoma in Young Women. When carcinoma of the endometrium does occur in young women, it appears that in 20 to 25 percent of cases there has been coexisting PCO. In view of the high probability that an abnormal, relatively unopposed type of estrogenic stimulation acting over a prolonged period is etiologically related to the development of endometrial carcinoma at any age (Chaps. 17 and 27), it is perhaps not surprising that patients with Stein-Leventhal syndrome, some of whom certainly exhibit signs and symptoms of prolonged, unphysiologic estrogen exposure, are predisposed to endometrial hyperplasia, atypicalities, and ultimately malignant change.

Ovarian Hyperthecosis
(Diffuse Ovarian Stromal Luteinization)

Although in some instances there are marked differences between ovarian hyperthecosis and Stein-Leventhal syndrome in terms of symptomatology and ovarian anatomy, there is more often an obvious general resemblance and a frequent overlap in the clinical features as well as in the gross and microscopic changes in the ovaries.

Clinically the symptoms may appear shortly after the menarche and progress slowly. Less frequently, they appear abruptly in an older woman, not infrequently developing after one or more pregnancies. Sometimes the clinical picture is indistinguishable from that of the PCO syndrome, and it invariably includes amenorrhea or oligomenorrhea (less often, endometrial hyperplasia and dysfunctional bleeding and infertility). However, there is nearly always associated, often pronounced hirsutism and even virilization with clitoral enlargement, temporal balding, increased muscle mass, and voice changes. Manifestations suggesting a hyperadrenal state are also frequently present and include obesity, hypertension, disturbances in carbohydrate metabolism as indicated by an abnormal glucose tolerance test of the pattern seen in Cushing's disease, and often elevated serum DHEAS. Rarely, an associated endometrial carcinoma is found. As in the case of the PCO syndrome, the evidence favors an ovarian rather than an adrenal origin for these androgenic and adrenogenic effects.

Grossly, the ovaries may be somewhat enlarged and may resemble polycystic ovaries externally by virtue of a smooth, pale white capsule showing no evidence of ovulation. They tend, however, to be firm and solid, often sclerotic, rather than soft and cystic; and the small follicle cysts so typical of the PCO syndrome are frequently absent or few in number. As the term hyperthecosis suggests, the characteristic microscopic feature is the presence of nests of lipoid-laden, theca-lutein cells in the ovarian stroma, the latter being hyperplastic and usually forming a dense, tumor-like mass in the central portion of each ovary. When the ovaries are enlarged and polycystic, the stroma is nevertheless extensively luteinized, permitting differentiation from the Stein-Leventhal type of ovarian histologic appearance. The heavily luteinized stroma probably secretes abnormal steroids with androgenic and, at times, adrenogenic activity.

The differential diagnosis is similar to that of the Stein-Leventhal syndrome, although the clinical picture is often even more suggestive of an adrenal disorder or a masculinizing ovarian tumor, and both must be carefully excluded. The same diagnostic plan of study is employed. With regard to therapy, medical management as with PCO should be employed. If medical therapy is unsuccessful, bilateral wedge resection of the ovaries can be considered, but the success rates are less than with PCO.

Premature Menopause

The development of secondary amenorrhea and hot flashes, often preceded by an interval of gradually increasing menstrual irregularities, in a woman under age 40 (frequently in her late twenties or early thirties) with a history of normal menarche at the usual time and previously perfectly normal and regular ovulatory cycles strongly suggests the possibility of early menopause. If it occurs before age 35, the term *premature menopause* can be applied.

Often these patients are nulliparous, although some are multiparous. There are no other symptoms or signs suggestive of an underlying endocrine or local pelvic disorder (the breasts and external genitalia are normal, but the uterus and ovaries may be slightly smaller than normal). All laboratory studies show normal findings, with the exception of an elevated serum FSH level, which is similar to levels found during normal menopause. If laparoscopy is performed, the ovaries present the typical atrophic appearance of the normal menopausal state, but this finding is not invariably diagnostic.

Presumably, the quantity of original primordial ovarian follicles is deficient in these patients, possibly on a genetic basis, as in some instances a familial tendency has been noted. A few patients have been reported to have X chromosomal abnormalities, e.g., mosaicism (XO/XX/XXX/XXXXX), and an occasional patient is found to have unilateral or bilateral streak gonads; most of these patients have a normal chromosomal pattern, however. There is a high incidence of demonstrable circulating autoantibodies in these patients, and autoimmunity has been implicated as a basis for rapid destruction of the primordial follicles resulting in premature menopause.

There is no known curative treatment for this disorder. It represents, however, one of the most valid and definite indications for prolonged substitution therapy with estrogens to prevent the manifestations of a premature deficiency of the basic ovarian hormone.

GENERALIZED ENDOCRINE AND METABOLIC DISORDERS WITH SECONDARY GYNECOLOGIC MANIFESTATIONS

Generalized endocrine and metabolic disorders with secondary effects on the reproductive system are many and varied and, in most instances, relatively uncommon. Because they are extrapelvic in origin and not primarily gynecologic in nature, no attempt is made here to consider them in great detail. However, insofar as possible, they are completely enumerated; and, where indicated, the highlights of their clinical features and their diagnosis and treatment are presented in outline form.

Thyroid Gland Disorders

Hypothyroidism or hyperthyroidism may ultimately lead to anovulatory cycles and menstrual irregularities, including hypomenorrhea, menorrhagia, menometrorrhagia, oligomenorrhea, or complete amenorrhea. Obesity is often associated with hypothyroidism

but not invariably, especially in the early stages of hypothyroidism. In mild cases, menstrual abnormalities may be minimal or absent, with infertility or repeated abortion representing the principal gynecologic symptom; the diagnosis is often apparent on the basis of the rest of the clinical picture, although studies of thyroid function are obviously needed for confirmation (Chap. 2). They should be part of any evaluation of patients with persistent menstrual disorders of this type, as mild hypothyroidism is common and often not readily recognizable clinically.

The primary treatment is aimed at correcting the thyroid disease. The objective and subjective responses to thyroid medication in these patients are often dramatic.

Adrenal Disease

Adrenogenital Syndrome. Adrenogenital syndrome is produced by an acquired form of adrenal hyperplasia limited to the androgen-producing zone of the adrenal cortex. It is characterized by male-type hirsutism usually progressing to virilization, without accompanying hypertension or alterations in glucose or electrolyte metabolism and with ovarian inhibition causing oligomenorrhea and eventually amenorrhea secondary to the pituitary inhibition induced by rising androgen levels. In addition to amenorrhea and masculine hirsutism, other signs of virilization may include acne, breast atrophy, clitoral hypertrophy, deepening of the voice, and a male type of muscular development and weight distribution. In its mildest forms, the only manifestation may be anovulatory menstrual disturbances, with or without moderately elevated androgens. The syndrome may be caused by a tumor (adenoma or carcinoma) or by diffuse, bilateral hyperplasia. The latter is due to a congenital or acquired deficiency in the hydroxylating enzymes (most commonly 21-hydroxylase) necessary for the synthesis of cortisone.

In addition to the frequently characteristic clinical features of adrenogenital syndrome, a number of laboratory determinations and other studies may be diagnostic. There is a moderate elevation of serum androgens and usually normal pituitary gonadotropins. The ACTH stimulation test (40 units in an 8-hour intravenous infusion) and the dexamethasone suppression test (2 mg daily for three days) may help to distinguish between adrenal tumor and adrenal hyperplasia. Thus 0.5 to 1.0 mg of dexamethasone produces a fall in serum androgens in the presence of adrenal hyperplasia, but no effect is observed if the disorder is due to an adrenal tumor. A stimulatory dose of ACTH may produce elevation of the androgens in the presence of either hyperplasia or tumor, but this response is more likely with the former. Computed tomography (CT) scan or magnetic resonance imaging (MRI) reveals most adrenal tumors (except for very small ones).

Treatment of the adrenal tumor is resection. For hyperplasia, cortisone is given, e.g., cortisone 25 to 50 mg daily or equivalent dosages of other corticosteroid drugs.

Congenital Adrenal Hyperplasia. For a discussion of congenital adrenal hyperplasia (female pseudohermaphroditism), see Chapter 8.

Mild Adrenal Hyperplasia. Mild adrenal hyperplasia presents a PCO type of clinical picture except for moderately elevated serum DHEAS. The differential diagnosis is the same as for adrenogenital syndrome and as discussed in the section on PCO syndrome. Treatment consists in 0.5 mg of dexamethasone once or twice a day or 5 mg of prednisone daily at night.

Cushing's Disease. In Cushing's disease, the abnormal overproduction of adrenal steroids primarily involves the corticoid compounds having to do with carbohydrate, protein, and electrolyte metabolism; the androgens are involved to only a slight extent. Again, the hyperadrenal state may develop either as the result of diffuse, bilateral adrenal hyperplasia (50 to 60 percent of cases), sometimes in association with and possibly secondary to a basophilic adenoma or diffuse "basophilism" of the pituitary, or as the result of an adrenal adenoma (30 to 40 percent of cases) or adrenal carcinoma (5 to 10 percent of cases).

The characteristic clinical features of classic Cushing's disease include the following: obesity of the trunk with associated "buffalo hump" and moon face, amenorrhea, hirsutism, acne, osteoporosis, hypertension, purple striae of the skin (particularly of the abdominal wall, the so-called skin fractures), polycythemia, a plethoric appearance, and rarely true virilization. Note that mild forms of the disease frequently are accompanied by only some of the usual clinical symptoms and signs, many of which may be atypical and equivocal. Also in many hyperadrenal states, whether due to tumor or hyperplasia, there is a wide spectrum of clinical and biochemical abnormalities that include features of both Cushing's syndrome and the adrenogenital syndrome and reflect the varying disturbances present in the particular type of tumor or hyperplastic glandular tissue.

There are certain laboratory findings in Cushing's disease that help in the diagnosis: Serum cortisol, especially free cortisol, is elevated; the glucose tolerance test results are diabetic in type; and the skeletal radiographs show osteoporosis. Serum ACTH is elevated if the Cushing's disease is due to a pituitary adenoma. CT scan or MRI should show or locate the tumor in the adrenal or pituitary.

Addison's Disease. Addison's disease (adrenal failure) invariably leads to amenorrhea. It ordinarily does not pose any diagnostic problem.

Hypothalamic-Pituitary Disorders

Pituitary Insufficiency or Failure. Pituitary insufficiency or failure is usually secondary to severe postpartum hemorrhage with thrombosis and necrosis or infarction of the pituitary (Sheehan's syndrome). Occasionally, it is due to a chromophobe adenoma or a suprasellar cyst.

Symptoms include amenorrhea, occasionally persistent galactorrhea, progressive atrophy of the uterus and vagina, muscular weakness, and an initial weight gain followed by progressive cachexia (Simmonds' disease), as thyroid and adrenal functions also become depressed.

Laboratory studies show a low basal metabolic rate, low protein-bound iodine level, and depressed levels of T_3, T_4, TSH, FSH, LH, prolactin, cortisol, DHEAS, and estradiol. Failure of response to GnRH administration or to clomiphene or human menopausal gonadotropin stimulation is to be expected.

Treatment is by replacement therapy for thyroid, adrenal, and gonadal insufficiency.

Pituitary Tumors. Pituitary tumors include eosinophilic adenomas (acromegaly) and basophilic adenomas (Cushing's disease), which lead to amenorrhea with or without galactorrhea; there are associated headaches, visual disturbances, and other symptoms. Diagnostic techniques include x-ray cone down views of sella turcica to detect enlargement; CT scan or MRI of the pituitary gland; serum FSH, LH, and prolactin levels; and special neurologic studies, including visual fields, preferably the visual evoked response (VER) visual field test.

An unusual and uncommon condition of unknown cause, referred to as the *empty sella syndrome,* is seen most often in obese adult women, many of whom also have hypertension and diabetes. The pituitary gland is actually present but is severely compressed and flattened against the sella floor, the sella being filled primarily with cerebrospinal fluid and appearing empty on radiographic examination. Levels of pituitary, adrenal, and ovarian hormones as well as plasma testosterone levels are usually normal, although some of these patients have been reported to have had associated hirsutism and menstrual irregularities. This entity is important only from the standpoint of differential diagnosis and the need to distinguish it from abnormalities of the sella accompanying pituitary tumors or cysts. The empty sella syndrome can be easily distinguished from the true pituitary tumors by CT scan or MRI of the pituitary gland.

Treatment is by medical therapy with the dopamine agonist bromocriptine or L-dopa for cases of acromegaly. Surgical removal (transsphenoidal resection) is performed in patients with Cushing's disease or acromegaly. Pituitary irradiation is sometimes employed.

Amenorrhea-Galactorrhea Syndromes. Amenorrhea-galactorrhea syndromes result from a specific type of endocrine disturbance of pituitary or hypothalamic origin and are characterized by amenorrhea accompanied by galactorrhea (excretion of milky fluid from the breast, as during lactation). These disorders result from inappropriate hypersecretion of prolactin, by ei-ther a prolactin-secreting tumor of the pituitary or a hypothalamic-pituitary disturbance giving rise to deficient production of prolactin-inhibiting factor (PIF). The excessive prolactin is directly responsible for the galactorrhea and indirectly responsible for the amenorrhea. The disorder is often encountered after delivery in otherwise normal postpartum women (*Chiari-Frommel syndrome*), and it occurs occasionally in nonpregnant women with prolactin-secreting pituitary tumors (*Forbes-Albright syndrome*). The syndrome is also seen in the absence of either pregnancy or pituitary adenoma, when it is presumably due to some form of specific pituitary or hypothalamic dysfunction resulting in excessive prolactin or inadequate PIF secretion. This disorder is referred to as the *Ahumada-Argonz-del Castillo syndrome.*

Far more commonly, a similar, physiologic type of amenorrhea-galactorrhea encountered in patients receiving antihypertensives and tranquilizers (e.g., reserpine, phenothiazines, or tricyclic antidepressants), as well as in patients who have discontinued oral contraceptive usage after some duration and then not only failed to resume normal, spontaneous menstrual cycles but also noted the onset of persistent lactation ("post-pill galactorrhea-amenorrhea syndrome" or "oversuppression syndrome"). The typical, almost diagnostic clinical features include amenorrhea, which is often permanent, and a constant milky breast discharge (galactorrhea) that is usually chronic, often lasting for years, in association with large, engorged breasts and profound atrophy of the ovaries, uterus, and vagina. The diagnosis is confirmed by finding markedly reduced pituitary gonadotropin (FSH and LH) excretion and low or undetectable estrogen levels. Both endometrium and vaginal mucosa are atrophic. As indicated by clinical and laboratory evidence of normal thyroid, adrenal, and pancreatic function, no other fundamental pituitary dysfunction is present. Thyroid function (serum TSH) particularly should be carefully evaluated in all patients with the Chiari-Frommel variant of the syndrome, as hypothyroidism, especially when it develops postpartum, can cause amenorrhea-galactorrhea and is easily treated by administration of thyroid hormone.

Spontaneous recovery with return of normal menses and cessation of lactation has been observed only occasionally. Treatment with clomiphene citrate is employed in patients with amenorrhea-galactorrhea disorders if the patient wishes to conceive. Ovulation with resumption of menses can be established. A more specific and effective therapy for hyperprolactinemia is with the ergot alkaloid bromocriptine, which is a dopamine agonist. Bromocriptine inhibits pituitary secretion of prolactin and restores normoprolactinemia, with resumption of menstruation and ovulation; complete cessation or lactation is much more slowly and less completely achieved.

If the pituitary tumor is 10 mm or larger, it is referred to as a *macroadenoma;* a tumor less than 10 mm is a *microadenoma*. Whereas a patient with microadenoma can be allowed to become pregnant with little risk of complications during pregnancy, a patient with macroadenoma is best treated definitively prior to attempting conception, as there are significantly increased pituitary-related complications during pregnancy. Macroadenomas can also be conservatively treated; if such therapy is unsuccessful, surgical removal or, less frequently, irradiation may be employed.

Pituitary "Dysfunction" or Hypothalamic Amenorrhea. The "diagnosis" of pituitary "dysfunction" hypothalamic amenorrhea is based on depressed serum FSH and LH levels and an apparent pituitary insufficiency in the absence of any obvious cause (e.g., absence of pituitary tumor or possibility of postpartum necrosis and lack of apparent underlying psychosomatic factors, nutritional factors, or associated chronic disease such as tuberculosis or nephritis).

Diabetes Mellitus. Frequently, the various metabolic disturbances in *diabetic* women are reflected in an increased incidence of anovulatory menstrual irregularities, including dysfunctional bleeding, oligomenorrhea, amenorrhea, infertility, and premature menopause. Dietary and insulin management of the diabetes is of the greatest benefit. Other routine diagnostic and therapeutic measures such as are used for management of any kind of menstrual dysfunction or infertility problem can be of additional help.

HIRSUTISM AND AMENORRHEA

The two most frequent symptoms of a gynecologic endocrine disorder are (1) hirsutism (sometimes accompanied by virilization) with or without obesity and menstrual irregularities (usually) and (2) amenorrhea (or oligomenorrhea). The differential diagnosis for each of these two symptomatic features is presented below in outline form. The diagnostic study plan employed in patients with hirsutism has been covered in Chapters 2 and 8 and is not reviewed here, but a diagnostic approach that can be used for evaluation of patients with amenorrhea is suggested.

Hirsutism

Virilization, obesity, and menstrual irregularities may be present in patients with hirsutism. The differential diagnosis includes the following.

1. *Idiopathic:* congenital, familial, racial. (Normal ovulatory menses with elevated plasma testosterone are found in a significant number of these patients.) Probably due to a familial tendency to excessive androgen sensitivity of the hair follicles and sebaceous glands at certain times, especially during puberty, menopause, or pregnancy.
2. *Adrenal disease.*
   a. Mild congenital hyperplasia: unrecognized until primary amenorrhea and hirsutism with virilization appear.
   b. Adrenal tumors (adenoma or carcinoma) or hyperplasia: acquired adrenogenital syndrome.
   c. Cushing's disease (hyperplasia or tumor).
   d. Mild hyperplasia with a syndrome resembling Stein-Leventhal syndrome.
3. *Ovarian disorders.* The most common cause of female hirsutism. Ovarian causes include the following.
   a. Stein-Leventhal syndrome.
   b. Ovarian hyperthecosis.
   c. Ovarian tumors (Chap. 18).
      (1) Arrhenoblastomas (Sertoli-Leydig cell tumors).

(2) Hilus cell (pure Leydig cell) tumors or hyperplasia.

(3) Adrenal rest (lipoid cell) tumors.

(4) Gynandroblastomas (mixed granulosa-theca cell and Sertoli-Leydig cell tumors).

4. *Pituitary disorders.*

  a. Nonfunctioning tumors and cysts with pituitary destruction.

  b. Acromegaly (eosinophilic adenoma).

  c. Cushing's disease (basophilic adenoma).

5. *Miscellaneous disorders.*

  a. Postmenopausal hirsutism.

  b. Androgen therapy.

  c. Diphenylhydantoin (Dilantin) therapy.

  d. Some epileptic patients.

  e. Morgagni-Stewart-Morel syndrome: hyperostosis frontalis interna, obesity, mental retardation, and hirsutism of unknown cause. Diabetes mellitus, thyroid dysfunction, menstrual disorders, and hypertension are often present as well. There is usually no demonstrable disease in either the pituitary or the hypothalamus despite the many similarities to acromegaly and Cushing's disease. Androgen levels are usually normal.

Amenorrhea

Amenorrhea is usually classified into *primary* or *secondary amenorrhea,* albeit an artificial classification that is not usually helpful for the evaluation of amenorrheic women. *Primary amenorrhea* is the absence of menarche by the age of 16 years in girls who have never menstruated. *Secondary amenorrhea* is the absence of menstruation for three cycle lengths or more in women with past menses.

Amenorrhea is a symptom and indicates failure of the hypothalamic-pituitary-gonadal axis to induce cyclic changes in the endometrium that normally result in menstruation, but it can also result from absence of the end-organs (uterus, vagina) or obstruction of the outflow tract (Table 11-1).

Differential Diagnosis of Amenorrhea (or Oligomenorrhea)

PRIMARY AMENORRHEA

1. *Uterovaginal disorder.* About 20 percent of patients with primary amenorrhea prove to have a congenital müllerian duct anomaly of some type.

  a. Congenital anomalies (absent or hypoplastic uterus).

Table 11-1. Etiologic Mechanisms of Amenorrhea

Level	Factors or mechanisms	Hormone affected
Hypothalamus	Psychosomatic factors Obesity Brain tumor, cyst, toxic damage	GnRH
Pituitary	Nutritional, chronic disease Pituitary tumors or hypofunction Androgen antagonists: adrenal tumor or hyperplasia Estrogen antagonists: hormone-producing tumors	FSH, LH, prolactin
Ovary	Thyroid disorder Primary ovarian dysfunction Polycystic ovarian disease, hyperthecosis syndromes Gonadal dysgenesis, congenital absence Premature menopause	Estrogen, progesterone, androgens
Uterus	Congenital absence or hypoplasia Artificial factors (surgery, irradiation) Uterine disease (endometritis, Asherman's syndrome)	No hormone affected but endometrial response and bleeding absent

b. Imperforate hymen, transverse vaginal system, or congenital absence of the vagina.
2. Ovarian disorder.
   a. Primary gonadal disorder (e.g., gonadal dysgenesis, testicular feminization). About 40 to 50 percent of apparent females with primary amenorrhea have a sex chromosomal disorder. Of them, 75 percent have Turner's syndrome or mosaic forms of gonadal agenesis, and the other 25 percent have a 46,XY chromosome and either the testicular feminization syndrome or, less often, pure gonadal dysgenesis, mixed gonadal dysgenesis, or dysgenetic male pseudohermaphroditism (Chap. 8).
   b. Congenital absence of the ovaries.
   c. Hypogonadotropic hypogonadism associated with anosmia, probably of central nervous system origin. The hypogonadism responds to clomiphene or gonadotropin administration and most likely is due to hypothalamic dysfunction with a GnRH defect.
3. *Hypothalamic disorder.*
   a. Generalized hypothalamic defect, with deficiency of thyrotropic, adrenocorticotropic, and gonadotropin-releasing hormones.
   b. Isolated gonadotropin deficiency (low to absent LH, FSH, and estradiol) with normal TSH, ACTH, and growth hormone secretion. Again, the defect resides in the hypothalamus (lack of GnRH).
4. *Pituitary insufficiency (pituitary dwarfs).*
5. *Premenarchal occurrence of any of the disorders ordinarily producing secondary amenorrhea.* See below.

In 25 to 40 percent of patients with primary amenorrhea, the problem lies in the hypothalamic-pituitary-ovarian axis; 40 to 50 percent of cases are secondary to sex chromosomal disorders, and in the remaining 15 percent miscellaneous systemic, nutritional, and psychological factors are responsible.

SECONDARY AMENORRHEA

1. *Physiologic changes.*
   a. Pregnancy (signs and symptoms of pregnancy, positive test for hCG; still the commonest cause of secondary amenorrhea in premenopausal females).
   b. Postpartum (failure of menses to return within 18 months of delivery); usually responds to a three-month course of cyclic estrogen-progesterone. Rule out postpartum pituitary necrosis (Sheehan's syndrome) or Chiari-Frommel syndrome.
   c. Menopause (elevated FSH and LH levels are diagnostic).
2. *Pituitary or hypothalamic disorders.*
   a. Insufficiency or failure: Sheehan's syndrome, Simmonds' disease.
   b. Tumors (adenomas, cysts) of the pituitary gland, stalk, or suprasellar space.
   c. Chiari-Frommel syndrome and related amenorrhea-galactorrhea disorders.
3. *Ovarian disorders.*
   a. Dysfunction (anovulatory cycles with oligomenorrhea or amenorrhea).
   b. Neoplasms (Chap. 18).
      (1) Granulosa cell or theca cell tumors.
      (2) Arrhenoblastoma or hilus cell tumors.
      (3) Adrenal cell rest (lipoid cell) tumors.
   c. Stein-Leventhal syndrome.
   d. Ovarian hyperthecosis.
   e. Premature menopause (ovarian failure).
   f. Severe pelvic inflammatory disease or mumps oophoritis with bilateral ovarian destruction.
4. *Adrenal disorders.*
   a. Adrenogenital syndrome and related disorders.
   b. Cushing's disease.
   c. Addison's disease.
5. *Thyroid disorders.*
   a. Hyperthyroidism.
   b. Hypothyroidism.
6. *Diabetes mellitus.*
7. *Nutritional disorders.*
   a. Severe malnutrition.
   b. Marked obesity.
8. Chronic disease (e.g., tuberculosis, nephritis, rheumatoid arthritis).
9. *Psychosomatic and neurogenic (hypothalamic) disorders* (e.g., major psychoses, anorexia ner-

vosa, pseudocyesis, emotional shock, organic brain disease).

10. *Artificial causes,* e.g., hysterectomy and/or bilateral oophorectomy, radiation therapy, excessively traumatic curettage, severe endometritis, Asherman's syndrome (intrauterine adhesions).

Workup for Amenorrhea

PRIMARY AMENORRHEA. Although the diagnosis of primary amenorrhea is made if there is no spontaneous menstruation by the age of 16 years, diagnostic workup should be performed by the age of 15 years (1) if there is also no breast development (absence of secondary sexual characteristics) and (2) if there is no menstruation within 2 years of thelarche and development of other secondary sexual characteristics.

The diagnostic workup of primary amenorrhea can be clinically approached based on the absence or presence of a uterus and if there is breast development. The presence of breast development indicates a strong likelihood of adequate endogenous estrogen, reflecting probably adequate ovarian estrogen output at thelarche, whereas absence of breast development reflects low endogenous estrogen output due to failure or dysfunction of the hypothalamic-pituitary-ovarian axis at any level. The presence of a uterus with no anatomic obstruction of the outflow tract speaks against congenital müllerian tract anomalies as a cause of the amenorrhea. The absence of a uterus entertains the possibility of testicular feminization syndrome, congenital absence of the uterus, or enzyme deficiency (17,20-desmolase, 17α-hydroxylase). A systematic investigation approach to the diagnostic evaluation of patients with primary amenorrhea is summarized in Figure 11-4.

SECONDARY AMENORRHEA. Certain aspects of the history are particularly important for evaluation of a woman with secondary amenorrhea. They include (1) sudden weight changes (gain or loss); (2) stress factors (e.g., bereavement, loss, job-related pressures, educational pressures); (3) geographic change (e.g., moves across time zones); (4) radiation exposure or treatment, medication or drug intake (psychotropic drugs such as the tricyclic antidepressants,

haloperidol, estrogens, androgens, corticosteroids, phenothiazine compounds); (5) family history of premature menopause; and (6) presence of galactorrhea.

During the physical examination, attention should be especially directed to the following (1) breast development (Tanner staging) and presence of galactorrhea, spontaneous or expressible; (2) any change in voice; (3) the presence of a receding hairline; (4) body dimensions and habitus; (5) distribution and extent of terminal androgen-stimulated body hair (moustache area, face, between the breasts, pubic hair distribution); and (7) external and internal genitalia, especially for effects of androgens (clitoromegaly) and estrogens.

It cannot be overemphasized that during the workup of secondary amenorrhea pregnancy must be ruled out. Thus a reliable, sensitive pregnancy test should be done initially. Having ruled out a pregnancy, further laboratory or ancillary tests are performed as outlined for the workup of secondary amenorrhea in Figure 11-5.

Treatment of Amenorrhea and Induction of Ovulation. Amenorrhea is purely a symptom, and therefore proper therapy is directed at the specific underlying cause once the diagnosis is established. The plan of treatment for specific underlying disorders has been discussed in the previous sections. For most problems due to chronic anovulation secondary to a hypothalamic-pituitary-ovarian axis disturbance, ovulation induction is necessary if the patient is infertile. Details of medical induction of ovulation are given below. Five agents are currently used for induction of ovulation: (1) clomiphene citrate; (2) human menopausal gonadotropin; (3) human follicle-stimulating hormone; (4) gonadotropin-releasing hormone; and (5) bromocriptine.

CLOMIPHENE CITRATE. Clomiphene citrate (CC), closely related to chlorotrianisene (TACE) and diethylstilbestol (DES), has both estrogenic and antiestrogenic properties. It is a racemic mixture composed of cis-clomiphene and zur-clomiphene. CC acts on the estrogen receptors on the pituitary and hypothalamus, combining with these receptors and preventing their replenishment. In this way, CC prevents the positive feedback of rising estrogen levels on LH

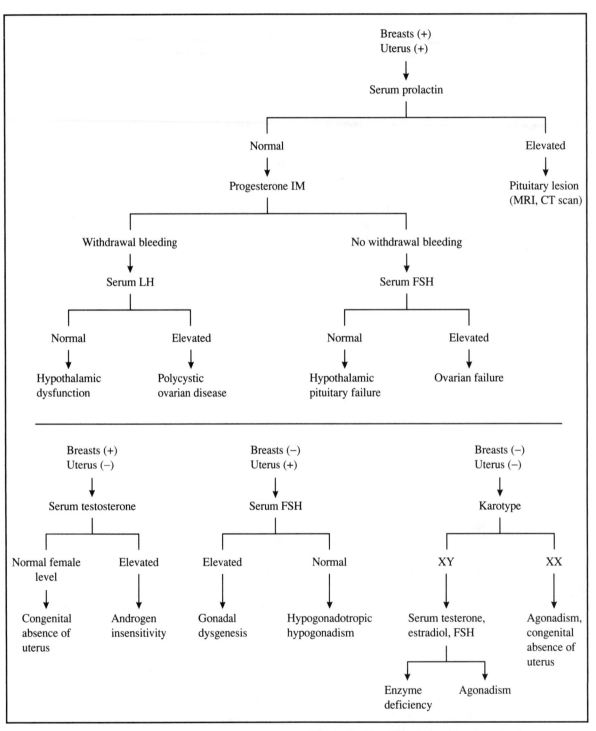

Fig. 11-4. Algorithm for the workup of primary amenorrhea based on the presence or absence of the uterus and breast development.

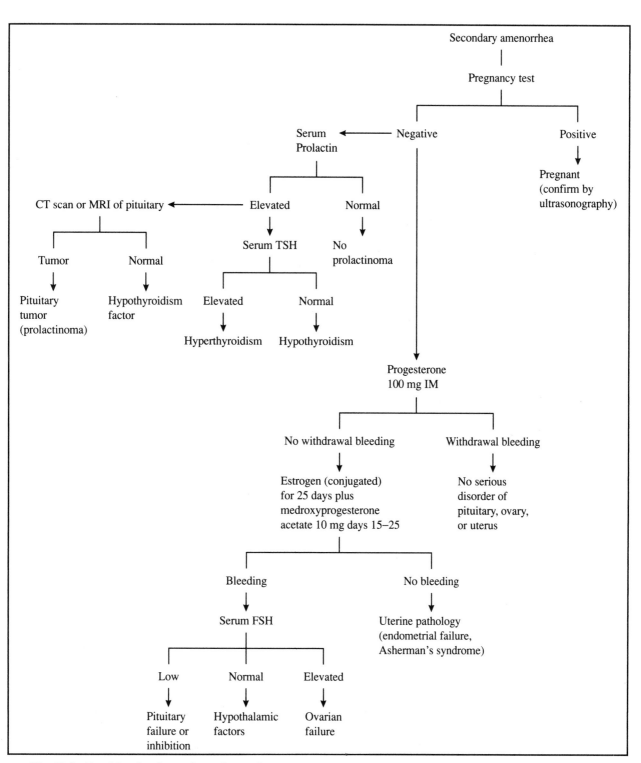

Fig. 11-5. Algorithm for the workup of secondary amenorrhea.

surges while allowing the pituitary to continue to secrete both FSH and LH, which in turn stimulate ovarian folliculogenesis. When appropriately given (dose and timing), CC is capable of inducing ovulation in 70 to 80 percent of cases of anovulation, including hypothalamic amenorrhea and PCO syndrome. CC effectively induces ovulation only in cases where the pituitary is still intact and the gonadotropes are capable of function. Thus CC cannot be used effectively if the pituitary has been resected, irradiated, or sufficiently infarcted (as in Sheehan's syndrome).

The usual starting dose is 50 mg daily for five days beginning on day 5, although it could be started on day 3 for controlled ovarian hyperstimulation to recruit more follicles (and therefore oocytes) for in vitro fertilization or gamete intrafallopian tube transfer. If the patient is sensitive to clomiphene citrate, one can start with 25 mg (half a tablet). If ovulation occurs, the dose is maintained and given for three cycles. The dose is increased by 50 mg daily if pregnancy does not occur after three ovulatory cycles up to a maximum dose of 200 mg daily.

Ovulation usually occurs three to nine days after the last dose of CC, usually on day 15 or 16 but can be from day 12 through day 18. Coitus daily or at least every other day is encouraged during this periovulatory phase. If pregnancy does not occur, hCG 5000 IU can be added to the CC treatment on days 15 and 17. This addition improves the pregnancy rates slightly. The untreated cycle following CC treatment can be fertile, and pregnancies are not infrequently reported to ensue during that cycle.

Pregnancy rates of 35 to 40 percent are produced by CC induction of ovulation. This discrepancy between the pregnancy rate and the ovulation rate is believed to be due to luteinized unruptured follicle, failure of the oocyte to be fertilized, inadequate implantation, or poor cervical mucus due to the antiestrogenic effect of CC. If there is evidence of poor cervical mucus due to CC treatment, estrogens (conjugated estrogens 0.3 mg or DES 0.1 mg) given daily from days 10 through 14 of the cycle should improve the cervical mucous quality.

Side effects of CC include nausea, vomiting, hot flashes, headache, disturbances of vision such as spots in the eye and blurring, multiple pregnancy, and ovarian hyperstimulation (10 to 20 percent). The rate of multiple pregnancy is about five- to eightfold higher than in unstimulated cycles, with twin pregnancies occurring in about 1 of 15 pregnancies (compared to a twinning rate of 1 in 90 pregnancies normally).

Varying degrees of ovarian hyperstimulation occur if the patient is sensitive to CC or if large doses of CC have been employed, although there is no direct evidence showing a dose-dependent risk of developing severe hyperstimulation syndrome. When ovarian hyperstimulation occurs, the only change may be slight enlargement of the ovary with multiple follicles or as extreme as severe massive ovarian multicystic enlargement extending up to the umbilicus accompanied by hemorrhage or torsion of the ovary, ascites, pleural effusion or pulmonary edema, hydrothorax, contraction of the circulating plasma volume due to fluid shift into the third space with consequent hypercoagulability, and intravascular coagulation. Severe ovarian hyperstimulation syndrome is less likely to occur if hCG has not been administered.

Management of this complication is essentially nonsurgical except when there is complication of the multicystic, severely enlarged ovaries (e.g., bleeding and torsion). Bed rest, correction of the contracted plasma volume with saline infusion to correct the hyponatremia, attention to electrolytes, and refraining from coitus are the mainstays of therapy, as the condition is often self-limiting and improves within 7 to 10 days. Diuretics should not be given as they only compound the problem of hypovolemia and hyponatremia.

HUMAN MENOPAUSAL GONADOTROPIN. Induction of ovulation in women was successfully carried out using pituitary FSH and LH extracted from human pituitaries. Except for one or two countries, the use of pituitary extracts of FSH and LH for induction of ovulation has now been replaced with use of human menopausal gonadotropin (Pergonal) derived from the urine of postmenopausal women who excrete elevated amounts of FSH and LH. The principal indications for the use of hMG are secondary amenorrhea, anovulatory oligomenorrhea, hypothalamic amenorrhea with abnormal serum FSH and LH levels, and Sheehan's syndrome or any condition involving destruction of the pituitary gland (surgery, irradiation, infarction). It is also used for multiple follicular recruitment for in vitro fertilization and for gamete intrafallopian tube transfer.

Unlike clomiphene citrate, it is not necessary to have an intact pituitary gland capable of functioning. However, the ovaries must be capable of responding, and therefore hMG is not effective in, and should not be given to, women with ovarian failure (e.g., premature menopause, gonadal dysgenesis, streak ovaries, and Turner's syndrome). Because of the expense involved, it is necessary to establish that at least one of the fallopian tubes is patent before embarking on hMG treatment.

Human menopausal gonadotropin is commonly given as an intramuscular injection on a daily basis beginning on either day 3 for controlled multiple follicular recruitment or day 5 for in vivo ovulation. Each ampule of hMG contains either 75 IU of FSH plus 75 IU of LH or 150 IU of FSH plus 150 IU of LH. The dose should be adjusted on a daily basis after the first four to five days of administration according to the patient's sensitivity to the medication and her ovarian response. A baseline serum estradiol level is measured, and subsequent monitoring of the ovarian response is done with a combination of serum estradiol and vaginal ultrasonography to determine the number and size of the follicles. For in vivo ovulation, a follicle size of 20 to 24 mm should be attained together with a preceding five days of increase in the serum estradiol level (by at least 50 percent each day over the level on the previous day). When these criteria are fulfilled, hCG 5000 IU is given to trigger ovulation and is repeated 48 hours later. The couple should have coitus every day over this three- to four-day period. The serum progesterone level can be measured during the midluteal phase to confirm that ovulation had occurred.

Ovulation is produced with hMG in 80 to 90 percent of cases, and cumulative pregnancy rates of up to 60 to 65 percent have been achieved. The pregnancy rates are higher with hMG induction of ovulation in women with amenorrhea than in those with oligomenorrhea.

Disadvantages of hMG induction of ovulation include the high cost of medication and treatment, the need for daily injections and to be seen frequently by the physician, the need for daily monitoring, and the increased incidence of multiple pregnancies and ovarian hyperstimulation syndrome. The rate of multiple births may be as high as 15 to 30 percent but can be kept low with good monitoring and experienced and skillful use of the medication. The risk of ovarian hyperstimulation syndrome is also higher than with CC and occurs in 15 to 20 percent of patients. The critical features of ovarian hyperstimulation syndrome are similar to those described when it occurs with clomiphene citrate treatment. It is noteworthy that the clinical manifestation of ovarian hyperstimulation occurs about three to five days after the first dose of hCG is given, and the condition runs its course over the next seven to ten days. Thus ovarian hyperstimulation syndrome can be avoided by withholding the hCG whenever there is monitoring evidence to indicate ovarian hyperresponse.

HUMAN FOLLICLE-STIMULATING HORMONE. Human follicle-stimulating hormone is a HMG preparation that has had its LH removed and only FSH remains in the preparation. It is marketed as Metrodin. Its use for ovulation induction is similar to that of hMG, but each ampule of hFSH costs almost twice that of an ampule of hMG. hFSH is probably best limited to use for ovulation induction in patients with PCO who have elevated serum LH levels. There is an unwarranted and scientifically unsubstantiated claim for its more liberal use in most indications for ovulation induction.

GONADOTROPIN-RELEASING HORMONE. The GnRH is a decapeptide secreted by the hypothalamus to the pituitary to induce secretion of FSH and LH. Consequently, GnRH is particularly useful and effective for inducing ovulation, with fewer side effects, in patients with hypothalamic amenorrhea and a functional pituitary gland. These patients generally have very low or subnormal levels of serum FSH and LH. Unlike hMG or hFSH, GnRH must be given in *pulses* to induce ovulation. GnRH is usually given subcutaneously but can also be given intravenously in pulses every 90 minutes through an automatic programmable pump that delivers the pulses at the dose and frequency set. These pulses are given on a continuing basis until follicular growth has reached a maximum of at least 20 mm (preferably 24 mm), at which time hCG 5000 IU is given to trigger ovulation. Thus the patients must have the pump and medication on them around the clock during therapy. The dose delivered in each pulse can be increased and adjusted based on the ovarian response to the GnRH stimulation.

Monitoring of ovarian response to GnRH is carried out with serum estradiol and vaginal ultrasound of the ovaries similar to that used for hMG (see above) but not as frequently. The risk of ovarian hyperstimulation with GnRH is much less than with hMG. Although the incidence of multiple pregnancies is slightly higher than with spontaneous pregnancies, it is much lower than with hMG-induced ovulation. It is less expensive than hMG.

GnRH, or usually its agonist, is also used to suppress pituitary gonadotropin secretion by down-regulation. When GnRH is used to suppress pituitary gonadotropin secretion, ovulation induction can be carried out with hMG, which acts directly on the ovaries to induce folliculogenesis. This method of ovulation induction is increasingly employed for in vitro fertilization (Chap. 13) and for patients with polycystic ovarian disease to suppress their pituitary LH secretion and thus overcome the risk of premature LH surge or premature luteinization of the developing follicles. When used in combination with hMG for this purpose, GnRH agonist is not given in a pulsatile fashion but as a subcutaneous injection, intramuscular injection, or intranasally. Apparently, better pregnancy rates are obtained with this controlled method of ovulation induction with GnRH agonist and hMG for in vitro fertilization than with hMG alone.

BROMOCRIPTINE. Ergot derivatives such as bromocriptine or the long-acting lergotrile mesylate lower prolactin levels. These drugs can be used for induction of ovulation in patients with hyperprolactinemia as well as for treatment of amenorrhea with or without galactorrhea due to hyperprolactinemia and with or without a demonstrable pituitary tumor. In the presence of microadenomas (pituitary tumors less than 10 mm), ovulation induction and pregnancy can be undertaken without significantly increasing risks of pituitary complications during pregnancy. However, macroadenomas (pituitary tumors 10 mm or more) should be treated with bromocriptine until sufficiently shrunk, or resected, before attempting pregnancy with whatever form of medical induction of ovulation is selected. Pregnancy in the presence of a macroadenoma is associated with a significantly increased risk of pituitary complications.

Bromocriptine and lergotrile mesylate are dopamine receptor agonists, which activate postsynaptic dopamine receptors in the hypothalamus and pituitary, thereby acting in a fashion similar to that of prolactin-inhibiting factor to bring about lowering of prolactin secretion by the pituitary lactotropes. To avoid the common and sometimes intolerable side effect of nausea and vomiting, it is best to start bromocriptine in the lowest possible dose, 1.25 mg (half a tablet) once a day (at bedtime) for a week, increase to 2.5 mg once a day for another week, and increase it again thereafter to 2.5 mg twice a day. The usual dose of bromocriptine is 2.5 mg twice a day. Daily basal body temperature charts should be kept and coitus timed to coincide with a rise in body temperature or when the urine LH dipstick test for preovulatory surge indicates a surge. The bromocriptine can be discontinued a couple of days after a definite shift in basal body temperature or other evidence of ovulation. Alternatively, bromocriptine medication is continued for another two weeks after ovulation and is discontinued if there is no menses when a blood pregnancy test is carried out.

Bromocriptine treatment of selected patients with hyperprolactinemia induces ovulation successfully in 80 percent of them, with good pregnancy rates and no significant increase in twin pregnancy rates. Congenital anomalies in the fetuses arising from successful ovulation induction are similar to those seen with spontaneous pregnancies.

In addition to nausea and vomiting, bromocriptine can produce symptomatic hypotension and muscle aches and pains; pulmonary infiltrates, pleural effusion, and thickening of the pleura have been noted with long-term therapy, albeit rarely. Bromocriptine should not be used in patients with uncontrolled hypertension or toxemia of pregnancy or in those who are sensitive to ergot alkaloids.

Bromocriptine is also given on a similar (as above) but continuous basis for six months or longer to treat pituitary tumors (micro- and macroadenomas) with or without amenorrhea and using barrier contraceptives to avoid pregnancy. If it is a small microadenoma without optic chiasma compression, it is probably not necessary to treat it other than with serial follow-up and observation because this tumor has been demonstrated to be very slow growing.

Visual fields compromised by tumor compression of optic chiasma are quickly restored with bromocriptine therapy in 75 percent of cases of galactorrhea and amenorrhea; the galactorrhea is completely or almost completely suppressed, and menses are restored. Re-initiation of menstruation usually occurs (within 6 to 8 weeks of therapy) prior to suppression of galactorrhea (usually 8 to 12 weeks after starting therapy). If pregnancy occurs and the pituitary reexpands, it can be induced to shrink with bromocriptine. Thus far, the fetus of pregnancies treated with bromocriptine for this reason do not appear to be at any significant risk with respect to congenital anomalies.

SELECTED READINGS

Chang, R. J. (Guest editor). Polycystic ovarian disease. *Semin. Reprod. Endocrinol.* 2:223, 1984.

Dawood, M. Y. Current approaches to dysfunctional uterine bleeding. *Diagnosis* 5:138, 1983.

Dawood, M. Y. Amenorrhea. In R. E. Rakel (Ed.), *1988 Conn's Current Therapy.* Philadelphia: Saunders 1988. P. 922.

DeVore, G. R., Owens, O., and Kase, N. Use of intravenous Premarin in the treatment of dysfunctional uterine bleeding—a double-blind randomized control study. *Obstet. Gynecol.* 59:285, 1982.

Holman, J. F., and Hammond, C. B. Induction of Ovulation with Clomiphene Citrate. In S. J. Behrman, R. W. Kistner, and G. W. Patton (Eds.), *Progress in Infertility* (3rd ed.), Boston: Little, Brown, 1988. Chap. 21, p. 499.

Judd, H. L., Rigg, L. A., Anderson, D. C., et al. The effects of ovarian wedge resection on circulating gonadotropin and ovarian steroid levels in patients with polycystic ovary syndrome. *J. Clin. Endocrinol. Metab.* 43:347, 1976.

Lunenfeld, B., Vardimon, D., and Blankstein, J. Induction of Ovulation with GnRH. In S. J. Behrman, R. W. Kistner, and G. W. Patton (Eds.) *Progress in Infertility* (3rd ed.), Boston: Little, Brown, 1988. Chap. 22, p. 513.

Marut, E. L., and Dawood, M. Y. Amenorrhea (excluding hyperprolactinemia). *Clin. Obstet. Gynecol.* 26:749, 1983.

Reindollar, R. H., and McDonough, P. G. Adolescent menstrual disorders. *Clin. Obstet. Gynecol.* 26:690, 1983.

Reindollar, R. H., Novak, M., Tho, S. P. T., and McDonough, P. Adult-onset amenorrhea: A study of 262 patients. *Am. J. Obstet. Gynecol.* 155:531, 1986.

Vorys, N. Menstrual dysfunction. In S. J. Behrman, R. W. Kistner, and G. W. Patton, *Progress in Infertility* (3rd ed.), Boston: Little, Brown, 1988. Chap. 16, p. 333.

12

Endometriosis

mechanism(s) involving infertility in endometriosis and the role of endocrine and surgical therapies. Current investigations on therapy with gonadotropin-releasing hormone agonists, antiestrogens, antiprogestins, and laser therapy permit improved choices for the management of endometriosis in individual patients.

DEFINITION

Historically, endometriosis and adenomyosis were thought to be similar. In 1895 von Recklinghausen applied the term *adenomyoma* to endometriotic lesions because most of his small group of cases were adenomyosis rather than endometriosis. Another 30 years passed before the differences between adenomyosis and endometriosis as two distinct unrelated disease processes were understood and accepted. Cullen (1897) was the first American to describe and discuss the occurrence of aberrant endometrial tissue within the uterine wall (adenomyosis). During the next 25 years his investigations ultimately defined adenomyosis and accurately demonstrated its true pathogenesis. Meanwhile, isolated reports of aberrant endometrium found in sites other than the uterus began to appear in the literature; Pfannenstiel (1897) reported a case involving the rectovaginal septum; Russell (1899) reported the first case documented in the ovary; and Meyer of Berlin (1909) reported the first recognized case of bowel endometriosis, the patient ultimately having a bowel resection performed by Mackenrodt.

In 1921 Sampson of Albany, New York, led the beginnings of comprehensive studies on endometriosis concerning its origins and significance. He reported on "perforating hemorrhagic [chocolate] cysts of the ovary" and subsequently on his theory of retrograde menstrual reflux and implantation for the pathogenesis of endometriosis. Blair-Bell of Liverpool first used the terms *endometriosis* and *endometrioma* to refer to the disease and the individual cystic lesion involving the ovary.

Considerable advances have been made in our understanding of endometriosis from the many studies performed over the last five decades. During the 1980s, advances in endocrinology and biochemistry have begun to shed light on our understanding of the

Endometriosis (endometriosis externa) may be defined as a disorder resulting from the presence of actively growing and functioning endometrial tissue (usually both glandular and supporting stromal elements) in locations outside the uterus. The precise mechanism by which the ectopic endometrium appears in its abnormal site is still not proved. Theories of origin are discussed here; but in view of the widespread anatomic locations in which endometriosis may be encountered, several etiologic mechanisms undoubtedly exist, as no single theory can satisfactorily explain its appearance at all the sites where it is known to occur.

In contrast, adenomyosis (endometriosis interna), though similar in histologic appearance, is a condition wherein islands of endometrial glands and stroma are found within the myometrium, interspersed between and surrounded by the smooth muscle fibers. A direct connection between these aberrant islands and the surface endometrium lining the uterine cavity can invariably be demonstrated, so it appears as an ingrowing of the endometrium into the myometrium. Thus the etiologic mechanism involved in the development of adenomyosis seems to be entirely different from that of endometriosis. The validity of the concept of adenomyosis and endometriosis as two disease entities, each with a different pathogenesis, is further supported by the fact that the former characteristically is found in older, multiparous patients, whereas the latter typically appears in the young, nulliparous woman. Although in the past the term *endometriosis interna* was used to refer to adenomyosis and *endometriosis externa* to "true" endometriosis, it is preferable that adenomyosis be referred to as adenomyosis, as it appears to be a different disease entity.

One other entity, *stromal endometriosis* (a variety

of other terms have also been used to designate this lesion, most of them more accurate and appropriate), should be mentioned for clarification. As suggested by the term, the aberrant tissue consists of endometrial stromal cells without glandular elements, but the primary lesion has never been found outside the uterus. Clinically, it behaves as a uterine neoplasm; and because it often pursues a highly malignant course, extrauterine and extrapelvic metastases and local extensions do occur. Obviously, "stromal" endometriosis bears no clinical resemblance to the "true" endometriosis under discussion here. Occasionally, in true endometriomas of long standing, repeated hemorrhage with necrosis or pressure atrophy may cause degenerative changes in the endometrial glands and produce a histologic picture in which glandular elements are absent and only stromal cells are found; this

situation also bears no relation to so-called stromal endometriosis. Although some believe the latter may be a variant of the commoner form of endometriosis, the majority opinion favors a different pathogenesis. (Stromal endometriosis is therefore considered a uterine malignancy and is discussed more fully in Chapter 27.)

SITES OF ENDOMETRIOSIS

The areas involved by endometriosis are widespread and usually multiple (Fig. 12-1). Within the pelvis, it is found most frequently in the ovaries and on the peritoneal coverings of the uterosacral ligaments, posterior cul-de-sac, and posterior wall of the lower uterine segment. It is also commonly encountered in the serosa of the fallopian tube, the anterior cul-de-sac

Fig. 12-1. Sites of occurrence of endometriosis.

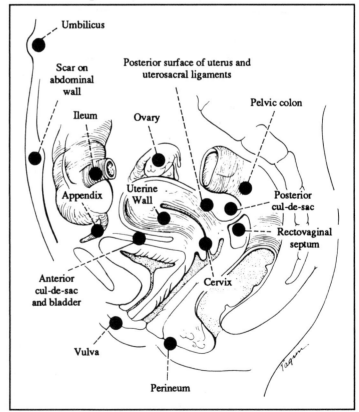

peritoneum and other pelvic peritoneal surfaces, the rectovaginal septum, the broad ligaments, the round ligaments including the portions within the inguinal canals, and the sigmoid colon. Less often, it involves the cervix, vagina, vulva, perineum, bladder (the actual vesical wall itself), and ureters or periureteral tissues. Elsewhere in the abdomen it occasionally involves the appendix, small bowel, umbilicus, and scars of previous anterior abdominal incisions, and there have even been isolated reports of endometriosis of the gallbladder, liver, and kidneys, though its presence within the peritoneal cavity above the level of the umbilicus is rare. It has been found in pelvic and inguinal lymph nodes; and, more rarely, it has been encountered in the pleura, lung, and skeletal muscle and bone of the extremities.

INCIDENCE

The incidence of endometriosis appears to be increasing. Such an increase is real as well as apparent. The real increase is probably due to the current trend of postponing conception well into the fourth decade of life. The apparent increase is due to both the frequent and indicated use of diagnostic laparoscopy as well as the heightened awareness of this disease complex by gynecologists.

In 1949 Meigs found that 5 to 15 percent of patients undergoing pelvic operations had endometriosis. This incidence increased to 18 percent of all gynecologic laparotomies as reported in 1978. Presently, it is estimated that one-third to one-half of all patients undergoing major gynecologic procedures have findings of endometriosis. From the early report of Meigs, it was noted that women who defer pregnancy to a later age and belong to higher socioeconomic groups were more frequently found in those who had endometriosis. Thus with increasing numbers of women working and pursuing careers and the accompanying deferment of pregnancies into the fourth decade of life, the incidence of endometriosis is likely to increase further.

Contrary to traditionally held views, endometriosis is more common in teenagers than hitherto believed. Endometriosis accounted for 65 percent and 47 percent of 43 and 140 symptomatic teenagers, respectively, who underwent laparoscopy.

Endometriosis has also been frequently found in women who have undergone elective tubal sterilization. Endometriosis was found in 21 percent of 54 women who had tubal ligation. In another study, endometriosis was found in 74 percent of women whose tubes were sterilized within 4 cm of the proximal end but in only 20 percent if the tubes were interrupted more than 4 cm from the proximal end. Although endometriosis generally regresses with the menopause when cyclic ovarian activity ceases, postmenopausal endometriosis was found in 1.3 percent of 903 patients operated on for endometriosis.

There is a familial incidence of endometriosis with a 7 percent relative risk of developing it if a first-degree female relative has it. The incidence of severe endometriosis in the familial group is higher (61.1 percent) than in the nonfamilial group (23.8 percent). Contrary to the former belief that endometriosis affects whites more often than blacks, it is now clear that black women are as frequently affected by endometriosis as their counterparts. Therefore endometriosis should be considered in black patients who present with pelvic pain but do not fit the diagnosis of pelvic inflammatory disease. Regardless of the origin of the disease, the lesion is more apt to occur and become clinically significant in women who have postponed childbearing, as prolonged cyclic ovarian function, uninterrupted by pregnancies, results in a continuous stimulus to proliferation and extension of the disease.

PATHOGENESIS

Many theories have been advanced, but the pathogenesis of endometriosis remains uncertain. At least twelve theories have been advanced, with the principal ones outlined in the following paragraphs.

1. *Retrograde menstruation and tubal reflux.* The most widely held explanation of the initiation of endometriosis is the retrograde flow of menstrual fluid with subsequent implantation of viable fragments of endometrium within the pelvic cavity. This hypothesis is known as Sampson's theory, as he favored this mechanism. In support of this theory is the observation that retrograde menstruation was found in women undergoing peritoneal dialysis during menstruation

and in women and rhesus monkeys undergoing laparoscopy during menstruation.

Blood may appear during the few days before menstruation and usually persists during the first day of menstrual flow. Retrograde menstruation can account for the frequent sites of endometriosis in the posterior aspects of the pelvis. Women with endometriosis often have a long history of dysmenorrhea. The excessive uterine contractions characteristic of primary dysmenorrhea may further contribute to a bidirectional menstrual flow from the uterus. However, Sampson's theory of retrograde menstruation does not explain the extrapelvic sites of endometriosis, such as endometriosis of the limbs, thoracic cavity, and elsewhere. Therefore retrograde menstruation per se is unlikely to produce endometriosis by itself. It is most probable that a genetic factor or susceptibility, as well as a favorable hormonal milieu are necessary for successful implantation and growth of the transported fragments of endometrium.

2. *Celomic metaplasia.* The celomic metaplasia theory was advanced by Meyer of Berlin and Ivanoff of Russia. All tissues in which endometriosis arises are embryologically derived from celomic epithelium. Chronic irritation of the peritoneum by menstrual blood may cause celomic metaplasia, which can subsequently result in endometriosis. Alternatively, müllerian tissue remnants trapped in the peritoneum could undergo metaplasia and be transformed into endometriosis. Repeated, cyclic ovarian stimulation that occurs after menarche induces histologic differentiation of the totipotential celomic epithelial cells into the metaplastic formation of functioning endometrial tissues in ectopic sites. This theory can account for all the sites of endometriosis that have so far been described in the literature, including rare instances of endometriosis of the lung, pleura, arm, thigh, and buttocks.

3. *Direct implantation.* According to this theory, endometrial tissues are displaced into an implant in the new sites. This theory is supported by endometriosis seen in scars as a result of direct seeding of the new sites of surgery. In rabbits, endometriosis is produced in the pelvic peritoneum by direct subperitoneal implantation of surgically excised endometrial tissue segments. This model has been employed for a number of studies on endometriosis. For successful implantation to occur, ovarian estrogens or exogenous estrogens are necessary. In rhesus monkeys, bilateral oophorectomy without estrogen replacement produced significantly less direct implantation of endometrium for production of endometriosis, whereas replacement with exogenous estrogens produced a significantly higher rate of induction of endometriosis. Although direct implantation may explain many of the endometriosis sites, it cannot explain the occurrence of endometriosis in the limbs and thoracic cavity.

4. *Genetic and immunologic factors.* There is a 5.8 percent familial incidence among immediate female siblings, an 8.1 percent risk if the mother has endometriosis, and a 7 percent risk if a female sibling has endometriosis. These figures suggest a polygenic and multifactorial inheritance for endometriosis. The genetic basis of endometriosis probably accounts for some patients with endometriosis who have a family history but not for most of those who do not.

Findings in monkeys with spontaneous endometriosis suggest that a defect of cellular immunity may be the basis for the ectopic tissue being allowed to grow in abnormal locations only in certain patients. It may explain why cervical endometriosis is rare despite regular exposure of the cervix to menstrual fluid.

5. *Luteinized unruptured follicle syndrome.* The luteinized unruptured follicle (LUF) syndrome reportedly occurs more commonly in women with endometriosis than in normal women. It is postulated that the high concentrations of steroid hormones in peritoneal fluid after ovulation inhibit and inactivate endometrial tissues reaching the peritoneum in normal women. In women with the LUF syndrome, the suboptimal content of peritoneal fluid steroid hormones reduces inhibition and inactivation of retrograde endometrial tissues, thereby promoting ectopic implantation of endometrial tissues. In monkeys and rabbits with experimental endometriosis, LUF has been found to be a common correlate of infertility, suggesting that the presence of pelvic endometriosis may cause an attenuation of follicular rupture.

6. *Elevated prostaglandin levels.* The ectopic endometrial implants have been found to have higher prostaglandin $F_{2\alpha}$ ($PGF_{2\alpha}$) concentrations in women with endometriosis. Indeed if the increased prostaglandins are present and could therefore alter tubal motility depending on the relative composition of the various prostaglandins, further retrograde showering of menstrual endometrial tissue into the peritoneal cavity may occur as a result of tubal dyskinesia. However, the early observation that peritoneal fluid prostaglandins and prostanoids are elevated in women with endometriosis has been refuted by several large, well controlled studies. Nevertheless, the increased production of $PGF_{2\alpha}$ by the ectopic endometrium itself could lead to exposure of the tube to increased local blood levels of prostaglandins.

7. *Lymphatic dissemination.* Halban suggested that normal endometrium might "metastasize" via lymphatic channels and thus spread to extrauterine sites where implantation and growth would produce the characteristic lesions of endometriosis. This theory is supported by the finding of benign endometriosis in pelvic lymph nodes, though conceivably the celomic metaplasia theory could also account for this finding.

8. *Vascular theory.* Navratil suggested the possibility of deportation of normal endometrium via venous channels, with vascular dissemination to remote areas of the body. Although both the vascular and lymphatic dissemination theories could explain the presence of endometriosis in distant sites such as limb buds and the thoracic cavity, they are not well supported by clinical observations or experimental data.

PATHOLOGIC FEATURES

The three diagnostic histologic features of endometriosis are (1) endometrial glands, (2) endometrial stroma, and (3) evidence of hemorrhage, either fresh (red blood cells and hemosiderin pigment) or old (hemosiderin-laden macrophages). The typical lesion also shows an abundance of inflammatory cells and fibrous connective tissue indicative of the intense reaction of the surrounding normal cellular elements to the presence of the functioning ectopic endometrial tissue.

Because of its precise microscopic resemblance to normal endometrium and its known responsiveness to ovarian hormonal stimulation, the functioning epithelium of an endometrioma sometimes duplicates closely the phases of the normal intrauterine endometrium, demonstrating proliferative change during the preovulatory portion of the menstrual cycle and secretory changes during the postovulatory or progestational phase. However, more often the ectopic endometrial tissues of the areas of endometriosis, particularly the more advanced lesions, are out of phase with the normal endometrium within the uterus and are found in the proliferative stage even during the secretory phase of the normal menstrual cycle. Presumably, this situation is due to the difference in blood supply and to the effects of the increasing tissue fibrosis surrounding the endometriosis. The altered responsiveness to the normal ovarian hormonal cycle occasionally results in a microscopic picture of cystic hyperplasia or even a pseudodecidual reaction in the ectopic endometrium of endometriosis. As previously mentioned, destruction of the glands by hemorrhage and pressure atrophy in lesions of long standing may occur, with only the endometrial stromal cells and evidence of old hemorrhage remaining as histologic guideposts to the true nature of the process.

During pregnancy a marked decidual reaction is noted microscopically, with softening and some gross shrinkage of the areas of endometriosis. At the conclusion of the pregnancy, with subsidence of the decidual reaction, microscopic atrophy and a pronounced tendency to regression of the visible and palpable gross lesions of endometriosis are usually seen. This beneficial effect of pregnancy on endometriosis is the basis of some forms of current medical treatment creating or employing "pseudopregnancy."

The characteristic gross anatomic appearance of endometriosis again differs somewhat with the location and duration of activity of the lesions. In the ovary the process is almost always bilateral, and the tendency is for the formation of cystic structures varying from tiny, bluish or dark-brown blisters to large chocolate cysts up to 20 cm or more in diameter. There is usually considerable fibrosis and puckering of the ovarian surface in the region of the cyst, as well as adherence to neighboring structures (sigmoid, uterus, broad ligament, or pelvic wall). It occurs because of the intermittent rupture (usually during or just after a period) and partial spillage of the contents of the endometrioma, with resulting local peritonitis and fibrosis, which seals off the leak and produces scar-tissue fixation. It is this scar tissue's puckering and dense adherence to its surroundings that is so indicative of endometriosis, not simply the chocolate contents of the cyst, as the latter may be encountered in hemorrhagic corpus luteum cysts or any cystic lesion of the ovary in which hemorrhage has occurred and old blood is present.

In the other most frequently involved areas, i.e., the uterosacral ligaments, cul-de-sac, posterior uterine surface—in fact, throughout the pelvic peritoneum—the lesions are smaller and often more numerous, consisting of multiple "blueberry spots" or "powder-burn" lesions surrounded by a stellate pattern of dense, fibrous scar tissue, the latter making up most of the bulk of the visible and palpable puckered nodules. The intense fibrotic response to the presence of active ("menstruating") ectopic endometrium in these areas is undoubtedly the limiting factor in the growth of the lesions. This same scar tissue contraction tends to draw up or down and create fixation of any and all of the neighboring structures (e.g., the uterus, which characteristically becomes fixed in a retroverted position, rectosigmoid, adnexa, and small bowel) with ultimate obliteration of the cul-de-sac and marked anatomic displacement and functional impairment of the pelvic viscera.

In some areas and organs the process may spread or "invade" in cancerlike fashion (e.g., the rectovaginal septum and posterior vaginal fornix, rectum, sigmoid, bladder, ureter, and small bowel). The endometriosis burrows in from the serosal surface, penetrating deeply into the muscular and submucosal layers of the walls of these structures, where it may spread further in a longitudinal direction but rarely involves the mucosa.

Intermittent bleeding into the gastrointestinal or urinary tract may result, usually coinciding with the menses, but it is due to periodic congestion of the overlying mucosa and not to actual mucosal ulceration. Eventually, the accompanying extensive fibrosis may produce a tumor-like mass indistinguishable grossly from carcinoma, particularly in the colon; and the resulting constriction of, and encroachment on, the bowel lumen may produce variable degrees of obstruction. Ureteral obstruction may occur in a similar way. Small-bowel obstruction may also result, but it is usually due to fixation and kinking rather than to narrowing of the lumen.

CLINICAL MANIFESTATIONS

It is apparent from the discussions of its pathologic features and probable etiology that endometriosis is a disease of the active reproductive life of women. It is unusual before the menarche and is most frequent in women in their twenties and thirties. Pelvic endometriosis in teenagers may be somewhat more common than has generally been appreciated. With increasing use of laparoscopy, endometriosis has been found more frequently in teenagers than was conventionally believed. In any case, the diagnosis should be considered, even in teenagers, if there are any suggestive physical findings or if the menstrual discomfort differs from that usually accompanying primary dysmenorrhea in terms of its nature, location, and response to standard therapy.

As would be predicted, it ceases almost entirely to be a problem after menopause because with cessation of cyclic ovarian function the lesions ordinarily atrophy and regress, leading to softening and almost complete disappearance of the secondary surrounding fibrotic nodules and scar tissue deformities. Occasional exceptions to the postmenopausal inactivity of the disease have been encountered and reported, but they are rare. In some cases, reactivation may have been induced by hormonal therapy. Occasionally, at the time of laparotomy for other causes in postmenopausal women, persistent scarring in the form of cul-de-sac obliteration, old adnexal adhesions, or pelvic tissue plane distortions may point to the probable prior presence of pelvic endometriosis, but microscopic proof is usually absent due to the total atrophy of the endometrial glands and stroma.

Thus the typical patient is in her twenties or early thirties, is either single or has married late and has voluntarily delayed childbearing, or is suffering from involuntary sterility. Many are nulliparous, and the rest usually have had one or two pregnancies.

SYMPTOMS

The symptoms and signs of endometriosis are summarized in Table 12-1. The classic history is *dysmenorrhea* (painful menstrual periods). This disorder is secondary dysmenorrhea; and although in some cases it can be remarkably similar to primary dysmenorrhea, more often than not the symptom is of recent or new onset, may not date back to the menarche, and may have recently increased in intensity. The dysmenorrhea is more likely to begin a day or two before the onset of menstrual flow, though the intensity of pain may increase during the early days of menstruation. In Sampson's original report, 50 percent of patients with endometriosis had dysmenorrhea. More recent reports indicate that, overall, dysmenorrhea occurs in about 63 percent of women with endometriosis. The frequency of severe dysmenorrhea in patients with endometriosis is 27 percent in mild disease, 26 percent in moderate disease, and 35 percent in severe disease.

Pelvic pain is another symptom of endometriosis. Such pain should not be confused with dysmenorrhea. With dysmenorrhea, the pain is confined to or around the time of menstrual flow. In contrast, pelvic pain in women with endometriosis tends to be a deep-seated aching or bearing-down pain in the lower abdomen, deep in the posterior part of the pelvis, vagina, and back. It often radiates to the rectal and perineal areas with rectal tenesmus and symptoms of bowel irritation. Such a distribution of the pain is secondary to the characteristic involvement of the uterosacral ligaments, cul-de-sac, and adjacent surfaces of the uterus and rectum, with or without vaginal septal disease. As the endometriosis progresses, the pain extends over the entire luteal phase, leaving only a few pain-free days postmenstrually. If one or both ovaries are affected by endometriomas, dull unilateral or bilateral lower abdominal pain, often with radiation to the thighs, may be noted.

Two additional points are noteworthy. First, not all patients with endometriosis have pain. Despite extensive disease palpable on pelvic examination or found at laparoscopy or laparotomy, about 30 to 35 percent of patients report no discomfort whatsoever, though they may suffer from other manifestations of the pathologic process, notably infertility or a pelvic mass. Some patients with extensive disease involving the cul-de-sac and both uterosacral ligaments as well as extensive pelvic adhesions found at laparoscopy or laparotomy report no pain whatsoever. Such a disparity between the extent of the pathologic findings and the absence of pain may be due to the denervation or neuropraxia that may accompany the disease process as it involves the pathway of the pelvic innervation. Second, the small "peritoneal implant" type of lesion may produce intense pain from stretching of the overlying peritoneum and tight constrictions produced by fibrosis. On the other hand, the presence of a large chocolate cyst of the ovary, which is accompanied by little if any fibrosis and is relatively free to expand, may produce little discomfort until the cyst becomes distended or ruptures. Thus the severity of the pelvic endometriosis is not necessarily directly related to the likelihood of pelvic pain.

The mechanisms for pelvic pain in endometriosis are poorly understood and probably multifactorial. They include adhesions, scarring, stretching of the peritoneum, alteration in pelvic blood flow, impingement of pelvic nerve pathways, and possibly pelvic

Table 12-1. Signs and Symptoms of Endometriosis

Symptoms	Signs
Common	Common
Infertility	None
Dysmenorrhea	Tender, enlarged
Pelvic pain	ovary
Dyspareunia	Pelvic nodularities
Less common	Pelvic thickenings
Premenstrual spotting	Fixed retroverted
Menstrual	uterus
dysfunction	Less common
Urinary symptoms	Intestinal obstruction
(dysuria, urgency,	Hemoperitoneum
hematuria)	Torsion of ovarian
Bowel symptoms	cyst
(tenesmus, melena,	Catamenial
vomiting)	pneumothorax

prostaglandins. The extent, vascularity, fibrosis, and distortion of pelvic structures caused by the adhesions secondary to the endometriosis are important factors in pelvic pain. With cryptic menstruation of ectopic endometrium in confined spaces between or underneath peritoneal layers, pelvic pain can result from peritoneal stretching and irritation, as indicated above. With healing and dense scarring of the endometrial implants, pain may arise secondary to scar tissue contraction and distortion of the surrounding structures or impingement on nerve pathways. Alteration of pelvic blood flow secondary to adhesions, scarring, elevated or altered prostaglandins, or inflammatory response to the ectopic endometrium can give rise to pelvic congestion and pelvic discomfort. Impingement of pelvic nerve pathways (e.g., those around the uterosacral ligaments, the ovarian nerve supply, and the hypogastric nerve plexus) by scarring, bleeding, or fibrosis can certainly give rise to pelvic pain. Prostaglandins E_2 and $F_{2\alpha}$ levels have been found to be increased in uterine endometrial tissues as well as endometriotic tissues. Although prostaglandins may contribute to some degree to the pelvic pain or dysmenorrhea of endometriosis, they are less likely to be a significant physiologic basis of the pain in most instances. Clinical trials with several nonsteroidal antiinflammatory agents have not produced significant relief of the pelvic pain in women with endometriosis.

Dyspareunia is another characteristic chronic symptom associated with pelvic endometriosis. The dyspareunia is usually deep-seated, and pain often intensifies with vigorous intercourse during rapid to-an-fro intravaginal movement of the penis. This symptom can be readily elicited by the presence of deep-seated tenderness on a bimanual pelvic examination. The dyspareunia probably arises from the tenderness elicited by the stretching of the structures in the cul-de-sac by the penis or by direct-contact tenderness. Thus the dyspareunia is sometimes relieved or eliminated by a change in coital position. In 27 percent of patients with endometriosis who reported dyspareunia, this symptom appeared to have no relation to the severity of endometriosis. This symptom is likely to be present if there is disease in the cul-de-sac, rectovaginal septum, uterosacral ligaments, or ovaries if they are situated or adherent in the cul-de-sac.

Menstrual irregularities have been noted in 12 to 14 percent of patients with endometriosis irrespective of the severity of their disease. Premenstrual spotting is found to be significantly more common in women with endometriosis than in those with luteal phase defects without endometriosis. Therefore regular premenstrual spotting in an infertile woman should be a helpful clue to the likelihood of endometriosis. With ovarian endometriotic cyst (chocolate cyst), menstrual disorder and lower abdominal pain were the two most common symptoms in 72 percent of the cases.

Other *chronic symptoms* varying with the anatomic areas involved and the extent of the disease, include cyclic bowel disturbances with painful defecation, rectal bleeding, and even some acute intestinal obstruction, as well as rare manifestations such as cyclic painful swelling (endometriosis of the round ligament, inguinal ligament, or inguinal peritoneum) and bladder irritability and hematuria (bladder wall involvement).

Infertility is a common initial complaint in patients with endometriosis. Their infertility may exist in the absence of any other symptoms or significant abnormalities on pelvic examination. Often the endometriosis is found only as a result of investigations for the infertility or at the time of laparoscopy for unexplained infertility after much of the office evaluation of the infertility has been completed and found to be normal. The frequency of infertility in women with endometriosis is difficult to assess, as many series have no matched controls. The incidence of infertility of more than 1 and 2 years' duration has been reported to be as high as 100 percent and 79 percent, respectively. The duration of infertility was unrelated to the severity of the endometriosis, and primary infertility was twice as frequent as secondary infertility. Other findings and our own experience has indicated that mild endometriosis in the absence of anatomic distortion of the reproductive tract or ovulation does not interfere with female infertility, and that pregnancy rates are similar with or without treatment by medication or surgery.

The physiologic basis for infertility in women with endometriosis is probably multifactorial. In some women, the mechanism(s) responsible for infertility are self-evident and readily explicable. Such etiologic factors include adhesions, tubal occlusion, interference with the tuboovarian mechanism for ovum pickup and transfer, ovulatory dysfunction, prostaglandins and tubal dyskinesia autoimmunity, decreased sperm transport, and finally increased spontaneous abortions. Ovulatory dysfunction includes anovulation, luteinized unruptured follicle (where the ovum is trapped in the follicle, which becomes luteinized), and luteal phase defects. There has been some suggestion that increased prostaglandin production by the endometriosis could give rise to abnormal tubal activity, thereby causing inappropriate tubal transit of either ovum or blastocyst and hence failure to implant.

Leakage or frank rupture of an enlarging ovarian endometrioma occurs not infrequently and may produce generalized *peritonitis* and an acute abdominal emergency. Spillage of old blood (the chocolate-like content of the endometriosis) produces an intense local irritation and inflammatory response, which results in a chemical peritonitis. As might be expected, the acute episode usually starts shortly after a menstrual period, rupture having been prompted by fresh bleeding into the chocolate cavity with resulting sudden increase in intracystic pressure. Although small leaks may have occurred previously, with rapid sealing-over and prompt subsidence of the local peritoneal reaction, most of the acute episodes require immediate laparotomy, the mortality of nonsurgically treated cases in the past having approached 50 percent. In some instances the leak can be adequately dealt with by laparoscopy and translaparoscopic attention to the chocolate cyst and peritoneal spillage.

PHYSICAL FINDINGS

The findings on pelvic examination are somewhat variable and occasionally are minimal or even absent during the early stages of endometriosis. However, the characteristic finding is the hard, fixed, fibrotic nodule usually felt as a beaded or shotty thickening in the uterosacral ligaments, cul-de-sac, or posterior surface of the lower uterine wall or cervix. The presence of such nodularity in these specific locations is virtually pathognomonic of endometriosis. Although these thickenings may be palpable vaginally, they are best appreciated on a rectovaginal examination, particularly in patients with minimal involvement with endo-

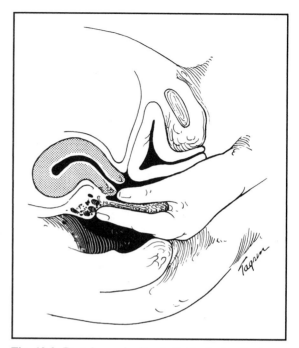

Fig. 12-2. Rectal examination in the typical patient with pelvic endometriosis. The tender nodularity of the uterosacral ligaments and cul-de-sac and the fixed retroversion of the uterus are almost diagnostic of the disease.

metriosis. The palpating finger can readily reach and explore these posterior structures (Fig. 12-2). Thus a rectovaginal examination is a *sine qua non* component of the pelvic examination. If the disease is sufficiently extensive, the cul-de-sac may have been completely obliterated, and the uterus is drawn back and adherent to the rectum in fixed retroversion. Other specific abnormalities to look for during the pelvic examination include the presence of tender enlarged ovaries, an adnexal mass (as is the case with ovarian chocolate cyst), and more rarely a bluish nodule or nodules present in the posterior vaginal fornix (best visualized on speculum examination). Tenderness and pain on motion of any of the involved structures is another characteristic feature, although not necessarily diagnostic. Such tenderness and pain are typically maximal just before and during each menstrual period. Less frequent findings may include torsion of an ovarian cyst, catamenial pneumothorax, hemoperitoneum from rupture of a chocolate cyst, and signs of intestinal obstruction in the bowel significantly infiltrated by endometriosis.

DIAGNOSIS

It is apparent that endometriosis is more common than generally realized. Unless thought of, endometriosis can be missed, with the diagnosis delayed or never made. In typical cases the correct diagnosis is often strongly suggested by the history alone; and even in patients with minimal involvement and mild symptomatology, a careful detailed history may raise the suspicion of endometriosis. Usually a presumptive diagnosis based on the characteristic symptoms and their chronologic relation to the menstrual cycle can be verified with almost absolute certainty if on vaginal and rectal examination the tender uterosacral ligament or cul-de-sac nodules are palpable and if there is associated fixed retroversion of the uterus.

Endometriosis should be differentiated from primary dysmenorrhea and other causes of secondary dysmenorrhea, pelvic inflammatory disease, and other causes of an adnexal mass. With primary dysmenorrhea, the pain usually begins immediately before the onset of menstruation, is usually gone within 48 hours, and is accompanied by nausea, vomiting, diarrhea, and tiredness. With endometriosis, however, the pain often starts several days before and persists throughout menstruation and even for a few days thereafter. The pain of primary dysmenorrhea is cramp- or labor-like, whereas the pain associated with endometriosis is usually dull, dragging, and referred to the rectum. Historically, primary dysmenorrhea begins at the time of or a few months after menarche, when ovulatory cycles are established; the dysmenorrhea of endometriosis, on the other hand, often begins a few years after the menarche. Nevertheless, in the absence of positive physical findings, the dysmenorrhea of endometriosis can mimic primary dysmenorrhea so strikingly that laparoscopy should be performed only when the patient fails to respond to cyclic oral contraceptives and to the nonsteroidal anti-inflammatory agents.

Endometriosis may present so subtly that it is not uncommonly confused with pelvic inflammatory dis-ease, with the patient then being given repeated courses of antibiotic therapy. This diagnostic trap is often true in patients with pelvic pain and those who have minimal pelvic tenderness and adnexal thickenings without fever or other signs. With florid acute pelvic inflammatory disease or an acute exacerbation, the diagnosis may be more readily apparent when there is a history of pelvic infection and the current presence of chills, fever, purulent vaginal discharge, adnexal masses (usually bilateral), and pelvic tenderness. Failure to respond to appropriate antibiotic therapy should arouse suspicion of endometriosis, especially if pelvic abscess has been ruled out. With pelvic infection, the adnexal masses, if present, are usually bilateral. Although a unilateral inflammatory adnexal mass has been shown to be present in some women using the intrauterine device, endometriosis also should be considered in the presence of a unilateral adnexal mass. Unless endometriosis is considered in patients with adnexal or pelvic masses, the diagnosis is often not made before surgery. In one series of 263 patients with ovarian endometriotic cysts, the diagnosis was made on admission and prior to surgery in only 7 percent of cases. Therefore in the presence of a unilateral adnexal mass in the premenopausal women, endometriosis should always be considered.

Endometriosis involving the bowel and urinary tract with bowel or urinary symptoms must be differentiated from other gastrointestinal and urinary tract symptoms.

Diagnosis by visual inspection is necessary before commencing therapy. Therefore laparoscopy is required invariably in all cases where endometriosis is suspected unless a laparotomy is indicated or if the endometriosis involves structures such as the skin, vagina, or cervix, which are readily visible on routine gynecologic examination. The gross appearance of endometriosis is so characteristic that histologic confirmation is generally unnecessary. The lesion within the pelvis is biopsied for histologic documentation only if the site of the lesion is not hazardous for such a biopsy to be performed.

The extent of the diagnostic workup depends on the stage of the disease and the structures involved. Intravenous pyelography or cystoscopy becomes necessary if ureteral or bladder involvement is suspected. Barium enema, sigmoidoscopy, and upper gastrointestinal series are indicated if the bowels are suspected to be involved with endometriosis. Endocrine evaluation is usually not helpful unless the patient is suffering from menstrual dysfunction, ovulatory dysfunction, or luteal phase defect. In such cases, either an endometrial biopsy or a midluteal phase serum progesterone assay can be helpful. Hysterosalpingography may be necessary in patients suspected of having tubal involvement but can be omitted if laparoscopy is performed.

At laparoscopy, the pathognomonic appearance of endometriosis is due to blood deposition into the tissues, which gives a rust-colored appearance with time. Older endometriotic deposits appear yellowish brown and even gray as the blood is resolved. Healed areas may show puckering with fibrosis and even adhesions (Fig. 12-3). With larger endometriotic deposits in the ovary the characteristic chocolate cyst may be seen. With severe disease, extensive adhesions may develop, with the cul-de-sac completely obliterated and the sigmoid and other loops of bowel stuck to the uterus. Peritoneal defects (Fig. 12-3) in women with pelvic pain have been found to be associated with endometriosis in 68 percent of cases. When these

defects are observed at laparoscopy, endometriotic deposits should be carefully sought. Nevertheless, these peritoneal defects have also been incidentally found in women with no pelvic pain, dysmenorrhea, or endometriosis at routine laparoscopy for other indications.

CLASSIFICATION

All cases of diagnosed endometriosis should be classified and staged as an aid to predicting prognosis, choosing therapy, and managing the disease. Several classifications have been introduced, with the Acosta classification most popularly used until recently. Currently, the official classification of the American Fertility Society is perferred. This classification has undergone revision, and the revised classification by the American Fertility Society is currently in use (Table 12-2).

MANAGEMENT

The management of endometriosis should be approached from the standpoints of both prevention and treatment.

Prevention

Because the potential for the development of endometriosis seems to be an intrinsic feature of the embryol-

Fig. 12-3. Characteristic findings of pelvic endometriosis at surgery (laparoscopy or laparotomy).

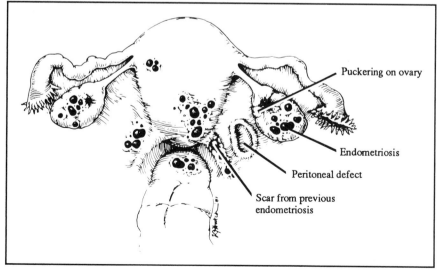

Puckering on ovary

Endometriosis

Peritoneal defect

Scar from previous endometriosis

Table 12-2. American Fertility Society Revised Classification of Endometriosis

Parameter	Points assigned for severity of finding							
	Peritoneum		Right ovary		Left ovary		Posterior cul-de-sac	Right or left tube/right or left ovary[a]
	Superf.	Deep	Superf.	Deep	Superf.	Deep		
Depth of endometriosis								
1 cm	1	2	1	4	1	4		
1–3 cm	2	4	2	16	2	16		
3 cm	4	6	4	20	4	20		
Degree of obliteration								
Partial							4	
Complete							40	
Adhesions								
⅓ Enclosure								
Filmy								1
Dense								4
⅓–⅔ Enclosure								
Filmy								2
Dense								8
>⅔ Enclosure								
Filmy								4
Dense								16

[a] Both the ovaries and the tubes are scored.

The scores are summed and the stage of endometriosis is assigned according to the following scale:

1–5 = Stage I (minimal)
6–15 = Stage II (mild)
16–40 = Stage III (moderate)
40 = Stage IV (severe)

ogy and physiology of the human female, prevention in the absolute sense may not be possible for most women, who have an inherited susceptibility to the disease. However, prophylaxis against occurrence of clinically significant endometriosis (extensive, progressively increasing involvement, disabling symptoms, and disorders of pelvic function including infertility) may be achieved by women who choose to avoid undue delay in childbearing and have several pregnancies at reasonable intervals (five years or more). Additionally, women who have a female sibling, mother, or maternal aunt with endometriosis should be encouraged not to defer childbearing to a late age because they have a 7 percent chance of having endometriosis. Furthermore, such women may be encouraged not to use tampons because of the theoretical possibility of further enhancing retrograde menstruation and reflux, thereby promoting the development of endometriosis. Although early childbearing may not reduce the incidence of endometriosis occurring at a later age, it can certainly obviate the tragedy of "voluntary" sterility.

Treatment

Endometriosis can be treated surgically, medically, or by combination of the two modalities. There is continuing controversy as to which type of therapy produces better results. However, it is clear that both medical and surgical therapies have their place in the management of the woman with endometriosis, depending on her age, reproductive status, presenting complaints, need for fertility, and extent and location of disease. The only method of treatment that offers permanent cure is castration, thus making it a treatment of last resort. All other methods are for temporary remission at best.

Surgical Management. For the management of endometriosis, surgery is clearly indicated in the following situations.

1. Diagnosis
2. Tubal occlusion; peritubal, pelvic, and ovarian adhesions (when fertility is required)
3. Chocolate cyst of the ovary

4. Intractable pelvic pain unrelieved by medical management
5. Failed medical management

However, when the patient is asymptomatic or the disease is mild or moderate, it is less clear if surgical ablative therapy gives better results than medical therapy. There are increasing data to indicate that with mild disease and in the absence of tubal occlusion pregnancy rates are similar with medical treatment, surgery, or even no treatment.

Definitive surgery for management of endometriosis can be either conservative surgery or complete extirpative surgery. The conservative surgical approach is indicated in women who want to become pregnant or who wish to preserve their reproductive function. Ovarian cystectomy is done for chocolate cyst, lysis of adhesions and salpingoplasty for tubal complications, and cauterization or laser vaporization for pelvic peritoneal lesions if they are not at critical sites. Microsurgical technique should be employed. With adhesive disease, plication of the round ligament, approximation of the uterosacral ligaments posteriorly, or even ventral suspension of the uterus may be necessary to prevent it from becoming adherent in the culde-sac or posteriorly; treatment should be individualized in each case.

Some of these procedures may be carried out with the laparoscope. Laser vaporization of endometriosis deposits using either the argon or the carbon dioxide laser can be employed and have been advocated enthusiastically by some. The advantages of laser photocoagulation of endometriosis through the laparoscope include (1) reduced morbidity; (2) less likelihood of postoperative adhesion formation, as the abdomen is not opened; (3) reduced tissue injury and necrosis; and (4) vaporization of the endometriosis including proteins, which are thought to be antigenic and to produce autoimmune changes in the patient. Such a treatment appears to extirpate the lesion completely and reduces the risk of autoimmunity. However, there are no good controlled studies to indicate that, in terms of restoring fertility or abolishing symptoms, laser vaporization of endometriosis produces better results than cauterization of such lesions through the laparoscope. Lysis of adhesions and cauterization of pelvic peritoneal endometriosis can also be performed through the laparoscope. It is prudent not to cauterize lesions that are close to or on critical structures, as undesirable postoperative thermal injury complications may arise. The carbon dioxide laser has also been used through the laparoscope for lysis of adhesions and neosalpingostomy in patients with endometriosis. If pelvic pain has been a significant symptom, presacral neurectomy is usually advisable at the time of laparotomy as a further means to prevent recurrence of the pain. In addition, division and partial resection of the uterosacral ligaments to denervate the autonomic nerve supply of Frankenhauser's plexus, which runs through this ligament, can be performed to interrupt the nerve. It can be done through either a laparotomy or through the laparoscope.

The results of conservative surgery have been satisfactory, and pregnancy rates of 50 to 65 percent may be achieved if the surgery is properly and meticulously done. Even if pregnancy does not occur, many of the women have relief of their symptoms.

Complete Extirpative Surgery. For women who have completed their families or if medical therapy has failed, radical surgery may be indicated. The surgery should include total hysterectomy and bilateral salpingo-oophorectomy. All gross endometriosis, including any ovarian endometriomas, should be removed. Oophorectomy is necessary to remove the source of endogenous ovarian estrogens, which are the cause of continuous stimulation and growth of the endometriosis. Although it has been advocated that women in their thirties undergo radical surgery for endometriosis, but have some ovarian tissue preserved, these patients often return for removal of the residual ovaries several years later because of recurrence of the symptoms of endometriosis. For patients with pelvic pain, presacral neurectomy may be included in the radical surgery.

Estrogen replacement therapy can be started for menopausal symptoms within a few days after surgery if all endometriotic tissue has been removed. The regimen employed is described in Chapter 23. Conjugated estrogens or ethinyl estradiol can be given orally, or estradiol can be given transdermally as a skin patch (Estraderm). Nevertheless, postmenopausal endometriosis has been reported in as many as 2 percent of patients with endometriosis, usually in association with either endogenous estrogen sources or exogenously administered estrogens. Therefore although the dose of estrogen used for postmenopausal estrogen replacement therapy is low, if there is any likelihood of endometriosis remaining or of restimulation of the endometriosis with estrogens the postmenopausal symptoms as well as the endometriosis can be readily controlled with a progestin, e.g., medroxyprogesterone acetate. Then, after three to six months estrogen replacement therapy may be initiated. Thus long-term prevention of osteoporosis can still be accomplished while immediate short-term relief of hot flashes and psychoemotional symptoms can be readily controlled with the initial progestin therapy.

Based on the retrospective analysis of only those patients who have repeat surgery for symptoms, the annual recurrence rate after surgery ranges from 0.9 percent during the first postoperative year to 13.6 percent during the eighth postoperative year, with accumulative three- and five-year recurrence rates of 13.5 and 40.3 percent, respectively. The latter cumulative recurrence rates are similar to those obtained after medical treatment. However, the nature of the problem of women with endometriosis is recurrent abortion. Because of the disease, surgery gives better results than medical therapy in terms of reducing the abortion rate. Therefore surgery is the preferred treatment in patients with endometriosis who have recurrent abortions due to it.

Combined Surgery and Medical Therapy. Combined surgery and medical therapies have been employed for the management of endometriosis. In this respect danazol (see below, under Medical Management) has been used in combination with surgery. The best means of combining the two remains uncertain, but danazol has been employed preoperatively for six weeks or more followed by surgery. It appears that danazol therapy induces regression of the endometriosis and renders surgical dissection easier. Additionally, conservative surgery following hormonal treatment permits lysis of adhesions that might have formed during healing of the disease. Medical therapy has also been employed postoperatively, especially when all the endometriosis could be technically removed at surgery.

Medical Management. Significant relief of endometriosis can be obtained with medical management. In addition to the established methods of medical treatment using oral contraceptives, danazol, and progestins, several new approaches to medical management based on advances in endocrinology are evolving. All medical management of endometriosis is thus far based on hormonal therapy.

Hormonal therapy is indicated (1) in patients whose endometriosis is not extensive; (2) when there is need to conserve reproductive function; (3) when the disease is located at critical sites and surgery could be damaging or technically difficult but there is a need to "reduce" the endometriosis; (4) to render the subsequent surgery easier; and (5) for relief of symptoms in young patients and for suppression or eradication of the endometriosis until the woman is ready for childbearing.

Two basic approaches to medical management of endometriosis are currently in use: pseudopregnancy therapy and pseudomenopause therapy. The ideal hormonal therapy is to induce pregnancy. The progesterone produced by the placenta and suppression of ovarian function during pregnancy induce regression of the endometriosis, but pregnancy is not always readily achievable in women with endometriosis, nor is it desired by some of them. Such hormonal therapy is aimed at: (1) suppressing ovarian function and thus reducing the growth-promoting effects of ovarian estrogen; (2) directly inhibiting endometrial growth; and (3) converting the endometrium to a secretory or pseudodecidual type of tissue with resultant glandular atrophy.

PSEUDOPREGNANCY THERAPY. Women can be rendered pseudopregnant through the use of one or several gestagens currently available, including norethindrone, oral medroxyprogesterone acetate (Provera), Depo-Provera, and 6-retroprogesterone (Duphaston). Medroxyprogesterone acetate and norethindrone are given orally, and the dose is progressively increased until symptoms are relieved or the patient is intolerant of the dose. The maintenance dose is then continued. Depo-Provera is given intramuscularly 100 mg every two weeks for four doses and thereafter maintained with 200 mg every month. Hormonal therapy should be continuous for six to nine months depending on the extent of the endometriosis, the rapidity with which relief is obtained after initiating therapy, and if intolerable side effects develop. Progestins inhibit pituitary gonadotropin secretion as well as induce excessive secretory and pseudodecidual changes of the endometrium, including the endometriosis, giving rise to glandular atrophy, increased macrophage activity, and fibrosis. Side effects of progestin therapy include water retention and weight gain, oily skin, acne, and infrequently mild hirsutism. If the dose of progestin is inadequate, breakthrough bleeding occurs. Spotting and breakthrough bleeding are common side effects of progestin therapy despite adequate dosage.

An alternative form of pseudopregnancy therapy uses oral contraceptives. Any oral contraceptive can be used, but one with a high progestin content is preferable. The oral contraceptive is given continuously rather than cyclically as used for birth control purposes. Continuous administration of oral contraceptive renders the patient amenorrheic and therefore pseudopregnant. Oral contraceptives suppress ovarian function, inhibit pituitary gonadotropins, and inhibit endometrial growth leading to an inactive and atrophic endometrium. Treatment is usually continued for 9 months. If pain or dysmenorrhea is unrelieved or if breakthrough bleeding occurs, the dose of the pill may be increased to 2 tablets or more per day. Side effects are usually associated with oral contraceptive therapy.

The results of pseudopregnancy treatment have been found to be satisfactory. With progestin-induced pseudopregnancy, symptoms improved in as many as 94 percent of patients. In general, the pregnancy rates are lower after pseudopregnancy treatment than after conservative surgery. However, corrected pregnancy rates as high as 90 percent have been reported with medroxyprogesterone acetate. Nevertheless, the usual pregnancy rate after pseudopregnancy therapy is 43 to 55 percent. Recurrence rates after pseudopregnancy therapy are similar, irrespective of the medication employed. The recurrence rate is 5 to 10 percent annually, with 17 to 18 percent reported one year after treatment.

II. Reproductive Endocrinology and Infertility

PSEUDOMENOPAUSE THERAPY. The term pseudo-menopause has been employed for treatment of endometriosis with danazol. However, it is a misnomer, as the endocrine changes induced by danazol are not similar to those of menopause. Danazol is one of the more effective hormonal therapies for endometriosis currently available, but it is expensive compared to the other hormones used. Danazol is a modified androgen, an isoxazol derivative of 17α-ethinyl testosterone (Fig. 12-4) and is therefore mildly androgenic and anabolic. It is an antigonadotropin and suppresses the pulsatile release of gonadotropin but not the basal secretion. Therefore ovulation is only suppressed by danazol. The usual dose is 800 mg daily given orally in two divided doses of 400 mg. It must be given in two divided doses to maintain an adequate blood level throughout 24 hours because of its pharmacokinetics.

Danazol binds to progesterone receptors and inhibits ovarian steroidogenesis at a point distal to the gonadotropin receptor action of the ovary by interfering with gonadotropin action. Danazol is also anti-estrogenic, inhibits the enzymes of steroidogenesis in the ovary and endometrium, and induces an atrophic endometrium similar to that in the postmenopausal

Fig. 12-4. Chemical formulas for various groups of hormones or hormone agonists (progestins, androgens, and gonadotropin-releasing hormone agonists) used for treatment of endometriosis.

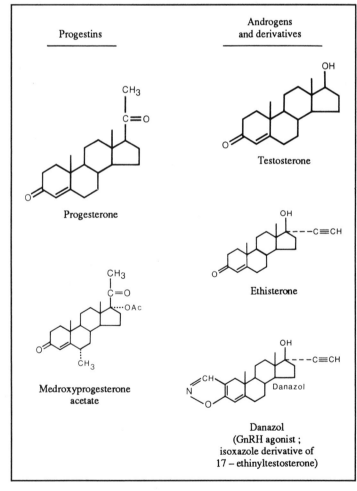

woman. Serum estrone, estradiol, and free estradiol concentrations are reduced to the low follicular phase range for premenopausal woman, but free testosterone levels are increased twofold secondary to marked suppression of sex hormone-binding globulin when danazol therapy is given.

Danazol therapy should be started on the first or second day of the menstrual cycle so that irregular bleeding and inadvertent exposure of an early conceptus to the drug can be avoided. Therapy should be continued for at least three months, but in most instances six to nine months of treatment is necessary depending on the extent of the endometriosis. The daily dose is 800 mg given in four divided doses because of the short plasma half-life (4½ hours). With lower doses of danazol (100 to 600 mg), the results of treatment for endometriosis have been variable, with a lower pregnancy rate and a higher rate of recurrence of symptoms within one year of discontinuation.

Effective treatment is marked by relief of symptoms, amenorrhea, and gradual decrease in the size of the lesions. If palpable lesions are present, the length of time for treatment may be guided by the time it takes for them to completely disappear. Danazol gives good relief of pelvic pain and dysmenorrhea. Symptomatic improvement occurs in 70 to 93 percent of patients, and improvement in pelvic findings can be noted in 80 percent. Similar improvement rates have been noted at laparoscopy after completing danazol therapy. The uncorrected fertility rate has been claimed to be 40 to 50 percent, whereas the correct fertility rate is estimated to be 76 percent after treatment with danazol. Hence the pregnancy rate compares favorably with that achieved with conservative surgery. Usually most of the conceptions occur within the first year after stopping medication. Early posttreatment conception appears to confer further protection from recurrence of endometriosis. Generally, conception is not recommended until at least one drug-free menstrual cycle has passed.

Danazol is often well tolerated, but a few side effects can occur. The side effects are usually due to the androgenic and antiestrogenic action of the drug as well as some idiopathic reactions. Androgenic side effects include acne (17 percent), edema (6 percent), weight gain (5 percent), hirsutism (6 percent), deepen-

ing of the voice (3 percent), and skin oiliness (3 percent). Antiestrogenic effects include hot flashes and sweats (15 percent), breakthrough bleeding (10 percent) especially with lower doses (less than 800 mg per day), decreased breast size (5 percent), decreased libido (5 percent), and atrophic vaginitis (3 percent). Idiopathic reactions include gastrointestinal disturbances (8 percent), muscle weakness and dizziness (8 percent), muscle aches or cramps (4 percent), skin rashes (3 percent), headaches (2 percent), and occasionally sleep disturbances. Recurrence of symptoms occurs in 5 to 15 percent of patients one year after completing treatment.

Androgen therapy employing testosterone and methyltestosterone have been used in the past and are highly effective in relieving the pain of endometriosis. The usual dose of methyltestosterone is 5 to 10 mg per day sublingually. Testosterone probably has a direct inhibitory action on the endometriotic lesions, as ovulation may not be inhibited by these doses. With low testosterone doses, side effects are infrequent but may include facial hair growth, acne, deepening of the voice, and infrequently jaundice. Conception rates tend to be higher with 10 mg of testosterone per day, but they decline to 8 to 30 percent when 5 mg of testosterone per day is given. Remissions tend to be transient; and when combined with the undesirable side effects of testosterone, the availability of danazol, and the emerging availability of gonadotropin-releasing hormone agonist, testosterone is seldom required for the treatment of endometriosis.

GONADOTROPIN-RELEASING HORMONE ANALOGS. Gonadotropin-releasing hormone (GnRH) analogs have been evaluated for the treatment of endometriosis, and there are several ongoing studies to further evaluate their efficacy in the treatment of endometriosis at the time of this writing. GnRH analogs that are agonists of GnRH can induce reversible medical oophorectomy and may therefore offer a less permanent and noninvasive form of ovarian ablation for endometriosis. The GnRH analogs currently being evaluated have a substitution of the amino acid in position 6 of the GnRH molecule so as to prolong its half-life.

One such potent long-acting GnRH agonist is D-TR^6_p-Pro-Net-LHRH. This analog is able to suppress ovarian function, follicle-stimulating hormone secretion, ovulation, and menstruation in monkeys as well as in women with endometriosis. Circulating estrogen levels are markedly suppressed by the GnRH agonist to concentrations normally found in oophorectomized women. Preliminary reports as well as ongoing clinical trials show that the potent long-acting GnRH agonists are as effective and perhaps more effective than danazol for relief of pain and regression of the endometriosis.

Our experience using the GnRH agonist buserelin (Fig. 12-4) indicates that patients with endometriosis who undergo 6 to 9 months of therapy with this peptide showed improvement or complete resolution of the endometriosis at laparoscopy performed immediately after completion of their treatment. Five of our patients who received buserelin have successfully become pregnant within six months of stopping treatment.

GnRH agonists can be given intranasally as a spray three times a day or by subcutaneous injections once a day. Another GnRH agonist that is effective against endometriosis is nafarelin. The long-acting depot preparation of a GnRH agonist (Lupron) is currently being evaluated and requires only a monthly injection.

When GnRH agonist is administered, there is an initial increase in pituitary gonadotropin secretion (for about 1 to 2 weeks) because of the stimulatory effect on the gonadotropins before down-regulation of the GnRH receptors on the pituitary takes place. After the initial stimulatory effect of GnRH agonist, pituitary gonadotropin secretion decreases to below normal levels secondary to down-regulation of GnRH receptors in the pituitary. The final result is ovarian suppression and low circulating estrogen levels.

The GnRH agonist treatment of endometriosis appears to have an advantage over danazol therapy: The androgenic side effects of danazol are obviated, and there are few side effects with GnRH agonist therapy. A common side effect is hot flashes similar to those experienced by postmenopausal woman. A potential long-term side effect is a decrease in trabecular bone density because of the "medical oophorectomy" and hypoestrogenemia induced by the GnRH agonist. However, this problem can be readily overcome by adding a progestin to the GnRH agonist treatment.

Such addition controls or eliminates the hot flashes and has also been shown to decrease bone loss in postmenopausal women.

RADIATION THERAPY. X-ray irradiation for castration is seldom employed today for the management of endometriosis. Rarely, in clinical situations in which patients are medically unable to undergo surgery, x-ray castration may be considered. However, as GnRH agonists become available for clinical use, x-ray castration may have little place in the management of the women with endometriosis.

ENDOMETRIOSIS IN LESS FREQUENT SITES

Rectosigmoid and Sigmoid Colon

Endometriosis of the bowel is infrequent, but failure to recognize it may lead to unnecessary radical operations because of confusion with malignant disease. In one series of 485 patients with endometriosis, the gastrointestinal tract was involved in 181 patients. In other studies the incidence of gastrointestinal endometriosis has been cited to be as low as 10 percent to as high as 67 percent. The pathology and symptomatology of endometriosis of the colon have already been mentioned. When typical endometriosis is present elsewhere in the pelvis, the diagnosis of endometriosis of the large bowel is often obvious. However, there are times when the clinical symptoms, the size and characteristics of the mass within the bowel wall, and the degree of obstruction it produces are such as to render the differentiation from carcinoma difficult, even at laparotomy.

Endometriosis usually begins on the serosal surface of the bowel; and with more extensive involvement there may be bleeding, healing, and eventual fibrosis, constrictions, and narrowing of the bowel. In most cases, endometriosis of the large bowel involves the rectum and sigmoid colon, and the lesion is therefore within the reach of the sigmoidoscope. Nevertheless, sigmoidoscopy does not usually permit a definite diagnosis of endometriosis because the lesion rarely involves the mucosa and is therefore not accessible for biopsy. Sigmoidoscopy, however, reveals the narrowed lumen if significant bowel wall involvement

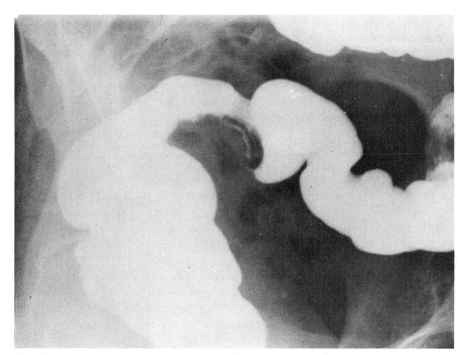

Fig. 12-5. Barium enema examination revealing the characteristic radiographic appearance of endometriosis of the rectosigmoid colon. Note the filling defect with sharply defined borders and a normal mucosal pattern throughout. During fluoroscopy the lesion was tender to palpation and relatively fixed. The patient was a 41-year-old nullipara who had been infertile during ten years of marriage. She had a nine-year history of increasingly frequent and troublesome bouts of lower abdominal cramps, diarrhea, and rectal bleeding, most of the episodes occurring premenstrually. The diagnosis of endometriosis was confirmed at laparotomy, at which time total hysterectomy and bilateral salpingo-oophorectomy were performed with subsequent complete relief of all symptoms.

and fibrosis has occurred. It is the presence of such a narrowed lumen in the absence of ulceration or a mucosal lesion at the constricted point that favors the diagnosis of endometriosis.

The radiographic findings on barium enema are usually so characteristic as to be almost diagnostic (Fig. 12-5). In typical cases, where the endometriosis is extensive, a filling defect of considerable length (4 to 7 inches) with sharply defined borders is seen, but the mucosal pattern is intact and normal throughout. An important associated feature is fixation and tenderness to palpation in the area of the lesion during fluoroscopic examination. It is possible that with magnetic resonance imaging diagnosis of such bowel endometriosis can be readily distinguished from malignant lesions.

In the older patients or those who have completed childbearing, management presents no problem, as bilateral oophorectomy produces complete regression with relief of all symptoms as well as the element of bowel obstruction. In this situation, bilateral oophorectomy is the treatment of choice; bowel resection should not be attempted. With the future approval and availability of GnRH agonist for the treatment of endometriosis, "medical oophorectomy" can be readily achieved without surgery and the bowel endometriosis should regress. In the rare instance of extensive rectosigmoid involvement in a young woman and when GnRH agonist or danazol therapy have failed and childbearing potential is needed, local resection of the involved segment of colon is occasionally indicated. Hormonal management employing pseudo-pregnancy is much less likely to be successful.

Small Bowel

Thirteen percent of women with endometriosis have some type of gastrointestinal involvement by endometriosis, 1 to 7 percent of which involves the small bowel. Endometriosis of the small bowel usually involves the appendix or the ileum, and, endometriosis of the ileum usually occurs only below the level of Meckel's diverticulum.

The average duration of the symptoms associated with endometriosis of the small intestine is about four years. Characteristically, the patient has recurrent attacks of nausea, vomiting, abdominal pain, and distention that occurs premenstrually or with the menstrual period. Some patients may have an intestinal obstruction, but perforation of the small intestine caused by endometriosis occurs rarely.

In the woman with classic symptoms of endometriosis of the pelvis, such as dysmenorrhea, dyspareunia, and infertility, the diagnosis is often readily apparent. Therefore special attention should be directed to relating the symptoms to the menstrual history so the necessary preoperative investigations are done. Once the diagnosis is made, a trial of medical therapy can be undertaken, if necessary.

Endometriosis of the ileum causes intestinal obstruction through four mechanisms: (1) The intestine may be kinked because of fibrous adhesions; (2) the fibrous reaction around the mural deposits of endometriosis may produce stenosis and constriction rings; (3) volvulus may occur because of adhesions; and (4) intussusception may arise.

An upper gastrointestinal series is usually helpful for the diagnosis of small bowel endometriosis. The roentgenographic examination should be performed during the intervals as well as at the time of menstruation because the endometriotic lesion on the intestine is responsive to ovarian hormonal changes during the menstrual cycle. Barium enema should also be done because the large and small bowel sometimes are jointly involved. The radiographic findings have already been described under endometriosis of the rectosigmoid and sigmoid colon. Sigmoidoscopy should

also be performed to rule out involvement of the rectosigmoid and the sigmoid colon.

Management of endometriosis of the small bowel is essentially similar to that of the large bowel (see above). If surgery is necessary, a laparotomy (not laparoscopy) should be performed. At the time of laparotomy, endometriosis of the small intestine must be differentiated from regional ileitis, carcinoid tumors, and carcinoma of the bowel. There are three important helpful differences between carcinoma and endometriosis of the intestine: (1) The endometriotic stricture does not tend to encircle the intestine as in carcinoma. (2) The tumor can be lifted up like a button on the intestinal wall and moves easily without moving the whole segment of the intestine. (3) Finally, there are usually no enlarged lymph glands in the adjacent mesentery. Because of the impact of malignancy, frozen sections of lesions not situated in the intestine are obtained preferably before definitive surgical excision.

It may be difficult to differentiate endometriosis from regional ileitis, as both conditions affect the distal portion of the ileum and may have extensive adhesions, fibrosis, stenosis, and ileal obstruction. However, if there is concomitant pelvic endometriosis found at laparotomy, the diagnosis is readily made.

Surgery is clearly indicated if there is intestinal obstruction, intussusception, volvulus, perforation of the intestine, small bowel endometriosis with no lesions elsewhere, obstructive fibrosis, or a need to confirm the diagnosis histologically. If the intestinal lesions are small and none of the above complications is present, nothing need be done about the lesion so long as there are no symptoms of intestinal obstruction or stenosis. If excision of the lesion is indicated, it can be done superficially without penetrating the mucosal layer because the lesions are usually confined to the serosal and muscular coat. Extensive involvement of the ileum with narrowing of the lumen may necessitate resection of the bowel with an end-to-end anastomosis.

Bladder and Ureter

Cyclic hematuria and other symptoms accompanying bladder involvement, e.g., dysuria, increased frequency of maturation, and recurrent cystitis, may occur when endometriosis is present in the urinary tract. Usually the bladder lesions are situated anteriorly on the bladder dome, away from the trigone. This problem is best treated by resection of the involved area if the involvement is extensive and can be simply and safely accomplished using a transabdominal approach, as the endometriosis usually starts from the serosal surface and works its way into the muscular coat of the bladder wall. If castration is contemplated, resection of the bladder lesion is usually not necessary.

Intermittent ureteral obstruction with cyclic renal colic related to the menstrual flow and more chronic, slowly progressive constriction of the lower ureter with increasing hydroephrosis above it and recurrent urinary tract infection have been reported. Such cases are relatively infrequent. Usually the obstruction is produced by constrictive scar tissue in the vicinity of peritoneal endometriosis at some point in the pelvis along the course of the ureter. Only rarely is the wall or lumen of the ureter invaded by the endometriosis. In such cases, cyclic hematuria may occur.

For the older patient, surgical castration is a treatment of choice and almost always results in return of normal ureteral anatomy and function. Only rarely is a direct attack on the ureter itself indicated or necessary, either in the form of lysis of adhesions or resection and reanastomosis.

Miscellaneous Endometriosis

Symptomatic endometriosis of the umbilicus, abdominal scars, groin, vulva, peritoneum, cervix, or vagina is uncommon. Endometriosis of the various cutaneous sites often seems to have occurred as a result of direct implantation, but in some instances lymphatic spread or possibly even metaplasia of adjacent coelomic epithelial derivatives better accounts for its appearance in these distant sites. The nature of the pathologic condition is often apparent from the obvious relation of the menstrual cycle with the symptoms and changes in size and appearance of the visible and palpable lesions. Treatment is simple excision for relief of symptoms as well as histologic confirmation of the diagnosis.

Endometriosis of the kidney is rare, fewer than a dozen cases having been reported. Back and flank pain with associated gross or microscopic hematuria are the usual clinical features, but only occasionally are the symptoms cyclic and related to the premenstrual phase. Intravenous pyelograms reveal a definite but nonspecific abnormality that often suggests renal cell carcinoma. Thus the correct diagnosis of endometriosis is invariably made only after histologic study of the nephrectomy specimen.

Rarely, involvement of the sciatic nerve sheath by areas of endometriosis lying deep underneath the broad ligament has been reported, with cyclic sciatica occurring in relation to the menses. Here again, in view of the serious nature of the potential disability, castration seems the wisest and most effective therapy, though local excision or hormone therapy might be attempted under exceptional circumstances.

Finally, there have been scattered case reports of thoracic endometriosis involving either the lung or the pleura. Thoracic lesions may produce either cyclic, recurring hemoptysis or recurring spontaneous pneumothorax, with symptoms coincident with menstruation.

Although cyclic external bleeding from areas of endometriosis located in extragenital sites such as the bladder, gastrointestinal tract, or thorax produces a type of "vicarious menstruation," this form of aberrant cyclic bleeding should be distinguished from a somewhat more common, truly functional type of vicarious menstruation. An example of the latter is vicarious nasal menstruation, which accounts for 30 percent of extragenital cyclic bleeding and is secondary to cyclic vascular congestion and hyperemia of the nasal mucosa induced by cyclic elevation of serum estrogen levels. Less often, these same estrogen-induced vascular disturbances occur in the oral cavity, bladder, stomach, retina, conjunctiva, or skin (especially on the hands) and result in vicarious menstruation from these sites.

MALIGNANT CHANGE

Although it rarely occurs, carcinoma may arise in the aberrant endometrium of endometriosis, just as it does in the endometrium lining the uterine cavity. The known frequency of endometriosis and the rarity of malignant change within it suggest that for various as yet unknown reasons malignant epithelial tumors are less likely to develop in areas of ectopic endometrium than in nonaberrant endometrium. When malignant change does take place, it invariably occurs in the ovary.

Sampson considered the possibility of the development of carcinoma in endometriosis and set forth the pathologic criteria for its recognition as follows: (1) Benign and malignant tissues must coexist in the same ovary and have the same histologic relation as for carcinoma of the body of the uterus; (2) the carcinoma must actually be seen arising in the benign tissue and not invading it from some other source.

Most of the reported cancers arising in ovarian endometriosis in which the evidence for this transformation was incontrovertible and Sampson's pathologic criteria had been satisfactorily fulfilled have been adenoacanthomas. These neoplasms are low grade malignancies and characteristically arise only in connection with endometrial or endocervical tissue; this same histologic type also accounts for 10 to 15 percent of the adenocarcinomas arising in the endometrial cavity. Adenoacanthomas are simply specific histologic variants belonging within the broader category of primary endometrioid carcinomas of the ovary, so termed because of their striking resemblance to primary carcinomas of the endometrium. The apparent origin of pure endometrioid tumors of the ovary (endometrial tissue-like adenocarcinomas without the malignant or metaplastic squamous cell elements that characterize adenoacanthomas) in areas of ovarian endometriosis has also been documented in a number of instances. Finally, the transition from ovarian endometriosis to malignancy has been established in some cases of the so-called clear cell adenocarcinomas of the ovary (formerly called mesonephromas); these tumors are probably of müllerian rather than mesonephric origin, however, and hence may well be simply another variant or near-relative of the endometrioid tumor category. Although endometrioid tumors of the ovary account for 10 to 15 percent or more of all primary ovarian malignant tumors, most endometrioid tumors appear to arise de novo; only a small number arise from malignant transformation of ovarian endometriosis.

It is apparent from the foregoing remarks that the possibility of malignant change in endometriosis is not a significant factor to be considered in the management of the overall problem in a given patient, and it is certainly no indication for prophylactic surgery. Far more significant from the clinical standpoint is the frequent need to distinguish an endometrioma from an ovarian tumor or to exclude the possibility of an ovarian tumor coexisting with pelvic endometriosis. In either circumstance, surgical exploration often becomes mandatory, even when the patient is asymptomatic.

SELECTED READINGS

Chalmers, J. A. Danazol in the treatment of endometriosis. *Drugs* 19:331, 1980.

Dawood, M. Y. Endometriosis. In J. J. Gold and J. B. Josimovich (Eds.), *Gynecologic Endocrinology* (3rd ed.). New York: Plenum Publishing Corporation, 1987. Chap. 18, pp. 387–403.

Dawood, M. Y. Endometriosis. In R. L. Nelson and L. M. Nyhus (Eds.), *Surgery of the Small Intestine.* Norwalk: Appleton and Lange, 1987. Chap. 29, pp. 345–350.

Dawood, M. Y., Khan-Dawood, F. S., and Ramos, J. Plasma and peritoneal fluid levels of Ca 125 in women with endometriosis. *Am. J. Obstet. Gynecol.* 159:1526, 1988.

Dawood, M. Y., Khan-Dawood, F. S., and Wilson, L., Jr. Peritoneal fluid prostaglandins and prostanoids in women with endometriosis, chronic pelvic inflammatory disease and pelvic pain. *Am. J. Obstet. Gynecol.* 148:391, 1984.

Dawood, M. Y., Lewis, V., and Ramos, J. Cortical and trabecular bone mineral content in women with endometriosis: Effect of gonadotropin-releasing hormone agonist and danazol. *Fertil. Steril.* 52:21, 1989.

Dawood, M. Y., Spellacy, W. N., Dmowski, W. P., et al. A Comparison of the Efficacy and Safety of Buserelin vs. Danazol in the treatment of Endometriosis. In B. Chada and V. C. Buttram (Eds.)., *Current Concepts in Endometriosis.* New York: Alan R. Liss, Inc., 1989.

Erickson, L. D., and Ory, S. J. GnRH analogues in the treatment of endometriosis. *Obstet. Gynecol. Clin. North Am.* 16:123, 1989.

Haney, A. F. (Guest editor). Pathophysiology of the infertility associated with endometriosis. *Semin. Reprod. Endocrinol.* 6:239, 1988.

Henzl, M. R., Corson, S. L., Moghissi, K., et al. Administration of nasal nafarelin as compared with oral danazol for endometriosis. A multicenter double-blind comparative clinical trial. *N. Engl. J. Med.* 318:485, 1988.

Kettel, L. M., and Murphy, A. A. Combination medical and surgical therapy for infertile patients with endometriosis. *Obstet. Gynecol. Clin. North Am.* 16:167, 1989.

Wheeler, J. M., and Malinak, L. R. Recurrent endometrio-sis: Incidence, management, and prognosis. *Am. J. Obstet. Gynecol.* 146:247, 1983.

Wheeler, J. M., and Malinak, L. R. The surgical management of endometriosis. *Obstet. Gynecol. Clin. North Am.* 16:147, 1989.

13

Infertility

Impaired fertility includes a wide range of anatomic and structural abnormalities: congenital anomalies, tumors, pelvic inflammation, and endometriosis as well as the various physiologic and endocrinologic disturbances of reproductive tract function. Indeed, the potential subject matter of the field of infertility runs the gamut of gynecologic physiology and pathology.

To avoid unnecessary repetition, the major emphasis in this chapter is on the approach to diagnosis and management of the couple who present to the physician primarily because of infertility. The general diagnostic plan is outlined and the techniques employed almost exclusively in infertility investigations are presented in some detail here. The methods of therapy for the various conditions responsible or contributing to the infertility are only briefly outlined in this chapter.

Whenever a specific condition is responsible for female infertility it is discussed in other chapters, and the reader should thus consult those chapters for further details. With respect to conditions responsible for male factors that contribute to the infertility of a couple, it is recommended that the reader consult monographs, reviews, or textbooks devoted to the subject for further details. However, the approach to evaluating the infertile couple discussed herein outlines the diagnostic tools and treatment methods available to the gynecologist for enhancing the couple's fertility as a reproductive unit.

DEFINITIONS AND EXTENT
OF THE PROBLEM

Infertility is defined from a clinical and practical standpoint as the inability of a couple to conceive after one year or more of intercourse without contraception. Not infrequently, if a couple has attempted conception for six months or more but less than a year, the couple may be considered *subfertile*. Infertility is often categorized as *primary infertility*, where the female partner has never conceived before and meets the criteria for infertility (above), or *secondary infertility*, where the woman has had a previous pregnancy irrespective of the final outcome of that pregnancy. This somewhat artificial division is useful sometimes for narrowing down or looking for the cause of the conception difficulty, but it offers little direction. It is noteworthy that among normal and ultimately fertile couples approximately 65 percent conceive within six months of trying for pregnancy and 80 percent after a year. The remaining 20 percent can be considered subfertile or relatively infertile rather than absolutely infertile.

Estimates have generally rated 12 to 15 percent of such couples as involuntarily infertile. Based on a report from the United States Office of Technology Assessment, the proportion of infertile couples, expressed as a percentage of married couples with females age 15 to 44 years, was 11.2 percent in 1965, 10.3 percent in 1976, and 8.2 percent in 1982. Based on these data, infertility affected an estimated 2.4 million married couples in 1982 in the United States. Although there does not appear to be an increase in either the number of infertile couples or the overall incidence of infertility in the population, there were increasing requests for infertility services during the 1980s. Office visits to physicians for infertility services rose from about 600,000 in 1968 to about 1.6 million in 1984. The increasing requests and use of infertility services are to a large extent contributed by the following: aging of the baby-boom generation who expects to control their own fertility but unfortunately cannot do so in many instances; delayed childbearing leading to more nulliparous women in higher risk age groups; childbearing condensed into shorter intervals during the reproductive years, often at later years; delayed conception due to prior use of oral contraceptives; heightened expectations and larger number of people in higher income brackets with infertility problems; larger number of infertile couples with primary infertility and decreased supply of infants available for adoption; more sophisticated diagnosis and treatment methods; evolution of new reproductive technologies such as in vitro fertilization, gamete intrafallopian tube transfer, and cryopreservation; and finally extensive media coverage. In 1987 Americans spent an estimated $1 billion on medical care for their infertility and as many as one-half of the infertile couples seeking treatment are ultimately unsuccessful despite trying many of the modalities available.

DIAGNOSTIC APPROACH TO INFERTILITY

At the outset of an infertility investigation it should be carefully explained to the couple that it is their reproductive capacity as a biologic unit that is under scrutiny and that therefore both husband and wife must be completely evaluated. The responsibility for initiating and supervising the study customarily falls to the gynecologist for several reasons: (1) the naturally predominant interest and concern of the female partner in the problem; (2) more widely known disturbances in the female reproductive tract anatomy and function adversely affecting fertility compared with reproductive system disorders in the man; and (3) the greater number of female factors that can be readily analyzed, studied, and successfully treated. The gynecologist should direct the preliminary investigation of the husband initially but then should refer him to either a urologist or a medical endocrinologist who deals with male infertility. There should be constant communication between the gynecologist taking care of the female partner and the physician who evaluates the male partner so that management of the couple's infertility can be coordinated and integrated. The gynecologist should, however, be completely familiar with the diagnostic aspects and general therapeutic principles of male infertility, as the status of the male partner obviously influences the course of study and therapy of the woman and information concerning both partners is essential to the gynecologist's role as principal counselor and chief administrator of the total diagnostic and treatment program. Hence for complete orientation in this chapter, the studies to be carried out in the male partner are briefly outlined.

The specific factors that must be studied and the various tests used to accomplish this end should be enumerated and described to the couple in advance to ensure their subsequent understanding and cooperation. It should be emphasized that multiple factors are often responsible for a couple's failure to conceive. The physician must bear this fact in mind because it is for this reason that the entire investigation must be carried through to completion before undertaking therapy for any obvious abnormality discovered early in the course of the evaluation. It should be pointed out initially that a proper study and any subsequently indicated therapeutic measures require time (often a year or more) and patience on the part of all concerned if success is to be achieved.

BASIC DIAGNOSTIC STUDIES FOR THE INFERTILE COUPLE

Both man and woman must initially be carefully assessed from the standpoint of the possible existence of any generalized disorders or conditions that might be major or contributing causes of their failure to achieve pregnancy. Therefore the major portion of the investigation is carried forward by more specific inquiry, examination, and special diagnostic studies focused on the inherent anatomic and functional status of both their reproductive tracts in order to assess the five principal factors involved in the process of conception: (1) seminal factor in the man; and in the woman (2) ovarian factor, (3) tubal factor, (4) cervical factor, and (5) peritoneal factor. Other less readily categorized aspects of the reproductive process, disturbances of which may result in impaired fertility, are evaluated simultaneously and may be considered as frequently significant miscellaneous factors.

A general idea of the relative frequency with which disturbances of the various factors are the major cause of infertility may be gained from the following composite estimates based on the reported experience of various individuals and clinics engaged in the diagnosis and treatment of sterility patients: male factor 30 to 40 percent; ovarian factor 15 to 25 percent (failure of ovulation in 10 to 20 percent; in 5 to 10 percent ovulatory dysfunction such as inadequate luteal phase, oligoovulation, defective ovulation, and irregular follicular length); tubal factor 25 to 35 percent (percentage may be higher in areas where there is an increased incidence of venereal disease, pelvic inflammatory disease, or tuberculosis); cervical factor 15 to 20 percent. In roughly 35 percent of infertile couples multiple factors are probably responsible for the problem; in 20 percent the infertility is the result of a combination of male and female factors.

General Evaluation

History and Examination. A complete general history is taken of both partners, and each has a physical examination and basic laboratory tests (blood count, urinalysis, serology, thyroid function studies) done to discover or rule out the following: obvious systemic disease, gross anatomic disturbances, generalized endocrine disorders (e.g., thyroid, adrenal, or pituitary), nutritional deficiencies, toxic exposures (e.g., male occupational exposures to heavy metals or radioactive substances, working in high temperature areas as in blast furnaces), and so on. A particular effort should be made to determine if prior illnesses, injuries, or surgical procedures in or near the genital tract might have resulted in impaired function. Examples of the latter include the following.

Male partner: previous mumps orchitis with testicular atrophy; a history of medications (a number of drugs, including some antibacterial agents such as the nitrofurantoins and a variety of psychotropic drugs, can cause oligospermia, sexual dysfunction, or both); previous venereal disease; varicocele; undescended testes; hypospadias or other congenital anomalies; chronic prostatitis; previous groin injuries or herniorrhaphies, in which possible damage to the vas deferens may have been sustained; a history of tuberculosis; use of recreational drugs (smoking marijuana and use of cocaine reduces sperm count; chronic alcoholism can cause oligospermia and sexual dysfunction).

Female partner: previous venereal disease, especially a history of symptoms suggesting prior pelvic inflammatory disease; history of appendicitis or appendectomy; prior abortions or miscarriages; obvious congenital anomalies of the uterovaginal tract; history of tuberculosis; history of contraceptive use of birth control pills and especially the intrauterine device.

Sexual and Psychological Factors. A detailed inquiry is made concerning marital adjustment; coital technique, frequency, and timing; and various psychosocial factors that may inhibit normal reproductive function. The importance of obtaining complete information along these lines by thoughtful, tactful questioning cannot be overemphasized, as coital infrequency, unsatisfactory and ineffective coital performance due to ignorance or psychic inhibitions, or tensions associated with inability to achieve a satisfactory overall marital adjustment often prove to be the sole or an important contributing factor in the failure to achieve pregnancy. Although this information should be sought reasonably early in the course of the sterility investigation, it is often wiser to postpone detailed discussion of these matters for a few visits until the physician–patient relationship is sufficiently well established to permit the patient or the couple to speak of them freely and openly. Less often, serious personality disturbances or even major psychiatric disorders may be discovered and prove to be the primary cause of sterility in one or the other of the marital partners.

Evaluation of the Male Partner (Seminal Factor)

Semen Analysis. At least two or three semen specimens should be examined, especially if the initial one is substandard. The specimen should be collected in a clean, dry jar (after at least three or four days of abstinence from ejaculation but preferably after four to six days), kept at room temperature, and examined within 2 to 4 hours with reference to the following.

1. *Volume:* Normally 2.5 to 5.0 ml, with an alkaline pH, and initially rather viscid.
2. *Liquefaction:* Normally complete within 10 to 30 minutes.
3. *Motility:* Normally at least 50 percent active, motile sperm at 4 hours or 60 to 80 percent at 2 hours. Examine a drop of semen on a slide with coverslip edges sealed with petrolatum.

4. *Cell count:* Use a white blood cell pipet, filling it with semen to the 0.5 mark and diluting to the 1:20 mark with tap water; using a red blood cell counting chamber, count the sperm in five small blocks (as for a red blood cell count). The total figure obtained yields a count in millions per milliliter. The average of several counts should be used for the final estimate. Normal range: 20 to 150 million per milliliter, with an average normal count of 60 to 100 million per milliliter. (Occasional pregnancies have occurred in the presence of sperm counts of 10 million to 20 million per milliliter or, rarely, even lower counts.) If the count is less than 20 million per milliliter, it is *oligospermic*. If there is no spermatozoon, the man is *azoospermic*. If azoospermia is encountered, the semen sample should be centrifuged and a sample taken from the pellet for microscopic examination to be sure it is indeed azoospermic.

5. *Cell morphology:* The semen smear is prepared in the same way as a routine blood smear. Stain with Wright's stain and evaluate and count several hundred sperm heads. Normal: 60 to 80 percent or more of the sperm heads should exhibit normal morphology. If fewer than 50 percent exhibit normal morphology, the test is reported as abnormal.

When evaluating the significance of semen analysis in the individual patient it should be kept in mind that, given a reasonable sperm count, the factors of motility and morphology are probably the most decisive ones with respect to fertility.

Testicular Biopsy. If complete absence of sperm is discovered on semen analysis or in the face of marked oligospermia, testicular biopsy may be indicated to differentiate between primary testicular failure and a mechanical block in the vas deferens or epididymis, or as a diagnostic and prognostic guide in the case of oligospermia.

Special Diagnostic Tests in the Female Partner

The gynecologic history—particularly with regard to menstrual function—together with the findings of the pelvic examination, may or may not be immediately suggestive of abnormal ovarian function or palpable disease of the uterus, adnexa, or both. In any case, detailed investigation of the three major female reproductive factors is carried out by the special tests described in the sections that follow.

Ovarian Factor and Endometrial Response. The procedures that follow are to establish if there is regular ovulation and production of a progestational endometrium satisfactory for implantation.

BASAL BODY TEMPERATURE CHART. The basal body temperature chart should be kept for three or more cycles, and it should include a record of coital frequency and timing. Typical biphasic temperature curves are indicative of regular ovulation. Irregular, monophasic curves indicate an anovulatory cycle or inadequate progesterone production about 95 percent of the time, but ovulation has been shown to occur in 2 to 5 percent of monophasic temperature charts. The lengths of the follicular phase (i.e., prior to the rise in temperature following ovulation) as well as the length of the luteal phase (after the rise in temperature following ovulation to the onset of menstrual flow) should be noted. An irregular follicular length may indicate poor or suboptimal folliculogenesis. The temperature rise following ovulation should be at least 0.5° F or more and remain at that level. A luteal phase length of ten days or less is abnormally short. Although a normal luteal phase length seems to indicate a normal ovulatory cycle, the luteal phase may actually be inadequate owing to inadequate progesterone secretion.

ENDOMETRIAL BIOPSY. Endometrial biopsy confirms the presence or absence of ovulation indirectly by evaluating the effect of progesterone on the endometrium. It determines if the development of a mature secretory endometrium is suitable for implantation and maintenance of a fertilized ovum during the cycle studied. For maximal information, endometrial biopsy should be done within 12 hours of the expected appearance of menstrual flow or at the most within a few days of the calculated onset of the period. (When performed at this time, it may also prove valuable in the discovery of unsuspected pelvic tuberculosis.) In practice, logistic difficulties may not allow biopsy at this time; but at any rate, the biopsy should be performed during the late luteal phase so that the maximum effect of the progesterone (produced by the corpus luteum, which develops from a follicle that has ovulated) has been exerted on the endometrium. A biopsy may also be done immediately following the onset of flow, but it is usually difficult for both patient and physician to arrange. Ovulation is indicated if microscopic study reveals a definite secretory endometrium. Furthermore, the degree of secretory maturation can usually be accurately estimated by histologic study and can serve as an index of whether progesterone production is adequate.

OTHER TESTS FOR OVULATION AND PROGESTERONE PRODUCTION. Not infrequently, determining the time of ovulation as precisely as possible may also be important, especially if studies reveal either that the man is subfertile, with a depressed sperm count or poor sperm motility, or that the quality of the woman's cervical mucus is poor and unresponsive to the usual methods of treatment. In such situations, more accurate estimates of the most fruitful time for coitus may improve the couple's chances for conception. (Precise timing of ovulation is also of obvious importance for determining the optimal period for therapeutic insemination.) The most useful methods for determining the time of ovulation with reasonable accuracy include observations of the thermal shift on the basal body temperature chart (ovulation is believed to occur 24 to 48 hours before the rise) and detection of the specific preovulatory and ovulatory changes in the vaginal cytologic smear, the cervical mucus fern test, the characteristics of the cervical mucus itself, especially the spinnbarkeit (see Cervical Factor, below), and the glucose content of the cervical mucus.

Tubal Factor. The tests described here are used to determine if the tubes are normal and patent. It should be emphasized again that not only must the tubes (or at least one tube) have a patent lumen, but the tubal anatomy and physiology must also be sufficiently normal to ensure that proper peristaltic and secretory activities are present to maintain viability and aid in the movements and function of the sperm and ovum, as well as provide a suitable milieu for the early days in the life of the zygote. Equally important, the fimbriated ends and distal portions of the tubes must be

sufficiently free within the pelvic cavity to come into normal apposition with the ovaries at ovulation time, and the surfaces of the latter and the intervening peritoneal space must not be separated from the tubes by adhesions that impede or completely block the passage of the ovum to the fimbriated tubal opening. Interference with the normal operation of this factor is encountered in the presence of local intraperitoneal adhesions secondary to such disorders as endometriosis, previous pelvic inflammation, or prior appendicitis. Thus complete assessment of tubal function involves not only determination of patency but also if the ovum transfer and pickup mechanism is unimpeded (peritoneal factor). Precise clinical assessment of the physiologic and biochemical performance of the fallopian tubes is not yet possible.

HYSTEROSALPINGOGRAPHY. Hysterosalpingography provides information not only about the patency of the tubes but also the outline of the cervical canal and the endometrial cavity. Therefore hysterosalpingograms can also detect uterine abnormalities that are of significance with regard to the infertility, e.g., submucous fibroids or congenital anomalies such as bicornuate or septate uterus. The procedure (injection of dye and fluoroscopic monitoring) should be done by the gynecologist to obtain the maximum information in relation to the clinical history and findings, which can be readily correlated.

TECHNIQUE. The procedure is most conveniently done in the radiology department on a special table such as is commonly employed for cystoscopy and retrograde pyelography. A nonradiopaque speculum is helpful though not essential.

The introitus, vagina, and cervix are thoroughly cleaned and sterilized with povidone-iodine (Betadine) solution, and the procedure is carried out in a sterile manner using sterile instruments. The anterior lip of the cervix is grasped with a tenaculum, and a uterine sound is passed to determine the direction and length of the uterine canal. An insufflation cannula is then introduced in the same manner as for tubal insufflation. A special adapter attached to the cannula permits the cervical tenaculum to be locked in place anterior to the cannula, mechanically applying countertraction and maintaining an airtight seal at the cervix, and has a Luer-Lok outer end for attaching the syringe containing radiopaque dye. The entire system should be filled with dye before inserting the cannula to avoid introducing air bubbles that might cause artifacts suggestive of intrauterine or tubal disease; either Ethiodol, an oil-based medium, or Sinografin, one of the aqueous-based media, is employed. Only 1 or 2 ml is injected initially because an excessive amount of dye at this point may mask intracavitary abnormalities, e.g., polyps submucous fibroids or intrauterine adhesions. Depending on the apparent size of the uterine cavity and the extent to which tubal filling has already been achieved, an additional 2 to 4 ml of dye is instilled and further observed on the fluoroscopy screen.

Patency of the tubes may be seen with the initial injection or the second instillation. If apparent cornual block is present, amyl nitrite inhalation may be tried or, better still, glucagon 10 mg intramuscular injection (more pleasant than the strong aromatic smell of amyl nitrite) to eliminate the possibility that the failure of tubal filling is due to temporary cornual spasm. Fimbrial occlusion may also already be suspected because of the demonstration of obvious dilatation of the tubal lumen and droplet formation of the dye (due to contact with the watery fluid contained in a hydrosalpinx or pyosalpinx in the fimbriated end). In any event, if Ethiodol or a similar oily medium has been employed, a third radiograph taken 24 hours later is usually advisable. This measure can definitely settle the question of whether dye has reached the free peritoneal cavity or has been trapped in diseased and occluded tubes. This delayed film is not necessary if patency has been visualized and demonstrated during the initial hysterosalpingography or if an aqueous medium such as Sinografin (preferred in many centers) is employed.

LAPAROSCOPY. Laparoscopy affords direct observation of the tubes during uterotubal instillation of an aqueous solution of methylene blue, indigo carmine, or a similar dye. This approach has frequently proved more accurate and is certainly often more informative than hysterosalpingography because it not only demonstrates tubal occlusion, if present, but permits visualization of the nature and anatomy of the pathologic process producing the block. It is especially useful when the results of hysterosalpingography together with the history and findings on pelvic examination are equivocal with respect to the presence or absence of tubal obstruction. In the presence of old appendicitis, endometriosis, or minimal chronic pelvic inflammatory disease, the tubes are frequently still patent; hence the hysterosalpingogram often shows patency of the tubes despite the peritubal pathologic condition present.

Perhaps most important, laparoscopy permits direct visual inspection of the adnexal regions, and often it is only by this means that one can detect interference with the normal transfer of ovum to tubes by periadnexal adhesions, with resulting restriction of normal tuboovarian mobility.

Parenthetically, it is worth pointing out that almost the entire basic female fertility study can be accomplished at a single laparoscopic procedure performed at the proper time during the menstrual cycle. Not only can the tubal (and peritoneal) factor be thoroughly investigated, but the status of ovarian function is readily apparent even to the point of demonstrating recent ovulation or the absence thereof. Certainly, if the other routine diagnostic maneuvers are not revealing and infertility persists after another year of study and attempted treatment, and assuming the male partner is found normal, most patients deserve to have laparoscopic examination. In many instances, an unexpected pathologic condition is discovered in this way.

Cervical Factor. Examination of the cervical mucus reveals whether it undergoes favorable changes at ovulation time, enabling penetration, survival, and normal progression of sperm.

POSTCOITAL CERVICAL MUCUS TEST (SIMS-HUHNER TEST). For a postcoital cervical mucus test the patient reports to the office within 2 to 6 hours after coitus on or within 24 to 48 hours of the day of the cycle that the basal body temperature or other tests have indicated is the probable time of ovulation. Without use of a lubricant, the cervix is exposed by speculum, and a sample of endocervical mucus is aspirated with a special plastic cannula from the *level of the internal os* and examined immediately using a clean glass slide with a coverslip. Another cervical mucus sample is obtained, smeared on a glass slide, and allowed to dry. A sample of vaginal secretion is examined for sperm to exclude the possibility of faulty coital technique in case the cervical mucus should be found to contain no sperm whatsoever. Normal findings are 5 to 20 motile sperm per high-power field at 2 to 6 hours after coitus.

In addition to the actual cervical mucus sperm count, simple observations of the volume and physical characteristics of the ovulatory cervical mucus usually yield valuable clues as to whether the normal, temporary changes favorable to sperm penetration and progression have occurred. The cervical secretion at this time (for a period of perhaps 48 to 72 hours) should be abundant in amount and appear crystal-clear, thin, and watery, yet with a characteristic consistency that permits it to be drawn in long threads (spinnbarkeit). It should be relatively free of leukocytes and epithelial cells on microscopic examination. A scoring system, summarized in Table 13-1, can be employed to assess the changes in the cervix and its secretions at the periovulatory phase. If the cervical secretion is scanty, cloudy, viscid, and cellular, an abnormal postcoital test is invariably obtained. Under these conditions the abnormal test can usually be assumed to be the result of poor ovulatory cervical mucus unless studies in the male partner suggest that a low sperm count or poor sperm motility is also a potential factor.

An abnormal test should be verified two or three times before it is considered conclusive. Excluding faulty coital technique or performance of the test on the wrong day of the cycle, an unsatisfactory test usually indicates one of the following abnormalities: (1)

poor sperm quality, (2) poor seminal fluid (e.g., chronic prostatitis), (3) poor quality cervical mucus owing to chronic endocervicitis, or (4) poor quality cervical mucus owing to inadequate estrogen effect or other hormonal imbalance.

That an abnormal postcoital cervical mucus test is the result of the poor quality of the cervical mucus itself may often be confirmed by performing a preovulatory cervical mucus fern test. If the fern phenomenon does not occur, the presence of either chronic cervicitis or a lack of adequate estrogen stimulation is probably the basis for the deficiency in the normal secretory activity of the endocervical glands and the resulting quantitative and qualitative abnormalities of the ovulatory cervical secretions that render them unsuitable for sperm penetration and survival.

SPERM HAMSTER OVA PENETRATION ASSAY. Until recently the only objective tests for male gamete assessment in the evaluation of the male partner are semen analysis and the postcoital test, which evaluate different aspects of the spermatozoa. Available today is the sperm hamster ova penetration assay, which measures the ability of the sperm to penetrate the egg, information provided by neither semen analysis nor postcoital test. Of course, the best test would be penetration of a human sperm into a normal human egg; however, because such a test is not ethically, morally, and logistically possible, zona-free hamster eggs are employed for the test.

Briefly, the test is conducted as follows. Female hamsters are given injections of pregnant mare serum

Table 13-1. Cervical Scoring Employed for Evaluating Cervical Factor

| Parameter | Degree of abnormality and the score (1–3) assigned | | | |
	0	1	2	3
Amount of mucus	None	Scant	Dribble	Cascade
Spinnbarkeit (cm)	0–2	3–6	7–10	10
Ferning	None	Linear (primary) branching	Secondary branching	Tertiary or quartenary branching
Viscosity	Thick	Medium	Slightly thin	Very thin and watery
Cervical os	Closed	Slightly dilated	Open	Gaping ("fish mouth")
Total score	0	5	10	15

on the first day followed by human chorionic gonadotropin on the third day. On the fourth day, the tubes and canulus are removed; the canulus is dispersed with hyaluronidase and the zona removed with trypsin digestion. Meanwhile, semen is collected from the male partner by masturbation on the third or fourth day of the hamster preparation. The spermatozoa are washed three times with buffer and capacitated in vitro, after which they are ready for use. The zona-free hamster ova are then inseminated with the capacitated human spermatozoa in a petri dish and incubated at 37°C for 2 hours, at which time the eggs are examined microscopically for sperm penetration.

If 10 percent or more of the hamster eggs are penetrated by the spermatozoa, the male fertility is adequate, as there is good correlation with fertility. Penetration of less than 10 percent of the hamster eggs *may* indicate reduced or absent fertilizing capability, but the correlation is not nearly as good as with the positive correlation with fertility when penetration is more than 10 percent. It is worth noting that this test is a bioassay, and so a negative finding (i.e., less than 10 percent penetration) may be due to variations and potential problems of the assay as well as the inherent qualitative or quantitative defects in the ability of the spermatozoa to penetrate ova. This conclusion is supported by the fact that up to 15 percent of men whose spermatozoa showed poor hamster egg penetration demonstrate satisfactory penetration and fertilization of ova removed from their female partners during attempts at in vitro fertilization. In some centers this test has been modified using a TEST-yolk buffer (containing TES buffer, tris buffer, chicken egg yolk, fructose or D-glucose, penicillin, and streptomycin) to allow spermatozoa to be transported and shipped by mail for testing in centralized laboratories. Such a transport buffer apparently preserves sperm motility and penetration.

Miscellaneous Implantation and Maintenance Factors. When considering female infertility, a fifth category must be added to the usual four to include certain disorders affecting female fertility that are less directly related to the basic physiology of reproduction and do not fall under any of the preceding four headings. Because these disorders concern abnormalities of uterine anatomy, this category might properly be termed the uterine factor. Some of these conditions may result in apparent primary infertility due to immediate failure of implantation (the onset of the next normal menstrual period is not delayed), but many of them result in occult abortions (missing the menstrual period by a few days, so the patient appears to have a delayed period) and repeated abortion (Chap. 16). Most frequent among such uterine conditions affecting fertility are submucuous or intramural fibroids, endometrial or endocervical polyps, traumatic intra-uterine adhesions (Asherman's syndrome), congenital uterine anomalies (primarily the various duplications, including bicornuate and septate uterus), and incompetent internal cervical os, an acquired defect (following obstetric or surgical trauma to the cervix) that is often the cause of repeated second-trimester abortions (Chap. 16). The diagnosis of these conditions rests primarily on the findings on pelvic examination supplemented by study of the anatomy of the uterus by hysterosalpingography and hysteroscopy.

IMMUNOLOGIC FACTORS IN INFERTILITY

Immunologic factors have been widely investigated to determine their contribution to infertility and difficulties in conception. Although a variety of antibodies have been demonstrated in biologic fluids of both the male and female partners and a variety of tests have been developed for evaluating the infertile couple, it should be remembered that the significance of abnormal test results and these findings are not well established. Furthermore, if one accepts the validity of these tests as beyond reproach, it is questionable if any *proved effective* therapy is currently available. Nevertheless, tests for possible immunologic factors accounting for a couple's infertility may be undertaken and offered when other, more readily treatable causes have been ruled out and the couple is appraised of the usefulness and limitations of the tests. The tests could provide a limited explanation and prognosis for the couple's infertility.

A clue to the presence of *antisperm antibodies* is the finding of (1) good quality cervical mucus in which spermatozoa are present and vibrating but do

Table 13-2. Types of Antisperm Antibodies and Tests to Detect Them

Type of test	Body fluid	Antibodies tested
Sperm agglutination		
Gelatin agglutination (Kibrick test)		
Microagglutination (Franklin-Duke)	Male serum, female serum, female cervical mucus	IgG, IgM, IgA[a]
Tray agglutination (Friberg)		
Complement-dependent		
Immobilization (Isojima)	Male serum, female serum,	IgG, IgM
Cytotoxic (Cytotox)	female cervical mucus	
Immunobead binding (Immunobead)	As above	IgG, IgM, IgA,[a] and subclasses
Mixed agglutination reaction	Semen only	IgG

[a]Detectable only in semen or cervical mucus (i.e., reproductive tract secretions only).

not exhibit progressive motility, (2) sperm agglutination in a semen analysis, and (3) otherwise unexplained infertility. The most common etiology for male antisperm antibodies is reversal of a previous vasectomy. Antibodies may be present in the serum of one or both partners, in the cervical mucus of the woman, or in the semen of the man. The types of antibodies and the tests that can be employed to detect them are summarized in Table 13-2.

It is preferable to perform the immunologic tests on the cervical mucus against the male partner's spermatozoa, as tests performed only on the serum may not truly reflect local antisperm activity in the female reproductive tract. Cervical mucus must be specially prepared for the test using Bromelin or another substance that puts the mucus into solution. It is also worth remembering that secretory immunoglobulin A (IgA) is present in reproductive tract secretions but not in serum, whereas IgM is so large that it might not cross from the serum into the female reproductive tract. Therefore results of sperm antibody tests in the serum can be misleading and have limited value.

TREATMENT

Disturbances of the Male Factor

Although detailed discussion of therapy for male infertility is beyond the scope of this book, a brief summary seems indicated.

1. If the sperm count is in the low normal range or sperm morphology, sperm motility, or semen volume or quality is poor (in the absence of infection or local anatomic or pathologic disorders), general empiric measures that may improve male fertility include the following: adequate diet, rest, exercise in moderation, and relaxation from a too strenuous living pace, as well as avoidance of excessive alcohol, tobacco consumption, and recreational drugs. In some couples, too frequent intercourse may result in sufficient reduction in the husband's semen quality and sperm count to prevent conception; if this situation is suggested by the results of repeated semen analyses following varying intervals of abstinence, a reduction in the frequency of intercourse and a period of abstinence just before ovulation may improve the chance of conception. Although previously employed to improve sperm counts and motility in otherwise normal men, testosterone or other similar steroid hormone preparations have so far not been shown to be of any benefit for either spermatogenesis or male fertility. Although a relatively uncommon cause of male infertility, male impotence may be discovered to be the source of the infertility. If hyperprolactinemia, a pituitary tumor, and hypogonadism have been ruled out, reassurance, psychotherapy, or sex therapy may be necessary and can be helpful.

2. Chronic prostatitis and cytourethritis often result in poor quality semen and sperm, and vigorous

treatment of the chronic infection may improve this situation and restore fertility.

3. Because of the importance of the heat-regulatory mechanism of the scrotum for maintaining an optimal testicular temperature for normal spermatogenesis, marked obesity, confining sedentary occupations, the wearing of excessively tight clothing (e.g., skintight jockey shorts or athletic supporters), frequent steam or sauna baths, or chronic occupational exposure to high temperature (bakers, furnace workers, certain industrial workers) may significantly affect sperm count and quality. Correction or elimination of these factors may improve fertility in the man. The presence of a significant degree of varicocele may also impair male fertility by interfering with scrotal thermal control (or possibly causing retrograde venous blood flow from the renal vein into the spermatic vein, with resulting abnormal hormonal or metabolic effects). Surgical repair of a large varicocele often improves the sperm count and motility in infertile oligospermic men, with return of normal fertility. Such surgical repairs are often followed with human chorionic gonadotropin therapy two to three times a week for six to twelve weeks. These results are particularly significant, as it is estimated that varicocele may be responsible for up to 20 to 25 percent of the cases of male infertility.

4. Although orchiopexy for bilateral undescended testes rarely results in normal spermatogenesis if carried out after puberty, it is nevertheless an important measure for the prevention of potential male infertility if performed in time.

5. Congenital or acquired anomalies of the penis and urethra, e.g., hypospadias, epispadias, phimosis, or urethral stricture—any of which may interfere with normal ejaculation and semen placement—are sometimes corrected by surgical measures.

6. If semen analysis reveals a complete absence of sperm, but testicular biopsy shows normal testicular histology and spermatogenesis, the epididymis or vas deferens is usually obstructed. Such obstruction can sometimes be relieved or bypassed by a surgical procedure, e.g., epididymovasostomy or resection of the area of block and reanastomosis in the case of an occluded vas deferens.

7. Rarely, a hypogonadal state in the azoospermic man with absent spermatogenesis on testicular biopsy and low or absent follicle-stimulating hormone (FSH) secretion may be due to a primary pituitary deficiency. This condition sometimes responds favorably to human menopausal gonadotropin and human chorionic gonadotropin therapy.

8. If there is complete azoospermia and testicular function is absent on testicular biopsy, the possibility of employing artificial insemination using semen from carefully selected donors should be considered and discussed with the couple. The legal implications for the resulting offspring may vary from state to state, but real problems are seldom encountered if the couple has been adequately counseled and wants this form of treatment. Frozen semen that has been screened and quarantined to rule out acquired immune deficiency syndrome in the donor, is employed rather than fresh semen, as was done in the past. Therapeutic insemination is now a well established procedure and has successfully brought the joys and satisfactions of parenthood to thousands of couples. The other alternative, of course, is adoption.

9. Artificial insemination using the husband's semen is employed if the semen analysis repeatedly shows borderline parameters (e.g., sperm count or sperm motility) or if there is a cervical factor (see below) that must be bypassed. Either the whole ejaculate can be employed or a split ejaculate is used for insemination. Split ejaculate is employed if the sperm motility is poor or borderline or the semen volume is large (more than 5 ml; semen volume of 7 ml or more is often associated with poor or questionable sperm motility). The male partner collects the first few drops of the ejaculate into a jar and the rest in another container. Both fractions should be examined to determine which has more motile spermatozoa. In 90 to 95 percent of instances, the first fraction is the better one to use.

Where there is failure of the semen to liquefy (e.g., due to agglutination—not infrequently seen in men who have undergone vasectomy and subsequent reversal), the semen can be made to disaggregate by forcibly pushing through a 22-gauge or smaller needle at the end of a syringe. The processed semen is then used for artificial insemination. Finally, semen with poor or borderline sperm motility can be washed in buffer, centrifuged, and the spermatozoa applied to an albumin column to allow the spermatozoa to swim up or down (depending on the site of application). The more progressively and forwardly motile spermatozoa are collected at the other end of the column, resuspended, adjusted for concentration, and used to inseminate the female partner. Varying degrees of success have been obtained with this method.

10. Artificial insemination using donor spermatozoa is also resorted to if the semen analysis and hamster ova penetration show poor results and if artificial insemination using the male partner's poor semen has been unsuccessful. In couples in whom the male partner has a genetic disease with a readily understood mode of transmission or a male sex-linked disorder, artificial insemination using donor semen can be employed.

Disturbances of the Ovarian Factor

The various disturbances in physiology that may result in female infertility include the basic endocrine diseases and the essentially functional disorders, discussed in Chapters 11 and 18, respectively. There is therefore no need to repeat the details of the diagnostic recognition and treatment here.

Most of the women with these disorders, however, have some form of ovulatory dysfunction. Either supplemental hormone therapy or induction of ovulation is thus necessary to restore and maintain ovulation and adequate luteal function. For anovulation, oligoovulation, or conditions such as inadequate luteal phase, induction of ovulation using clomiphene citrate, human menopausal gonadotropin with or without human chorionic gonadotropin (hCG), and bromocriptine (Parlodel) is employed for treatment. If there is hyperprolactinemia and no macroadenoma of the pituitary gland, ovulation induction is carried out with

bromocriptine, a dopamine agonist that restores normoprolactinemia. If a macroadenoma of the pituitary is present, it should be treated first and the tumor surgically removed as the risk of complications during pregnancy is significantly higher with macroadenomas than microadenomas of the pituitary. For induction of ovulation in women with hyperprolactinemic amenorrhea, bromocriptine 2.5 mg twice daily is given for four weeks after inducing withdrawal bleeding with intramuscular progesterone 10 mg. Alternately, bromocriptine 2.5 mg twice daily is given until the basal body temperature chart indicates ovulation has occurred or the urine luteinizing hormone (LH) self-test kit such as Ovustick or First Response indicates an LH surge. Pregnancy rates of 70 to 90 percent have been obtained with no increased incidence of spontaneous abortion or congenital malformations.

Clomiphene citrate, usually started in daily doses of 50 mg taken on days 5 through 10 of the cycle, is the ovulation-inducing agent of choice if the pituitary is intact. Clomiphene citrate is used for hypothalamic amenorrhea, chronic anovulation, and polycystic ovarian disease if fertility is desired. If the patient is amenorrheic, withdrawal bleeding is induced with intramuscular progesterone (see above) after ruling out a pregnancy. Ovulation can be expected on days 12 through 18, during which time coitus should occur frequently, at least every other day if not everyday. If ovulation occurs, the same dose (50 mg) of clomiphene citrate is maintained for three cycles. If there is no ovulation or if pregnancy does not occur after three cycles, the dose of clomiphene citrate is increased to 100, 150, 200, and finally 250 mg per day for five days as before. hCG 5000 IU may be given on days 14 and 16 or 15 and 17. It should be given with clomiphene therapy if the latter is being employed for treatment of a luteal phase defect.

Clomiphene citrate, a racemic mixture of a nonsteroidal substance with estrogenic and antiestrogenic properties, competitively binds with hypothalamic estrogen receptors and prevents their replenishment. Thus FSH and luteinizing hormone (LH) secretion is increased, whereas ovarian estradiol continues to build up without prematurely recruiting the estradiol-negative and estradiol-positive feedbacks on LH and FSH. Side effects of clomiphene citrate are minimal and usually tolerable. They include nausea, vomiting, headache, hot flashes, visual disturbance, rashes, ovarian hyperstimulation, and multiple pregnancy (five- to sevenfold increase, with twins occurring in about 8 percent). Ovarian hyperstimulation is infrequent and usually mild. Pregnancy rates with clomiphene are usually about 40 percent despite ovulation rates as high as 70 to 80 percent.

Induction of ovulation with human menopausal gonadotropins (hMG) is best left to physicians with special training or experience. It is indicated in infertile women who have failed to respond to clomiphene citrate, and it is the primary method of inducing ovulation if the pituitary is absent, nonfunctioning, or has been surgically ablated. For hMG to be effective the ovaries must be functional and have recruitable follicles. Usually two ampules of hMG (containing 75 IU FSH and 75 IU LH per ampule) are given intramuscularly daily, starting from day 5 or as early as day 3 of the cycle; the dose is adjusted from day to day. Beginning four or five days after starting hMG injections, the response is monitored with serum estradiol, cervical mucus examination, and ultrasonography of the ovaries to determine the number and size of the follicles developed. Serum estradiol should increase stepwise with a logarithmic increase of 50 percent each day over the last 5 to 6 days to reach levels of 600 to 800 pg per milliliter but not more than 1500 pg per milliliter. To avoid ovarian hyperstimulation, hCG should not be given if the serum estradiol level is 1500 pg per milliliter or more. The optimal follicle diameter is 18 to 25 mm. Pregnancy rates of up to 70 to 80 percent can be readily achieved if no other infertility factor exists. Sometimes clomiphene is used in combination with hMG to reduce the quantity of hMG required, thereby reducing the cost of treatment.

Gonadotropin-releasing hormone (GnRH) is useful for inducing ovulation in infertile women with hypothalamic amenorrhea. Treatment with GnRH is less expensive than with hMG and carries a lower risk of hyperstimulation and multiple pregnancies. GnRH is given subcutaneously in pulsatile doses every 90 minutes with an automatic programmable infusion pump.

The usual dose used is between 2.5 and 25.0 μg. Intravenous infusion has been used as an alternate route. Monitoring the response is required and is carried out in a manner similar to that for hMG therapy.

Luteal phase inadequacy can also be satisfactorily treated with supplemental progesterone therapy. Vaginal progesterone suppositories are inserted from days 18 through 28 of the cycle.

Although bilateral ovarian wedge resection has been widely used in the past for inducing ovulation in infertile women with polycystic ovary disease, it has limited use today. Bilateral ovarian wedge resection is often not necessary; it should be reserved for patients with extreme hirsutism and severe hypertestosteronemia in whom ovulation (not pregnancy) cannot be successfully induced. Wedge resection of the ovaries carries the potential risk of pelvic (specifically periovarian and peritubal) adhesions, which could themselves worsen the infertility status of the patient. Additionally, ovarian wedge resection does not permanently cure the anovulation due to polycystic ovarian disease. The ovulatory cycles are induced on average about 14 months; but by 28 to 36 months after resection the ovaries have become polycystic again and ovulatory dysfunction returns. If a wedge resection must be done, microsurgical techniques should be employed to reduce the chances of postoperative adhesions.

Advances in our ability to induce ovulation medically have clearly indicated that if pregnancy does not occur with clomiphene therapy for several cycles and up to the maximum doses used, a rest cycle or two is prescribed followed by a switch to hMG. If hMG therapy for six cycles or so is unsuccessful, treatment can be switched back to clomiphene after one or two rest cycles. Pregnancies have occurred with this nonsurgical and less invasive regimen. Details of medical induction of ovulation are also given in Chapter 11.

Disturbances of Tubal and Peritoneal Factors

Occasionally, repeated hysterosalpingograms or chromopertubations at laparoscopy are followed by pregnancy in previously infertile women in whom impaired tubal patency had been suggested by initial abnormal results in tests of tubal function. It is nearly always impossible to determine whether the successful outcomes are due to disruption of filmy tubal or peritubal adhesions, to dispersal of mucus plugs within the tubal lumens, or simply to overcoming chronic tubal spasm by the hydrotubation. They may merely be coincidental events. On the basis of such sporadic favorable experience, some have advocated hysterosalpingography as the initial approach in women with apparent impaired tubal function or during the initial workup of the infertile woman. Of course, such an approach cannot be successful if unequivocal bilateral tubal occlusion exists. Minimal pelvic tuberculosis with impaired tubal function, often first discovered during the course of an infertility investigation, perhaps represents an exception. The conservative treatment of this disease, with preservation of childbearing potential and an occasional subsequent successful pregnancy, is discussed in Chapter 15.

When anatomic distortion by a pelvic disease that produces a mechanical tubal block or interferes with the tubal ovum pickup and transfer mechanism exists, a reparative surgical procedure offers hope of restoring normal tubal function. As indicated in the following paragraphs, the nature and extent of the pathologic process determine the best procedure for surgical reconstruction of the tube.

1. Pelvic endometriosis with adherent uterus and adnexa and extensive peritubal adhesions, with or without fimbrial occlusion. *Treatment:* A conservative operation with excision of all gross areas of endometriosis; mobilization and suspension of the adherent uterus; mobilization of the adnexa with lysis of peritubal adhesions and fimbrioplasty, if necessary. (See Chapter 12 for a more detailed consideration of the indications and techniques of conservative surgical procedures and a discussion of hormonal therapy in certain selected patients with endometriosis accompanied by infertility.)

2. Uterine fibroids so situated as to cause tubal obstruction in the cornual regions. *Treatment:* Myomectomy, with care to avoid injury to the adjacent cornual portions of the tube.

3. Tubal occlusion secondary to previous pelvic inflammatory disease or salpingitis isthmica nodosa. The occlusion may involve either or both of the fimbrial and cornual ends of the tubes and is often associated with extensive pelvic adhesions. *Treatment:* One type of tuboplasty or a combination of the various types, which, depending on the site of block, may involve cornual resection and tubal reimplantation, midtube resection, and end-to-end anastomosis or fimbrioplasty (Fig. 13-1). The development and refinement of meticulous, atraumatic, microsurgical techniques, together with the employment of antibiotics and adjuncts for prevention of postoperative adhesions (e.g., hydroflotation with Hyskon, antiinflammatory agents, and corticosteroids) have tended to improve the results of these procedures in recent years. Microsurgical technique involves gentle atraumatic handling of tissues, prevention of tissue dehydration at surgery with constant irrigation using heparinized saline or heparinized Ringer-lactate solution, meticulous hemostasis to cut down fibrin deposition, loupes or operating microscope for careful apposition and realignment of the tubes, correct placement of sutures and easy use of microsutures (7-0 to 10-0 sutures), and nonirritating suture materials such as polyglactin (Vicryl or Dexon) or nylon sutures. With such techniques, the pregnancy rates after repairing diseased tubes (e.g., after pelvic inflammatory disease associated with extensive endometriosis) are about 30 to 40 percent. With distal tubal disease the pregnancy rates are lower (about 25 to 30 percent) than with proximal tubal occlusion if resection and end-to-end reanastomosis is performed (40 to 50 percent).

Because of the underlying damage to the tubal endothelium and muscular wall and the resulting impairment of normal secretory and peristaltic activity present in most of these cases, the percentage of patent tubes resulting from operative repair far exceeds the percentage of subsequent pregnancies. However, ectopic gestation is frequently encountered among the latter because of persistence of abnormal function despite restoration of patency. Thus in terms of the ultimate index of success, i.e., the occurrence of a normal intrauterine term pregnancy, favorable results following tuboplasty occur in 30 to 40 percent of cases, at best, if the tubes have been previously diseased. It is therefore important that the couple be made aware of the limited chances for success before

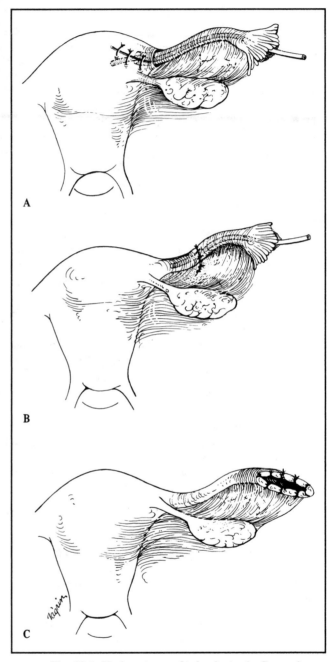

Fig. 13-1. Various types of tuboplasty. A. Cornual resection and tubal reimplantation. B. Partial tubal resection and end-to-end anastomosis over a splinting polyethylene catheter. C. Salpingostomy (or fimbrioplasty).

proceeding with tuboplasty. Nevertheless, the procedure is invariably worth attempting, as it usually represents the sole chance for restoration of fertility, and the risk and morbidity of the operation are small. On the other hand, if only lysis of peritubal adhesions is required to restore normal tubal function, the tubes themselves being basically normal, a 60 to 70 percent pregnancy rate can be anticipated. With previous tubal ligation, successful pregnancy rates of 80 percent or more can be readily obtained after microsurgical reanastomosis if the total tubal length is 5 cm or longer, the previous tubal ligation was not done by cauterization, and there are no additional infertility factors. The risk of ectopic pregnancy, however, is also increased after reversal of tubal ligation.

For any attempt at tuboplasty (both diseased tubes and reversal of tubal ligation), optimal results are obtained with the first repair and should therefore be undertaken by trained infertility surgeons who perform microsurgical tuboplasty on a regular basis. A second attempt at repairing tubes that have previously undergone tuboplasty generally carries a poor outcome, with pregnancy rates of, at best, 10 percent or even lower.

In vitro fertilization and embryo transfer (IVF), which was developed to enable pregnancies to be achieved by bypassing the tubes, especially for women with irreparably damaged tubes or absent tubes, can be offered if tuboplasty is not surgically possible or has not been successful. Currently this procedure has an average true pregnancy rate of 10 to 15 percent and at best 20 percent. The procedure involves inducing ovulation by recruiting multiple follicles with clomiphene, hMG, or both; retrieving the oocytes either by laparoscopy or vaginally by ultrasound guidance; culturing and fertilizing the oocyte in a dish using washed, capacitated sperms from the male partner; and subsequently using intrauterine transfer of the four- to eight-cell embryo via the vaginal route.

In vitro fertilization is now being employed to treat infertility due to reasons other than disturbed tubal factor as well, but it is questionable if the true success rates are any better than without such expensive treatment under these circumstances. Indeed some studies have indicated that the pregnancy rates among women to be treated with IVF were not remarkably different between those who underwent the treatment and those who became pregnant while waiting for it. One cannot help but wonder about the real indications for IVF in such patients, many of whom do not have a disturbed tubal factor. Thus comparison of success rates becomes unfathomable if the compared centers differ in terms of their criteria for IVF and the type of patients treated (e.g., disturbances of the tubal factor, peritoneal factor, or male factor), in addition to their technical expertise and other considerations.

Disturbances of the Cervical Factor

When thorough investigation of the male partner has eliminated his reproductive system as a factor, repeatedly poor results of postcoital cervical mucus tests, examination of the cervix itself, and additional studies of cervical secretions usually confirm that the difficulty stems from primary cervical disease (chronic infection) or inadequate secretory activity. Chronic vaginitis with its invariably associated cervicitis should be vigorously treated. If extensive congenital cervical erosion or chronic endocervicitis is found and appears to be the most likely cause of poor cervical mucus, careful cauterization of the cervix is indicated in an effort to eradicate the infection while preserving the normal secretory capacity in the uninvolved cervical glands.

In the absence of chronic cervicitis, poor cervical mucus (thick, opaque, and cellular instead of thin, clear, and watery) may be the result of inadequate estrogenic stimulation of the cervical glands during the critical preovulatory and ovulatory phases of the cycle. At times the resulting abnormal cervical factor is simply one of many manifestations of the abnormal physiology of anovulatory reproductive tract function, all of which are contributing to the resulting infertility, and treatment must be directed at the overall problem of ovarian dysfunction.

However, it is not uncommon to encounter women in whom ovulation with adequate progesterone production is occurring regularly but in whom preovulatory estrogen levels are apparently inadequate to bring about the normal quantitative and qualitative changes in cervical secretory activity necessary for the production of favorable cervical mucus at ovulation. In this situation, it is useful to give diethylstilbestrol in a dose of 0.1 to 0.2 mg daily from days 5 through 14 of the cycle for three or four cycles—a dose that does not interfere with ovulation but frequently improves both the quality and quantity of cervical mucus.

An alternative method is to give conjugated estrogens (Premarin) 0.3 mg daily by mouth from days 10 through 14 of the cycle (i.e., the last five days before expected ovulation). This approach is also not infrequently employed in the small percentage of women who develop poor cervical mucus during clomiphene therapy despite good follicle recruitment and estradiol levels, presumably because of the antiestrogenic effect of clomiphene being exerted on the cervix.

Robitussin cough syrup may also be taken by some patients in place of estrogen to successfully improve cervical mucus secretion. In patients with adequate mucus that is, however, viscid despite correct timing of the postcoital factor and the cycle being ovulatory, douching with baking soda solution (one tablespoon of baking soda to one quart of water) can improve the cervical mucus quality (presumably through a change in pH) and the postcoital test.

At times, a persistently poor postcoital test may be due to premature semen loss from the vagina or inadequate cervical contact with the seminal pool secondary to faulty coital technique or minor vaginal anatomic variations. If this problem is suggested on the basis of the history, pelvic findings, and failure to demonstrate any abnormality of the semen or of the cervix and its secretion, the use of special plastic vaginal tampons (Fertilopak) that the patient inserts immediately after intercourse may be tried in an attempt to facilitate retention of the semen in close apposition to the external cervical os.

Finally, if despite the various therapeutic efforts that have been described satisfactory sperm penetration of the cervical canal cannot be achieved in the usual way, artificial insemination using the husband's semen should be considered. The semen can be introduced by placing it in a snug-fitting plastic cap that is then applied to the cervix or, by careful direct injection, into the cervical canal or intrauterine cavity. In any case, the optimal time for insemination is of course selected as accurately as possible on the basis of the basal body temperature chart, other indexes of ovulation, or both. If intrauterine insemination is performed, only a drop or two of the semen is instilled, with the rest being instilled into the endocervical canal. This technique avoids or reduces the likelihood of severe uterine cramping.

Miscellaneous Factors Responsible for Implantation and Maintenance Failures (Uterine Factor)

The treatment of abnormal uterine factors implicated in infertility is as follows.

1. Intramural and submucous fibroids: myomectomy.
2. Endometrial or endocervical polyps: dilatation and curettage (D&C) with excision of polyps.
3. Asherman's syndrome (traumatic intrauterine adhesions): surgical removal of intrauterine adhesions by curettage or hysterotomy followed by estrogen therapy for three to six months to stimulate regeneration and growth of the endometrium throughout the endometrial cavity.
4. Congenital anomalies and their treatment.
   a. Complete duplications: unification operation of Strassman (Fig. 8-5), Tompkins, or Jones.
   b. Uterine septa: resection of septa (done through laparotomy or through hysteroscopic resection).
   c. Rudimentary uterine horn: resection of rudimentary horn.
   d. Bicornuate uterus: unification operation of Strassman.
5. Incompetent internal cervical os with repeated second-trimester abortions (Chap. 16).
   a. If discovered during pregnancy but before abortion: surgical closure of the internal os (McDonald procedure or Shirodkar procedure; Fig. 16-2).
   b. If discovered between pregnancies: Shirodkar procedure.
6. T-strain *Mycoplasma* infection of the cervix, vagina, or endometrium. There is some evidence that the presence of mycoplasmas within the

lower genital tract may be responsible for some cases of infertility and perhaps an even larger number of repeated spontaneous abortions. Administration of tetracycline or doxycycline (Vibramycin) to affected infertile women has seemed to increase fertility in some and appears to reduce the number of spontaneous abortions in women who had previously shown a high rate of spontaneous abortion.

"Unexplained" Infertility

Despite a thorough and complete workup for their infertility, no readily explicable and identifiable cause can be elicited in 10 to 15 percent of cases. For such couples, advances in reproductive technology have provided forms of therapy other than adopting a child.

For example, gamete intrafallopian tube transfer (GIFT) can be offered to such couples if the woman has normal healthy tubes that have not undergone surgery before. GIFT is essentially similar to IVF except that the oocytes are allowed to be fertilized in the fallopian tube instead of a petri dish in a laboratory incubator. The female partner undergoes ovarian stimulation to recruit multiple follicles, which are harvested by laparoscopy or through a minilaparotomy. The oocytes are then prepared as for IVF and the male partner's spermatozoa, which have been washed, capacitated, and selected for good motility (by a swim-up or swim-down technique on an albumin column), are mixed in a small volume of incubation medium. The mixture of male and female gametes are then placed into the fimbrial opening of the fallopian tube at about the region of the ampulla at the same operative setting as for retrieval of the oocytes. Pregnancy rates with GIFT have been encouraging (60 to 70 percent success rates have been claimed) and better than those with IVF. As more experience is being accumulated at various centers, however, the true success rates are being challenged and may be somewhat lower than the initial enthusiastic claims.

Modern Approaches to Treatment of Infertility

With the availability of reproductive technologies such as IVF and GIFT, manipulations and variations of the original technique are being explored and employed for treatment in patients. Some of these variations are not technical but merely social challenges or experimentation of socially and conventionally established and accepted customs.

In vitro fertilization and GIFT have been employed using donor semen instead of semen from the male partner of the couple when the man's semen is poor or after six or more artificial inseminations with either the partner's or the donor's semen have been unsuccessful.

Similarly, not only donor male gametes (spermatozoa) have been used for GIFT and IVF, but donor oocytes have been tried to a limited extent. For this procedure, a female donor is inseminated with the spermatozoa of the husband of the putative embryo recipient. The resulting embryo is then lavaged out of the female donor uterus and transferred transvaginally via the cervix into the uterine cavity of the recipient, who is at the same phase of the menstrual cycle as the donor.

Finally, surrogates have been employed instead of transferring the embryo as described. For surrogate pregnancy, a contracted female donor is inseminated with the spermatozoa of the husband of the couple, who will receive the child at birth. This procedure is usually a financially arranged contract, and the donor is reimbursed for her services. Many moral, legal, and ethical questions are raised with a surrogate pregnancy. Indeed, contractual disputes leading to prolonged legal wrangling for the custody of the child as a result of change of mind have occurred and have been brought to court in the United States. In some western countries, surrogate pregnancy is not permitted; and in the United States some states have already instituted legislation to ban it.

The technical variation introduced into IVF and GIFT include cryopreservation of the embryos and subsequent transfer into the same woman or donated to another infertile woman. Cryopreservation of embryos is still an imperfect science or art and is at an early stage of development. If cryopreservation becomes more successful, it can reduce costs for IVF and cause surgery to be avoided in subsequent cycles when only embryo transfer of the thawed frozen embryos is all that is required.

RESULTS OF THE STUDY AND TREATMENT OF INFERTILITY

It is estimated that by careful study and treatment between 25 and 50 percent of all infertile couples can be cured of their involuntary sterility and helped to achieve one or more successful pregnancies. An adequate therapeutic program may require several years of continuing investigation and may involve prolonged or repeated treatment of various factors with all the potentially helpful measures. The great variation in the percentage of favorable results and the length of time required to achieve them is of course markedly influenced by the age of the couple, the nature of the disease or functional disorder present, and if multiple factors are responsible for the infertility. For example, the results in terms of subsequent fertility and normal pregnancy following the surgical treatment of the infertile woman with the Stein-Leventhal syndrome are favorable in 85 to 90 percent of patients (the normal fertility range), whereas successful pregnancy following tuboplasty occurs in 30 to 40 percent of patients. Conservative surgery for infertility due to pelvic endometriosis restores fertility in approximately 50 to 60 percent of patients. Most patients suffering from infertility do not require operative therapy; and although it is difficult to assess the percentage of favorable results following the various forms of medical therapy, or even to be certain that the treatment was responsible for the successful outcome, persistent and patient efforts are rewarded by successful pregnancy in 40 to 50 percent of this large group.

Although there is no absolute upper age limit above which couples should be advised that the study and attempted treatment of their infertility are unlikely to be worth the effort, the woman in her late thirties or early forties should understand that the chances of achieving a successful pregnancy are considerably less than in the case of women under age 35. This fact is in part a reflection of the decline in fertility experienced after age 30 even with no fertility problems. Furthermore, there tends to be an increased incidence of serious organic disease in the group of women over 35 who suffer from infertility: extensive endometriosis, multiple fibroids, chronic pelvic inflammatory disease, or previous pelvic surgery that has resulted in

the loss of an ovary or both one tube and ovary. Nevertheless, many couples with infertility of long standing can be helped to have children by careful treatment of the often multiple factors that a thorough investigation shows to be contributing to their impaired fertility. Therefore they should not be unduly discouraged from embarking on a standard program of study and therapy.

MANAGEMENT FOLLOWING UNSUCCESSFUL THERAPY

If it is soon obvious that an incurable barrier to conception exists, or if after a period of years the program of therapy has failed to achieve pregnancy, the possibility of adopting children should be considered seriously. It is part of the physician's responsibility to help the couple reach this decision, to refer them to adoption agencies known to the physician to be reliable and ethical, and to cooperate fully in helping them secure a child. The other alternative—artificial donor insemination—may also be considered if, as previously discussed, the sterility is based solely on an abnormal male factor.

Even if incorrectable impairment of fertility is ultimately demonstrated, a thorough sterility investigation accomplishes a worthwhile purpose: It is only by a complete study of the problem and an adequate trial of all known therapeutic measures that a couple is assured that everything possible has been done, is willing to abandon further anxiety-ridden and fruitless efforts, and is able to achieve the peace of mind necessary to accept and live with the final reality of the situation. The couple is then in a position to proceed with adoption or with a mature readjustment of their marital goals.

SELECTED READINGS

Asch, R. H., Balmaceda, J. P., Ellsworth, L. R., et al. Preliminary experiences with gamete intrafallopian tube transfer (GIFT). *Fertil. Steril.* 45:366, 1986.

Boer-Meisel, M. E., te Velde, E. R., Habbema, J. D. F., et al. Predicting the pregnancy outcome in patients treated for hydrosalpinx: A prospective study. *Fertil. Steril.* 45:23, 1986.

Grimes, E. M. (guest editor). Management of the infertile couple. *Semin. Reprod. Endocrinol.* 3:93, 1985.

Kovacs, G., Baker, G., Burger, H., et al. Artificial insemination with cryopreserved donor semen: A decade of experience. *Br. J. Obstet. Gynaecol.* 95:354, 1988.

Lalos, A., Lalos, O., Jacobsson, L., et al. Depression, guilt and isolation among infertile women and their partners. *J. Psychosom. Obstet. Gynaecol.* 5:197, 1986.

Mosher, W. D. Fecundity and infertility in the United States. *Am. J. Public Health* 78:181, 1988.

Schulman, J. D., Dorfman, A. D., Jones, S. L., et al. Outpatient in vitro fertilization using transvaginal ultrasound-guided oocyte retrieval. *Obstet. Gynecol.* 69:665, 1987.

Smarr, S. C., Wing, R., Hammond, M. G. Effect of therapy of infertile couples with antisperm antibodies. *Am. J. Obstet. Gynecol.* 158:969, 1988.

Sogor, L. (guest editor). Pathophysiology of male infertility. *Semin. Reprod. Endocrinol.* 6:309, 1988.

Vermesh, M., Kletzky, O. A., Davajan, V., et al. Monitoring techniques to predict and detect ovulation. *Fertil. Steril.* 47:259, 1987.

Wallach, E. E., Moghissi, K. S. Unexplained infertility. In S. J. Behrman, R. W. Kistner, and G. W. Portton (eds.), *Progress in Infertility* (3rd ed.), Boston: Little, Brown, 1988. P. 799.

Williams, T. J. Surgical procedures for inflammatory tubal disease. *Obstet. Gynecol. Clinics North America* 14:1037, 1987.

III

General Gynecology

14

Benign Disorders and Infections of the Lower Genital Tract

VAGINA

Vaginitis

Vaginal and vulvar infections and inflammatory processes are common and represent the most frequently encountered diagnostic and therapeutic problem in gynecologic office practice. Because vaginal discharge and vulvar irritation are such frequent complaints and often, though by no means always, indicative of an underlying vaginitis, it is well to begin by considering the most common causes of vaginal discharge.

Evaluation of Vaginal Discharge

HISTORY. The main points to be covered in the history are the following.

1. Presence or absence of associated symptoms, e.g., burning, itching, pain, bleeding. The mucoid discharge of a cervical ectropion or the physiologic increase in normal secretions at midcycle or premenstrually are asymptomatic, as is the pubertal monthly mucoid discharge of young girls. This picture is in sharp contrast to that of *Candida* or *Trichomonas* vaginitis, in which pruritus is intense, or atrophic vaginitis, in which a burning discomfort is often the most prominent symptom.
2. Relation to menses. Symptoms of trichomoniasis invariably have their onset or become worse just after a menstrual period, whereas those of *Candida* vaginitis are often worse just before a period.
3. Relation to other features of the history. Candidiasis is common in pregnant women and diabetic women, after therapy with broad-spectrum antibiotics, after estrogen therapy, and after therapy for trichomonal vaginitis.

PHYSICAL EXAMINATION. Check for an associated vulvitis or other vulvar lesion that might be responsible for the symptoms. Check for the presence of visible vaginal inflammation, cervicitis or cervical erosion, or a retained foreign body. Determine the status of the vaginal mucosa with regard to estrogen effect. Rule out sexually transmitted disease, malignancy (cervical, endocervical, and endometrial biopsies if necessary, as well as routine Papanicolaou smears), or pyometrium (probe the cervix).

EXAMINATION OF THE DISCHARGE

1. Gross appearance, color, consistency, odor, pH.
   a. *Trichomonas:* yellow, thin, foamy, malodorous, alkaline (e.g., pH 5.0 to 6.0).
   b. *Candida:* white, thick, flaky, cheesy, usually not malodorous, often acidic (e.g., pH 3.0 to 4.0).
   c. Bacterial vaginosis: thin, watery, malodorous ("fishy" or "musty"), alkaline (e.g., pH 5 to 6).
   d. Atrophic vaginitis: scant, yellowish or brownish, occasionally blood-tinged.
   e. Malignancy: bloody, often malodorous.
   f. Retained tampon: often bloody and malodorous.
   g. Cervicitis: mucoid or mucopurulent.
2. A wet smear (Chap. 2) is usually diagnostic for trichomoniasis and bacterial vaginosis, and of considerable help in the diagnosis of vaginal candidiasis and atrophic vaginitis.
3. Cultures: Routine for bacterial vaginosis, special for *Candida, Chlamydia,* gonorrhea, and herpes (Chap. 2).
4. Papanicolaou smears for cytologic study.

Trichomonas Infection. Trichomonas vaginitis is caused by a unicellular anaerobic flagellated protozoan (*Trichomonas vaginalis*) that inhabits the lower genital and urinary tract of women (and men). Until the discovery of an effective treatment (metronidazole) a quarter of a century ago, this disease was typified by a chronic irritation and copious discharge in many women. It is estimated that there are approximately 3 million new cases diagnosed annually in the United States.

The disease is clearly sexually transmitted, with

the finding that nearly three-fourths of male sexual partners, although asymptomatic, are also culture-positive for *T. vaginalis*. In men, *T. vaginalis* resides in the urethra and prostate. Many women are asymptomatic: Approximately 15 percent of asymptomatic gynecology patients are culture-positive for *T. vaginalis*.

Trichomonas vaginitis is most often diagnosed in women of reproductive age. The low pH (high acidity) of the vagina makes it usually resistant to *T. vaginalis*. However, with changes in the vaginal pH leading to a more basic environment, which may be caused by other vaginal pathogens or menstrual blood, the endemic *Trichomonas* organisms may overgrow. The symptoms of *Trichomonas* vaginitis are a profuse yellow to yellowish-brown vaginal discharge that is often accompanied by an unpleasant odor. Vulvar erythema and edema, usually limited to the vestibule and labia minora, is often noted. Only approximately 25 percent of patients with asymptomatic *Trichomonas* vaginitis complain of vulvar pruritus. Because of the increased pH following a menstrual period, the signs and symptoms of *Trichomonas* vaginitis are usually worse postmenstrually.

Examination of the patient with *Trichomonas* vaginitis may reveal vulvar erythema and edema. The vaginal discharge usually appears yellow, gray, or green and may have a bubbling appearance. This frothy appearance, however, is not specifically diagnostic of *Trichomonas* vaginitis. The characteristic "strawberry" appearance of the vagina and cervix (reddened, punctate epithelial papillae) is apparent in only 10 percent of patients.

The diagnosis of *Trichomonas* vaginitis is most frequently made by microscopic examination of the vaginal discharge. It is best to obtain the specimen from high in the posterior vaginal wall or from secretions on the posterior blade of the vaginal speculum. Examination of the discharge specimen mixed with normal saline on a miscroscope slide with coverslip is recommended. No specific stain is needed. *T. vaginalis* is a flagellated organism that is oval to spherical in shape and slightly larger than a white blood cell. Three to five flagella are apparent, arising from one end of the unicellular organism. Specimens warmed to body temperature usually show active movement of the flagella and propulsion of the protozoan. The microscopic background may be heavy in white blood cells and vaginal epithelial cells that are reacting to the *T. vaginalis* infection. The diagnosis may also be suggested by the Papanicolaou smear, although relatively high false-positive and false-negative rates have been noted with this diagnostic method. An adjunct to the microscopic examination is a simple test of vaginal pH. *T. vaginalis* organisms usually require a pH of 5 to 7 and are rarely noted with more acidic pH. A culture for *T. vaginalis* is rarely needed to make the diagnosis.

The cornerstone of therapy for *T. vaginalis* infection is metronidazole (Flagyl). Because *Trichomonas* may inhabit the vagina, cervix, anus, and urethra, and the prostate of the male partner, systemic therapy is strongly recommended. Metronidazole is available as a 250 mg tablet that is readily absorbed after oral administration. Metronidazole is also available in intravenous form for severe anaerobic infections. The standard regimen recommended for the treatment of *Trichomonas* vaginitis is metronidazole 250 mg orally every 8 hours for seven days. A single-dose regimen (2 gm by mouth in one dose) has been found to be as effective as the traditional regimen. The advantage of the single-dose regimen is that it is less expensive, seems to have fewer side effects, and has better patient compliance. Both regimens are approximately 90 percent effective in eradicating *T. vaginalis* from the lower genital tract. Because of the venereal nature of this disease, it is recommended that male sexual partners of women with symptomatic *Trichomonas* vaginitis be treated at the same time. If a male partner is not treated, the reinfection rate of the treated woman is approximately two to two and a half times greater. The same regimen that is used for the woman is recommended for treatment of the male partner.

Side effects of metronidazole are minimal. Approximately 5 percent of patients have nausea associated with its use. Metronidazole may have a disulfiram-like effect if taken with alcohol, and patients should be warned to avoid ethanol intake while on metronidazole therapy. Because metronidazole has been found to be teratogenic in some animals, it is contraindicated during the first trimester of pregnancy and should be used during the second and third trimesters only in severe cases. There is no evidence that metronidazole is carcinogenic in humans.

Recurrent *T. vaginalis* infections are not uncommon and are most often due to reinfection from either a male partner or reinfection from the patient's own *Trichomonas* reservoir in the lower genital tract. Usually retreatment with the standard regimens is sufficient therapy, and attention should be paid to treating male partners. Resistant strains of *T. vaginalis* have been identified that appear to be successfully treated with higher doses of metronidazole (1 to 2 gm daily for seven days). Patients allergic or intolerant of metronidazole may be treated with povidone-iodine douches daily for seven days or topical clotrimazole cream for seven days.

Candida Vaginitis. Vaginitis caused by an overgrowth of *Candida albicans* occurs in approximately 30 percent of women. The incidence of this disease is doubled during pregnancy and is increased in other clinical circumstances that alter host factors leading to increased *Candida* growth. *C. albicans* and other *Candida* species are part of the normal vaginal flora in approximately 25 percent of women. This ubiquitous gram-positive fungus is even more prevalent in the rectum and the oral cavity. Changes in the vaginal pH or a decrease in the population of lactobacilli allow *C. albicans* to become an opportunistic pathogen.

In contrast to *Trichomonas vaginalis, Candida* should not be considered a sexually transmitted disease. Investigation of male partners of women who have symptomatic *Candida* vaginitis rarely reveals urethral *Candida* growth, and therefore the male partner does not require treatment.

Host factors associated with increased *Candida* growth include a change in the hormonal milieu, decreased immunity, antibiotic use, and diabetes mellitus. As noted previously, *Candida* vaginitis is nearly doubled in frequency during pregnancy when a high estrogenic state exists. Symptomatic *Candida* vaginitis is often noted immediately preceding or immediately after a menstrual period and has also been noted to be increased with use of oral contraceptives containing high doses of estrogen. On the other hand, modern combination oral contraceptives, which contain much lower doses of estrogen than before, are not

associated with an increased incidence of *Candida* vaginitis. Conditions that decrease cell-mediated immunity (including corticocosteroid use, chronic illness, and use of cytotoxic agents for neoplasms) and the use of broad-spectrum antibiotics, especially those that eliminate lactobacilli from the vaginal flora, predispose to overgrowth of *C. albicans* and subsequent symptomatic vaginitis. The first symptom leading to the diagnosis of diabetes mellitus may be a fluminant *Candida* vulvovaginitis, and it is quite clear that diabetics and women who are obese (and have glucose intolerance) have an increased incidence of *Candida* vaginitis. If possible, elimination of these compounding factors is important to the primary treatment of *Candida* vaginitis as well as to its decreased recurrence rate. Although *Candida* is an endemic species of the vaginal flora, it is only the symptomatic patient who requires evaluation and treatment.

Most frequently, patients present with a vulvovaginitis and complain of intense pruritus and vulvar burning, dysuria from urethral irritation, and dyspareunia. Pelvic examination often reveals an erythematous, edematous vulva, which in fulminant cases may involve the entire labia minora and majora. Inspection of the vagina reveals a white to whitish gray, thick discharge that is adherent to the vaginal wall. This discharge is often typified as "cottage cheese" in consistency. Usually there is no associated odor unless the patient has a concurrent infection with *T. vaginalis* or *Gardnerella*.

The diagnosis is usually made by microscopic examination of the vaginal discharge. In order to lyse the white and red blood cells in the vaginal discharge, the discharge is mixed with 10% potassium hydroxide (KOH preparation). The material is covered with a coverslip and examined microscopically, which reveals filaments, hyphae, and pseudohyphae. Diagnosis based on microscopic examination alone is correct approximately 65 percent of the time. When in doubt, or in cases of recurrent vaginitis of uncertain etiology, cultures should be obtained and plated on Nickerson's medium.

The current treatment of *Candida* vaginitis is with the topical application of one of the synthetic imidazoles (miconazole, chlortrimazole, or butoconazole). These agents are available as either a vaginal suppository or cream applied by a vaginal applicator. Randomized trials have shown that a three-day course (applied once a day) of these medications is as effective as a seven-day course. Ninety percent of the time symptoms of *Candida* vaginitis are eliminated by this regimen. In the past, nystatin was the primary therapy, given daily for a ten- to fourteen-day course. However, cure rates are lower with nystatin than with the imidazoles. Povidone-iodine douche is also effective for some patients with *Candida* vaginitis.

Unfortunately, and to the frustration of many patients and physicians, recurrence is frequent after apparent cure. Patients with recurrent symptoms suggestive of *Candida* vaginitis should be reevaluated, and a culture or KOH preparation should be done for microscopic analysis to confirm reinfection.

Other causes of symptoms, including sensitivity to the vaginal medication, should be considered. Patients with recurrent infection should be screened for occult diabetes mellitus. Occasionally, cultures reveal other *Candida* species, including *C. glabrata* and *C. tropicalis*. These two *Candida* species are best treated with topical application of 1% gentian violet solution applied on three occasions, at approximately three- or four-day intervals. More frequent application may lead to a chemical vaginitis from the topical gentian violet.

In resistant cases of *Candida* vaginitis success has been achieved with the use of ketoconazole (400 mg PO daily for six months). This intense regimen should be reserved for patients who have had resistant *Candida* vaginitis with multiple recurrences. Liver toxicity is an important side effect that must be evaluated periodically by liver function tests.

Bacterial Vaginosis. Bacterial vaginosis is the most frequently diagnosed symptomatic vaginitis in American women. The condition is caused by an increased growth of both anaerobes and *Gardnerella vaginalis* in an apparent symbiotic relationship. In the past, this vaginitis was referred to as a "nonspecific vaginitis" and was thought to be associated with increased growth of *Hemophilus* or *Corynebacterium vaginale*. The offending bacterium has more recently been identified as a gram-negative bacillus and has been named *Gardnerella vaginalis*. This bacillus is present in 30 to 40

percent of asymptomatic women. Because of the current understanding that symptoms are caused by a symbiotic infection, the condition is now called "bacterial vaginosis."

Symptoms associated with bacterial vaginosis are usually a thin, watery vaginal discharge that is malodorous. The odor is described by many patients as "fishy" or "musty." Vulvitis is relatively infrequent.

The diagnosis of bacterial vaginosis is primarily made by wet-preparation microscopic examination. Microscopically, clumps of bacteria and vaginal epithelial cells with adherent bacteria, called "clue cells," are noted. Microscopic examination, especially when compared with wet preparations of a patient with *Candida* vaginitis or *Trichomonas* vaginitis, shows a relative lack of inflammatory cells. The vaginal pH is usually between 5 and 6.

The treatment of bacterial vaginosis has changed. The most effective regimen is metronidazole taken as 500 mg by mouth b.i.d. for seven days. This regimen achieves a 90 to 95 percent cure rate. A single-dose regimen of metronidazole, as is recommended for treatment of *Trichomonas* vaginitis, is not as effective for bacterial vaginosis. Treatments utilized in the past, including sulfa creams and suppositories, oral ampicillin, or tetracycline, result in only a 60 to 70 percent success rate. The male partners of patients with resistant or recurrent bacterial vaginosis should also be treated. This recommendation is somewhat controversial, although it is recognized that 90 percent of male sexual partners of women with bacterial vaginosis also culture positive for *G. vaginalis*.

Atrophic Vaginitis. Vaginitis in menopausal women is most commonly secondary to an infection of susceptible, easily traumatized atrophic vaginal epithelium. With estrogen withdrawal (at menopause, due to surgery, or following radiation therapy) vaginal atrophy occurs, leading to a decrease in vaginal thickness and subsequent diminution of vaginal rugae. This process, as it affects the remainder of the genital tract, is discussed in Chapter 23. The atrophic vaginal epithelium is thin and easily traumatized with intercourse or douching; it is also susceptible to infectious agents.

Symptoms of atrophic vaginitis include vulvar and vaginal pruritus, vaginal burning, dyspareunia, and scant bleeding. Because these symptoms may be related to other etiologies (e.g., endometrial or cervical cancer) all women with these complaints should be examined to establish a definitive diagnosis. Examination usually reveals atrophic changes in the lower genital tract, including changes in the vulvar and periurethral skin. The vaginal epithelium appears thin and transparent with decreased rugal folds. It may be easily traumatized with gentle speculum examination and may appear reddened. The vaginal discharge is often thin, watery, and blood-stained. Microscopic examination of the vaginal discharge reveals some inflammatory cells and epithelial cells. Most often, a dominant organism is not identified. Should a specific infectious agent be found (e.g., *Trichomonas vaginalis* or *Candida*) it is treated in addition to treating the atrophic vaginitis.

Atrophic vaginitis is treated by estrogen replacement, the management of which is outlined in detail in Chapter 23. To treat specifically the symptoms of atrophic vaginitis, we have found that topical application of intravaginal estrogen cream produces the fastest resolution of symptoms. Intravaginal application of estrogen does lead to systemic absorption, however, and so must be considered contraindicated in patients in whom systemic estrogen is contraindicated. The long-term prevention of atrophic vaginitis is through the continued use of estrogen replacement, usually systemically. In most cases, even when a specific infective organism is found, estrogen replacement therapy of the atrophic vaginitis improves vaginal epithelial health, making it more resistant to overgrowth of pathogens.

Toxic Shock Syndrome

Toxic shock syndrome is an acute febrile illness that may result in multiple system failure, hypotension, and death in 2 to 8 percent of cases. Toxic shock syndrome is discussed in the context of vaginal disease because it is most often associated with infection of *Staphylococcus aureus* in the vagina. *S. aureus* produces a specific exotoxin that is absorbed across the vaginal mucosa, leading to subsequent systemic insult. This infection is associated with use of intravaginal tampons or other foreign bodies (contracep-

tive sponges, diaphragms, cervical caps) that promote increased growth of *S. aureus* and may traumatize vaginal epithelium, allowing easier passage of the exotoxin.

The toxic shock syndrome was first described in 1978, and most subsequent cases have been reported in healthy women under age 30. Much less commonly, toxic shock syndrome is associated with a cutaneous staphylococcal infection postpartum or following surgery.

The responsibility for reduced mortality with this disease lies heavily with the clinician for early diagnosis. In most cases of death, the patient had been under treatment for another presumed illness. Toxic shock syndrome is usually preceded by a prodromal flu-like illness following menses. Nausea, vomiting, sore throat, and high fever are the early signs. Many of these symptoms are mild or vary in severity. A more fulminant form of the illness is seen in patients who develop a high fever and skin rash. The rash initially appears as an intense "sunburn" over the entire body, which evolves over the next few days to a macular rash. Over the next ten to fourteen days there is generalized desquamation and exfoliation of the skin over the palms and soles of the feet. Hypotension and systemic organ failure may also ensue resulting in a critically ill patient.

Recognition of the signs and symptoms of toxic shock syndrome and a high index of suspicion in patients with less severe symptoms is the keystone to early diagnosis. Cultures should be obtained from the cervix and vagina, searching for *S. aureus,* which is present in most patients with toxic shock syndrome. Conversely, blood cultures are rarely positive and clearly should not be relied on to establish the diagnosis. Remember that it is the exotoxin that is thought to be the pathogenic agent in this disease. The pathophysiology of this process is not clear, however, although it appears to be secondary to an intravascular exotoxin, leading to increased vascular permeability and loss of intravascular volume in two-thirds of patients.

Management of the severe form of the syndrome is with aggressive fluid replacement, supporting the intravascular volume. Central monitoring with a Swan-Ganz catheter is highly recommended in an intensive care setting. Antibiotics (β-lactamase-resistant penicillins) should be administered intravenously for ten to fourteen days. The administration of corticosteroids is controversial at this time. Further supportive care of adult respiratory distress syndrome (shock lung) may require mechanical ventilation. The early recognition of toxic shock syndrome and appropriate management in an intensive care setting is paramount to prevention of death from this disease.

Recurrences have been noted in up to 33 percent of patients who have not been given antibiotics. Prevention of this syndrome has been aided by the elimination of superabsorbent tampon materials from the market, as well as patient education. Patient awareness as to the signs and symptoms of toxic shock syndrome should be part of a physician's discussion regarding menstruation and the use of tampons. Vaginal tampons should be changed every 4 to 6 hours, and the use of external perineal pads for part of the menstrual period (e.g., while sleeping) may be encouraged.

Vaginal Cysts

Cysts of the vagina may arise at any location and may represent inclusion cysts from vaginal trauma, mesonephric duct remnants, or urethral diverticulum. Consideration of these cysts is important for proper management.

Inclusion Cysts. The most common cyst of the vagina is an inclusion cyst, which usually arises on the posterior or lateral walls in the lower vagina. Typically, these cysts range in size from a few millimeters to 3 cm and are usually noted following childbirth. It therefore seems most likely that they arise from the inclusion of vaginal epithelium from an episiotomy or laceration. Typically the cysts are entirely asymptomatic unless they grow to a large enough size to cause dyspareunia or pressure symptoms. Excision of a cyst reveals a lining of squamous epithelium. Surgical therapy, however, is not necessary unless the cyst is symptomatic.

Gartner Duct Cysts. Gartner duct cysts are usually found on examination of the upper one-half of the vagina (Fig. 14-1). These cysts may be single or mul-

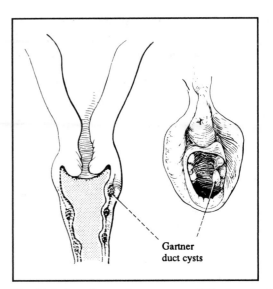

Fig. 14-1. Location and appearance of Gartner duct cysts of the vagina.

tiple and are generally arranged in a linear fashion along the axis of the vagina. They usually are a few millimeters to a few centimeters in diameter and are most often asymptomatic. Symptoms associated with the larger cysts include dyspareunia and pressure in the vagina. These cysts are usually located on the anterolateral vaginal wall and frequently appear bilaterally. They may occur as frequently as one in every 200 women examined. The etiology of these cysts is the failure of full regression of the mesonephric ducts. If symptoms of dyspareunia, pain, or urinary tract pressure are noted, surgical excision is recommended.

Urethral Diverticulum. Urethral diverticulum may initially present as a vaginal wall cyst. Confusing it with a Gartner duct cyst might result in urinary tract injury at the time of excision. Approximately 3 percent of women develop a urethral diverticulum, usually late in life. Symptoms most frequently associated with urethral diverticulum are those of recurrent urinary tract infection with urgency, frequency, and dysuria. Some patients dribble small amounts of urine or have dyspareunia.

The diagnosis of urethral diverticulum may be elusive, and physical findings on pelvic examination may not show a cystic structure in the anterior vaginal wall underneath the urethra. Therefore it is important to suspect urethral diverticulum in patients with chronic urinary tract symptoms and recurrent urinary tract infections. Urethral diverticula may be 3 mm to 3 cm in diameter and are most frequently found in the midurethra. Palpation of this region may express a purulent or bloody material from the diverticulum that is noted at the urethral meatus. A voiding cystourethrogram or cystourethroscopy is usually required to visualize the urethral diverticulum. An intravenous pyelogram should also be obtained to ensure that the ostia noted on radiologic or cystoscopic examination is not an ectopic ureter.

Urethral diverticulum must be managed surgically, with the preferred approach being a transvaginal excision and closure of the urethra and vagina in layers. The procedure is complicated by urethrovaginal fistula in approximately 1 percent of cases.

Endometriosis

Endometriosis may be found in the vagina, implanted in either an old episiotomy scar or a laceration following childbirth, or it may erode through from the posterior cul-de-sac into the posterior upper vagina. This direct extension of intraperitoneal disease is of concern, as it may appear similar to a vaginal or cervical cancer. Biopsy of such lesions is necessary. The usual management of endometriosis is discussed further in Chapter 12.

Adenosis

The identification of a complex of gynecologic anatomic abnormalities associated with intrauterine exposure to diethylstilbestrol (DES) has now been fully documented. The specter of clear cell adenocarcinoma of the vagina or cervix secondary to intrauterine DES exposure is discussed in Chapter 29. Women who are exposed to DES before the twenty-second week of pregnancy have a 30 to 40 percent chance of having vaginal adenosis found on pelvic examination. Adenosis is nothing more than columnar epithelium arising in the vagina, usually as patchy areas in the upper vagina. Adenosis has also been noted to have spontaneously arisen in women who were not exposed to DES.

The condition may be relatively asymptomatic, although some patients have a mucoid discharge or vaginal spotting. Over time, these areas of glandular epithelium are replaced or covered by squamous metaplasia, much as occurs during the natural history of the normal cervix. Malignant transformation of true vaginal adenosis is rare, but adenosis should be fully evaluated as part of the comprehensive evaluation of the DES-exposed woman. It should include a careful history and physical examination with Papanicolaou smear, as well as colposcopy of these areas to assess the possibility of intraepithelial neoplasia or a frankly invasive lesion. Biopsy should be done of any areas that are suspicious, although as previously noted adenosis carries a minimal possibility of developing subsequent invasive carcinoma.

The other vaginal lesions associated with DES exposure in utero are transverse vaginal ridges, which occur in approximately 25 percent of patients exposed to DES during early pregnancy. They are usually located in the upper one-third of the vagina.

Vaginal Trauma

Trauma to the vagina is usually identified by profuse vaginal bleeding and pain. The most frequent cause of vaginal laceration is sexual intercourse, followed by straddle injuries, insertion of foreign bodies, sexual assault, and waterskiing. Speculum examination of the vagina is required to evaluate the extent of the lesion, which is usually a tear in the posterior or lateral fornices of the vagina. Profuse vaginal bleeding may occur because of laceration of one of the vaginal arteries. Comprehensive evaluation of the patient with a vaginal laceration is important so as to be certain that urinary or gastrointestinal tract injury is not coincidental. In fact, large lacerations in the posterior vagina may lead to evisceration of small bowel. Simple suturing of the vaginal laceration is usually adequate therapy, although with deeper penetrating lesions exploratory laparotomy, cystoscopy, proctosigmoidoscopy, or laparoscopy may be required for full evaluation.

Tampon-Related Trauma. The frequent use of tampons for menstrual hygiene leads to occasional problems that bring a patient to the physician's attention.

Toxic shock syndrome, the most dramatic of these problems, has been discussed separately. Prolonged use of tampons may lead to epithelial drying and microulceration, and even gross ulceration of the vaginal mucosa. These ulcers may be asymptomatic or may bleed and cause vaginal discharge. They are nearly always due to the drying and pressure necrosis caused by the tampon. A similar condition may be seen with the chronic use of a contraceptive diaphragm or pessaries. Conservative therapy is recommended with removal of the offending foreign body. A Papanicolaou smear should be obtained from the ulcer upon initial evaluation to be certain that no evidence of malignancy or neoplasia is noted. If the ulcer does not heal within a week or two, biopsy should be obtained to exclude the possibility of a vaginal cancer.

Occasionally, tampons are forgotten in the vagina and the patient presents with the classic signs and symptoms of a foul vaginal discharge. Simply removing the tampon, which may be high in the upper vagina, is sufficient therapy.

VULVA

Detailed knowledge of the specialized physiology and cytochemistry of vulvar skin is scanty, but it is important to bear in mind that there are unquestionably significant differences from other areas of the body and special features. Moreover, it must be remembered that the vulva represents a skin organ, not just another area of general body integument. The following are three obvious gross anatomic peculiarities.

1. The vulvar skin and subcutaneous tissues are highly vascular, being supplied by the dorsal artery and vein of the clitoris and the bilateral internal pudendal arterial and venous systems. The organ is, at least in part, an erectile one.

2. The vulvar structures are heavily innervated, receiving a bilateral somatic sensory and motor supply from the pudendal nerves and another sensory supply, largely to the skin of the labia majora and mons veneris, from the femoral, genitofemoral, and ilioinguinal nerves bilaterally. There is also an extensive autonomic nerve supply, the plexus cavernosus, with the sympathetic components derived from the sympathetic trunk and the inferior mesenteric ganglion, and the parasympathetic components originating in the second, third, and fourth sacral nerve roots and sacral ganglia. Undoubtedly, the rich cutaneous sensory innervation explains why itching is a prominent symptom of almost all vulvar diseases and why, even in the absence of local organic disease, severe pruritus of the vulvar skin may also accompany a variety of psychosomatic disturbances as well as certain generalized metabolic disorders with cutaneous manifestations.

3. The lymphatic supply to the vulva is one of the most extensive of any of the surface areas of the body. There is a rich, delicate network of local lymphatics, many cross-pathways between the two sides of the vulva via anterior and posterior "commissure" anastomotic channels or via the communicating network of channels in the mons veneris, and abundant collecting trunks passing anteriorly within the boundaries of the labiocrural folds and draining into the regional nodes of the inguinofemoral region. This extensive lymphatic supply is responsible for many of the gross pathologic characteristics of local vulvar diseases and is, of course, important in connection with the natural history and proper treatment of vulvar carcinomas (Chap. 29).

The functions of the vulva are largely supportive and protective. The skin and subcutaneous structures, including the secretory glands and hair-bearing appendages, serve the twofold purpose of adequately supporting and protecting this sensitive and delicate area, much of the time sealing it off from a potentially injurious external environment, while at the same time permitting and facilitating normal sexual and reproductive function. In this regard, its lubricative function and its mating function—the latter being particularly obvious in lower animals—suggest that vulvar physiology is probably to some extent linked to the female steroid hormone cycle and that the vulvar skin and its appendages may be responsive to variations in steroid metabolism.

An awareness of the specialized anatomy of the vulva and its specific histologic components is most helpful for understanding the nature and origin of the various vulvar disorders as well as for their clinical recognition. This information is outlined in the following sections.

Specialized Anatomy of the Vulva

1. *Gross anatomic components:* mons veneris, labia majora, labia minora, clitoris, vestibule, accessory glands (Bartholin's, Skene's)
2. *Histologic components of the vulvar skin organ*
   a. Epidermis
   b. Dermis
   c. Glandular elements
      (1) Hair follicles
      (2) Sebaceous glands
      (3) Sweat glands
          (a) Eccrine glands
          (b) Apocrine glands
3. *Normal underlying tissues:* fat, muscle, fibrous tissue, lymphatics, blood vessels, nerves
4. *Aberrant tissues:* accessory breast tissue, paramesonephric (müllerian) and mesonephric (wolffian) duct remnants, endometriosis
5. *Gross anatomic abnormalities:* pudendal and inguinal hernias

Histologic Origin of Certain Vulvar Diseases

1. *Epidermis-dermis:* epidermoid carcinoma, malignant melanoma, vulvar dystrophy, lichen sclerosus, and many other common dermatologic disorders
2. *Glandular elements*
   a. Hair follicles: folliculitis
   b. Sebaceous glands: seborrheic dermatitis; rarely, carcinoma
   c. Sweat glands
      (1) Eccrine: hidradenoma
      (2) Apocrine: hidradenitis suppurativa, Paget's disease, Fox-Fordyce disease
3. *Normal underlying tissues:* lipoma, fibroma, sarcomas, hemangiomas
4. *Aberrant tissues:* ectopic breast tissue (rarely, adenocarcinoma), vulvar cysts, endometriosis

Vulvitis and Common Dermatologic Disorders of the Vulva

Vulvitis is not a specific disease or even group of diseases. Rather, vulvar inflammation may arise in connection with a number of underlying disorders, both local and generalized in nature.

1. It may be the first manifestation of a systemic disease (e.g., the specific type of vulvitis seen in diabetes) or part of a generalized dermatologic disorder (e.g., psoriasis, syphilis).
2. It may be entirely secondary to a specific vaginitis, the irritating discharge from the latter producing vulvar inflammation (vulvovaginitis), as seen with trichomonal or candidal vaginitis.
3. It may represent a secondary inflammatory reaction arising in a potentially far more serious vulvar lesion (e.g., vulvar dystrophies, carcinoma in situ, Paget's disease, or even early invasive carcinoma).
4. It may be an accompanying manifestation of a specific local dermatologic condition or a venereal disease.

It is therefore obvious that a thorough, detailed history, complete physical examination and careful pelvic evaluation, and appropriate laboratory studies, including vaginal smears and cultures and urine and blood tests to investigate the possibility of an underlying disease, are essential to accurate diagnosis and proper management. If the presence of a malignant or premalignant vulvar lesion is suggested, a vulvar biopsy should be done.

Vulvar Infections. There are a variety of dermatologic and infectious conditions of the vulva frequently evaluated and managed by the gynecologist or dermatologist. Some of these diseases are similar to dermatologic conditions found elsewhere on the body, whereas others are unique to the vulva. Infections of the vulva often coexist with an infection of the vagina, and therefore the term *vulvovaginitis* is used frequently. In this section, infections that present with primarily vulvar symptoms are reviewed. Other infections were discussed under the section on vaginitis in this chapter.

For purposes of classification, vulvar infections may be divided into nonulcerative or ulcerative lesions.

NONULCERATIVE LESIONS

CONDYLOMAS. Condylomata acuminata, commonly called "genital warts," is caused by a sexually transmitted virus. An estimated 3 million cases are diagnosed annually in the United States. The incidence increased to epidemic proportions during the 1980s, with an estimated 400 percent increase in visits to physicians because of symptomatic vulvar condylomas. Although clearly a sexually transmitted disease with 60 to 80 percent of male partners also infected, it is not currently reported to public health authorities. Condyloma acuminatum is caused by a DNA-containing human papilloma virus. Of the many subtypes of this virus identified to date, subtypes 6 and 11 are most frequently found in these condylomas. Because growth of this virus has not been accomplished in the laboratory to date, subtyping is based on DNA probing of the viral genome in the human cell. Following exposure to the human papilloma virus, incubation before clinical evidence of condyloma acuminatum may vary significantly, but on average it is approximately three months. The peak age at diagnosis of condyloma acuminatum is between 15 and 25 years in sexually active women. This age distribution is similar to that of other sexually transmitted diseases, e.g., gonorrhea and *Chlamydia* infection; and in many instances more than one sexually transmitted disease is found to coexist in the same patient.

Condylomas frequently infect the entire lower genital tract including the vulva, vagina, urethra, and anus. However, the warts are usually first brought to medical attention because of external vulvar or anal lesions easily identified by the patient. Condylomas of the vulva usually cause pruritic irritation and occasional bleeding. The warts may become moist and macerated, and are prone to secondary bacterial infection. The course of condyloma acuminatum may be indolent with frequent spontaneous regression, recurrences, and reinfection. The spontaneous regression rate of condyloma acuminatum has been estimated at approximately 33 percent within six months of initial infection.

Because of the high frequency of repeat clinical infections, treatment of condyloma acuminatum is frequently frustrating to the patient and the physician. Unfortunately, until a systemic therapy specifically directed at eradication of the human papilloma virus is developed, it is likely that this frustration will continue to exist to a greater or lesser degree. Additionally, there is evidence that the human papilloma virus is associated with the development of cervical, vaginal, and vulvar epidermal (squamous) carcinoma, although types 6 and 11 (which cause condylomas) are not as frequently associated with malignancy as are the other human papilloma virus types (Chap. 25).

To a large degree, the clinical course and natural history of condylomas depend on the host's defense and cell-mediated immunity. Patients with altered cell-mediated immunity, especially immunosuppressed renal transplant patients or patients receiving systemic chemotherapy, are at a much higher risk for developing condyloma acuminatum. Other states with altered immunity, including pregnancy, diabetes, and oral contraceptive use, may increase the frequency of clinical infections. A pregnant patient with condyloma acuminatum presents a significant challenge in that large condylomas of the vulva or vagina may obstruct or impede labor or may lead to significant postpartum hemorrhage that is difficult to control as the condylomas are torn with vaginal and vulvar dilatation at the time of vaginal delivery. Important to the infant is the occurrence of laryngeal papillomas, which are associated with delivery through a vaginal canal infected with condyloma acuminatum. The incidence of this occurrence, fortunately, is relatively low, and at the present time cesarean section is not recommended for routine prophylaxis of laryngeal papillomatosis.

The diagnosis of condyloma acuminatum is usually easily made based on clinical examination. The acuminate wart has a raised papillary or spiked surface. Early in the course of infection, small 1- to 5-mm lesions may be identified. As the disease progresses, pedunculated polypoid growths appear that may flatten and extend over large areas of the vulva and vagina. Most of these warts are white to gray, although those involving mucosal surfaces of the vagina or cervix may be pink to purple. Small warts may be more easily identified by the colposcope (Chap. 25). It is not usually necessary to biopsy "classic" condylomas, but biopsy is clearly indicated for lesions whose appearance is not as clear-cut or for those that have had an indolent course of recurrences or a poor response to standard therapy. Lesions that sometimes mimic condyloma acuminatum include carcinoma in situ of the vulva or verrucous carcinoma. Verrucous carcinoma, however, is usually seen in older women not of the age group where condylomas are most prevalent. Evaluation of the patient with condyloma acuminatum should also include a search for perianal, vaginal, urethral, and cervical warts. In the vagina and cervix the condylomas may appear flat (flat wart) or may have the more traditional appearance of "tiny cauliflowers." A Papanicolaou smear should be obtained from the cervix, as patients with condylomas have a high incidence of cervical intraepithelial neoplasia, often induced by the human papilloma virus.

The most successful treatment of condyloma acuminatum is local destruction of the lesion with an attempt to eradicate viral particles in adjacent skin. Small lesions are often easily treated with 25% podophyllin in tincture of benzoin. Podophyllin should be applied to epidermal surfaces only. The patient is instructed to wash the remaining podophyllin and tincture of benzoin away with soap and water 4 to 6 hours later. Treatment should be repeated at weekly intervals, and usually three or four treatments are sufficient to eradicate small lesions. Podophyllin should not be used on large lesions or in the vagina and cervix, as systemic absorption may lead to significant neurotoxicity, liver failure, and possible death. It should also not be used during pregnancy, as absorption may lead to congenital anomalies or fetal death. Trichloracetic acid may also be applied topically to the wart, although the initial application may be slightly more painful than podophyllin.

5-Fluorouracil cream (Efudex 5%) has also been used with success to treat vulvar and vaginal condylomas. This treatment is especially attractive for treating diffuse condylomas in the vagina, as it may be applied high in the vaginal canal with a vaginal applicator and applied directly to the condylomas on the vulva. Treatment should be on a daily basis for ap-

proximately ten days; repeat treatment may be required if the warts recur. Widespread and prolonged application of Efudex to the vulvar skin may lead to painful ulceration, however.

A large condyloma acuminatum lesion requires a more aggressive surgical approach. The carbon dioxide laser is now the current surgical treatment of choice because of the advantages of laser vaporization (precise vaporization of tissues, minimal thermal damage, and therefore less scarring of the vulva). When condylomas are vaporized from the vulva, an additional 0.5 to 1.0 cm of clinically apparent normal skin adjacent to the wart should also be vaporized to eradicate latent virus in this region. In the past, vulvar condylomas have been eradicated using electrocautery or cryotherapy, although both lead to more scarring and are probably associated with a slightly higher recurrence rate.

Unfortunately, with whatever treatment modality is chosen, the condylomas recur in at least 20 percent of patients. Therefore before treatment is instituted the patient should be forewarned about this possibility to minimize later frustrations.

Adequate therapy of condyloma acuminatum includes treatment of the patient's male sexual partner. As previously noted, 60 to 80 percent of male sexual partners of women with clinically obvious condyloma acuminatum are found to have warts on the penile shaft, scrotum, or medial thighs. Men should be evaluated by a dermatologist or a urologist interested in managing this disease process. Until both partners are adequately treated and in remission, condoms should be used during sexual intercourse.

Because of the chronic nature of condyloma acuminatum in some patients, other therapies are being evaluated, including the use of interferons and autologous vaccines. Initial results of interferon therapy are encouraging, especially realizing that patients participating in these experimental trials have failed many previous conventional therapies. The exact dose and optimal route of administration (topical, intralesional, or parenteral) are currently being evaluated.

BARTHOLIN'S GLAND CYSTS AND ABSCESS. Batholin's gland is a mucus-secreting gland located bilaterally in the lower pole of the labium majus, connected to the surface by a transitional cell-lined duct that opens just external to the hymeneal ring. The function of Bartholin's gland appears to be to moisten the vestibule, but it is clearly not significantly important in terms of lubrication for sexual function. Most diseases of Bartholin's gland are caused by obstruction of the duct, which may follow trauma, infection, or epithelial hyperplasia; or the obstruction may be due to a relative congenital atresia or narrowing. When the duct is obstructed, a mucus-filled cyst of Bartholin's gland (Fig. 14-2) may subsequently form.

Many of these cysts are asymptomatic, remain small (1 to 2 cm), and require no particular therapy. On the other hand, drainage of a Bartholin's gland cyst is clearly indicated if it is large enough to cause symptoms in the patient (commonly dyspareunia or vulvar pressure), is rapidly enlarging, is painful, becomes infected, or has developed in a woman over age 40.

The most common problem with Bartholin's gland, which brings patients to the physician's attention with acute symptoms, is a Bartholin's gland abscess. This abscess is typified by acute onset of pain, swelling, exquisite tenderness, and associated cellulitis of the vulva. Dyspareunia is frequently reported, and the patient often has difficulty walking.

The treatment of a Bartholin's gland abscess follows the basic surgical principle that an abscess must be drained. An additional treatment principle is to establish a permanent fistulous tract between the epithelial cell-lined abscess or cyst and the vulvar epithelium. Simple incision and drainage is frequently followed by recurrent abscesses or cysts. Therefore marsupialization is recommended (Fig. 14-3), which can usually be accomplished under local anesthesia in the office. Some clinicians have chosen to use the Word catheter, which is a small catheter with an inflatable balloon that is positioned inside the cyst or abscess cavity, thereby establishing drainage. The catheter is left in the cavity for four to six weeks while an epithelialized tract develops. Usually, however, simple marsupialization is sufficient.

Because *Neisseria gonorrhoeae* is found in approximately 10 percent of Bartholin's gland abscesses, a specimen for culture should be obtained when the abscess is drained. On the other hand, unless *N. gonorrhoeae* is isolated, antibiotic therapy is generally not necessary, as the infection is usually adequately treated with drainage of the abscess. Warm sitz baths several times a day following marsupialization reduce pain and speed the healing process.

Bartholin's gland abscesses developing in a diabetic patient are particularly worrisome, as these patients have a relatively high frequency of developing secondary necrotizing fasciitis, which may be fatal in a high percentage of the patients. Aggressive surgical drainage with antibiotic coverage should be the initial treatment with close surveillance for any signs of a necrotizing fasciitis.

Also of concern is a Bartholin's gland cyst that arises in a woman over age 40. In this case, Bartholin's gland carcinoma must be suspected and the diagnosis excluded by biopsy or excision of the cyst. In younger women, however, excision of Bartholin's gland cysts or abscesses should be avoided as it is usually unnecessary.

In rare cases where recurrent cysts or abscesses are

Fig. 14-2. Gross clinical appearance of a Bartholin cyst of the vulva.

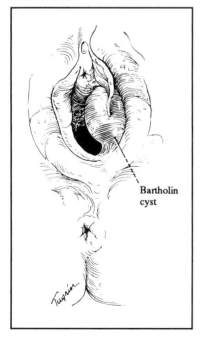

Bartholin cyst

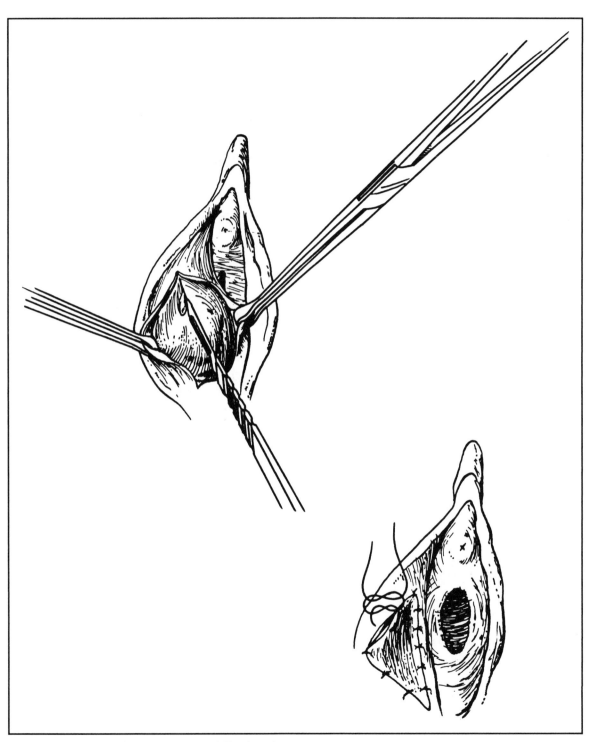

Fig. 14-3. Incision, drainage, and marsupialization of a
Bartholin abscess.

formed, excision of the cyst may be indicated, although the surgeon must be aware that because of the extensive vascularity in this area, what appears to be a simple procedure may be associated with a reasonably high blood loss. Excising a Bartholin's gland cyst or abscess may be associated with later chronic pain due to vulvar scarring.

CANDIDA VULVITIS. *Candida* vulvitis is a common problem that is usually associated with a vaginal infection. Because the vagina is usually the primary site of infection, *Candida* infection is discussed in more detail under the section on vaginitis.

Diabetics are prone to develop *Candida* vulvitis; and, in fact, approximately one-half of all patients who have fulminant *Candida* vulvitis are diabetic. Patients who are not known to be diabetic should undergo blood glucose screening for glucose intolerance, as *Candida* vulvitis may be the first symptom suggesting diabetes mellitus. Usually patients with *Candida* vulvitis have severe pruritus and burning with secondary excoriation and ulceration. The skin of the labia major, labia minora, and the labial crural fold is often entirely involved.

On examination, the vulva is intensely erythematous and moist, and satellite pustules are often found at the periphery. Examination of the vagina may reveal the classic "cottage cheese"-appearing, grayish-white, thick vaginal discharge. Microscopic examination of a wet preparation aided by the application of potassium hydroxide is usually diagnostic, although culture on Nickerson's medium may be indicated when the diagnosis is not apparent or in recurrent cases.

The therapy for vulvar candidiasis is directed at treating the vaginal *Candida* infection, as discussed in the section on vaginitis, utilizing an imidazole cream or suppository regimen. Gentian violet 1% may be painted on the vulva weekly but is usually reserved for refractory cases. Diabetic control is clearly indicated to minimize the recurrence of *Candida* vulvitis.

PEDICULOSIS PUBIS. Pediculosis pubis, or crab louse (*Phthirus pubis*), is transmitted by close contact or by contaminated towels or linen shared with an infected person. This species is different from the head and body louse and is usually confined to pubic hair. Pediculosis may be found in pubic hair in any of three stages: the egg stage (nit) usually around the base of hair follicles, the nymph, and the adult form. The adult is an approximately 1-mm, dark gray, slow-moving insect.

Symptoms are usually constant pubic itching with irritated pubic skin secondary to scratching. Examination with the naked eye or aided by colposcopic magnification usually reveals the nits or adult forms. Skin scrapings studied under the microscope may show the typical crab louse.

Treatment of pediculosis must include disinfection of contaminated linens and clothes. All family members should be treated, including showering and shampooing using lindane (Kwell) shampoo, followed by application of lindane lotion to affected areas. The lotion should be allowed to remain on the skin for 12 hours before washing and is reapplied on a second consecutive day.

SCABIES. Scabies, or the itch mite (*Sarcoptes scabiei*), is transmitted by close personal contact with an infected person. In contrast to localized disease noted with pediculosis, scabies usually is found to be widespread over the entire body, not confined to the hair. The female mite burrows underneath the skin to lay her eggs, leaving a characteristic lesion. Severe itching, papules, vesicles, and burrows result and can be seen on examination. The burrow may be excavated using a needle and the contents studied microscopically, searching for the offending mite. Treatment of scabies is identical to that for pediculosis, though lindane lotion should be applied to the entire body, rather than just to the affected area of the pubic hair.

MOLLUSCUM CONTAGIOSUM. Molluscum contagiosum is a poxvirus that is spread by close contact with an infected person and by autoinoculation. In contrast to other infections, molluscum contagiosum is only mildly contagious. After exposure the incubation prior to clinical evidence of the infection varies from two to seven weeks. Most patients are entirely asymptomatic; they usually seek medical advice for the management of small nodules on the vulva that are usually not pruritic.

On examination, small domed papules approximately 1 to 5 mm in diameter are noted. The center of the papule is umbilicated and underneath is a nodule filled with a white, waxy material that can be easily removed with a curet. Diagnosis of molluscum contagiosum is based on the microscopic examination of the waxy material from the "water wart." The material is smeared on a slide and stained with Wright's stain or Giemsa stain. Microscopic examination reveals intracytoplasmic molluscum bodies that are characteristic of this disease.

Therapy is usually excision with local anesthesia. A sharp dermal curet can be used to excise the nodule. The base of the nodule is then treated with trichloracetic acid or Monsel solution. In a similar fashion, the base of the nodule may be treated with cryotherapy, electrocautery, or laser vaporization.

ULCERATED LESIONS. Ulcerated lesions of the vulva are frequently caused by primary vulvar infections or secondary infections of traumatized or abraded vulvar skin. Because many primary vulvar ulcers are due to venereal disease (herpes, syphilis, lymphogranuloma venereum, granuloma inguinale, chancroid) physicians and other health care personnel must take adequate precautions to minimize transmission of these communicable diseases to other patients, health care personnel, or even autoinoculation of the patient herself. It is important to establish a definite diagnosis as to the etiology of the ulcer. The patient, her consorts, and society at large should not be left with the uncertainty as to whether the patient truly has a venereal disease. Confirming the presence of venereal disease includes the obligation to identify and treat sexual partners and to provide proper counseling. Furthermore, finding one venereal disease suggests the probability that the patient has a second sexually transmitted disease of the lower genital tract. Therefore, when the question of sexually transmitted disease is raised, full screening that includes cultures and a serologic evaluation is recommended.

Some sexually transmitted diseases are associated with a high incidence of epithelial neoplasia of the vulva, vagina, and cervix. Papanicolaou smear screening of the cervix and vagina are clearly appropriate when a vulvar infection is found, and biopsy specimens for histologic evaluation should be obtained from any vulvar ulcer or lesion in which a diagnosis cannot be confirmed by other means or that does not improve with therapy.

HERPES INFECTION. Infection of the vulva by herpes simplex virus (HSV) currently is the most common cause of vulvar ulcers. As with other sexually transmitted diseases, herpes has become epidemic, with an estimated 2 million cases being diagnosed annually. Herpes simplex virus is an enveloped DNA-containing virus that can be subgrouped into two varieties. HSV-1 is usually associated with oronasal infections ("cold sores"), and HSV-2 usually causes infections of the vulva, vagina, cervix, and anus. However, either type may be found in either location of the body; HSV-1 is found in 10 to 30 percent of pelvic infections.

Herpes simplex virus infection is clearly a sexually transmitted disease and is highly contagious. The infected sexual partner may or may not have active lesions and may be entirely asymptomatic yet be actively shedding viral particles. After exposure the incubation period is 48 hours to seven days before the onset of a primary herpes infection. The infection may be preceded by a prodrome of malaise, fever, inguinal adenopathy, and tingling of the vulvar skin. Subsequently, vesicles develop on the vulva that rupture after several days, leaving shallow ulcers. These ulcers may become confluent and are often painful.

Ulceration of the urethra causes dysuria and may lead to urinary retention, requiring urinary catheter drainage by either a transurethral Foley catheter or a suprapubic catheter. Four to eight percent of patients develop meningitis caused by the herpes, and rare patients develop encephalitis—an ominous sign associated with an approximately 50 percent mortality rate.

During the primary infection the ulcers persist for approximately one to three weeks and then heal spontaneously without leaving a scar. The ulcers may become secondarily infected with bacteria, leading to more pain and slower resolution of the infection. Viral shedding may persist for two to three weeks after complete resolution of the lesions. This scenario is usual for the primary, or first, HSV infection. An occasional patient has a relatively asymptomatic infection that is not recognized, though the HSV antibody titer is elevated.

The natural history of herpes simplex vulvar infection is described as recurrent episodes at unpredictable times. The herpes virus is latent and resides in the dorsal root ganglion of S2, S3, and S4 and within the autonomic nerves along the uterosacral ligaments.

Recurrences seem to be associated with stress or emotional upheaval or with immunosuppressions, as is found during pregnancy, in patients being treated with cytotoxic chemotherapy, or in leukemic patients. Because of the recurrent and chronic nature of this infection, many patients have significant psychological trauma, requiring counseling and emotional support. Feelings of social isolation and being infected with an "incurable disease" are common problems. Many communities have support groups and counseling centers to aid patients who have herpes infections.

Symptoms of recurrent infections are usually milder and have a shorter duration than during the primary infection. However, vesicle formation followed by a painful ulcer remains characteristic. Many patients have a vulvar prodrome five to ten days prior to the development of vesicles described as a tingling of the vulvar skin or pruritus. Patients who have this prodrome should abstain from sexual contact throughout the prodrome, during the active phase of the lesions, and for a week following the disappearance of the lesions in order to minimize exposure of sexual partners to active viral particles.

Genital herpes infections have been associated with the development of severe dysplasia and invasive cervical carcinoma, although a cause-and-effect relation has not been proved. Because these patients do seem to be at higher risk for the development of cervical neoplasia, a Papanicolaou smear should be obtained at least annually.

Genital herpes infection during pregnancy also raises the specter of a severe neonatal infection. Neonates infected with HSV often develop profound neurologic injury and have a high mortality rate. Patients who have had previous herpes infections should include this information in their prenatal history so that they undergo close surveillance with cultures throughout the third trimester of pregnancy and so the clinician will be suspicious of lesions found on the vulva or cervix during pregnancy. Patients who are actively shedding herpesvirus or who have lesions should have cesarean section deliveries, preferably before the amniotic membranes are ruptured, to reduce the risk of neonatal herpes encephalitis.

Aside from the physical findings of vesicles or small or confluent ulceration of vulvar skin, culture is the most sensitive method to detect herpes infection. Herpesvirus culture has an approximately 80 percent sensitivity but varies depending on the state of the active lesion. Herpesvirus growth is much more frequent when a culture specimen is obtained from vesicles rather than from the crusted ulcers later in the course. Papanicolaou smear may be used to detect giant cells associated with herpes infections, although a 30 percent false-negative rate is expected. Serologic tests for herpes demonstrate only if the patient has been exposed in the past, although acute-phase and convalescent titers may be used to support the diagnosis of a resolving infection.

To date there is no active antiviral medication that can eradicate the herpes infection and forestall recurrences. Current treatment is primarily aimed at providing symptomatic pain relief with the use of oral and topical analgesics, cold wet compresses of Burow's solution, or artificial seawater sitz baths. Patients who have severe pain, urinary retention, malaise, hepatic or central nervous system involvement require hospitalization for more intensive therapy.

The most significant breakthrough in herpes therapy has been the development of acyclovir, which is provided in topical, oral, or intravenous forms. Intravenous use is reserved for patients with severe systemic infections and those necessitating hospitalization. In general, acyclovir therapy can reduce the duration of viral shedding, the time to healing, the duration of symptoms, and the clinical course of the disease. With primary infections, the use of oral acyclovir given as 200 mg tablets five times a day for five to seven days reduces the clinical course by approximately one week. The use of topically applied acyclovir ointment in primary infections seems to reduce the course somewhat, although not as well as the oral regimen. Treatment of recurrent episodes is of less benefit unless the treatment can be initiated within two days of the onset of lesions. In a patient who has a vulvar prodrome prior to the onset of lesions, the use of oral acyclovir with a dosing schedule similar to that used for primary infections may shorten the clinical course by approximately 1 to 2 days. Continuous treatment with acyclovir (200 mg orally two to five times daily) is suggested for prophylaxis of patients with frequent recurrent herpes vulvar infections. This regimen, used over a six-month period, appears to reduce the frequency of recurrent infections by at least 75 percent among patients who experience frequent recurrences (at least six times a year). Following discontinuation of chronic treatment with acyclovir, the frequency of infections appears to return to that experienced previously. Acyclovir should not be used in women who may become pregnant or who are pregnant, as its safety has not been established. Finally, the chronic use of acyclovir may promote selection of resistant strains of HSV. Clearly, optimal treatment for genital herpes has yet to be established, although research into the development of a vaccine holds the most promise for the prevention of this disease.

SYPHILIS. Despite ready means for diagnosis and simple and effective methods of treatment, syphilis remains an important sexually transmitted disease in the United States today. Approximately 280,000 cases are reported annually in the United States. A full discussion of the multiple manifestations and ramifications of syphilis is presented in Chapter 15. This section discusses only the vulvar manifestations of syphilis.

Infection of the vulva by the spirochete *Treponema pallidum* leads to vulvar ulceration with both primary and secondary syphilitic infections. The initial contact of the spirochete may lead to a primary chancre of the vulva, vagina, or cervix. Actually, the primary chancre may appear at any point the spirochete has broken through the skin; therefore it may be found on the mouth, tongue, or elsewhere on the body. The vulvar primary chancre is classically described as a single, firm, painless ulcer with an indurated base. More often, however, the chancre is multiple and may be painful if secondarily infected with bacteria. Classically, a chancre becomes clinically apparent approximately three weeks after inoculation (ten- to ninety-day incubation) and heals spontaneously within approximately one to six weeks without any therapy. Inguinal adenopathy, which is usually nontender, may be apparent at the time of the primary chancre.

Evaluation of a lesion suspected to be a primary chancre should include darkfield microscopic examination of a wet preparation from the ulcer. Visualization of *Treponema* is diagnostic. The VDRL test is positive in approximately 70 percent of cases of syphilis at this stage of the disease. If the VDRL is negative, it should be repeated weekly for four weeks before assuming that the patient does not have syphilis.

Secondary syphilis develops after hematogenous dissemination of the spirochete, with clinical symptoms becoming apparent three weeks to six months after the primary chancre. Vulvar findings of secondary syphilis include soft papules or mucus patches that may be erosive. In contrast to lesions due to genital herpes, the secondary syphilitic lesions are usually larger, raised, and much less tender. At this juncture, VDRL serology is positive in these patients, aiding in diagnosis. Left untreated, these secondary lesions resolve within two to six weeks.

The vulvar manifestation of tertiary syphilis—condyloma latum—is a large, flat, grayish white area involving a large amount of the vulva. Papules may appear on moist surfaces, and they may become confluent and ulcerated but are relatively painless. Adenopathy with bubo formation is also noted at this stage of the disease.

Having confirmed the diagnosis of primary, secondary, or tertiary syphilis based on serologic testing or darkfield examination, the patient should receive appropriate therapy as recommended by the Centers for Disease Control. Primary, uncomplicated syphilis may be adequately treated with benzathine penicillin G 2.4 million units given intramuscularly as a single dose. Alternatively, for patients with penicillin allergy, tetracycline 500 mg orally every 6 hours for fifteen days or erythromycin 500 mg orally every 6 hours for fifteen days is adequate. The other recommendations for treatment of various stages of syphilis are discussed in detail in Chapter 15.

OTHER VENEREAL DISEASES OF THE VULVA. Granuloma inguinale, lymphogranuloma venereum, and chancroid are sexually transmitted diseases that present initially as vulvar ulcers. Historically, they have been included in gynecologic textbooks. These diseases were much more frequent in the United States prior to the advent of antibiotics and careful reporting and surveillance of communicable and venereal diseases. Fortunately, they are now rare, and even a gynecologist with an active practice sees them infrequently. On the other hand, these diseases are found not infrequently in Third World countries and in the tropics.

Granuloma Inguinale. Granuloma inguinale is a chronic, ulcerative bacterial infection of the skin and subcutaneous tissue of the vulva caused by a gram-negative intracellular nonmotile rod (*Calymmatobacterium granulomatis*). Although the disease is relatively common in the tropics and the Caribbean islands, fewer than 100 cases were reported in the United States during 1988.

Granuloma inguinale is spread via sexual intercourse and close sexual contact, although it is not highly contagious. The incubation time from exposure to clinically obvious infection is approximately one to twelve weeks. Initially, an asymptomatic nodule is noted on the vulva that becomes progressively ulcerated. The ulcer is typified by a beefy-red lesion with fresh granulation tissue at its base. These ulcers may grow in size and coalesce, destroying normal vulvar architecture. Unless secondarily infected, the ulcers remain relatively painless, however. During this stage of the infection, inguinal adenopathy is infrequent unless the patient suffers from a secondary bacterial infection. Left untreated, the disease results in significant scarring and lymphedema of the vulva, giving the vulva an engorged, thickened, leathery appearance.

The diagnosis of granuloma inguinale is based on the histologic or cytologic finding of Donovan bodies in smears from the ulcerated lesion or a biopsy specimen stained with Giemsa or Wright stain. Donovan bodies appear as clusters of dark bacteria found in the cytoplasm of large mononuclear cells. Because it is difficult grossly to distinguish the ulcerated lesion from squamous cell carcinoma or basal cell carcinoma, a biopsy is recommended to exclude invasive cancer.

The treatment of granuloma inguinale is simple: tetracycline 500 mg orally every 6 hours until complete response of the vulvar lesions is noted (usually two to three weeks). Parenteral aminoglycosides may be used for refractory cases.

Lymphogranuloma Venereum. Lymphogranuloma venereum, a classic venereal disease, is now relatively rare in the United States, with fewer than 500 new cases reported annually. The disease results in a chronic infection of lymphatic tissues of the vulva, perineum, anus, and inguinal and pelvic lymph nodes caused by *Chlamydia trachomatis,* serotype L. Fol-

lowing an incubation period of one to four weeks, the patient develops nonspecific symptoms of fever and malaise associated with a vulvar papule that undergoes ulceration but heals spontaneously. Approximately four weeks later, tender inguinal adenitis or pelvic lymphadenitis develops and evolves into buboes that may ultimately rupture and drain. These buboes are similar to those found with secondary syphilis, and both venereal diseases must be considered in the differential diagnosis. Most often, unilateral lymph nodes are involved with the disease. Gradually, the inguinal, vulvar, and anorectal structures fibrose and cause stricture. This phase leads to the "groove sign" in the genitocrural fold, which is a depression between inflamed lymph nodes. Sinus tract formation on the vulva and the perineum and rectovaginal fistulas are common in advanced, late, untreated disease.

The diagnosis of lymphogranuloma venereum is made either by a complement fixation test (LGV-CFT) or by monoclonal antibody identification of *Chlamydia trachomatis.* The VDRL may be falsely positive in 20 percent of cases, and therefore fluorescent treponemal antibody absorption (FTA-ABS) test should be done to confirm the diagnosis of syphilis.

Therapy of lymphogranuloma venereum is with tetracycline 500 mg orally every 6 hours for a minimum of three weeks or until resolution of the disease. Alternative treatment with sulfamethoxazole 1 gm orally twice a day provides adequate antibiotic therapy. Buboes in the inguinal region should be aspirated with a large-bore needle but should not be incised and drained, as it would lead to worsening of the inguinal scarring and deformity. Management of late, advanced cases following antibiotic therapy often requires surgical excision and vulvar, perineal, and anal reconstruction. In some intractable cases a colostomy is advised.

Chancroid. Chancroid is another rare cause of acute vulvar ulceration. Approximately 1500 cases of chancroid are reported to the Centers for Disease Control annually, with most occurring in men. In contrast to a syphilitic chancre, the chancroid ulcer is always painful and most often soft. Chancroid is caused by a small gram-negative rod that is a facultative anaerobe (*Hemophilus ducreyi*). It presents clinically as solitary or multiple ulcers on the vulva and, less frequently, on the vagina or cervix. The ulcer is often covered by a necrotic gray exudate, and approximately 50 percent of patients have tender inguinal lymph nodes. *H. ducreyi* is difficult to culture. Therefore Gram stain and biopsy are usually required to find the classic streptobacillary chains of the gram-negative rod, classically described as a "school of fish," in an extracellular location.

Therapy for chancroid is with a combination of trimethoprim 160 mg and sulfamethoxazole 800 mg orally every 12 hours for ten days. Erythromycin 500 mg orally every 6 hours for ten days provides excellent coverage for patients allergic to sulfa drugs.

HIDRADENITIS SUPPURATIVA. Hidradenitis suppurativa is a chronic recurrent infection of the apocrine sweat glands of the vulva, groins, and axillary skin and subcutaneous tissue. The etiology of this disease is unknown, but it is not a sexually transmitted disease. The bacteriology of the abscesses and draining sinuses reveals a wide range of flora, mostly endemic to the vulva and vagina. Infections with *Staphylococcus* and *Streptococcus* are common. Early in the course of the disease, small, raised lesions that ulcerate and drain may be inadvertently diagnosed as folliculitis or a furuncle; but as the disease progresses, the true nature of hidradenitis becomes apparent with multiple chronic draining abscesses and sinus tracts involving the vulva, medial thighs, and groins. Subsequent scarring of the subcutaneous tissue and skin with palpable subcutaneous "cords" is classic. Late in the course of hidradenitis suppurativa the chronically indurated and draining sinuses may mimic lymphogranuloma venereum, Crohn's disease, granuloma inguinale, or vulvar tuberculosis. In many patients axillary sweat glands are similarly involved.

Symptomatic therapy with careful local hygiene and systemic and topical antibiotics may provide some relief, though usually not a permanent cure. In most cases, surgical excision of involved tissues or incision and drainage of the sinus tracts offers the best hope for significant resolution of symptoms. In advanced cases partial vulvectomy with vulvar reconstruction using a split-thickness skin graft or other plastic reconstructive procedures should be considered.

MISCELLANEOUS ULCERATIVE CONDITIONS OF THE VULVA. There are myriad other causes of vulvar ulcerations,

most of which are relatively rare and usually are a manifestation of a more widely disseminated systemic disease.

For example, vulvar ulcerations may be the first manifestation of *Crohn's disease,* preceding by months or years the recognition of the gastrointestinal manifestations of this disease. The vulvar ulcers of Crohn's disease are usually linear in appearance and are typified as a "knife cut" on the labia majora. These ulcers are classic and are unlike any other ulcers of the vulva. Further involvement of the perineal and perianal areas by Crohn's disease results in edema, draining sinuses, and rectovaginal fistulas. Crohn's disease must be considered prior to undertaking surgical therapy of perineal sinuses or rectovaginal fistulas, as the surgical result is doomed to failure if Crohn's disease is not adequately treated and in a quiescent state.

Tuberculosis of the vulva is exceedingly rare, especially in the United States. In patients with systemic disease, tuberculosis may present as draining sinus tracts from pelvic tuberculosis located in deep pelvic locations. Cultures of these draining sinus tracts yield the acid-fast bacillus. Vulvar tuberculosis responds equally well to appropriate systemic antimicrobial therapy.

Behçet's disease is characterized by primary symptoms of relapsing oral and genital ulcerations and ocular inflammation. Minor criteria for the disease include ulcerative colitis, thrombophlebitis, acneiform skin eruptions, arthritis, and neurologic aberrations. An autoimmune etiology has been proposed but not proved for this disease. The vulvar manifestations of the disease are usually a highly destructive, tender vulvar lesion leading to fenestration of the labia minora, scarring, and a loss of vulvar tissue. The diagnosis of Behçet's disease is based on finding major symptoms and at least one minor criterion. It is primarily a diagnosis of exclusion once herpes, syphilis, Crohn's disease, and pemphigus have been excluded.

Pemphigus and *pemphagoid* are autoimmune diseases causing bolus lesions of the skin and mucous membranes. They are rarely confined to the vulva. As the bullae erupt, the skin appears ulcerated in the affected area. Diagnosis is confirmed by biopsy of the lesion and with staining for immunoglobulin G (IgG). Intracellular deposition of IgG identifies pemphigus, whereas IgG found on basement membranes at the dermoepidermal junction identifies pemphigoid. The management of pemphigus and pemphigoid of the vulva is similar to the current recommended treatment for other dermatologic and systemic involvement and should be carried out by a physician skilled in the care of this disease.

Pyoderma of the vulva is manifested as furuncles, abscesses, and possibly necrotizing fasciitis secondary to pyogenic bacterial infection. It is almost always due to poor perineal hygiene, causing irritation, scratching, and subsequent infected ulceration. Draining sinus tracts are relatively rare with pyoderma. The therapy for pyoderma is primary cleansing and use of antibiotics systemically and topically. Cultures of the ulcerated areas may help to select a specific antibiotic.

Finally, and most important, ulceration of the vulva may represent an *invasive vulvar cancer.* Squamous cell carcinoma and basal cell carcinoma of the vulva may appear initially as an ulcer with an appearance no more worrisome than that of many of the ulcers previously noted in this chapter. Important to the early diagnosis of vulvar cancer is timely vulvar biopsy. Even when another etiology for the vulvar ulcer has been identified with culture, serology, or cytology, a persistent or unresponsive ulcer should be rebiopsied to exclude the possibility of invasive cancer.

VULVAR DYSTROPHIES. Vulvar dystrophies are a group of diseases of the vulvar skin that have been inadequately evaluated and treated. Because of confusing terminology, which described the gross vulvar lesion rather than vulvar histology, delay in diagnosis and inappropriate therapies have abounded. It is unfortunate because vulvar dystrophies comprise the most common disease found on the vulva. Vulvar dystrophies can be chronically disabling, confining the patient to home with severe and chronic pruritus and vulvar pain. Accurate diagnosis and appropriate therapy may avoid these problems in many patients in the future.

Paramount to the evaluation and management of vulvar dystrophies is the histologic diagnosis of the disease process, which must be based on vulvar biopsy results. Because the vulvar biopsy technique is so simple (Chap. 29) it should be readily available and performed liberally by any physician caring for the gynecologic problems of women. Delays in diagnosis and inaccurate diagnoses can be eliminated with a simple vulvar biopsy performed in the office under local anesthesia.

Further simplifying the management of vulvar dystrophy is a new nomenclature developed by the International Society for the Study of Vulvar Disease (ISSVD). The system is based on the clinical and histologic characteristics of a lesion rather than the gross or clinical descriptive factors used in the past. For example, the term vulvar "leukoplakia" was used to describe any white-appearing lesion on the vulva. White lesions, however, make up a large group of varying diseases. If a white lesion were carcinoma in situ, it would indeed carry a potential premalignant connotation. However, because of the myriad other white lesions of the vulva that have no premalignant potential, the diseases must be clearly distinguished histologically before recommending therapy that might include vulvectomy.

The ISSVD nomenclature proposed and currently used subdivides vulvar dystrophies into three groups: (1) atrophic dystrophies (lichen sclerosus); (2) hyperplastic dystrophies; and (3) mixed dystrophies (atrophic and hyperplastic). The hyperplastic and mixed dystrophies can be further subdivided as to whether they contain cellular atypia (Table 14-1).

LICHEN SCLEROSUS. Lichen sclerosus is the most common of the vulvar dystrophies. It is typified grossly by a thinning of the vulvar skin in which gradual dissolution of the labia minora and agglutination of the prepuce ultimately bury the clitoral shaft. Further scarring of the vulva leads to a decreased diameter of the introitus and eventual inability to accomplish coitus. Lichen sclerosus usually appears diffusely over most of the vulva, resulting in a pale, shiny, thin epithelium with a "wrinkled parchment" appearance. Symptoms associated with this process are primarily pruritus that may be intense, resulting in significant scratching and rubbing of the vulva, with ultimate ulceration. Continued scratching produces areas of hyperplasia, which then lead to a mixed dystrophy.

Lichen sclerosus may occur at any age and does not appear to be related to levels of systemic estrogens. The disease is seen in children, menstruating women, and most commonly postmenopausal women. The

Table 14-1. Classification of Vulvar Dystrophies Adopted by the International Society for the Study of Vulvar Disease

Vulvar dystrophy	Clinical criteria	Histologic criteria
Lichen sclerosus	Pruritic, thin parchment, "atrophic," introital stenosis	Thin, loss of rete, homogenization inflammatory infiltrate
Hyperplastic[a]	Pruritic, thick, gray or white plaques, skin, or mucosa	Acanthosis, hyperkeratosis, inflammatory infiltrate
Mixed[a]	Areas compatible with both forms present at the same time	

[a]Atypia may accompany hyperplastic dystrophy and is graded mild, moderate, or severe.

etiology of the disease is unknown, although a genetic or autoimmune hypothesis has been proposed.

Diagnosis of lichen sclerosus is often based on a fairly typical examination, as previously described. However, vulvar biopsy should be done to confirm the diagnosis before undertaking treatment. Ulcerated areas are biopsied, and toluidine blue staining may aid in the detection of areas of mixed dystrophy with atypia. Raised, thickened areas should also be biopsied to exclude the possibility of carcinoma in situ. Histologically, lichen sclerosus has a thin squamous epithelium with loss or blunting of the epithelial folds (rete ridges). The dermis is acellular and homogeneous in appearance with chronic inflammatory cells deep in this zone.

Treatment with topical 2% testosterone propionate seems to give the best results. During the acute and most symptomatic phase of the disease, testosterone should be rubbed into the affected vulvar skin three times a day. After three to four weeks the applications can be used daily for another month, as symptoms resolve. If after two months of therapy symptoms have not resolved, repeat biopsy should be done to reevaluate the disease status. It takes much longer for the cutaneous changes to regress. Lifetime maintenance therapy for lichen sclerosus is advised, applying testosterone twice weekly. For patients who cannot tolerate testosterone because of its side effects or hypersensitivity, topical progesterone cream has also been used effectively. Surgery has no role in the treatment of this disease.

HYPERPLASTIC DYSTROPHIES. Hyperplastic dystrophies are most often diagnosed in reproductive-age and menopausal women. The primary symptom of the disease is vulvar pruritus that is so intense the patient is compelled to scratch. The skin changes found on the vulva are proportional to the duration and degree of scratching.

Examination of the vulva shows foci of thickened, often excoriated skin. Further distinguishing this disease from lichen sclerosus are the findings that the clitoral prepuce and labia minora are not obliterated.

Vulvar biopsy should be done to confirm the diagnosis and to exclude the possibility of cytologic atypia or carcinoma in situ. Classically, histologic examination of hyperplastic dystrophy reveals thickened epithelium (hyperkeratosis) with enlarged rete pegs (acanthosis) and dermal inflammation. The pathologist's report may subdivide the hypertrophic dystrophies into such other diagnoses as lichen simplex chronicus, hypertrophic vulvitis, chronic reactive vulvitis, lichen planus, or neurodermatitis. Clinically, such subdivision is relatively unimportant, as the therapy and response to therapy are nearly identical for all of these processes.

Key to the treatment of hypertrophic dystrophy is the goal of stopping the chronic itch–scratch cycle. It requires a comprehensive program that is rarely successful unless most or all of the key elements are employed simultaneously. First, potential irritants to the vulva are eliminated. All perfumes, deodorants, synthetic fabrics and fibers, hygiene sprays, douches, laundry detergents, and dyes are removed from the vulvar environment. The patient is instructed to wear loosely fitting clothing and cotton undergarments. No pantyhose should be worn. The vulva must be kept clean and dry, washing with a mild soap and blowing dry the vulva with the cool setting on the hair dryer. Aveeno oatmeal baths two or three times a day help sooth the vulvar skin and reduce itching. A neurotranquilizer such as hydroxyzine (Atarax or Vistaril) should be taken at bedtime and possibly during the waking hours if the desire to scratch is overwhelming. Cotton gloves should be worn to bed at night, as many patients unconsciously scratch during their sleep. Finally, topical application of hydrocortisone cream to the affected areas two or three times a day is advised. It may be combined with crotamiton (Eurax) because of the latter's antipruritic nature. Topical corticosteroid therapy should continue for four to eight weeks before reevaluation.

Because of the chronic nature of this disease, it may take many weeks before symptoms are eliminated and the vulvar skin begins to appear normal. Usually, however, with the adequate therapy program outlined above, dramatic results can be obtained. Unless scratching is reinstituted, hypertrophic dystrophies may remain quiescent. Any persistent disease or recurrences should be reevaluated with biopsy.

MIXED DYSTROPHIES. Mixed vulvar dystrophies are established by gross examination and biopsy. As the term implies, areas of lichen sclerosus plus hyperplastic dystrophy are found and account for approximately 15 to 20 percent of all vulvar dystrophies. Mixed dystrophies are more likely to contain areas of cellular atypia, and therefore it is important to establish a diagnosis by vulvar biopsy. Treatment of mixed vulvar dystrophies requires the use of both corticosteroids and testosterone to treat the two disease processes. The fastest route to resolution of the mixed dystrophy appears to be sequential use of corticosteroids for approximately six weeks and then testosterone propionate to treat the lichen sclerosus. Testosterone propionate must be used chronically to keep the lichen sclerosus in remission. Others have managed mixed dystrophies by the alternate-day use of testosterone and corticosteroids, although this regimen seems to be a slower route to resolution.

VULVAR DYSTROPHY WITH ATYPIA. Finding cellular atypia on vulvar biopsy usually combined with a hyperplastic or mixed dystrophy causes some concern about malignant potential. The natural history of mild to moderate atypia is unknown, although it appears to have a limited potential for progression to worse disease. Usually treating the underlying dystrophy appropriately eliminates the atypia without the need for surgery.

Severe dysplasia and carcinoma in situ, on the other hand, if left untreated, do appear to carry the potential to develop into invasive squamous cell carcinoma. The management of carcinoma in situ of the vulva is discussed in detail in Chapter 25. Current terminology for vulvar atypia parallels that of cervical dysplasia, utilizing the term vulvar intraepithelial neoplasia (VIN). Mild atypia involving one-third or less of the epithelium is classified as VIN I. Moderate atypia reveals atypical cells in the lower half of the epithelium and is classified as VIN II. Finally, full-thickness dysplasia or atypia of the vulvar epithelium is classified as VIN III, or carcinoma in situ and severe dysplasia. The management of these lesions is discussed in Chapter 25.

REACTIVE VULVITIS. Intense inflammation and pruritus of the vulvar skin may be due to physical or chemical irritants. The list of such irritants is lengthy and includes chemical irritants in laundry detergent, perfumed oils, hygiene sprays, vaginal contraceptive creams or foams, douches, and even dyes in toilet tissue. Synthetic fabrics in undergarments may cause a reaction of the vulvar skin, as may medications applied to the vulva for therapy, e.g., podophyllin or fluorouracil (Efudex).

The patient usually complains of intense pruritus and pain. Examination reveals an erythematous, diffuse involvement of the vulvar skin. If the dermatitis is severe, vesicles and ulceration may also appear.

Key to the management of reactive vulvitis is elimination of the offending agents. A cleaning and drying regimen and other methods to break an itch–scratch cycle should be employed and are discussed in the next section. Oral analgesics may be necessary initially to ease the pain of the acute inflammation. Wet compresses with Burow's solution mixed in a concentration of 1:20 may also relieve the discomfort initially. In severe cases of reactive vulvitis oral therapy with prednisone 50 mg daily for seven to ten days may be of help.

VULVAR PRURITUS AND PAIN (VULVODYNIA). There

are multiple causes of vulvar pruritus and pain, several of which have already been discussed. Their common denominator is pruritus, which usually invokes an itch–scratch cycle: Scratching the pruritic vulvar skin leads to its breakdown with subsequent excoriation. Later, during the healing process, further itching occurs that leads to more scratching. The patient thus is held captive to a vicious cycle that must be interrupted to achieve adequate resolution of the symptoms.

The term *vulvodynia* has been coined to describe chronic vulvar discomfort typified as a "rawness," burning, and stinging of the vulva. This situation can be frankly disabling for women who are unable to achieve relief of these symptoms. Because of the need to constantly scratch the vulva and perineum these women are afraid to leave the house for fear of severe discomfort.

Relief of vulvodynia rests essentially on the diagnosis of the condition and appropriate therapy. Delay in diagnosis because of hesitation to perform vulvar biopsy or even to examine the patient is to be condemned. It is the unfortunate women who have had an incorrect initial diagnosis who ultimately have the worst problems, as the itch–scratch cycle then becomes established and even more difficult to break.

A general regimen to improve local vulvar hygiene along with interrupting the itch–scratch cycle is recommended as part of the initial treatment before vulvodynia becomes a chronic process. All other potential irritants to the vulva should be removed from the vulvar environment, including laundry detergents, perfumes, hygiene sprays, douches, and other potential chemical irritants. The patient's vulva should be kept clean, dry, and cool. Cotton underwear should be worn and pantyhose or tightly fitting clothing that constricts or obstructs air circulation in this area proscribed. Itching may be reduced by the use of systemic Atarax at bedtime and, in severe cases, during the daytime hours. The vulva should be kept clean; Aveeno oatmeal baths seem to be of help in this regard because they also are soothing. The vulva should be dried with a hair dryer on the cool setting. Topical application of hydrocortisone cream is appropriate three times a day; triamcinolone (Aristocort) and fluocinolone acetonide (Synalar) are this author's prefer-

ences. Eurax cream should also be used to reduce pruritus. A comprehensive program using all of these modalities has been found to be effective and leads to rapid relief of symptoms.

SMALL VULVAR CYSTS

EPIDERMAL INCLUSION CYSTS. Small inclusion cysts are frequently found on the vulva. In general they are asymptomatic and are of no clinical significance to the patient unless they become infected. These cysts are often small (less than 1 cm), multiple, and most often found on the anterior labia majora. Most cysts are round with a firm, shotty texture and are nontender. Upon distending the vulvar skin over the cyst, the contents appear to be white or yellow. These small cysts are slowly growing and, on examination, freely mobile and nontender. Incision or aspiration of the cysts reveal a thick, yellow-white, cheesy material.

Epidermal inclusion cysts are caused by the enfolding of the squamous epithelium or occlusion of pilosebaceous ducts. Histologically, they are lined by a layer of keratinized squamous epithelium, and the cheesy contents are composed of cellular debris. Because most of these cysts are asymptomatic and are easily identified, no biopsy or therapy is necessary. Should a cyst become infected, local therapy with heat (sitz baths or hot soaks) and incision and drainage of the infected cyst are the keys to appropriate therapy.

VESTIBULAR CYSTS. Vestibular cysts arise between the hymeneal ring and the labia minora and are caused by obstructed ducts of the minor vestibular glands. In contrast to epidermal inclusion cysts, vestibular cysts are usually singular; however, they are also small, often less than 1 cm in diameter. Vestibular cysts are always confined to the vestibular ring and contain mucus. On palpation they feel much more cystic (unlike the hard epidermal inclusion cyst) and are blue or yellow in appearance. These cysts are usually asymptomatic and require no further therapy. An enlarged cyst may lead to difficulty with urination or dyspareunia and should be excised if symptomatic.

HIDRADENOMA. Hidradenoma is most frequently found on the labia as a single isolated cyst. Hidradenoma appears to arise from apocrine sweat glands. Hidradenomas are usually about 1 cm in diameter and may ulcerate with increased intracystic pressure. Biopsy of the cyst reveals an irregular papillary formation making up the cyst wall. This irregular formation has been confused with adenocarcinoma, although careful study of the individual cells show no atypia or other malignant features. Hidradenoma must be considered in any case of a small vulvar lesion diagnosed as adenocarcinoma, and review of the slides is mandatory before recommending or undertaking a radical vulvectomy. Excision of the hidradenoma is key to the appropriate diagnosis and suffices as adequate therapy.

VULVAR HERNIA. Hernia of the vulva is a relatively rare occurrence but must be considered during the evaluation of a vulvar mass so that appropriate therapy can be offered. *Pudendal hernia* may present as an asymptomatic mass of the labia majora. It arises from a defect in the levator sling with progression of the hernial sac down the lateral vaginal wall and onto the vulva. Palpation of a pudendal hernia reveals that the sac is easily reduced, which is the key to diagnosis. *Inguinal hernia* arises from an incompetent external inguinal ring with progression of the hernial sac to the vulva by way of extension along the round ligament. Inguinal hernia may present as an inguinal mass and should not be mistaken for other mass lesions in this region. Finally, a *cyst of the canal of Nuck* is synonymous with the hydrocele in the male scrotum. It is present as a cystic vulvar mass, and in such cases this diagnosis should be considered before deciding to excise the mass. Repair of a hernia, especially a pudendal hernia, may be a surgical challenge and requires both an intraabdominal and a transperineal approach.

MISCELLANEOUS VULVAR LESIONS. Essentially any cutaneous lesion found elsewhere on the body has been found, diagnosed, and treated on the vulva. In most instances the signs and symptoms, diagnosis, and treatment are virtually the same as for the condition when it is found elsewhere on the body. Several conditions that, although not unique to the vulva, are found with some frequency there, are discussed in the following sections.

HEMANGIOMA. Small hemangiomas are frequently found on the labia majora of postmenopausal women. Usually they are 2 to 3 mm in diameter, red to purple, and asymptomatic. Because an infarcted or thrombosed hemangioma may appear darker and raise the specter of melanoma, any unusual lesion should be biopsied. Hemangiomas occasionally bleed, which can often be controlled by cautery or topical application of silver nitrate. Most hemangiomas are asymptomatic, however, and no therapy is needed.

ACCESSORY BREAST TISSUE. The labia majora are in the milk line and therefore on occasion contain breast tissue. The diagnosis of accessory breast tissue is usually made during pregnancy when the breast tissue is stimulated, leading to enlargement of the labia majora by a subcutaneous mass. Usually the symptoms are no more than a fullness or a mass effect, with minimal discomfort. The diagnosis should be considered in any patient developing these symptoms during pregnancy. Treatment of accessory breast tissue in the vulva usually is excision of the tissue, which is best performed in the postpartum state when the tissues are less vascular.

ENDOMETRIOSIS. Endometriosis may be found anywhere on the body and is fully discussed in Chapter 12. Suffice it to say that endometriosis may also be found on the vulva. In particular, endometriosis is most frequently found in the midline of the perineum, which suggests implantation of endometrial tissue at the time of episiotomy closure. Symptoms and signs may vary from a tender nodule that is red to purple to cyclic bleeding from this lesion. Treatment of endometriosis of the vulva is local excision.

NEUROFIBROMA. Neurofibromatosis (von Recklinghausen's disease) may produce cutaneous manifestations on the vulva. In nearly all cases this diagnosis is suspected because the patient had been previously diagnosed with the disease. It is rarely first identified on the vulva. No therapy for neurofibromatosis of the vulva is necessary.

FOX-FORDYCE DISEASE. Fox-Fordyce disease is typified by tiny papules on the vulva that cause intense pruritus. These papules are not associated with the erythema noted with folliculitis. It is hypothesized that Fox-Fordyce disease is caused by the obstruction of apocrine sweat glands, which produces retention vesicles and subsequent clinical lesions and itching. It may also be diagnosed at the same time in the axillae. The disease is nearly always found in menstrual and postmenopausal women. Historically, it has been noted that the disease goes into remission during pregnancy and in women taking oral contraceptives.

The treatment for Fox-Fordyce disease in young women is oral contraceptives, which may suppress apocrine activity. It is one of the few vulvar diseases that may be relieved by topical application of estrogen cream. Both medications should be tried to relieve the severe pruritus that accompanies the disease.

VARICOSE VEINS. Varicose veins are most often diagnosed during pregnancy and are noted in approximately 2 percent of pregnant women. Varicosities are worst during pregnancy owing to pelvic venous stasis, which may lead to symptoms of pressure, engorgement, or pain. Usually these symptoms are mild and require no therapy. On occasion, though, a varicosity thromboses, causing severe pain and discomfort. In this situation excision ligation of the varicose vein is appropriate treatment. It is preferable to attempt to treat symptomatic vulvar varicosities in the postpartum state, after resolution of the pelvic venous engorgement. Support garments for the vulva may offer some temporary relief during pregnancy, especially if swelling and pressure are the primary symptoms. In addition to ligation and excision, sclerosing agents have been injected in these varicosities, as elsewhere in the body, with some success.

HEMATOMA. Trauma to the vulva may cause hematoma, which may result in considerable pain, swelling, and discomfort. Management of vulvar hematoma in the adult is similar to that recommended for the child, as discussed later in this chapter.

TUMORS OF FIBROCONNECTIVE TISSUE. Fibroma, leiomyoma, and lipoma may be found in the vulva, although they are relatively infrequent conditions. The lesions are moderate to large in size, usually a few centimeters in diameter. Usually the lesions arise on the labia majora and are asymptomatic except for the symptoms of a mass effect and rarely pain. Classically, lipoma is a softer lesion than is a fibroma or a leiomyoma. Evidence of rapid enlargement or pain should raise the specter of potential malignancy, e.g., a vulvar sarcoma, which requires immediate attention. Symptomatic connective tissue tumors are treated by excision.

VESTIBULAR ADENITIS. Minor vestibular glands may be found circumferentially in the region between the hymen and the labia minora. These mucus-secreting glands are infrequently seen. However, should they become inflamed, they lead to pain, pruritus, and erythema in this area. Diagnosis of vestibular adenitis is based on biopsy showing mucus-secreting glandular epithelium with evidence of acute and chronic inflammatory reaction. Local application of estrogen and antibiotic creams for vestibular adenitis has been relatively ineffective. Surgical excision with advancement of the vaginal mucosa to cover the defect or laser vaporization to a depth of 1 to 2 mm seems to offer the best long-term results.

DARK LESIONS ON THE VULVA. Any dark lesion of the vulva should raise the specter of vulvar melanoma and requires excision and histologic evaluation for diagnosis. Although vulvar skin comprises only 1 percent of the total body surface area, 5 to 10 percent of all melanomas are found on the vulva in women.

Only approximately 2 percent of all dark lesions on the vulva are melanomas. The most frequently diagnosed lesion is lentigo, which comprises approximately 36 percent of vulvar hyperpigmented lesions, followed by carcinoma in situ (22 percent) and nevi (21 percent). Less frequently seen dark lesions include reactive hyperpigmentation and seborrheic keratosis. Because signs and symptoms are not necessarily typical for any of these lesions, biopsy is strongly advised to establish a firm diagnosis before instituting any therapy.

LENTIGO. Lentigo is the most common dark lesion of the vulva and is usually diagnosed during adult life. Lentigo is an asymptomatic, flat, dark lesion of the vulvar skin or mucous membrane. Most typically, lentigo appears to be a freckle, although it is obviously not on a sun-exposed area. Because lentigo may be associated with superficial melanoma, excision and careful histologic study are recommended.

NEVI. Nevi on the vulva are relatively frequent and are usually asymptomatic. Nevi may be either junctional, compound, or intradermal in location, as they are elsewhere on the skin of the body. These dark, discrete lesions are usually round, flat macules. Occasionally a nevus ulcerates or bleeds, which is an ominous sign suggesting possible malignant transformation to melanoma. In fact, approximately 30 percent of melanomas arise in an area of preexisting nevi. It is therefore recommended that nevi be excised for histologic study and possibly to prevent malignant transformation.

CARCINOMA IN SITU AND MELANOMA. Other important hyperpigmented lesions of the vulva include carcinoma in situ and melanoma. These entities are discussed in Chapters 25 and 29, respectively.

CERVIX

Relative to the multiple benign diseases discussed with regard to the vulva and vagina, the cervix seems to have few pathologic processes. Benign conditions, including cervicitis, cervical polyps, nabothian cysts, and anomalies associated with diethylstilbestrol exposure, are discussed in this section. Reaching epidemic proportions today is cervical intraepithelial neoplasia (CIN), which is discussed at length in Chapter 25. Carcinoma of the cervix, although decreasing slightly in frequency, remains an important gynecologic oncology subject and is reviewed in Chapter 26. Chapter 8 discussed the congenital anomalies of the cervix.

Although the cervix has an embryologic origin similar to that of the uterus and is grossly an extension of the uterine fundus, it behaves essentially as an independent anatomic and physiologic organ. Histologically, the cervix contains both columnar (glandular) epithelium of the endocervical canal and squamous epithelium that covers the exocervix. It is from this squamous epithelium that most diseases of the cervix arise. The stroma of the cervix is primarily fibroconnective tissue, which seems to serve its primary function by providing cervical competence throughout pregnancy and then controlled dilatation at the time of vaginal delivery.

Nabothian Cysts

Nabothian cysts are a frequent, benign, asymptomatic condition of the cervix noted only on visual inspection of the cervix. A nabothian cyst is nothing more than a dilated retention cyst on the exocervix caused by obstruction of an endocervical gland by squamous metaplasia. These mucin-filled cysts usually grow to a few millimeters in diameter and are easily identified on the cervix as yellow to whitish, domed protrusions from the exocervix. On rare occasion they reach 1 cm in diameter. They are often multiple and are usually found in women of childbearing or premenopausal years. These cysts are most often asymptomatic and require no therapy.

Cervical Polyps

Cervical polyps are common benign growths of the cervix that may arise either in the endocervical canal or from the exocervix. The etiology of cervical polyps is thought to be chronic inflammation leading to focal hyperplasia and cellular proliferation. Characteristically, they are smooth, soft, red polypoid lesions that are easily recognized on speculum examination of the cervix. Polyps may be single or multiple and usually achieve several millimeters in diameter and length, although some may be as large as 4 to 5 cm in diameter. The base of the polyp may be a narrow stalk or broad-based. It is sometimes difficult to ascertain the exact origin (exocervix, endocervical canal, or endometrial cavity) on gross physical examination. Polyps may be associated with intermenstrual and postcoital bleeding, or may cause a mucinous vaginal discharge. Many cervical polyps are asymptomatic.

True cervical polyps are not a premalignant lesion, nor are they associated with cervical carcinoma. On the other hand, polyps protruding through the cervix from the endometrial cavity may represent a uterine sarcoma and therefore should be excised and studied histologically. Excision of polyps can most often be accomplished in the office setting, as most cervical polyps are on a narrow stalk and may be removed with a biopsy forceps or other grasping instrument. Occasionally, formal dilatation and sharp curettage is necessary to remove broad-based cervical polyps. Histologic study shows that most cervical polyps arise from columnar epithelium and are covered by metaplastic squamous epithelium. Chronic inflammation is usually noted histologically with ulceration of the polyp surface.

Cervical Myoma

In most respects, myomas (leiomyomas) arising in the cervix are similar to those arising in the uterine fundus (Chap. 17). Cervical myomas commonly present as either a large protruding mass exiting the cervical canal or as a mass expanding the cervical stroma. Myomas protruding through the cervix may actually be pedunculated submucosal leiomyomas arising from the uterine fundus that are delivered through the cervical canal. True cervical myomas are usually small and asymptomatic, although on occasion they enlarge to cause pressure symptoms on the bladder or rectum, dyspareunia, vaginal discharge, or intermenstrual and postcoital bleeding.

Any mass of the cervix should be evaluated histologically to exclude the possibility of cervical cancer or sarcoma. Once the diagnosis of cervical myoma is established, the lesion should be managed with treatment similar to that for uterine myomas: If the myoma is essentially asymptomatic and small, it may be left untreated. On the other hand, if significant symptoms are noted, abdominal or vaginal hysterectomy may be the treatment of choice. In a woman wishing to retain fertility, myomectomy may be considered. However, myomectomy of the cervix is a more difficult surgical procedure, primarily because of the close anatomic proximity of the cervix to the ureters and bladder, as well as its location deep in the pelvis.

Cervical Stenosis

Cervical stenosis is most often an acquired condition resulting in narrowing and obstruction of the cervical canal. The obstruction usually occurs at the level of the internal os, although after surgical manipulation it may occur at the external cervix. Cervical stenosis is most frequently found following cold knife conization, cryotherapy, or electrocautery of the cervix. Cervical stenosis may also occur spontaneously during menopause owing to atrophy of the cervix. During menopause, however, the stenosis must be considered to be associated with cervical malignancy, which may be causing obstruction of the cervical canal. Finally, radiotherapy, especially intracavitary brachytherapy, for cervical carcinoma may lead to profound cervical stenosis.

In many instances cervical stenosis is asymptomatic, although when it occurs in the premenopausal woman the patient may first note oligomenorrhea or amenorrhea caused by the obstruction of the cervical canal. As menstrual fluids fill the uterus and cannot exit through the cervix, uterine cramping or more severe dysmenorrhea may be noted. Therefore cervical stenosis must be considered in the differential diagnosis of secondary amenorrhea or dysmenorrhea. Symptoms are rare in postmenopausal women, although the uterus may fill with blood (hematometra), purulent material (pyometra), or clear secretions (hydrometra). An enlarging uterine mass may be the first symptom of cervical stenosis. In the postmenopausal woman, cervical and endometrial carcinoma occluding the cervical canal must be excluded, requiring endocervical and endometrial biopsies or fractional dilatation and curettage (D&C).

If cervical surgery (cold knife conization) has been performed, the uterine sound should be passed into the cervical canal approximately four weeks after surgery to ensure patency. Thereafter patency should be checked until the cervix is entirely healed.

Diethylstilbestrol-Related Anomalies

The most infamous change in the cervix induced by intrauterine exposure to diethylstilbestrol (DES) is clear cell adenocarcinoma, which is discussed in Chapter 26. The frequency of clear cell carcinoma arising in the cervix is approximately 1 in 1000 to 2000 exposed women; other benign cervical anomalies occur much more frequently. The most frequent structural anomalies of the cervix associated with DES exposure are gross anatomic changes, e.g., cervical collars, hoods, cock's combs, hypoplasia, and pseudopolyps. One or more of these findings are noted in approximately 25 percent of women who were exposed to DES during the first or second trimester of their fetal life. The frequency of these changes is clearly related to the dose, duration, and timing of DES exposure in pregnancy.

Cervical ectropion is noted in a large portion of

women exposed to DES and correlates closely with vaginal adenosis. Essentially, cervical ectropion appears grossly to be a large area of reddened epithelium extending onto the exocervix. Histologically, it is nothing more than columnar epithelium in continuity with the endocervical canal, which has developed farther out onto the exocervix than is normally found. With time, the cervical anatomy changes, with squamous metaplasia occurring across the ectropion. Similar changes have also been noted with vaginal adenosis. In approximately 75 percent of women the ectropion disappears by the time the women reaches her midthirties. To date, there has been no clinical significance associated with the presence of an ectropion, although it was hypothesized that this large transformation zone undergoing squamous metaplasia might make these women at high risk to develop cervical intraepithelial neoplasia. Based on our understanding of cervical intraepithelial neoplasia, this concept is sound. However, cohort studies to date have not shown an increased incidence of CIN in this patient population.

Finally, it has been suggested by at least one author that the cervix of a woman exposed to DES is more likely to become stenotic following surgical manipulation or cryotherapy. This problem may be due to some inherent change in the cervical stroma, and it is therefore recommended that the cervix be manipulated surgically only when it is absolutely required for therapy of premalignant disease. The carbon dioxide laser may lead to less scarring and less stenosis than cold knife conization or cryotherapy.

Condylomas

Condylomas may infect the cervix and appear clinically as a cauliflower lesion, although they may be clinically occult. They are detected only by cytologic findings on Papanicolaou smear. Condylomas of the cervix are most frequently associated with coexisting condylomas of the vulva and vagina and represent the clinical manifestation of diffuse human papilloma virus infection of the lower genital tract. Flat condylomas of the cervix are often associated with cervical intraepithelial neoplasia (Chap. 25).

Because of their potential association with preinvasive disease, Papanicolaou smears should be obtained from all patients with cervical condylomas, and patients with the findings of CIN should be evaluated and treated as discussed in Chapter 25. Treatment of isolated condyloma of the cervix may include local destructive therapy with cryotherapy or carbon dioxide laser vaporization. Topical application of 5-fluorouracil (Efudex) cream has been helpful for treating extensive vaginal and cervical disease, which is nearly impossible ablate with more locally destructive therapy such as laser vaporization.

Cervical Ectropion

Anatomic variations of the cervix occasionally lead the inexperienced clinician to be more concerned than is necessary. One of these frequent findings is cervical ectropion, or what has been termed *cervical erosion*. In most cases this entity is nothing more than an anatomic variation in the location of the squamocolumnar junction (the junction between the squamous epithelium and the columnar epithelium of the cervix). When visualizing the exocervix, the squamocolumnar junction of menstrual-age women who are nulliparous is usually located at the external cervical os, whereas in patients who have delivered vaginally the squamocolumnar junction may lie farther out on the exocervix. Cervical ectropion is columnar epithelium that rests farther out on the exocervix, making the cervix appear red and more granular than the smooth, pink squamous epithelium that normally covers the exocervix. This normal anatomic variant is found in 15 to 20 percent of normal young women and is noted more frequently in women taking oral contraceptives.

Cervical ectropion is usually asymptomatic and of no clinical importance. A large ectropion may be associated with a vaginal discharge of mucus, which can be bothersome and may be further aggravated by chronic cervicitis. Usually, however, no therapy is required or necessary. In the face of an infection, such as with *Trichomonas vaginalis,* the cervical ectropion may become friable and bleed easily on contact.

Treatment of the primary infection usually resolves symptoms. Cervical ectropion is not associated with cervical intraepithelial neoplasia or malignancy and usually regresses over time by transformation of squamous metaplasia.

Cervicitis

Because the cervix is in the environment of the normal vaginal flora, chronic inflammation and cervicitis are normal findings in most women. It is an asymptomatic condition but is often found during histologic evaluation of the cervix or on cervical biopsies. The organisms found comprise a mixed bacterial flora that are normally in the vagina and most often do not cause a frank infection. Bacterial cervicitis is not associated with the occurrence of cervical cancer.

On the other hand, the cervix may become infected with pathogens that cause problems, including viral, protozoa, and fungal organisms. Most frequently, the cervix is infected with the same organisms that cause clinical vaginitis (e.g., *Trichomonas* or *Gardnerella*). Infections of the cervix that most frequently produce significant symptoms are caused by *Neisseria gonorrhoeae, Chlamydia trachomatis,* herpes simplex virus, and human papilloma virus. These infections are sexually transmitted diseases and should be treated appropriately in both the patient and her male sexual partner (Chaps. 15, 25).

Mucopurulent Cervicitis. Mucopurulent cervicitis, a pathologic process in most patients, by definition requires that a yellow mucopurulent material be found on swabbing the endocervical canal and more than ten polymorphonuclear leukocytes per high power field on Gram stain of the endocervix. Approximately 40 percent of women with sexually transmitted disease have mucopurulent cervicitis, although most are asymptomatic. A vaginal discharge, cervical discharge, dyspareunia, and postcoital bleeding suggest the possibility of mucopurulent cervicitis. Such patients should be evaluated with a simple Q-tip test and Gram stain.

The most frequent infecting organism in patients with mucopurulent cervicitis is *Chlamydia trachomatis,* accounting for approximately 50 percent of cases. Herpes simplex virus infection and gonorrhea are other frequent causes. Appropriate cultures should be obtained to establish a diagnosis and to guide therapy. Treatment for *C. trachomatis* infection is tetracycline 500 mg by mouth every 6 hours for seven days or doxycycline 100 mg by mouth twice a day for seven days. The male sexual partner should be treated also.

VULVOVAGINAL DISEASE IN INFANTS AND CHILDREN

Vulvovaginitis

Vulvovaginitis is the most common reason for children to visit a gynecologist. In many instances the child is much less concerned about the signs and symptoms than is her mother. Nonetheless, children with a vaginal discharge or vulvar irritation should be thoroughly evaluated utilizing most of the same examination steps applied to the adult.

In the premenarchal child, the lack of estrogen causes the vaginal epithelium to be thin and prone to inflammation and infection. Moreover, the neutral vaginal pH is an ideal culture medium for a variety of organisms. Most childhood vulvovaginitis is due to irritation of the vulva and then secondary involvement of the lower third of the vaginal canal. This vulvovaginitis is due to a nonspecific infection caused by the inoculation of gastrointestinal tract bacteria onto the vulva and vagina, which is then further aggravated by scratching, breaks in the skin, and a difficult to treat itch–scratch cycle. Inadequate local hygiene of the young child is the most common cause of this nonspecific infection. Approximately 25 percent of vulvovaginitis is secondary to a specific organism, which should be sought by specific culture methods. The identification of *Neisseria gonorrhoeae, Trichomonas, Chlamydia,* or herpes raises the question of sexual abuse.

The most common entities noted during infancy and childhood are discussed in the following sections.

Neonatal Leukorrhea. Neonatal leukorrhea is a physiologic vaginal discharge seen in female newborns. The discharge occurs in response to high levels of circulating maternal estrogens stimulating mucoid secretions and desquamation of cornified vaginal epithelial cells from the vagina and cervix of the newborn. Neonatal leukorrhea is transient and ordinarily subsides within a few weeks after birth as the influence of maternal estrogens is withdrawn.

Nonspecific Vulvovaginitis. Frequently vulvovaginal infection in children is a nonspecific infection due to normal gastrointestinal flora. It occurs as a result of poor toilet hygiene following bowel evacuation, the child wiping anal and perineal areas in a posteroanterior direction. A mixed-bacterial flora of colonic origin is thus introduced onto the vulva and into the vaginal canal. Tight-fitting underclothing and lack of proper bathing may further contribute to this problem.

The child with vulvar irritation may ultimately present with ulcerated excoriation secondary to itching. The discharge is usually thin and nonbloody. Once the mixed-bacterial, nonspecific nature of the infection has been established by careful examination and bacteriologic studies, therapy is directed toward improvement of local vulvovaginal and perineal hygiene.

Nonspecific vulvovaginitis may also be caused by irritative agents such as bubble bath, harsh soaps, or laundry detergents. Elimination of these irritative agents along with improved local hygiene usually resolve the acute problem. The pain and pruritus secondary to these infections and excoriations may be treated symptomatically with sitz baths composed of lukewarm bath water and two tablespoons of baking soda. Aveeno oatmeal baths may soothe the intense vulvar pruritus and interrupt the itch–scratch cycle. The vulva must be kept clean and dry, and loose-fitting cotton undergarments should be worn. Occasionally, oral antibiotic therapy is necessary to resolve the infection. Antibiotic therapy should be directed by specific culture and sensitivity methods and be used in a limited course of seven to ten days. In resistant cases, estrogen cream may be used to improve cornification of the vaginal and vulvar epithelium, leading to improved host defenses and elimination of the infection. Nightly application of estrogen cream to the vulva and lower vagina should be limited to a maximum of fourteen days so as to minimize systemic absorption of the estrogen. Intense cases of pruritus

may be treated with 0.5% hydrocortisone cream applied topically.

Vaginal Foreign Body. The innate curiosity of infants and young children leads to the not infrequent insertion of objects into the vaginal canal. Perhaps the commonest cause of vaginal discharge is the presence of a foreign body, not noticed by the mother and even forgotten by an older child. The discharge, due to secondary inflammation and infection of the vagina, may be purulent and bloody. The foreign body may be any object small enough to be inserted into the vagina, including small toys, tissue paper, or crayons. Foreign bodies can usually be discovered and removed during a simple office examination. The possibility of a vaginal foreign body must be kept in mind in any child presenting with a vaginal discharge or bleeding. The associated secondary irritation or infection usually subsides rapidly after removal of the foreign body.

True Vulvovaginitis. Approximately 25 percent of vulvovaginitis during childhood is due to a single specific organism. Although the etiology for some of these infections is obvious, other infections are usually venereally transmitted, and sexual abuse must be seriously considered during the evaluation.

Candida Vaginitis. Vulvovaginitis due to a *Candida albicans* infection is uncommon during infancy and childhood. It is most often encountered following intensive antibiotic therapy or in a juvenile diabetic patient. It should be remembered that the appearance of *Candida* vulvovaginitis may be the earliest manifestation of occult diabetes, and children with such infections without other identifiable causes should be screened for diabetes mellitus. The thick vulvovaginal discharge associated with intense pruritus and inflammation should be evaluated and treated in a fashion similar to that employed for the adult patient.

Bacterial Vaginitis. Bacterial organisms causing vulvovaginitis in children may be of the coliform, streptococcal, staphylococcal, or pneumococcal type; more rarely, they are typhoid, paratyphoid, or diphtherial in origin. The inflammatory process and symptomatology are usually acute in onset and of short duration. Diagnosis rests on accurate identification by culture of the specific organisms and treatment with the appropriate antibiotic as indicated by sensitivity studies, together with attention to any deficiencies in local hygiene and the possible presence of more generalized factors, including poor nutrition or systemic illness.

Identification of *Trichomonas vaginalis, Neisseria gonorrhoeae,* or *Chlamydia* as the etiologic agent of vulvovaginitis in the child should prompt treatment similar to that for the adult patient. Because these infections are often associated with child abuse, the child should be carefully evaluated from both a physical and a psychological perspective (Chap. 20). Consultation with appropriate pediatric, social work, and law enforcement agencies is clearly appropriate for the child's welfare.

Parasitic Vulvovaginal Infestations. Various intestinal parasites, most commonly the ubiquitous pinworm (*Enterobius vermicularis*), may cause vulvar pruritus, irritation, and discharge. Less commonly found is the roundworm (*Ascaris lumbricoides*) or the whipworm (*Trichuris trichiura*). These organisms are transferred anteriorly into the vulvovaginal region through poor local hygiene and improper toilet habits. The pinworm in particular migrates from the rectum and anus to the perianal skin at night to lay its eggs. The intense itching and resultant scratching produces vulvar inflammation, excoriation, and secondary bacterial vulvovaginitis.

Diagnosis is best made by inspecting the anal and perineal skin with a flashlight at night while the child is sleeping or by pressing a piece of cellophane adhesive tape against the perianal area in the early morning to recover the typical parasitic ova, which can be identified by microscopic examination. Management involves the current therapeutic programs for elimination of these common intestinal parasites, and treatment of the entire household is indicated.

Physiologic Discharge in Premenarchal Girls. Cyclic "leukorrhea" in premenarchal girls is similar to the neonatal leukorrhea previously mentioned. It is fre-quently a source of concern to both the young girl and her mother. The cyclic nature of this discharge, which is rarely accompanied by symptoms of irritation, is physiologic in nature. Examination with a wet preparation reveals abundant epithelial cells without identifiable pathogenic organisms. This discharge is simply the earliest manifestation of the beginning cyclic ovarian activity and cyclic estrogen secretion. Treatment should be reassurance that it is a normal physiologic process.

Recurrent Vulvovaginitis in Children. Most children with vulvovaginitis can be readily treated and the condition resolved without subsequent recurrence. Recurrent vulvovaginitis should be carefully and thoroughly reevaluated; treatment should not be based on a previously presumed diagnosis. The possibility of a foreign body should be reconsidered, and if it cannot be excluded by office examination, examination should be performed under anesthesia. Examination and culture of stool for ova and parasites may be used to detect occult parasitic infections. Urologic evaluation, searching for an ectopic ureter, should also be considered in rare cases of recurrent vulvovaginitis. An ectopic ureter is infrequently apparent on a routine examination, as it usually releases only a small amount of urine during the examination. Finally, child abuse must be considered in all cases of recurrent vulvovaginitis.

Labial Agglutination

Although often termed "vulvar fusion," the common adherence of the labia minora of infants and young children is not accompanied by any anatomic union of the deeper tissues. Therefore it is not a true anatomic congenital anomaly but, rather, an acquired postnatal condition resulting in the simple sticking together of the epithelial surfaces that normally lie in close apposition to each other in the young female. Labial agglutination may be promoted by vulvar inflammation and excoriation. It is therefore important to recognize the situation for what it is and to distinguish it from imperforate hymen, congenital absence of the vagina, or the anomaly of congenital adrenal hyperplasia without the need for elaborate diagnostic procedures. Such distinction should not be difficult, as only the labia minora are involved and a careful examination reveals the genital tract to be normal.

Adherent labia frequently cause no symptoms, and normal separation usually occurs spontaneously as the infant or young child grows older. Although parents may be seriously concerned about this abnormality and wish it to be corrected, the labial adhesions rarely require forcible separation. Occasionally, if the extent of agglutination is considerable, leading to difficulty voiding or dysuria with local vulvovaginal irritation due to constant presence and accumulation of small amounts of urine and vaginal secretions in the area, the labia are carefully separated by a physician. Should symptoms recur, the mother is instructed to keep the labia separated by occasional genital manipulation at home until a tendency to be adherent is no longer present. Permanent separation in patients with recurrent symptoms may be achieved by a brief course of topical application of estrogen cream to the labia minora nightly. In any event, the condition ultimately disappears completely during later childhood.

Vulvovaginal Trauma

Because of the highly protected location of the vulvovaginal soft tissue, traumatic injuries might be expected to be uncommon, and in fact are rare in adults. However, in young girls a specific type of vulvar trauma is encountered with relative frequency. It invariably occurs as a result of a straddle-type injury, most often caused by a fall while bicycling or when climbing fences, walls, or jungle gyms. The vulva often absorbs almost the entire force of the impact of such falls, as the child lands astride the object. Soft tissue lacerations of varying severity may occur, requiring careful evaluation and management. Penetrating injuries of the vulva and vagina may be associated with deeper internal injury. The bladder, rectum, and intra- and retroperitoneal structures should be carefully evaluated. Examination under anesthesia with cystoscopy and proctoscopy may be warranted. Débridement of the laceration and ligation of bleeding vessels is often required. Children with penetrating soft tissue injuries should receive a tetanus toxoid

booster if they have not had one for more than five years.

More common and troublesome is the development of a massive perineal hematoma. It is an almost inevitable phenomenon in view of the great vascularity and rich lymphatic supply of the soft tissue in this area. Hematoma usually results in excruciating pain and often leads to acute urinary retention due to occlusion of the urethral meatus. As the hematoma expands in the closed space of the vulva, venous pressure is usually exceeded, and the size of the hematoma stabilizes. Rarely is it necessary to incise and drain a hematoma or search for an arterial bleeding point. Acute management of hematoma therefore is elevation of the pelvis and application of ice packs to the vulva and perineum. It is also frequently important to anticipate the development of urinary retention by placing an indwelling Foley catheter for 48 to 72 hours until the edema has begun to subside.

SELECTED READINGS

Butler, E. B., and Stanbridge, C. M. Condylomatous lesions of the lower female genital tract. *Clin. Obstet. Gynecol.* 11:171, 1984.

Copenhaven, E. H. *Surgery of the Vulva and Vagina.* Philadelphia: Saunders, 1981.

Dawson, S. G. *Gardnerella vaginalis* and nonspecific vaginitis. *Br. J. Hosp. Med.* 29:28, 1983.

Felman, Y. M., and Nikitas, J. A. Lympho-granuloma venereum. *Cutis* 25:264, 1980.

Fidian, A. P., Holsos, A. M., Kinge, B. R., et al. Oral acyclovir in the treatment of genital herpes. *Am. J. Med.* 73:335, 1982.

Fleury, F. J. Adult vaginitis. *Clin. Obstet. Gynecol.* 24:407, 1981.

Friedrich, E. G., Jr. *Vulvar Disease.* Philadelphia: Saunders, 1981.

Gall, S. A., Hughes, C. E., and Trofatter, K. Interferon for the therapy of condylomata acuminatum. *Am. J. Obstet. Gynecol.* 153:157, 1985.

Gordon, S. W. Hidradenitis supporativa: a closer look. *J. Natl. Med. Assoc.* 70:239, 1978.

Grissmann, L., deVilliers, E. M., and Zurhausen, H. Analysis of human genital warts (condylomata acuminata) and other genital tumors for human papilloma virus type 6 DNA. *Int. J. Cancer* 29:143, 1982.

Hart, W. R., Norris, H. H., and Helwig, E. B. Relation of

lichen sclerosus et atrophicus of the vulva to the development of carcinoma. *Obstet. Gynecol.* 45:369, 1974.

Heath, J. Methods of treatment for cysts and abscesses of Bartholin's gland. *Br. J. Obstet. Gynecol.* 195:321, 1988.

Huffman, J. W., Dewhurst, C. J., and Capraro, V. J. Premenarchial vulvovaginitis. In: *The Gynecology of Childhood and Adolescence* (2nd ed.). Philadelphia: Saunders, 1981.

International Society for the Study of Vulvar Disease. New nomenclature for vulvar disease. *Obstet. Gynecol.* 47:122, 1976.

Jacobsen, P. Marsupialization of vulvovaginal (Bartholin) cysts. *Am. J. Obstet. Gynecol.* 79:73, 1960.

Jones, I. S. C. Assessment of vulvar pigmentation. *N.Z. Med. J.* 89:348, 1979.

Kaufman, R. H., and Faro, S. Herpes genitalis: clinical features and treatment. *Clin. Obstet. Gynecol.* 28:152, 1985.

Korting, G. W. *Practical Dermatology of the Genital Region.* Philadelphia: Saunders, 1981.

Kuberski, T. Granuloma inguinale. *Sex. Transm. Dis.* 7:29, 1980.

Larsen, B., and Galask, R. P. Vaginal microbial flora composition and influences of host physiology. *Ann. Intern. Med.* 96:926, 1982.

McLellan, R., Spence, M. R., Brockman, M., et al. The clinical diagnosis of *Trichomonas. Obstet. Gynecol.* 60:30, 1982.

Rein, M. F. Current therapy of vulvovaginitis. *Sex. Transm. Dis.* 8:316, 1981.

Vontver, L. A., and Eschenbach, D. A. The role of *Gardnerella vaginalis* in nonspecific vaginitis. *Clin. Obstet. Gynecol.* 24:439, 1981.

15

Upper Genital Tract Infections and Sexually Transmitted Diseases

Infections and inflammatory processes that remain localized to the vulva, vagina, or cervix (the external genitalia and lower reproductive tract) are, with the exception of the specific sexually transmitted diseases, discussed in Chapter 14. Two common sexually transmitted disease syndromes in women—vaginosis (vaginitis due to *Gardnerella vaginalis*) and trichomoniasis—also are considered in Chapter 14, however, because they are confined almost exclusively to the vagina and cervix.

The pelvic infections remaining to be considered are those that tend to spread to or involve primarily the internal genitalia or upper reproductive tract, particularly the fallopian tubes (salpingitis). However, the uterus (endometritis) and its adjacent supporting tissues with their accompanying vascular and lymphatic channels (parametritis, pelvic cellulitis, septic pelvic thrombophlebitis, and pelvic lymphadenitis), the ovaries (oophoritis, tuboovarian abscess), and the pelvic peritoneal cavity itself (pelvic peritonitis, pelvic abscess) are frequently also involved.

In many instances a more or less generalized abdominal peritonitis may exist, particularly in the early acute phases. Despite varying etiologies, this general type of pelvic infection is usually termed *pelvic inflammatory disease,* a description that connotes an infectious process within the pelvic cavity and, for the most part, outside the uterus. Initially, a pelvic inflammatory disorder appears as an acute process, but as the inflammation subsides or with repeated flareups or reinfections a chronic stage of the disease develops with its own symptomatology, findings, and complications.

Infection with gonococci is responsible for up to 65 to 75 percent of all pelvic inflammatory disease. Other pyogenic organisms gaining access to the pelvis as the result of septic abortion or puerperal infection account for another 20 to 30 percent of cases. Finally, tuberculous salpingitis and endometritis are present in approximately 5 percent of patients with pelvic inflammation.

GONORRHEA

Gonorrhea is caused by the gonococcus *Neisseria gonorrhoeae*. Uncomplicated gonococcal infection may be defined as gonorrhea that remains localized to the site of initial inoculation, does not cause disabling symptoms, and if promptly and correctly treated rarely causes sequelae. It is one of the most common sexually transmitted diseases.

The true incidence of gonorrhea is difficult to determine because only a few countries have reporting systems for this disease. In the United States the number of reported cases has increased from about 170 to 180 cases per 100,000 population in 1965 to 443 cases per 100,000 population in 1980, when 1,004,029 cases were reported. An additional 1.0 million to 1.5 million cases are diagnosed each year but not reported, so that annually 2.0 million to 2.5 million cases are probably diagnosed in the United States. Forty-one percent of the reported cases are in women. The incidence of gonorrhea is partially age-dependent, with 83 percent of cases in 1979 in the United States occurring among those 15 to 29 years of age, the peak incidence being 38 percent in those 20 to 24 years old. Thus the incidence has risen sharply in youths and those below 25 years of age, perhaps a reflection of the increasingly earlier sexual experience in teenagers. Thus gonorrhea is almost twice as high in sexually active 15- to 19-year-old girls as in 20- to 24-year-old women. Other risk factors for gonorrhea include low socioeconomic level, urban residence, early onset of sexual activity, unmarried marital status, male homosexuality, and previous history of gonorrhea.

The rate of transmission of gonorrhea depends on the anatomic sites infected and exposed. Hence, whereas the organism is rarely present in men without producing symptoms, 50 to 80 percent of women with gonococcal infections are asymptomatic carriers. After a single episode of vaginal intercourse with an infected woman, the risk of acquiring urethral infection for a man is 20 percent and increases to 60 to 80 percent after four exposures. The prevalence of infection in women who were secondary sex contacts of men with gonococcal urethritis is 90 percent, but there is no information on the relation to number of exposures. Transmission of pharyngeal infection to other sites is uncommon, but transmission of infection from the genitalia to the pharynx and anal canal may not be uncommon depending on the sexual practice of the population. Transmission by nonsexual contact is rare.

In adults, only mucous membranes lined by non-squamous epithelium are normally susceptible to gonococcal infection. Mediated by pili and other surface proteins, the gonococci adhere to the mucosa, invade the latter, and are between the epithelial cells within 24 to 48 hours. In the fallopian tube, endotoxins (which are lipopolysaccharides) impair ciliary motility and destroy the epithelial cells. Progressive colonization by the gonococci is followed by a strong polymorphonuclear leukocytic response, submucosal microabscess formation, and exudates in the lumen of the infected organ. Untreated, the cellular inflammatory response is replaced by mononuclear cells and eventually abnormal round cell infiltration, at which point the gonococci can no longer be isolated.

Acute Gonorrhea

The endocervical canal is the primary site of urogenital gonococcal infection. Other sites at which it may infect the female lower reproductive tract during the acute infection include the urethra, Skene's glands (periurethral gland), and Bartholin's glands; but invariably the cervix is also concomitantly infected unless the cervix has been removed, e.g., after hysterectomy. Urethral colonization is present in 70 to 90 percent of infected women. Hence culture material for isolating gonococci should be taken from the endocervical canal and urethra while massaging Skene's glands. Rectal mucosa is infected in 35 to 50 percent of women, the organism gaining access to the rectal crypts.

Acute gonorrhea is usually readily recognized on the basis of the typical clinical features, including the following: (1) a history of exposure (sometimes the patient knows that the sexual partner was infected); (2) the incubation period (variable in women but usually seven to ten days); (3) the characteristic profuse, creamy, rather thick, highly irritating urethral and vaginal discharge; (4) urethral burning, dysuria, bladder irritability, and often accompanying vulvovaginitis; and (5) obvious evidence of inflammatory involvement of the urethra and cervix, and often of Skene's and Bartholin's glands as well, seen on pelvic examination. Signs and symptoms of gonorrheal pharyngitis (10 to 20 percent incidence), which includes sore throat, fever, and cervical lymphadenopathy, may also be present. At this stage of the disease, prior to the phase of ascending infection, there are essentially no lower abdominal symptoms or findings.

The diagnosis can sometimes (in 50 to 60 percent of infected females) be confirmed by identifying the gram-negative intracellular diplococci on a gram-stained smear of (1) urethral, vaginal, or cervical discharge, (2) secretions milked from Skene's glands in the paraurethral area, or (3) material from rectal crypts obtained via anoscopy. However, a definite and unequivocal diagnosis of gonorrhea can best be made by culture (urethral, endocervical, anal, and when indicated pharyngeal swabs), streaking the material directly and immediately on Thayer-Martin medium (which yields rapid and highly reliable results in 90 percent or more of infected females), and incubating under increased carbon dioxide tension in a candle-jar. If a laboratory is not close at hand, Transgro (Difco), a transport medium with the proper ingredients and already charged with carbon dioxide, can be used to facilitate the preparation and transport of cultures. Subsequent further confirmation, if necessary, can then be done by subculture on special carbohydrate media that permit even more specific identification of the gonococcus. Additional confirmation can be obtained by a direct fluorescent-antibody staining technique. Complete bacteriologic studies should be carried out in all cases, even though the diagnosis may be obvious clinically, as the disease is a reportable one in most states. In addition to potential medicolegal problems once the diagnosis is officially made, contact tracing and the need for sexual partners to be examined for gonorrhea is imperative socially, epidemiologically, and for prevention.

Penicillin has been and remains the antibiotic of choice for the treatment of gonorrhea, as most strains of *N. gonorrhoeae* remain susceptible in vitro to a broad range of antibiotics, including penicillins, tetracyclines, cephalosporins, rifampicin, and macrolides. Cultures convert to negative within 12 hours, and symptoms resolve within three days. Single-session treatment is traditionally preferred to eliminate the compliance problem, but some multidose regimens have important advantages. Until 1950 there was little gonococcal resistance to penicillin, but by the 1970s studies from different parts of the world reported that 18 to 90 percent of strains showed diminished susceptibility to penicillin. Fortunately, this resistance is, for the most part, not absolute. However, the recommended dosage of penicillin has been increased considerably.

In the United States, current therapy for acute gonorrhea is based on the regimens recommended by the Centers for Disease Control in Atlanta. The various regimens are summarized in Table 15-1. For primary treatment of uncomplicated infection caused by β-lactamase-negative gonococci, procaine penicillin G plus

Table 15-1. Regimens Recommended by the Centers for Disease Control for Treatment of Adults with Uncomplicated Gonorrhea

Drug regimens of choice[a]
1. Tetracycline hydrochloride[b] 0.5 gm PO four times daily for 7 days
2. Aqueous procaine penicillin G 4.8 million units IM + probenecid 1.0 gm PO
3. Ampicillin 3.5 gm PO in a single dose + probenecid 1.0 gm PO
4. Amoxicillin 3.0 gm PO in a single dose + probenecid 1.0 gm PO

Recommended combination regimen
   Ampicillin 3.5 gm PO or amoxicillin 3.0 gm PO + probenecid 1.0 gm PO in a single dose; followed by tetracycline hydrochloride 0.5 gm PO 4 times daily for 7 days

Alternative regimens
1. Spectinomycin 2.0 gm IM
2. Cefoxitin 2.0 gm IM + probenecid 1.0 gm PO

---

[a]The order of presentation does not indicate preference.
[b]Doxycycline hyclate may be substituted in a dose of 100 mg PO twice daily for seven days. All tetracyclines are contraindicated for pregnant women.

probenecid, ampicillin plus probenecid, amoxicillin plus probenecid, and tetracycline regimens are recommended. Probenecid given 30 to 60 minutes before one of the penicillin-type antibiotics blocks the renal tubular reabsorption of penicillin and thereby delays excretion and maintains elevated blood levels of the antibiotic.

If the patient is allergic to penicillin or if drug resistance is encountered despite adequate dosage of aqueous penicillin G (as much as 8 million units has been given), tetracycline may be used, giving 1.5 gm orally as an initial dose followed by 0.5 gm four times daily for four days. Unfortunately, increasing numbers of tetracycline-resistant strains are being reported. If resistance is a problem, spectinomycin or cefoxitin (Table 15-1) can be employed successfully. Spectinomycin is recommended for patients who cannot tolerate any of the regimens of choice, for those in whom previous treatment with any of the primary regimens failed to eradicate the infection, or for those who are known or suspected to be infected with penicillinase-producing *N. gonorrhoeae*. The cefoxitin–probenecid combination is recommended for patients infected with spectinomycin-resistant strains of penicillinase-producing *N. gonorrhoeae*.

Because 2 to 3 percent of patients with gonorrhea have also been infected with syphilis, and because the antibiotic therapy for the gonorrhea may not have been adequate for the incubating syphilis (if intramuscular penicillin has been used, it is simultaneously curative for any incubating syphilis), it is important that all patients treated for gonorrhea by other than the standard intramuscular penicillin regimen have follow-up serologic tests for syphilis during the next four months. Obviously, follow-up physical examination, smears, and cultures are indicated to be certain the gonorrhea has been eradicated.

Acute Gonorrheal Pelvic Inflammatory Disease

If treatment of the primary phase of the gonorrheal infection is delayed or inadequate, ascending surface spread of the organism may take place, usually toward the end of or just after the next menstrual period. At this time the normal barrier of the impenetrable cervical mucous plug is temporarily absent, and the menstrual blood provides an excellent medium for bacterial growth. The end result is the development of an acute salpingitis and pelvic peritonitis.

The patient then presents with an acute abdominal complaint that must be distinguished not only from other acute gynecologic disorders (e.g., ectopic pregnancy, twisted ovarian cyst, ruptured corpus hemorrhagicum or corpus luteum cyst, ruptured endometrioma, twisted or degenerating fibroid) but also from appendicitis, diverticulitis, or other intraabdominal disorders associated with peritonitis; occasionally, it must be distinguished from acute urinary tract conditions (infection and calculi).

Diagnosis. Acute gonococcal pelvic inflammatory disease is suggested if there is a typical history of vaginal discharge preceding the onset of fever and abdominal pain during or just after the next period. Gastrointestinal symptoms are often completely absent or minimal despite obvious and often diffuse peritonitis (in contrast to such symptoms with appendicitis, for example).

PELVIC FINDINGS. A urethral or cervical discharge may still be present and permit identification of gonococcal organisms by smear or culture, although if antibiotics have been administered it is often impossible. Pelvic tenderness is bilateral and exquisite, and the cervix is painful on motion. There may or may not be palpable adnexal swelling or thickening.

ABDOMINAL FINDINGS. Tenderness and muscle spasm may be generalized but are usually maximal in the lower abdomen and, again, are bilateral and diffuse. Rarely, perihepatitis develops (Fitz-Hugh-Curtis syndrome) owing to spread of purulent fluid above the liver, giving rise to upper abdominal pain and tenderness especially in the right upper quadrant. Intestinal peristalsis is often relatively normal, and the patient may even be hungry and thirsty despite considerable evidence of peritoneal irritation (in contrast to appendicitis, for example).

A high temperature (102° to 103°F) and marked leukocytosis (white blood cell count of 20,000 to 30,000 per cubic millimeter with a shift to the left) are often present; despite this finding the patient rarely appears very ill (in contrast to the patient with the peritonitis of appendicitis, diverticulitis, perforated ul-

cer, pancreatitis, and so on, who usually appears toxic). The characteristically mild clinical manifestations of gonococcal pelvic inflammatory disease are a reflection of the relatively noninvasive potential of the gonococcus, an organism that tends to remain localized to mucosal and serosal surfaces and to not penetrate deeper tissues or spread via the bloodstream or lymphatics. Thus the clinical picture contrasts sharply with that of peritonitis due to a ruptured appendix or similar acute general surgical conditions, as well as with that of acute pelvic inflammatory disorders caused by highly virulent and invasive organisms such as *Streptococcus, Staphylococcus, Escherichia coli,* and other related gram-negative bacilli commonly present in cases of puerperal or postabortal sepsis.

In the other acute gynecologic situations to be distinguished, the process is usually unilateral and more localized than in gonorrhea, and the clinical picture only rarely suggests infection. Laparoscopy is a useful diagnostic procedure if there is any doubt about the diagnosis. The minimum criteria employed for diagnosing pelvic inflammatory disease at laparoscopy should include (1) *erythema* of the fallopian tube, (2) *edema* and *swelling* of the fallopian tube, and (3) *seropurulent exudate* from the fimbriated end or on the serosal surface of the fallopian tube. A simple scoring system has been suggested and may be clinically useful.

Mild: presence of the minimum criteria described above together with tubes freely movable and patent

Moderate: minimum criteria as above but more marked plus tubes not freely movable and patency uncertain

Severe: an inflammatory mass or masses present

Laparoscopy should probably be done routinely, as several studies have shown that the accuracy of diagnosing acute pelvic inflammatory disease is only 50 to 60 percent when checked against laparoscopy. Such a routine can (1) save the cost of hospitalizing and treating those not having pelvic inflammatory disease, (2) offer correct, prompt treatment of other acute abdominal emergencies requiring laparotomy, and (3) permit definitive diagnosis and staging of the pelvic inflammatory disease. Furthermore, it is important that patients never be labeled as having had pelvic inflammatory disease on equivocal clinical grounds because further management—in particular, evaluation and therapy of future episodes of abdominal pain—invariably becomes fixed and stereotyped based on and prejudiced by what may have been an entirely erroneous clinical impression of the nature of the initial acute illness.

Although much less common than the direct contiguous spread of gonococcal salpingitis and peritonitis, blood-borne metastatic spread of the gonococcus is far more serious and should be sought in any patient with acute gonorrheal disease. The most common entities that result are migratory gonococcal arthritis, usually polyarticular (e.g., wrists, knees, ankles, hands, feet), and septicemia, with fever and associated skin lesions (initially hemorrhagic bullae); meningitis and endocarditis, myocarditis, and pericarditis also occur. These remote complications of the acute disease usually require and respond well to intensive, high-dose intravenous penicillin therapy.

Treatment. Although mild, subacute cases of salpingitis without significant pelvic peritonitis may sometimes be treated on an outpatient basis with oral tetracycline, oral ampicillin, or intramuscular aqueous penicillin G plus probenecid, the management of acute gonorrheal pelvic inflammatory disease in which the patient is ill enough to be hospitalized includes the following.

1. *Peritonitis regimen:* Infrequent pelvic examinations once a definite diagnosis is established, bed rest, low or medium Fowler's position; restriction of oral intake, depending on the degree of ileus (rarely, intestinal intubation), with intravenous fluids as indicated
2. *Antibiotics:* Aqueous penicillin G 20 million units intravenously daily for several days, shifting to oral ampicillin when clear-cut improvement has occurred; or other specific chemotherapy as indicated by the results of cultures and sensitivity studies and by the patient's response

During the acute phase of an initial attack of the disease, the clinical response to therapy is usually rapid and dramatic, with subsidence of fever and discomfort within 24 to 48 hours. If a prompt response is not forthcoming, look for more chronic manifestations of the disease with unresolved sepsis (pyosalpinx, tuboovarian abscess, cul-de-sac abscess) or suspect some other diagnosis (e.g., appendicitis or diverticulitis with abscess or a twisted, gangrenous ovarian cyst).

Good management includes hospitalization for seven to fourteen days, with gradual ambulation and oral chemotherapy with ampicillin (0.5 gm four times daily) for five to seven days after the temperature becomes normal. If an intrauterine device is present, it probably should be removed, as its continued presence tends to favor persistence of bacterial infection in both the fallopian tubes and the endometrium. Prolonged restriction of activities with adequate rest and nutrition and occasionally continuation of antibiotics at home are indicated for several months. Proper care and gradual return to normal activity may increase the number of patients who recover with minimal permanent tubal damage and preservation of normal tubal function. It is a favorable sign if adnexal swelling or induration does not occur or if it is detected only during the acute phase and rapidly subsides thereafter. Symptoms and fever that clear promptly and do not recur also are encouraging signs. When the patient is completely asymptomatic, has a completely negative pelvic examination, and has had several subsequently normal menstrual periods, she can be considered to have completed her convalescence and can be allowed more activity.

In the case of a mild, acute, first attack of salpingitis with prompt response to early treatment, subsequent fertility may run as high as 70 percent. After two or three attacks, however, it becomes 10 to 20 percent at best; and once the chronic, recurring phase is reached, permanent sterility is the rule.

It should also be emphasized that in almost every state reporting of all cases of diagnosed venereal disease is required by law. This information is considered confidential and cannot be revealed even to the spouse without the patient's permission. Only by each physician's fulfilling this legal obligation to report all cases of venereal disease can adequate measures be taken to trace all contacts and treat them adequately.

A vigorous public health program of this type is needed if the rising venereal disease rate in the United States is to be halted and reversed.

Prognosis After Salpingitis. There is a significantly higher incidence of infertility and ectopic pregnancy in women who have had acute pelvic inflammatory disease. The incidence of involuntary infertility in women who have had acute pelvic inflammatory disease is 21 percent compared to 3 percent in normal controls. The risk of being infertile increases with the number of attacks of pelvic inflammatory disease and with age of the woman. In those 15 to 24 years of age, one previous episode causes 9.4 percent infertility; with two episodes it is 20.9 percent; and with three episodes it is 51.6 percent. In those 25 to 34 years of age, one previous episode produces 19.2 percent infertility; two episodes cause 31.0 percent infertility; and with three episodes it is 60.0 percent. Tubal occlusion likewise increases with the number of episodes of pelvic inflammatory disease.

Chronic Gonorrheal Pelvic Inflammatory Disease

Clinical Features. Typical symptoms and findings of chronic gonorrheal pelvic inflammatory disease include the following: persistent pelvic pain, usually aggravated during menstrual periods—an acquired type of dysmenorrhea; dyspareunia; recurrent bouts of acute pain and fever; infertility; often dysfunctional uterine bleeding secondary to involvement and poor function of the ovaries; and palpable adnexal disease (e.g., dilated, tortuous hydrosalpinx or pyosalpinx, tuboovarian abscesses, periadnexal adhesions, ovarian cysts, chronic parametrial induration).

Pathologic Features. The initial acute salpingitis and chronic inflammatory process that so often follow are invariably bilateral. However, the severity and extent of the involvement, as well as the type of secondary chronic pathologic manifestation, may vary considerably on the two sides. During the acute phase there is marked inflammation of the tubal mucosa, with edema of the walls of the tubes and a tremendous outpouring of an abundant purulent exudate that fills the tubes and spills into the peritoneal cavity. The exudate and its contained organisms are highly irritating to the serosa of the parietal peritoneum, and acute peritonitis results. It is often confined to the pelvis at first; but not infrequently, with continued exudation, there is more widespread and generalized peritonitis as the exudate is dispersed more widely through visceral and body movements.

The visceral peritoneum of adjacent organs (uterus, ovaries, rectosigmoid, small bowel) also becomes inflamed, and there is a tendency for these structures, together with the omentum, to be drawn down to the region of the fimbriated ends of the tubes, from whence flows the noxious exudate as the body attempts to wall off the primary sites of the infection. As body defense mechanisms, with or without the aid of antibiotics, begin to localize and ultimately to control the acute infection, it is this walling-off process, together with the organization and eventual fibrosis of the areas where the inflammatory exudate has collected, that produces the secondary complications of the chronic phase of the disease. Such complications are distortion of normal anatomy, gross and microscopic, and chronic infection due to a superimposed, secondary bacterial invasion by organisms other than the gonococcus. The gonococci usually survive for only a limited time during the acute phase and only rarely are present during the chronic stages of the disease.

In regard to the tubes, by the time the acute infection has subsided, the tubal mucosa is often irreparably damaged, with destruction of the ciliated epithelium and narrowing or occlusion of the lumen. The damage is due either to inflammatory fibrosis of the tubal walls by localized or diffuse organization and fibrosis of the intraluminal exudate or to peritubal and fimbrial adhesions and blockade—again either as a result of the organized, fibrotic exudate or due to adherence to the neighboring visceral surfaces, which have also become involved by the inflammatory process. Thus even if some degree of tubal patency remains, tubal function is usually seriously impaired owing to mucosal destruction, thickening and rigidity of the wall, and peritubal fixation. More often than not, however, tubal occlusion occurs at the fimbriated or cornual end or, in many instances, at both ends. The specific type of chronic, inflammatory fibrosis of the tubal wall—nodular in gross appearance and restricted to and producing obstruction at the cornual ends of the tubes—is commonly referred to as *salpingitis isthmica nodosa.*

Regardless of the site of block, sterility is usually inevitable and complete. Furthermore, the damaged, obstructed tubes are not only the site of a low grade, symptomatic, chronic infection but also are susceptible to recurring secondary acute infectious flare-ups. Such flare-ups often develop during or just after a period, when secondary bacterial invaders from the vagina (e.g., *Streptococcus, E. coli*) gain access to the cervix and ascend to the tubes, where a perfect culture medium and a local environment ideal for their further growth awaits them. Such is the pathogenesis of recurring attacks of chronic pelvic inflammatory disease.

If the tubes are blocked at both fimbrial and cornual ends, the accumulating mucus and inflammatory secretions eventually fill and distend the tubes, leading either to a hydrosalpinx or, if the material is or becomes infected, to a pyosalpinx on one or both sides—the *retort tubes,* so named because of their gross resemblance to the glass retorts of the chemistry laboratory (Fig. 15-1). At times, secondary hemorrhage occurs in a hydrosalpinx or pyosalpinx, producing a hematosalpinx.

If the fimbriated end of a tube and its adjacent ovary have been fused together as part of the "wall" of an artificial abscess cavity, a chronic tuboovarian abscess results and may attain a considerable size (varying from a few centimeters to 30 to 40 cm in diameter). Often the rectosigmoid, uterus, lateral pelvic wall, and loops of small bowel form other portions of the wall of such a chronic tuboovarian abscess (see Fig. 15-1). It is likely that the ovary becomes extensively involved because organisms gain entrance to its deeper substance through the corpus luteum at the time of ovulation, when a defect in the serosal barrier is present.

As is already apparent, neighboring viscera may also be distorted by the adhesions that result from organization of the original acute exudate. The uterus is commonly drawn back into the hollow of the pelvis, and the adjacent small bowel (or even more distant loops elsewhere in the abdomen) may become fixed,

Fig. 15-1. Findings associated with chronic pelvic inflammatory disease, including tuboovarian abscess, adhesions, pyosalpinx, and an abscess located in the posterior cul-de-sac.

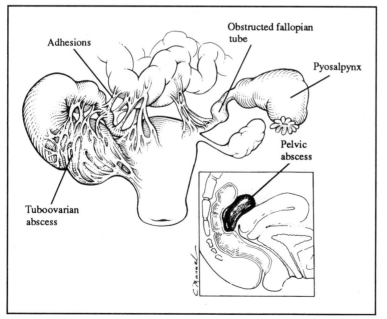

Adhesions

Obstructed fallopian tube

Pyosalpynx

Pelvic abscess

Tuboovarian abscess

kinked, or both, often leading to intestinal obstruction years later. The classic "violin-string" adhesions that form between the upper surface of the liver and the overlying diaphragm are such frequent and characteristic sequelae of the disease as to permit a diagnosis in retrospect whenever they are found at the time of laparotomy performed for whatever reason.

Management. In a young woman suffering her first or second recurrent attack of chronic gonorrheal pelvic inflammatory disease, a conservative program should again be tried, although the chances of resolution of the disease process with return of normal function in the face of repeated acute attacks and persistently palpable adnexal involvement are increasingly slight. Appropriate antibiotic therapy appears, in some patients at least, to facilitate the resolution of the chronic adnexal inflammation, chronic pelvic cellulitis, and parametritis frequently present. Disappearance of symptoms, with marked reduction in the amount of palpable induration, and even occasionally successful pregnancies can occur.

If the disease fails to respond permanently after one or two attempts at conservative therapy, surgical resection (total hysterectomy and bilateral salpingectomy) is often necessary and advisable as the only means of avoiding continued and increasingly frequent acute flare-ups with repeated hospitalizations, prolonged incapacity, and chronic pelvic pain. If the ovaries are markedly involved by the chronic inflammatory process, they too should be excised lest symptoms recur, with the patient requiring reoperation later. If one or both ovaries are totally uninvolved, they can and probably should be preserved in young women. When procedures less than total hysterectomy with bilateral salpingo-oophorectomy are performed, a calculated risk of recurrent difficulties must be accepted by both patient and physician.

A particularly serious complication of chronic pelvic inflammatory disease is the sudden, spontaneous rupture of a tuboovarian abscess, with massive flooding of the peritoneal cavity with its purulent contents. This acute abdominal emergency is rapidly fatal if not treated surgically; and even when surgical exploration is done, the mortality is high, approaching 50 percent if the correct diagnosis is not made immediately and operation carried out within 12 to 24 hours of the rupture. Therefore this diagnosis should be entertained first whenever an acute abdominal disorder develops in a patient with known or suspected chronic pelvic inflammatory disease. Temporizing management, even with massive antibiotic therapy, invariably leads to a fatal outcome. The treatment of choice is a short (6- to 8-hour) course of large intravenous doses of several broad-spectrum antibiotics to cover potential gram-positive, gram-negative, and anaerobic organisms, followed by immediate laparotomy with excision of the tuboovarian abscess and drainage of the peritoneal cavity. It is usually best accomplished by total hysterectomy and bilateral salpingo-oophorectomy, provided laparotomy is done promptly. If there has been prolonged delay in establishing the correct diagnosis and embarking on surgery, the patient's general condition may have deteriorated to the point where only life-saving salpingo-oophorectomy can be done. If there is widespread intraperitoneal sepsis, it may be necessary to explore and drain abscesses in various parts of the upper abdominal cavity as well as in the pelvis and lower abdomen. In such cases, subsequent reoperation and pelvic cleanout are necessary after recovery from the acute episode. Postoperatively, appropriate chemotherapy and other indicated supportive measures to combat shock and infection should be utilized. Because of the great danger posed by this acute complication of a chronic tuboovarian abscess, earlier elective surgical intervention should be seriously considered when this particular type of chronic pelvic inflammatory disease is believed present.

Occasionally, the inflammatory process subsides completely but the damaged tubes are functionally impaired, and the patient is infertile because of tubal occlusion or adherent tubes and ovaries. Although tubal occlusion can be demonstrated by hysterosalpingography, laparoscopy again provides an even more informative diagnostic approach. Not only can the presence of chronic pelvic inflammatory disease be definitely confirmed in this way but the extent and severity of the pathologic process can be accurately evaluated in terms of the chances of success of a trial of conservative management or the indications for some type of corrective surgery. If an infertility investigation of both husband and wife is otherwise normal and satisfactory, and if it is clearly understood that tuboplasty and mobilization of the adnexa successfully restores fertility in at best 20 to 30 percent (lower in many instances of badly diseased tubes), this type of reparative surgery may be suggested to the patient.

Special techniques for salpingostomy (fimbrioplasty), resection and tubal anastomosis, and cornual reimplantation have been developed using microsurgical techniques and adhesion-preventive adjuncts such as high-molecular-weight dextran (Hyskon) (Chap. 13).

CHLAMYDIA INFECTION

In industrialized western society, almost all *Chlamydia trachomatis* infections are sexually transmitted. *Chlamydia* must be considered a pathogen at all times, as the organism is an obligatory intracellular parasite and can survive only by a repetitive cycle that results in death of the infected host cells. Despite being a pathogen *Chlamydia* does not always produce clinically apparent infections.

Chlamydia trachomatis has been recognized as a genital pathogen responsible for many clinical syndromes that closely resemble infections caused by *Neisseria gonorrhoeae*. In women, it is unfortunate that chlamydial infections are difficult to diagnose clinically and so escape detection. Few or no symptoms are produced, and indeed the symptoms and signs that are produced are often nonspecific. The unavailability of ready access to good facilities for isolation of *C. trachomatis* further compounds the diagnostic difficulties and adds to the rise and spread of chlamydial infection because of nondetection and therefore no treatment and contact tracing.

Among populations of men attending general medical clinics, sexually transmitted disease clinics, and student health centers, the prevalence of chlamydial urethral infections is 3 to 5 percent of the asymptomatic men in the general medical settings and 15 to 20 percent of all the men attending the sexually transmitted disease clinics. Prevalence and site of mucosal infection correlate with age and sexual preference; in sexually transmitted disease clinics, 5 percent of homosexual men and 14 percent of heterosexual men

had positive urethral cultures for *Chlamydia;* serologic evidence of chlamydial infection increased with age in heterosexual men but not in homosexual men. Finally, chlamydial infection is infrequent in sexually inexperienced individuals. Prevalence of chlamydial infection in women ranged from 3 to 5 percent in asymptomatic women to more than 20 percent in women attending sexually transmitted disease clinics. Cultures positive for *Chlamydia* have been obtained in 5 to 7 percent of pregnant women and in up to 21 percent of inner-city black pregnant women. Increased risk factors for chlamydial infection include nonwhites (high in blacks), young age (tissue culture isolation of *Chlamydia* is higher in 15- to 21-year-olds, but serum antibody titers to *Chlamydia* increase until age 30), oral contraceptive users with cervical ectopy, and sexual activity. There is poor or no information on the incidence and transmissibility of *Chlamydia* in women. Among partners of men with either chlamydial or gonococcal urethritis, the female partners were infected 45 and 80 percent of the time, respectively; when the men had both infections, 45 and 64 percent of the women had chlamydial and gonococcal infections, respectively.

Chlamydial Cervicitis

Women with chlamydial infection may have no apparent clinical signs. Sites likely to be involved are the endocervical canal, urethra, and rectum. In general, *C. trachomatis* strains appear to be restricted to columnar and transitional columnar cells for their growth. The clinical manifestations of genital infections caused by *Chlamydia* closely parallel those due to *N. gonorrhoeae*. According to a large scale survey of women seen for genital tract complaints, half of the infections with *Chlamydia* were clinically not apparent. The usual finding in most women is an endocervicitis with mucopurulent discharge (37 percent of women). Hypertrophic cervical ectopy (an area of edema, congestion, and friability over the cervix) is found in 19 percent of women. Cervical ectopy may expose a greater number of susceptible columnar epithelial cells to *Chlamydia,* thereby making infection more likely. Because oral contraceptives tend to promote cervical ectopy, risk of *Chlamydia* infection is increased with oral contraceptive use only if cervical ectopy is also present. Colposcopically, cervical follicles can be seen with chlamydial infection but are uncommon. Women with signs of chlamydial cervicitis yield greater numbers of inclusion-forming units on primary isolation in tissue cultures than those without cervicitis.

Clinical recognition of chlamydial cervicitis rests on a high index of suspicion for the condition and a careful cervical examination. A mucopurulent discharge combined with friability and edema over an area of ectopy are findings highly suggestive of chlamydial cervicitis. Differential diagnosis should include gonococcal endocervicitis, salpingitis, endometritis, and intrauterine device-induced cervicitis. If these causes are not evident, a mucopurulent cervical discharge strongly suggests chlamydial cervicitis. Gonococcal endocervicitis can be distinguished after definitive culture results but may occur concomitantly with a chlamydial infection. Gram stain of the cervical discharge of a woman with chlamydial cervicitis usually shows many polymorphonuclear leukocytes, absence of gonococci, and only occasional bacteria. Nevertheless, clinical examination alone cannot distinguish most women with chlamydial infection from uninfected women. Nearly all women with endocervical chlamydial infection develop serum antibodies to *C. trachomatis,* but only 20 to 30 percent exhibit immunoglobulin M (IgM), suggesting that often the cervicitis was not recent.

Chlamydial cervicitis is often associated with cytologic atypia (including reactive and metaplastic atypia) and changes suggestive of dysplasia. There is a two- to fivefold greater risk of developing cervical dysplasia with chlamydial infection of the cervix.

Chlamydial Urethritis

Of women cultured for *Chlamydia trachomatis* at both the cervix and urethra, 50 percent with positive cultures yield the organism from both sites and 25 percent from either site alone. Although most of these patients are asymptomatic, women with chlamydial urethritis may have dysuria, frequency, and pyuria with no bacteriuria. Therefore sterile pyuria with urinary frequency and dysuria should raise the possibility of chlamydial infection of the urethra.

Because of the asymptomatic nature of chlamydial urethritis in many women, the diagnosis should be suspected in those with mucopurulent cervicitis and edematous, friable cervical ectopy. Chlamydial infection should also be strongly entertained in a sexually active young woman with frequency and pyuria or dysuria, especially if her sex partner has a nongonococcal urethritis or she had a new sex partner during the last month or so. Other useful clues supporting chlamydial urethritis include dysuria of more than seven to ten days, lack of hematuria, absence of suprapubic tenderness, and use of birth control pills. A urethral Gram stain showing ten or more polymorphonuclear leukocytes per oil immersion field in women with dysuria further supports the diagnosis of *Chlamydia* infection, although this result may also be found with gonorrheal or trichomonal infections.

Bartholin's duct gland infection with *Chlamydia* produces a purulent exudate similar to that seen with gonococcal infection and has a high incidence of concurrent gonococcal infection of the gland; seven of nine *Chlamydia*-positive women with bartholinitis had concurrent gonorrhea infection. Thus gonorrhea should also be sought when chlamydial bartholinitis is suspected or diagnosed.

Chlamydial Endometritis and Salpingitis

Chlamydia trachomatis may cause endometritis by an ascending infection from the cervix via canalicular spread through the endometrial cavity eventually involving the fallopian tubes. Studies have shown that in patients from whom *C. trachomatis* was isolated from uterine aspirates there was concomitant salpingitis, suggesting that the endometritis was responsible for the intermittent vaginal bleeding observed in patients with chlamydial salpingitis.

It is not clear what proportion of acute salpingitis is due to *C. trachomatis*. Of seven patients with salpingitis who had positive chlamydial cervicitis, six had positive cultures from their fallopian tubes. As many as 80 percent of women with acute salpingitis had antibodies to *C. trachomatis*, with 37 percent serologically indicative of acute chlamydial infection. Recovery of the organism declined with high antibody titer, suggesting that the immune response interferes with recovery of the organism. Thus many seropositive women with negative cultures may actually have chlamydial salpingitis.

Chlamydial infection may also be associated with perihepatitis, perhaps even more commonly than is *N. gonorrhoeae*. Therefore perihepatitis should be suspected in young, sexually active women who develop right upper quadrant pain, fever, nausea or vomiting, with or without evidence of salpingitis. Bronchitis, pneumonia, and endocarditis can be produced by *C. trachomatis,* often in immunocompromised patients who have had an organ transplant.

Diagnosis

Because patients with genital tract *Chlamydia trachomatis* infection are often asymptomatic or the symptoms are similar to those of other sexually transmitted diseases (e.g., gonorrhea), diagnosis of *C. trachomatis* requires confirmation by cytologic, tissue-culture, and serologic methods.

For successful isolation of *C. trachomatis* by culture the following conditions are essential.

1. Collect a specimen containing as many epithelial cells as possible.
2. Prevent bacterial overgrowth of the specimen during transport by adding antibiotics to the transport medium.
3. Centrifuge the specimen to maximize contact between initial bodies and the tissue-culture monolayer.
4. Use an antimetabolite or irradiation to inhibit replication of the tissue monolayer cells.
5. Use iodine, Giemsa, or immunofluorescence staining to detect mature inclusions in infected cells.

An obligate intracellular pathogen, *Chlamydia* is best isolated from cell scrapings rather than from discharges, secretions, or urine. Mucus and debris are removed and an adequate number of cells scraped from the cervix or urethra using rayon- or cotton-

tipped swabs with either an aluminum or plastic shaft (not wooden-shafted swabs because they reduce the number of inclusion-forming units stored in the transport medium). Specimens obtained are placed immediately in sucrose-phosphate transport medium (containing antibiotics—usually gentamicin, vancomycin, and nystatin), refrigerated, and inoculated preferably within 24 hours. Untreated patients give 70 to 80 percent repeatedly positive results or serial cultures, whereas negative patients remain negative. Because of the time, expense, and limited access to tissue culture on which the isolation of *Chlamydia* depends, confirmatory diagnosis of *C. trachomatis* is not widely available.

Serologic tests have not been used routinely for diagnosing chlamydial infections of the genital tract other than for lymphogranuloma venereum because: (1) there is a high baseline prevalence of antibody in sexually active populations likely to be at risk for the infection; (2) the seropositivity increases with age and sexual activity; (3) there is a high seropositivity in culture-negative, asymptomatic patients, presumably from old infection; and (4) the absence of abrupt onset of symptoms leads to inappropriate timing for demonstrating appropriate antibody rise or fall.

Therapy

Antibiotics effective against *Chlamydia trachomatis* in vitro include rifampin, the tetracyclines, macrolides, sulfonamides, and clindamycin. Penicillin, ampicillin, and spectinomycin in single-dose regimens for treatment of gonorrhea usually do not eradicate concomitant chlamydial infection, but tetracyclines or macrolides given for seven days or more can usually eradicate *Chlamydia*. Therefore patients having both gonorrheal and chlamydial infections should be treated for the two organisms by separate antibiotic regimens.

The effectiveness of antimicrobial treatment for uncomplicated cervical, urethral, or endometrial chlamydial infection in women has not been fully assessed. Tetracycline 500 mg twice a day for seven days has successfully eliminated *Chlamydia* from the cervix through three weeks of follow-up. Doxycycline 100 mg twice a day for ten days also successfully eradicated *Chlamydia* from the cervix and urethra of women with the acute urethral syndrome. At present, the relation between elimination of *Chlamydia* from the cervix and clinical cure of salpingitis or eradication of the organism from the fallopian tube has not been established. In practice, it is prudent to treat chlamydial genital tract infections with doxycycline 100 mg twice a day for at least ten days and preferably for two weeks.

PUERPERAL AND POSTABORTAL PELVIC INFLAMMATORY DISEASE

Acute postabortal or puerperal pelvic sepsis accounts for 15 to 20 percent of all pelvic inflammatory disease. Acute pelvic sepsis following abortion has been a serious problem with 3 percent or more mortality especially among those in whom septic shock develops. However, with legalization of abortion and availability of powerful antibiotics, especially against gram-negative anaerobes, the mortality is being reduced.

For a number of reasons, acute puerperal infections or acute pelvic inflammations associated with or immediately after induced, infected abortions differ considerably from the acute phases of gonorrheal pelvic inflammation in terms of their course, complications, and clinical manifestations. Furthermore, they are potentially far more serious from the standpoint of their threat to life and require even more careful, vigorous management if extreme morbidity and high mortality are to be avoided.

To begin with, the gravid or postpartum uterus and the adjacent pelvic soft tissues are vulnerable to infection, the uterine contents being an excellent medium for the growth and survival of bacteria as a focus of continuing systemic contamination. Second, the placental site, the edematous, congested, highly vascular uterine wall nearby, and the parametrial areas characteristic of the pregnant state offer little in the way of a barrier to bacterial invasion coming by way of both lymphatic and venous channels as well as by direct penetration of tissue planes, so that a diffuse pelvic cellulitis and a generalized septicemia are common. Finally, the nature of the bacteria usually involved has a profound influence on the course of the disease. This type of pelvic sepsis is frequently due to a mixed infection. Formerly, hemolytic streptococci and staphylococci were the chief offenders; today, in roughly two-thirds of these cases, gram-negative bacteria are the predominant organisms (*Escherichia coli, Pseudomonas, Proteus, Klebsiella,* and allied gram-negative enteric pathogens). Occasionally, members of the *Clostridium* group (notably *Cl. welchii* and less often *Cl. tetani*) are the principal organisms involved, producing even more local necrosis, sepsis, and overwhelming toxemia.

Because the pathogens usually encountered in septic abortions are highly virulent, invasive bacteria, the rapid local invasion and more generalized septic course are readily understandable. The gram-negative organisms, when permitted to propagate undisturbed in degenerating, necrotic uterine contents or in the wall of the uterus or adjacent parametrial tissues, may produce and liberate into the general circulation massive quantities of bacterial endotoxin, which may lead to a specific, highly lethal type of circulatory failure, termed *gram-negative endotoxemic shock.* When not promptly recognized and vigorously treated, endotoxemic shock has been associated with a mortality of 50 to 80 percent. With proper early treatment, however, mortality can be kept to 5 percent or less.

Pathogenesis of Septic Shock

The endotoxin present in the cell walls of gram-negative bacilli is a lipopolysaccharide or lipoprotein–carbohydrate complex. When large quantities enter the bloodstream, the most important adverse effect is generalized intense vasoconstriction, primarily at the microcirculatory level. The vasoconstriction leads to a marked increase in peripheral vascular resistance with a corresponding marked decrease in tissue perfusion. Intense vasospasm results in part from a direct effect on the microcapillaries and in part from the release of catecholamines from sympathetic nerve endings and the adrenal medulla, both endotoxin-induced. Even a superficial examination of the patient in the early phases of endotoxemic shock suggests the underlying vasospastic and sympathomimetic effects of endotoxin: There is cutaneous vasoconstriction and increased perspiration; and the patient's skin is pale, cold, and clammy despite the raging fever that is often present.

The ensuing generalized hemodynamic changes produce a "stagnant anoxia" that results in direct tissue damage as well as a metabolic acidosis due to defective oxygen delivery and metabolism. Ultimately, a hypovolemic state develops because of shunting and pooling of intravascular fluid beyond the constricted portion of the microcirculation (possibly significant pooling occurs in the splanchnic bed also) as well as plasma losses into areas of capillary congestion and local tissue damage. Hypotension soon follows and increases in severity as the metabolic lacticacidosis, together with decreasing venous return, begins to impair cardiac function. (The increasing impairment of cardiac function may even result in electrocardiographic changes suggestive of acute coronary occlusion.) Increasing hypotension, coupled with the intense vasoconstriction and impaired tissue perfusion, rapidly leads to failing renal function, with oliguria and eventually anuria.

The pulmonary microcirculation is equally vulnerable to these endotoxin effects, and the impaired pulmonary oxygenating capacity is often manifested clinically by cyanosis as well as by a striking tachypnea. Ultimately, acute pulmonary edema may appear, the end result of both cardiac and pulmonary failure.

The neurotoxic effects of the endotoxin, together with the generalized anoxia, are reflected clinically by the appearance of mental confusion and even a semicomatose state in the late stages. Liver damage due to intense vasoconstriction of the hepatic microcirculation occasionally leads to the appearance of jaundice in the late stages. When the gram-negative endotoxemic shock syndrome has entered the irreversible phase, complete vasomotor collapse with generalized vasodilatation may occur as a preterminal event.

With prolonged duration of endotoxin shock, especially in association with the pregnant state, disseminated intravascular thromboses in the kidneys, liver, lungs, and adrenals are prone to occur (*generalized Shwartzman reaction*), usually leading to progressive renal, cardiac, liver, and pulmonary failure, irrevers-

ible shock, and death. The diffuse intravascular coagulation results from stagnation of blood within the microcirculation, producing intimal damage, fibrin deposition, and an initial hypercoagulability with rapid conversion of fibrinogen to fibrin and generalized thrombosis in the smaller vessels. The most devastating effect of this sequence is the deposition of fibrin in the glomeruli, resulting in acute renal cortical necrosis, irreversible kidney damage, complete anuria, and eventually death due to uremia. In addition, the resulting hypofibrinogenemia, depletion of platelets and other clotting factors, and secondary fibrinolysis (generalized fibrinolytic systems are activated when disseminated intravascular thrombosis occurs) may rapidly lead to a state of hypocoagulability and abnormal bleeding of serious proportion, further complicating the clinical management of the desperately ill patient. (It is this predilection for the development of the generalized Shwartzman reaction that increases the risk of death from gram-negative endotoxemic shock in the pregnant patient.)

Septic shock may also accompany overwhelming gram-positive bacterial infection; usually hemolytic streptococci or staphylococci are the responsible organisms because they are among the few gram-positive bacteria that produce an exotoxin. Gram-positive toxemic shock is much less common, and the associated mortality is much lower. The circulatory abnormality is usually one of generalized vasodilatation. Hence the resulting shock is of the normovolemic type, and the patient appears warm and flushed. Vasoconstrictor drugs are therefore frequently indicated for treatment of gram-positive septic shock, whereas they are rarely beneficial and usually deleterious if used for gram-negative endotoxemic shock (see below).

Clinical Features

The clinical course is similar whether the infection follows a septic induced abortion, spontaneous premature rupture of the membranes with resulting chorioamnionitis and placentitis, or normal delivery (postpartum puerperal infection). It is characterized by high fever, rapid pulse, and shaking chills; and the general appearance of the patient is one of extreme toxicity. Examination reveals the typical picture of generalized peritonitis and septicemia; pelvic pain and tenderness are often extreme, and there is usually a purulent discharge from the cervix. In the presence of septic abortion there may be obvious retained placental fragments within the dilated cervical canal, and bleeding may complicate the picture. The accompanying leukocytosis is usually marked.

Later there may be a sudden, dramatic change in the picture, often ushered in by shaking chills, a sudden marked rise in temperature, or both, with the rapid development of vasomotor collapse, profound hypotension, and oliguria, all of which are resistant to the usual therapy and out of all proportion to any blood loss, dehydration, or plasma depletion that may have occurred. During the initial phases of this septic, bacteremic, and gram-negative endotoxemic shock, the patient may remain alert, highly perceptive, and restless, with a feverish, flushed skin and a full, bounding pulse despite marked hypotension. Her appearance at this point is deceptive, however, as within a few hours or even minutes she may rapidly become pulseless, have a subnormal temperature with pale, cold, clammy skin, become dyspneic and cyanotic, and exhibit mental confusion. With more prolonged duration of the endotoxemic shock phase, especially if diffuse intravascular thrombosis occurs, the patient may enter a near-moribund, totally anuric, semicomatose state that invariably implies irreversible shock and a fatal outcome. It is therefore essential that the true nature of the situation be clearly recognized and that vigorous, aggressive therapy be started long before this preterminal phase.

Septic pelvic thrombophlebitis with the development of septic pulmonary infarcts is another complication that may lead to the appearance of a shock-like picture. These events usually occur later in the course of the disease, however, after the septicemia has subsided and the infection has become localized, so that the danger or likelihood of septic endotoxemic shock has passed. When there is clinical and roentgenologic (chest films) evidence of septic pulmonary infarction, anticoagulant therapy is indicated; if repeated infarcts occur, vena caval and bilateral ovarian vein ligations usually prove necessary to prevent a fatal outcome.

Diagnosis and Management

The typical clinical features and the circumstances under which the pelvic infection arose usually render the diagnosis obvious, although other causes of peritonitis must occasionally be considered (e.g., perforated appendicitis). In the case of septic abortion, the physician should not be misled by the patient's refusal to admit that interruption of the pregnancy has been attempted, either by herself or another person, as it is common for patients to deny attempted abortion vigorously. Fever or other evidence of infection in the presence of obvious abortion should warrant substantial treatment immediately. If possible, learn the method and agent (mechanical or chemical) employed to induce the abortion. If a chemical agent has been used (soaps, bleaches, detergents, formalin), the likelihood of extensive uterine necrosis as well as systemic chemical toxicity (hemolysis, renal tubular damage, liver and adrenal injury) is great; and the likelihood of an associated, serious gram-negative or clostridial infection is markedly increased. Hence this situation is also one in which prompt hysterectomy is often indicated to prevent an otherwise uniformly fatal outcome.

From the standpoint of diagnosis, one of the most important steps, as soon as feasible, is the specific identification of the offending bacterial organisms, so that the most effective antibiotic can be employed. Immediate gram-stained smears of fresh cervical discharge are sometimes helpful, particularly for recognition of the *Cl. welchii* bacillus, which can often be identified by its characteristic capsule. Cultures and sensitivity studies of the cervical discharge and peripheral blood should be initiated immediately, as they ultimately provide the most valuable and reliable guides to antibiotic therapy.

Equally important is an immediately instituted, continuous record of frequent observations (at least every 30 to 60 minutes until the period of acute danger has passed) of the vital signs (blood pressure, pulse, respirations) and urine output (hourly measurements are indicated at first); for the purpose of the latter, an indwelling Foley catheter is usually essential. This regimen permits constant appraisal of the patient's condition and response to therapy and serves to give immediate notice of any sudden change that would indicate the need for reevaluation and alteration of the therapeutic program.

Treatment of Simple, Uncomplicated Septic Abortion

Fortunately, in most simple, uncomplicated cases of septic abortion seen early (pregnancy of less than three months' duration, no chemical agent used, no occurrence of uterine perforation, absence of clostridial organisms), bacterial invasion of the uterine wall and beyond is either negligible or completely absent. Therefore the key to successful treatment lies in evacuating the infected uterine contents before there is significant bacterial spread to the uterus itself. However, this goal is best achieved and morbidity and mortality best avoided by a 6- to 12-hour delay in emptying the uterus (unless continuing severe hemorrhage forces earlier intervention) while appropriate preoperative antibiotic therapy is begun. For broad-spectrum antibiotic coverage, penicillin and chloramphenicol are currently the drugs of choice. To obtain prompt, effective blood levels, penicillin 10 million to 20 million units and chloramphenicol 1.0 to 2.0 gm should be given in a continuous intravenous infusion during the preliminary 6- to 12-hour period, together with blood and fluid replacement as indicated. Thereafter, with both local and systemic control of the infection well under way and the patient preferably afebrile, the uterus can be emptied of all retained infected and necrotic tissue in as gentle and atraumatic a fashion as possible.

Cervical dilatation is ordinarily unnecessary, and the uterus can usually be emptied manually with the finger or using placental forceps. Unduly vigorous curettage is to be avoided at all costs, lest further systemic dissemination or even uterine perforation result. However, light anesthesia is necessary, and the uterus should be completely emptied as meticulously as possible by this atraumatic technique, removing all potential foci of infection that might serve as a source for continuing septicemia and gram-negative endotoxemia, ultimately leading to septic shock and a fatal outcome.

In this way the infection can be controlled and erad-

icated in most instances before it has spread beyond the confines of the uterine cavity; and parametritis, perisalpingitis and perioophoritis, pelvic and generalized peritonitis, pelvic abscesses, and septic pelvic thromboembolic complications, as well as overwhelming septicemia and endotoxemia, can be avoided. Early evacuation of the uterus after a preliminary 6- to 12-hour period of antibiotic therapy and restoration of normal blood volume and fluid and electrolyte balance appear to be the most important factors for reducing mortality and morbidity when dealing with septic abortions, particularly when the patient is seen relatively soon (within 24 hours) after induction.

Treatment of Septic Abortion Complicated by Impending or Early Endotoxemic Shock

Progression to the dangerous stage of septic abortion occurs in roughly 3 percent of patients, and it is a medical emergency of the highest order. It usually is the result of long delay by the patient in seeking medical attention or failure on the part of her physician to recognize the existence and serious nature of the potential complications inherent in any septic abortion, premature delivery, or puerperal infection and to anticipate and prevent their development by prompt institution of proper treatment. The mortality has ranged from 30 percent to as high as 80 percent in some reported series.

Once the acute process has progressed to the phase of incipient or early bacteremic shock, first heralded by the appearance of mild hypotension and relative oliguria (hence the importance of continuous and frequent observations of blood pressure and urinary output throughout the treatment), the following additional measures should be instituted immediately: monitoring, laboratory and diagnostic studies, massive intravenous antibiotic therapy, intravenous fluid therapy, drug therapy in support of the circulation, removing the source of infection, other supportive measures, and prevention or treatment of disseminated intravascular coagulation.

Monitoring. A central venous pressure (CVP) catheter should be placed in the superior vena cava via the antecubital or external jugular vein for continuous monitoring of the central venous pressure. This measurement is the best indicator of cardiac status as well as of the effective circulating blood volume. The normal CVP range is 8 to 12 cm H_2O; a CVP of 5 cm or less is indicative of hypovolemia, and a CVP of 15 cm or more is a sign of circulatory volume overload, impending cardiac failure, or both. Frequent, regular observations of the CVP, hourly or half-hourly measurement of urine output (an indwelling Foley catheter should be in place: an hourly urine volume of 25 ml is a reasonable satisfactory minimum), and regularly recorded vital signs (blood pressure, pulse pressure, pulse, respirations every 15 to 30 minutes) are reliable indexes of renal and cardiovascular function as well as of the circulating blood volume. They are also the best guides to fluid and vasoactive drug therapy. Clinical observations of the state of the peripheral circulation may also prove helpful: peripheral pulses, state of the neck veins, auscultatory chest findings (possible incipient pulmonary edema), and status of the cutaneous circulation (patient's skin warm, dry, and flushed; cold, clammy, and pale; or cyanotic).

Laboratory and Diagnostic Studies. Laboratory and diagnostic studies to be initiated as treatment gets under way include the following.

1. Complete blood cell count and hematocrit. These tests may indicate the need for administering blood or plasma.
2. Serum electrolytes (Na, K, Cl, CO_2) and blood urea nitrogen. These tests guide fluid and electrolyte replacement as well as correction of the metabolic acidosis frequently present owing to the increased anaerobic cellular metabolism that accompanies endotoxemic shock.
3. Cultures (both aerobic and anaerobic) and sensitivity studies on cervical discharge, placental tissue, and peripheral blood if not already done.
4. Gram-stained smears of the cervical discharge if not already done. The results can provide immediate identification of *Clostridium,* if present, and sometimes help to distinguish between the more frequent predominantly gram-negative and the less common primarily gram-positive mixed infections.
5. Radiographic studies: abdominal scout film (kidneys, ureters, bladder) to detect foreign bodies or free peritoneal air, indicating uterine perforation; chest films, in search of signs of septic pulmonary emboli.
6. Confirmatory cul-de-sac aspiration. This procedure is indicated if the findings on vaginal and rectal examinations raise the suspicion of a pelvic abscess.

Massive Intravenous Antibiotic Therapy. Rapid institution of massive antibiotic therapy is best done as an intermittent ("piggyback") intravenous infusion. Effective blood levels are achieved and help to avoid the problem of fluid overload in the presence of impaired cardiovascular function and oliguria. Initial antibiotic programs of choice, pending the results of cultures and sensitivity studies of the specific organisms present in the individual case may vary from hospital to hospital depending on local patterns of antibiotic resistance. However, the program should provide coverage for a polymicrobial infection, in particular with fatal gram-negative anaerobes. Suitable programs that have been employed include the following.

1. Penicillin 40 million to 60 million units (total 24-hour dosage) in combination with chloramphenicol 3.0 to 6.0 gm (total 24-hour dosage), each given by the intermittent intravenous infusion technique. They can be supplemented by streptomycin 250 to 500 mg given intramuscularly every 6 hours. If the patient is allergic to penicillin, large doses of cephalexin monohydrate (Keflex) can be used instead. Currently one of the cephalosporins is often used in place of penicillin.

2. If the urine output is satisfactory, 250 mg of kanamycin can be given intramuscularly every 6 hours in place of chloramphenicol and streptomycin. Kanamycin is particularly effective for *Proteus* infections, but the *Pseudomonas* organism has proved resistant to it. Furthermore, it is nephrotoxic (the dosage should never exceed 1 gm daily even under ideal circumstances), so that its use is probably best avoided, particularly if oliguria is present.

3. Gentamicin plus clindamycin and either a cephalosporin or ampicillin is a triple antibiotic combina-

tion often used for severe pelvic inflammation. The combination provides adequate coverage for most of the polymicrobial flora encountered in such pelvic infections. Metronidazole, given intravenously, has been employed also for severe pelvic infections.

4. A shift to another antibiotic program may be indicated if a favorable clinical response is not obtained or if sensitivity studies reveal the organisms to be more sensitive to other agents. Gentamicin sulfate administered intramuscularly or intravenously (60 to 80 mg every 8 hours) may prove useful because it is active against both *Pseudomonas* and *Proteus* as well as against virtually all other gram-negative pathogens including *E. coli* and *Klebsiella-Aerobacter* species. However, it too is associated with potential nephrotoxicity as well as ototoxicity; hence it should never be used in combination with kanamycin, streptomycin, polymyxin, or colistin. Serum gentamicin levels should be monitored. Gentamicin should be employed with caution in the presence of oliguria and impaired renal function and then should be used only if the infection has failed to respond to the usual agents. If sensitivity studies indicate that a favorable response can be expected, tetracycline can be safely used intravenously in a total daily dosage of 2 gm, even in the presence of impaired renal function. Other antibiotics known to be effective against gram-negative organisms (e.g., ampicillin, colistin, neomycin, polymyxin, paromomycin) may be indicated by sensitivity studies in individual cases. If *Bacteroides* organisms (*B. fragilis* is the most common anaerobe in this group) are detected, or if their presence is suspected on the basis of delayed clinical response or a particularly foul-smelling, effusive purulent drainage, chloramphenicol or clindamycin should definitely be administered, as these agents appear to be the most effective antibiotics against these anaerobic species, with tetracycline and lincomycin somewhat less so.

a. A booster dose of tetanus toxoid or tetanus antitoxin (100,000 units) should also be given; and if clostridial infection has been proved or is suspected, polyvalent gas gangrene antitoxin (100,000 units) should probably also be given intravenously, although its value is questionable.

b. During the initial phases of antibiotic therapy one must be on the alert for a possible increase in the severity of signs and symptoms of septic shock that may follow the rapid lysis of gram-negative organisms with release of more endotoxin.

Intravenous Fluid Therapy. Electrolyte and fluid replacement should include sodium bicarbonate solutions and should preferably be lactate-free (Ringer's solution with added sodium bicarbonate is probably ideal) to correct more effectively the metabolic lacticacidosis. Correction of dehydration also helps by reducing the abnormally elevated viscosity of the blood pooling in the constricted microcapillaries. Plasma may be needed to restore a normal circulating extracellular fluid volume because the previously discussed generalized plasma losses that occur during the early endotoxemic shock phase may be large. Some advocate the use of dextran 40 as a volume expander because of its potential beneficial effect of decreasing blood viscosity. Whole blood is less often indicated because it may further aggravate the problem of increased blood viscosity, but it may be needed if external blood losses have resulted from continued uterine bleeding. The best guides to the total volume as well as to the rate of fluid replacement are the central venous pressure, hourly urine output, and hematocrit, together with the regular blood pressure and pulse observations. It is important to avoid overloading the circulation. On the other hand, it is necessary at times to increase the rate of fluid replacement, especially if vasodilator drugs are employed (see below).

Drug Therapy in Support of the Circulation. Before administering vasoactive drugs, restoration of circulating blood volume and correction of acidosis should be well under way or nearly complete.

1. *Corticosteroids* should be given in so-called pharmacologic doses to all patients, regardless of the degree of hypotension and oliguria. They are not given for their usual physiologic effects because there is no evidence that an adrenal insufficiency per se develops during septic shock. In large doses, however, corticosteroids have an effect resembling that of α-adrenergic blocking agents in that they diminish vasospasm and thus tend to reverse the abnormal circula-

tory dynamics in endotoxemic shock by decreasing peripheral vascular resistance and increasing cardiac output. There is also evidence that corticosteroids exert a direct protective effect against endotoxin at the cellular level, possibly preventing damage to the cell membrane and thus avoiding increased capillary membrane permeability. Finally, it is also possible that corticosteroids provide specific protection against the development of bacterial hypersensitivity and subsequent anaphylactic reaction after the sudden release of endotoxic antigen triggered by the antibiotic treatment of the bacteremia.

Intravenous hydrocortisone 1 gm or its equivalent (e.g., Solu-Medrol 250 mg every 4 to 6 hours) is given immediately; and depending on the clinical response, the same dose may have to be repeated in a few hours. A daily dosage of 2.0 to 5.0 gm may be necessary for as long as five days in some patients.

2. When hypotension and oliguria persist after a few hours of the previously outlined therapeutic program, trial of a *vasoactive drug* is indicated. The question as to whether vasoconstrictor or vasodilator drugs should be used was at one time highly controversial. Because there may be alternating periods of vasoconstriction and vasodilatation during the early phases of endotoxemic shock, both may be useful in individual cases. Nevertheless, because the fundamental and ultimately the principal deleterious effect of endotoxin is widespread vasospasm, and the typical patient is cold and clammy despite an adequate central venous pressure and increasing hypotension, a vasodilator is usually the agent of choice.

a. Isoproterenol (Isuprel) has both *vasodilating and cardiac stimulant actions*, thereby increasing tissue perfusion as well as tending to increase cardiac output and blood pressure. It therefore seems to be ideal for correcting the hemodynamic alterations of endotoxemic shock and far more appropriate than a vasoconstrictor drug in the cold, clammy, hypotensive, oliguric patient in whom intense vasoconstriction is obviously already present. Isoproterenol is administered intravenously in a solution of 2.5 to 5.0 mg dissolved in 500 ml of 5% dextrose in water (D/W), adjusting the rate of infusion at 0.5 to 1.0 ml per minute, depending on the response as evaluated by the effects on blood pressure, urine output, central venous pressure, and general condition of the patient. If necessary, either the concentration or the rate of flow may be doubled. When vasodilators are used, the central venous pressure must be watched closely. A significant decrease indicates that fluid replacement with blood, plasma, and electrolyte solution has been inadequate and that the volume and rate of fluid therapy must be increased. Because of its positive inotropic effect on the myocardium, isoproterenol can produce significant tachycardia or cardiac arrhythmia, which should be monitored.

b. A heart rate of 120 beats per minute or more or the appearance of a cardiac arrhythmia (in both cases cardiac output decreases rather than increases) contraindicates the initial or continued use of isoproterenol. In this situation, other *vasodilating drugs* should be used instead, e.g., intravenous chlorpromazine (Thorazine) 5 mg or 10 to 15 mg if necessary, given at intervals in accordance with the effects on the central venous pressure and skin temperature, or phenoxybenzamine (Dibenzyline) 1 mg per kilogram of body weight, also given intravenously at intervals depending on the response.

c. Much less often in gram-negative septic shock, but fairly characteristically in the occasional patient with gram-positive bacterial shock, the clinical picture (hypotension, low central venous pressure, adequate urine output, warm and dry skin) suggests a generalized decrease in vascular tone; thus a *vasoconstrictor* may be tried instead. Metaraminol bitartrate (Aramine) affects both the myocardium and peripheral arterioles directly, producing an elevation of both systolic and diastolic blood pressures and increasing the blood flow through the cerebral, renal, and coronary vasculature. It is administered intravenously in a solution of 100 mg dissolved in 1000 ml of 5% D/W at a rate of roughly 20 mg per hour, adjusting the dose as necessary to maintain the systolic blood pressure in the 90 to 100 mm Hg range. If the amount of drug required increases, the central venous pressure rises abnormally, or oliguria develops, a prompt switch to a vasodilator is indicated.

3. General cardiovascular (and pulmonary) supportive measures include oxygen therapy (and endo-

tracheal intubation or tracheotomy if maintenance of an adequate airway is in doubt) and rapid digitalization if the central venous pressure rises above 15 cm H_2O or if signs of congestive failure appear.

Removing the Source of Infection. Eradication of the source of the continuing infection is the keystone of successful treatment. In most cases it can be accomplished by careful and complete evacuation of the uterus. In the presence of endotoxemic shock, evacuation should be done reasonably soon after the preceding supportive measures have been taken, usually within 4 to 6 hours. In the presence of clostridial infection, hysterectomy without a preliminary dilatation and curettage (D&C) is indicated. Occasionally, if the pregnancy is of three to four months' duration, the D&C can be facilitated by administering oxytocics beforehand to aid in evacuating the uterus. Oxytocics should be used cautiously, however, as the resulting increase in uterine contractions may, in the presence of significant myometrial necrosis or infection, lead to flooding of the circulation with large numbers of bacteria and additional endotoxin. If effective support of the circulation and adequate antibiotic therapy have been given preoperatively and are continued for as long as necessary postoperatively, the favorable clinical response after removal of all retained necrotic and infected uterine contents by a D&C is often dramatic.

However, in about 10 percent of cases, the infection has spread beyond the confines of the uterine cavity and its contents, and a D&C cannot adequately deal with the local source of infection. This situation should be recognized as early as possible, because an aggressive approach involving emergency hysterectomy may be the only hope of saving life. Because these patients are usually young, may require further childbearing, and usually recover with proper medical treatment combined with early uterine evacuation, it is difficult to decide if and when hysterectomy is necessary to save life. In the presence of endotoxemic shock, hysterectomy is nearly always indicated under the following circumstances.

1. *Clostridium perfringens* infection. Although clostridial organisms are responsible for only 1 to 2 percent of all septic abortions (3 to 5 percent of those

involving gram-negative bacteria), the infection is highly lethal unless promptly and properly treated, in which case the mortality can be held to 5 to 10 percent or less. These anaerobic organisms produce tissue-necrotizing and hemolyzing toxins, hyaluronidase (which permits rapid tissue invasion), and a copious amount of gas that permeates the tissues (characteristic of these "gas gangrene" infections). Clostridial infection is often suspected on the basis of the following clinical picture: extreme toxicity, high fever, rapid pulse, and marked leukocytosis; a tender, boggy uterus; occasionally palpable soft-tissue crepitus or radiographic evidence of gas in the tissues; early oliguria; occasionally hemoglobinuria, hemoglobinemia, and jaundice due to hemolysis; and a strikingly euphoric, placid appearance of the patient despite her grave condition. The diagnosis can be rapidly established by gram-stained smear of the purulent discharge taken directly from the cervix, revealing large gram-positive encapsulated rods; there should be no treatment delay for confirmation by culture. Prompt hysterectomy with bilateral salpingo-oophorectomy, *without* a preliminary D&C, should be done; if an attempt at medical management supplemented by D&C alone is made, mortality approaches 100 percent.

2. History of induction of abortion by corrosive, chemical, or toxic douches (formalin, soaps, Lysol, detergents, bleaches). Uterine necrosis with secondary infection of the uterine wall is invariably present, so that simple evacuation of the uterus cannot possibly eradicate the septic focus. The overwhelming infection and chemical injury that almost invariably accompany septic abortions induced by chemical solutions should usually be treated in the same fashion as a clostridial infection (i.e., by adequate initial medical therapy followed by prompt hysterectomy) if the almost universally fatal course that otherwise usually follows in this situation is to be prevented. Only occasionally does conservative management by intensive antibiotic therapy and simple evacuation of the uterus suffice and permit hysterectomy to be avoided. If an initial conservative approach is adopted, the patient must be followed closely and carefully, so that hysterectomy can be done immediately at the first sign of deterioration of her condition.

3. Evidence of an intraabdominal foreign body, uterine perforation, pelvic abscess. (Cul-de-sac aspiration yields pus under these circumstances.)

4. Uterus larger than three to four months' size. Here again a D&C is usually inadequate to the task of completely eliminating the source of the infection, which is vital to prevent mortality in the face of established endotoxemic shock.

5. Palpable adnexal abscess (also indicating clearly that sepsis has spread beyond the uterine cavity).

6. Assuming that adequate preliminary supportive therapy has been given, additional indications for prompt hysterectomy are as follows: (1) failure of the patient to improve within 4 to 6 hours after a D&C; (2) sudden deterioration of the patient's condition during or immediately following a D&C; (3) the finding of little or no retained products of conception at the time of curettage; or (4) progressive oliguria.

In other, less specific situations, only constant, close supervision of the patient's course and response to medical therapy as indicated by changes in vital signs, local findings, urine output, and so on enable the physician to make the timely decision that hysterectomy is indicated as an emergency lifesaving measure. It is important to make the decision and act on it promptly (preferably within 6 to 12 hours of the onset of shock) before the preterminal stage of irreversible shock has developed. Each case must be considered individually.

Hysterectomy should nearly always be accompanied by bilateral salpingo-oophorectomy, as microabscesses of the ovaries are often present despite a normal external appearance. Prophylactic vena caval ligation and high ligation of both ovarian veins should also be considered at the time the hysterectomy is performed and should definitely be done if recurrent septic pulmonary embolism has already occurred.

Other Supportive Measures. Hypothermia (reduction of body temperature to as low as 90°F) has been employed by some physicians, partly to control the frequent raging fever (103° to 105°F is not uncommon in the early stages of septic shock) but primarily to reduce tissue oxygen requirements in the face of prolonged hypotension in a desperately ill patient. *Hyperbaric oxygen* chambers have been utilized by others for this same purpose. *Hemodialysis* may be indicated and may have to be repeated several times during the recovery period in patients who have experienced acute temporary renal failure and who may be essentially anuric for as long as seven to ten days.

Prevention or Treatment of Disseminated Intravascular Coagulation. Although the generalized Shwartzman reaction with the formation of diffuse intravascular thrombi throughout the microcirculation can be one of the most serious, life-threatening complications of endotoxemic shock, the question of whether to give prophylactic therapy remains controversial. Intravenous heparin would be the appropriate drug, in a dosage of 60 mg every 6 hours, to maintain the clotting time at roughly twice normal until the infection is completely controlled. However, if there is definite evidence that disseminated intravascular coagulation (DIC) is occurring, heparin therapy is indicated, should be instituted promptly, and may prove lifesaving.

Clinically, the first manifestation of DIC may be the appearance of an abnormal bleeding tendency (*consumption coagulopathy*). The onset of DIC can also be recognized by simple laboratory tests, as it is accompanied by an obvious fall in platelet count and serum fibrinogen level and an increase in both prothrombin and partial thromboplastin times. Examination of a thin blood smear is helpful not only for estimating the platelet count but also for finding malformed red blood cells (helmet cells, comma cells, and burr cells—misshapen because they have been stripped away from partially thrombosed capillary walls), which are essentially diagnostic of DIC.

Heparin can be given either by (1) continuous intravenous infusion with a starting bolus dose of 5000 to 10,000 units followed by a maintenance infusion dose of 1000 to 2000 units per hour or (2) intermittently in a dosage of 5000 to 10,000 units every 4 to 6 hours. The aim is to obtain a prothrombin time two and one-half times that of controls (normal). Heparin prevents further progress of the intravascular coagulation process, and only occasionally is it necessary to give platelet transfusions, fibrinogen, and fresh frozen plasma or whole blood, as platelets, fibrinogen, and other depleted coagulation factors (e.g., Factors V and VIII) are rapidly replaced once the pathologic clotting process is halted. In any case, heparin should definitely be administered first; and unless a severe hemorrhagic problem is encountered, platelets are given only if the platelet count remains depressed for more than 12 hours. Although fibrinogen replacement is considered only if the fibrinogen level persists at less than 100 mg per deciliter, it is better to give *fresh* blood or *fresh* frozen plasma, which replaces most of the clotting factors consumed by the DIC.

Chronic Postabortal or Puerperal Pelvic Inflammatory Disease

The course and features of the chronic phase and the principles of management of chronic postabortal or puerperal pelvic inflammatory disease are in general similar to those for chronic pelvic inflammation following gonorrheal salpingitis. However, because of the deeply invasive propensities of the usual original causative bacterial organisms, a chronic woody, or "ligneous," pelvic cellulitis and parametritis are frequently encountered, with the result that the uterus and adnexa are literally frozen in place by the extensive chronic inflammatory reaction and fibrosis that surround them. On the other hand, pyosalpinx, hydrosalpinx, and tuboovarian abscess are somewhat less common, as the initial acute adnexal infection is frequently perisalpingitis and perioophoritis; and the resulting peritonitis, though intense, is not accompanied by the profuse, thick exudate so characteristic of acute gonorrheal salpingitis, the latter being primarily an ascending, surface infection of the tubal endothelium.

TUBERCULOUS PELVIC INFLAMMATION

Tuberculous salpingitis, with or without accompanying secondary involvement of the endometrium, once constituted 5 to 10 percent of all pelvic inflammatory disease, but it is becoming less frequent in the United States. Between 40 and 50 percent of patients suffering from pelvic tuberculosis are asymptomatic except for "unexplained" infertility. Tuberculosis is found to be responsible for approximately 5 percent of all cases of female infertility in the United States. In other areas of the world, the percentages are higher, e.g., India 20 percent and Europe 10 percent.

The remaining 50 to 60 percent of patients who are symptomatic have one or more of the following symptoms and signs: pelvic and abdominal pain and dysmenorrhea; low grade fever; fatigue and weight loss; occasional menstrual irregularity (less common than with other forms of chronic pelvic inflammation); slightly tender adnexal masses; rarely, ascites secondary to tuberculous peritonitis; and rarely, ulcerations and sinus tracts involving the external genitalia. The tuberculin skin test is usually strongly positive.

Pathologic Features

The fallopian tubes are the primary site of pelvic tuberculosis in all cases. The disease is nearly always bilateral, and spontaneous healing is rare. The endometrium is involved secondarily in fewer than half the patients with tuberculous salpingitis and associated pelvic inflammatory disease. The tubal lesion always develops as the result of spread via the bloodstream from a primary focus elsewhere, usually the lung. In this respect, tuberculosis of the reproductive tract is similar to urinary tract tuberculosis, which is also invariably a blood-borne infection; not infrequently, both develop in the same patient.

During the early phases of the disease the tubes may appear grossly normal or only slightly injected and imperceptibly swollen and edematous, even though definite histologic evidence of tuberculosis is already present and smears and cultures readily reveal the presence of acid-fast bacilli. It is this deceptively normal gross appearance during the early stages and the lack of symptoms, even when moderately advanced lesions are present, that often makes the disease difficult to recognize. However, even in the early, microscopic stage, infertility may already have resulted owing to the mucosal damage and impaired tubal function. In fact, in well over half the cases it is the complaint of sterility that prompts the patient to seek medical advice and ultimately leads to establishing the presence of pelvic tuberculosis. The occasional occurrence of ectopic pregnancy is probably also a complication of minimal, early disease, or of disease arrested by therapy, for in either case tubal function is often impaired.

As the pathologic process advances, the typical gross lesions of tuberculosis make their appearance, and the tubes often become filled with and distended by caseous material, resembling the "retort tubes" of chronic gonorrheal salpingitis with pyosalpinx. Peritubal adhesions, which are characteristically dense, form and encase the tube and ovary together in a solid mass of fibrocaseous reaction. The tubal fimbriae become agglutinated, and eventually complete fimbrial occlusion occurs. Often tubercles are visible on the serosal surfaces of the tubes as well as on the adjacent parietal and cul-de-sac peritoneum, rectosigmoid, and nearby loops of ileum; adhesions between these structures and the adnexa may also form.

Occasionally, with advanced pelvic tuberculosis before tubal occlusion has occurred, the outpouring of caseous exudate may result in a generalized tuberculous peritonitis, with tubercles and intense serosal inflammation present over a widespread area of the general peritoneal cavity. There is often accompanying ascites, the peritoneal fluid having a characteristic "ground-glass" appearance and yielding a positive diagnostic result when submitted for culture and guinea pig inoculation. A similar discharge of infected material into the endometrial cavity is presumably the cause of the usually superficial infection of the endometrium that is present in fewer than half the cases. The ovaries are involved in 10 to 15 percent of cases, and this situation together with the debilitating systemic effects of the infection may lead to menstrual irregularities and amenorrhea.

Although fortunately rare, one of the most serious complications of the disease is the occurrence of pregnancy in untreated patients: The possibility of acute fatal miliary dissemination is great, occurring in approximately one-third of such patients.

Diagnosis and Evaluation

In patients with minimal pelvic tuberculosis who are asymptomatic except for infertility and who have essentially negative pelvic examinations, the diagnosis may be suggested unexpectedly by the findings of hysterosalpingography, laparoscopy, or routine endometrial biopsy (typical tubercles noted on microscopic examination), all of which are procedures frequently done during the course of a routine sterility investigation. Diagnosis can and should be confirmed by bacteriologic studies performed on menstrual discharge (smear stained for acid-fast bacilli, tuberculosis cultures, and guinea pig inoculations).

In patients with a suggestive history and positive physical findings (e.g., tuboovarian masses)—in other words, advanced pelvic tuberculosis—the diagnosis can be made and confirmed by any or all of the preceding studies. If the diagnosis is suspected, curettage or hysterosalpingography should be avoided, as an acute flare-up of the usually low grade tuberculous salpingitis frequently occurs after either procedure due to secondary pyogenic bacterial invasion.

All patients should have chest roentgenograms and sputum cultures and smears. (Pelvic tuberculosis invariably is the result of blood-borne spread from a primary pulmonary focus, usually currently inactive.) An intravenous pyelogram, cystoscopy, acid-fast smears and cultures, and guinea pig studies of the urine should also be done to rule out concomitant tuberculosis of the urinary tract.

Treatment

Minimal Pelvic Tuberculosis. In addition to ensuring adequate diet and rest and the initiation of other general health measures, specific chemotherapy for tuberculosis should be given: isoniazid 100 mg orally three times daily for twelve months with dihydrostreptomycin 1 gm intramuscularly twice weekly for three to six months. It is important to use two or more antituberculosis drugs or antibiotics because of the frequency and rapidity with which drug-resistant strains develop when one one chemotherapeutic agent is employed. There should be a careful, prolonged followup period with premenstrual endometrial biopsies and menstrual cultures at intervals of four to six months for several years following cessation of treatment.

Complete, permanent cures and occasionally even normal pregnancies and deliveries have been reported following the use of this program in women with minimal disease. However, the chances for restoration of fertility are poor because, although the infection may be completely arrested and tubal patency maintained, impairment of tubal function is often unrelieved and ovum pickup and transfer remain unsatisfactory. Therefore the incidence of subsequent tubal pregnancy has been high.

If the disease recurs at any time, as indicated by positive menstrual cultures or endometrial biopsies or by the development of clinical symptoms or palpable adnexal disease, the patient should receive another course of chemotherapy followed by surgical removal of the uterus, tubes, and ovaries because the process has now reached the stage of advanced disease. Today, with adequate and specific systemic chemotherapy available, hysterectomy and bilateral salpingo-oophorectomy are necessary in only a small percentage (about 20 percent) of patients, provided the disease is discovered and drug treatment instituted during the early phases.

Advanced Pelvic Tuberculosis. With advanced pelvic tuberculosis, the institution of general measures, including bed rest, are even more important than in the earlier phases. Specific chemotherapy, as follows, is indicated for even longer periods: isoniazid 100 mg by mouth three times daily for twelve to eighteen months with dihydrostreptomycin 1 mg intramuscularly two to three times weekly (or if there is sensitivity to streptomycin, paraaminosalicylic acid 3 gm four times daily) for six to twelve months. The course of treatment should be longer if a pronounced systemic reaction (e.g., fever, weight loss) was present initially. Adnexal masses may become temporarily smaller, though they rarely disappear, and the patient usually shows a favorable general response. At the end of this time, total hysterectomy and bilateral salpingo-oophorectomy are carried out, and then the antituberculosis chemotherapy is continued postoperatively for another nine to twelve months.

The diagnosis of pelvic tuberculosis is sometimes first made at laparotomy. If so, total hysterectomy with bilateral salpingo-oophorectomy should be done, if feasible, and the operation followed by chemotherapy for nine to twelve months. Occasionally, the diagnosis is totally unsuspected even at laparotomy and is

not apparent until after histologic examination of part or all of the pelvic organs resected for what was believed to be chronic pelvic inflammatory disease of gonococcal or postabortal origin. If the operation was a complete one (total hysterectomy and bilateral salpingo-oophorectomy), postoperative chemotherapy should be given according to the preceding schedule. If the operation was incomplete, the patient should have specific chemotherapy for three to four months and then reoperation with removal of the remaining potentially involved pelvic structures.

OTHER CAUSES OF SALPINGITIS AND PELVIC INFLAMMATORY DISEASE

Nonspecific Infections

Although considerably less common than the infections discussed so far, nonspecific pelvic infections sometimes occur and may be caused by other pyogenic organisms (e.g., *Streptococcus, Staphylococcus*) or by the mixed bacterial flora present in the vagina and anogenital region. The organisms may ascend superficially through the endometrial cavity to produce an endometritis, salpingitis, and pelvic peritonitis; or they may gain direct access to the deeper parametrial areas by invading venous and lymphatic channels in the wall of the cervix or fundus to produce diffuse pelvic cellulitis and, ultimately, often peritonitis, perisalpingitis, and periooophoritis. These nonspecific pyogenic infections are invariably secondary to some form of local trauma, either acute or chronic, that disrupts the normal barrier or resistance of the vaginal mucosa and endocervix to ascending or invasive infection. Circumstances under which it may occur include the following.

1. Operative trauma, e.g., curettage, cervical biopsy or cauterization, and various local diagnostic or therapeutic procedures such as endometrial biopsy or hysterosalpingography. Fortunately, such complications are rare. (Pelvic sepsis following major pelvic surgery is discussed in Chap. 5.)
2. Abnormal uterine drainage situations, with retained secretions acting as a nidus for ascending infection, e.g., cervical stenosis, usually second-

ary to previous surgery or improper cauterization, or congenital anomalies of the uterus, particularly the various duplications.

3. Trauma and chronic infection associated with the old-fashioned cervical contraceptive stem pessary, less often in connection with improperly fitted or neglected vaginal pessaries.
4. Improper (high-pressure) douching, particularly if chemically irritating solutions are used.
5. Infected tumors, e.g., cervical or endometrial carcinoma, carcinosarcoma of the uterus, necrotic polyps, or fibroids.

The course and symptomatology of these nonspecific pyogenic infections are much the same as are encountered with postabortal pelvic inflammatory disease. However, in the absence of pregnancy the process is more likely to be mild, and fulminating septicemia and toxemia are only rarely encountered. Conservative treatment with antibiotics and general supportive measures usually rapidly bring these secondary infections under control, although occasionally the infection progresses to the formation of a pelvic abscess that requires drainage. Even rarer causes of acute or chronic salpingitis and associated diffuse pelvic inflammation and peritonitis include infection with the typhoid-paratyphoid group of organisms, actinomycosis, and parasitic infestations such as *Enterobius vermicularis* (pinworms) and schistosomiasis (common in Caribbean waters as well as in Egypt and South Africa).

Intrauterine Contraceptive Devices

Intrauterine contraceptive devices have been widely employed, and their use has been accompanied by acute and chronic pelvic inflammatory disease (endometritis, salpingitis, parametritis, and pelvic peritonitis) in a significant number of patients. The usual pyogenic organisms are the ones commonly involved, but actinomycosis infections have also been reported (Chap. 22). Another common association of the intrauterine device is with unilateral tuboovarian abscess.

Pelvic and Ovarian Vein Thrombophlebitis

Pelvic and ovarian vein thrombophlebitis should be mentioned, not only as inflammatory disorders in

their own right but also because they tend to simulate pelvic or lower abdominal inflammatory processes of a purely infectious type. Flagrant septic pelvic thrombophlebitis with or without septic embolization may occur as a complication of any of the acute pelvic infections previously described and is usually easily recognized, especially if pulmonary emboli occur. Such a septic thrombophlebitis should be treated with both antibiotics and anticoagulants, together with eradication of the primary septic focus within the pelvis and usually ovarian vein and vena caval ligations as well, especially if septic emboli are occurring.

A more benign type of pelvic phlebitis may develop in a postpartum or postoperative gynecologic patient and present diagnostic difficulties. Pelvic pain and a febrile course with the absence of positive findings other than tenderness on physical examination are characteristic and suggest low grade pelvic inflammatory disease. The sudden occurrence of a small pulmonary infarct may be the first clue to the real nature of the pelvic disorder.

In the case of ovarian vein thrombophlebitis, which occurs most frequently in postpartum patients (presumably because of the pelvic venous stasis and hypercoagulability present at term), the pain is unilateral and most often in the right lower quadrant (the venous flow on the right is often antegrade and hence more prone to stasis, whereas it is always retrograde in the left ovarian vein), thus frequently raising the question of appendicitis or twisted ovarian cyst. If thrombosis of the ovarian veins is extensive, the dilated mass of clotted veins and the swollen ovary, congested by venous obstruction, may present as a palpable, rope-like, tender pelvic or lower abdominal mass.

Despite the febrile course and occasionally positive blood cultures, antibiotic therapy by itself invariably has no effect on the clinical course of the disease. However, if the diagnosis is suspected on the basis of the typical sequence of events, and there is no obvious indication for exploratory laparotomy, institution of anticoagulant therapy usually produces a prompt response, with disappearance of pain, fever, and leukocytosis within a few days. Frequently, laparotomy proves necessary before a definite diagnosis can be established, particularly in the case of ovarian vein thrombophlebitis. In this situation, the thrombosed veins should be resected, preserving the adnexa when possible but otherwise carrying out unilateral salpingo-oophorectomy; anticoagulant therapy is then given postoperatively. If an episode of embolization occurs, anticoagulation should be instituted and maintained for an appropriate length of time. If there are recurring small pulmonary infarcts, ligation or plication of the inferior vena cava as well as bilateral high ovarian vein ligation are indicated.

OTHER VENEREAL DISEASES

In addition to gonorrhea and chlamydial infection, there are four other major specific sexually transmitted diseases involving the reproductive tract: syphilis, chancroid, lymphogranuloma (lymphopathia) venereum, and granuloma inguinale. Several minor diseases of the lower genital tract, including trichomoniasis, condyloma acuminatum, herpes progenitalis, and *Hemophilus vaginalis* infections, are also of venereal origin. Some believe that pediculosis pubis should be considered a sexually transmitted disorder. (The minor venereal diseases are discussed in Chap. 14.) Although these sexually transmitted diseases are less frequently encountered today, they are considered briefly here because when they do occur they are customarily treated by the gynecologist. They can pose problems diagnostically, and it is important that they are promptly recognized, appropriately treated, and referred for treatment if indicated.

Syphilis

Infection with the spirochete *Treponema pallidum* invariably occurs by direct genital (occasionally oral-genital) contact with an actively infected sexual partner. Rarely, accidental direct bloodstream infection can occur following transfusion with blood from an infected donor (hence the vital necessity for routine serologic tests for syphilis in all prospective blood donors). The disease is occasionally transmitted to a woman during impregnation by a man who is in the tertiary phase of the disease, the maternal bloodstream ultimately becoming infected via the fetal-placental-maternal circulatory pathways. The child of such a union is frequently born with congenital syphilis. For some years, syphilis was erroneously believed to be declining in incidence and therefore importance.

The reproductive tract is involved for the most part only during the initial or primary stage of the disease, serving essentially as the portal of entry. Thereafter and following the brief secondary phase, the prolonged (usually lifelong, unless discovered and successfully treated) tertiary stage of the disease is a generalized systemic infection that may be latent or silent or have widespread and highly protean manifestations throughout the body.

In women the primary lesion is a chancre that appears three to four weeks after exposure and most often is located on the labia majora. It may also develop elsewhere on the external genitalia or occasionally on the cervix, where it often resembles a simple "erosion" and frequently passes completely unnoticed. Even the vulvar lesions may be tiny, presenting only as small "abrasions" or superficial erosions or fissures that easily escape detection or go unrecognized. The classic lesion, however, is a deeper ulceration surrounded by a painless zone of induration. A few weeks later, a nontender, nonsuppurating, rubbery-firm inguinal lymphadenopathy appears, usually bilaterally. In addition to the primary chancre and associated lymphadenopathy, other symptoms and signs include a leukorrheal discharge and abnormal bleeding, particularly if the cervix is involved, and moist, ulcerating, coalescing, papular lesions of the vulva and adjacent skin of the perineum and thighs, the condylomata lata, which are probably manifestations of the secondary stage. Tertiary lesions of the reproductive tract are uncommon, although gummas of the cervix have been reported.

Diagnosis. Recognition of syphilis in the acute early primary stage is accomplished by dark-field examination of the clear serum that can be expressed from the ulcerated surface of the lesion and direct microscopic visualization of the spirochetes. The organisms can usually also be identified in the discharge from condylomata lata, so biopsy excision of a condyloma may be done and a histologic diagnosis of syphilis made. Finally, the serologic tests for syphilis (e.g., Wassermann, Hinton, VDRL) are usually strongly positive by five to six weeks. It is therefore important that any patient who has not received the standard penicillin treatment for acute gonorrhea be recalled in six weeks to have a serologic test for syphilis and be followed at intervals for another three to four months to be certain that any masked incubating syphilis is detected. The two diseases are not infrequently transmitted simultaneously; but unless penicillin has been used, the drug therapy for the gonorrhea may mask or prevent development of the primary luetic lesion, even though it is inadequate treatment for syphilis, and the latter could therefore easily go unrecognized and progress silently to the tertiary phase. A fluorescent treponemal antibody-absorption test is now available and is of considerable value for eliminating the possibility of a false-positive test in all patients with reactive serologic tests for syphilis. Each of these diagnostic maneuvers is helpful, often essential, in the differential diagnosis of suspicious ulcerated or papular lesions of the external genitalia that may be caused by any of the venereal diseases as well as by various other infectious processes or by certain neoplasms.

Treatment. Penicillin therapy remains the treatment of choice, and treponemal resistance has not been observed. The antibiotic therapy of syphilis as recommended by the Centers for Disease Control is summarized in Table 15-2. For acute infectious syphilis, the recommended therapy is 2.4 million units (1.2 million units in each buttock) of long-acting benzathine penicillin G (e.g., Bicillin) in a single session. Thus the standard treatment for gonorrhea is also curative for incubating syphilis. The standard course of treatment for late syphilis consists in a total of 6 million to 9 million units of procaine penicillin given in divided doses of 3 million units once every seven days over a period of fourteen to twenty-one days. The patient must be carefully followed, and at least a year should elapse with maintenance of negative serologic tests before she can be pronounced cured. If the patient is allergic to penicillin, treatment with large doses of tetracycline, erythromycin, or cephaloridine must be employed. Every potential contact should be traced, investigated, and treated when indicated.

Table 15-2. Drug Regimens for Treatment of Syphilis

Early syphilis (primary, secondary, or latent syphilis of <1 year's duration)
1. *Benzathine penicillin G* 2.4 million units IM.
2. If allergic to penicillin, *tetracycline hydrochloride* 500 mg PO 4 times daily for 15 days.
3. If penicillin-allergic but cannot tolerate tetracycline, either
   a. *erythromycin* 500 mg PO 4 times daily for 15 days if compliance and serologic follow-up ensured *or*
   b. If compliance and serologic follow-up cannot be ensured, refer to venereal disease consultant.

Syphilis >1 year (except neurosyphilis)
1. *Benzathine penicillin G* 2.4 million units IM once a week for 3 successive weeks (7.2 million units total).
2. If allergic to penicillin, *tetracycline hydrochloride* 500 mg PO 4 times daily for 30 days. Compliance is essential.
3. If penicillin-allergic but cannot tolerate tetracycline, same as for early syphilis (see above) except duration of *erythromycin* is 30 days instead of 15.

Neurosyphilis (no regimen adequately studied)
1. *Aqueous crystalline penicillin G* 12–24 million units IV per day (2–4 million units every 4 hours) for 10 days, followed by *benzathine penicillin G* 2.4 million units IM weekly for 3 doses *or*
2. *Aqueous procaine penicillin G* 2.4 million units IM daily plus probenecid 500 mg PO 4 times a day, both for 10 days; followed by benzathine penicillin G 2.4 million units IM weekly for 3 doses *or*
3. Benzathine penicillin G 2.4 million units IM weekly for 3 doses. For penicillin-allergic patients, refer to a venereal disease consultant.

Syphilis during pregnancy
1. *Penicillin* as indicated above for the particular stage of syphilis.
2. If penicillin-allergic, use *erythromycin* as above. Avoid tetracycline because of effect on fetus.

Chancroid (Soft Chancre)

Chancroid is a highly contagious infection caused by Ducrey's bacillus (*Hemophilus ducreyi*), a small, gram-negative, coccus-like bacillus. The principal manifestation is the development of a painful, tender, ulcerated, maculopapular lesion of the external genitalia usually three to ten days after sexual exposure (there is often considerable surrounding inflammation but never the hard induration that nearly always accompanies the primary chancre of syphilis), usually followed shortly thereafter by the unilateral or bilateral appearance of enlarged inguinal nodes that frequently suppurate. The ulcerated lesion is accompanied by a profuse, purulent, malodorous discharge.

Diagnosis is ordinarily made readily by gram-stained smears and cultures prepared from the discharge from the ulcerated lesion or, perhaps more reliably, on material aspirated from the swollen inguinal glands. An antigen skin test is also available but is rarely required. Dark-field examination should also be done to exclude the possibility of syphilis, and the specific diagnostic tests for the other granulomatous venereal diseases (discussed below) are also in order.

Treatment consists in a two-week course of sulfonamides or streptomycin, either of which is specific and highly curative. With regard to management of the suppurative lymphadenitis, simple aspiration is highly preferable to open incision and drainage, as the latter usually lead to troublesome secondary infection with extensive ulceration and prolonged healing.

Lymphogranuloma Venereum

Lymphogranuloma venereum, which is caused by a filterable virus, is essentially a disease of tropical or subtropical climates. An increased incidence of lymphogranuloma venereum has been noted in the United States. The infection and associated inflammatory process involve primarily the lymph channels and lymph nodes in the genital, inguinal, perianal, and anal regions—hence the name.

The clinical manifestations begin with a transient and inconspicuous initially external genital lesion that usually appears as a small vesicle seven to twenty-one days after exposure to an infected sexual partner and then rapidly fades away. Initially, there may be symptoms of systemic infection, including fever, malaise, headache, and arthralgia. A low grade, invariably unilateral inguinal adenitis appears two to three weeks later. The inflammatory process in the groin then steadily progresses until all the inguinal lymph nodes and surrounding soft tissues are involved and a firm,

tender, bulging inguinal mass, the bubo, is produced. Necrosis frequently occurs, leading to multiple fistulas and extensive ulceration and scarring in the groin. Further extension along lymphatic channels typically leads to involvement of the deeper nodes and lymph trunks of the pelvic wall, parametrium, and broad ligaments and particularly of the lymphatic tissues in the region of the perineum, anus, rectum, and sigmoid. As a result of the latter, chronic rectal and anal strictures and mucosal ulcerations are common sequelae of the disease. Vulvar elephantiasis due to chronic lymphatic blockade is also a frequent and exceedingly troublesome manifestation.

Diagnosis. Diagnosis can usually be made by means of a specific antigen skin test, the *Frei test,* which becomes positive ten to fourteen days after the appearance of the initial lesion and remains positive for the life of the patient. A complement-fixation test is also available. Again, the gamut of procedures to exclude the possibility of one or more of the other venereal diseases is in order. Where chronic anorectal lesions are concerned, proctoscopy and biopsy are essential to rule out carcinoma.

Treatment. Treatment involves a twenty-one-day course of either a sulfonamide, chlortetracycline, or chloramphenicol, each of which is effective during the early phases of the disease even though the disease is of viral origin. The inguinal buboes should be aspirated in preference to surgical drainage if suppuration occurs and breakdown seems imminent. Colostomy may ultimately prove necessary for the management of extensive anal or rectal strictures with complete or nearly complete obstruction, although sometimes repeated dilatation suffices.

Granuloma Inguinale

Unlike the situation with lymphogranuloma venereum, the inflammatory process accompanying granuloma inguinale spreads through the skin rather than via lymphatic channels. This chronic, ulcerating, granulomatous infection is caused by the microorganisms of *Donovania granulomatis,* which can be identified on the basis of their appearance as encapsulated inclusion bodies, the characteristic Donovan bodies, which are visible in the large mononuclear cells accompanying the chronic inflammatory process. The disease tends to be limited to blacks.

After sexual contact with an infected person, the initial lesion usually appears on the vulva, perineum, or vagina (less commonly in the groin and rarely on the cervix) as a small, circumscribed, elevated area of soft granulation tissue. Ulceration and secondary infection rapidly follow, and there is an accompanying profuse and malodorous discharge. Thereafter chronic and progressive spread of the ulcerated area occurs with marked proliferation of masses of granulation tissue. The process tends to be limited to the skin and immediate subcutaneous tissues of the external genitalia and inguinal areas, although the presence of severe secondary infection deep penetrating ulcers may form, and a secondary bacterial lymphadenitis may result in lymph node enlargement in the groins and elephantiasis of the vulva. In the absence of secondary infection, pseudobuboes may form in the groin that actually represent perilymphadenitis due to involvement of the soft tissues surrounding the nodes by the granulomatous process itself. There is little tendency to spontaneous healing; rather, the lesion slowly enlarges and advances peripherally to involve the groins (by direct extension, not by lymphatic spread), vagina, urethra, anus, and perineum. Local discomfort is often severe, and intercourse, urination, defecation, and even sitting or walking may become painful if not impossible.

Diagnosis. Diagnosis is made by obtaining smears or biopsy specimens directly from the ulcerating surface, staining them with Wright's or hematoxylin-eosin stain, and identifying the pathognomonic Donovan bodies within the huge, phagocytic mononuclear cells that are the most outstanding histologic feature of this chronic granulomatous process. The various clinical and laboratory tests for all the other venereal diseases should also be done, not only as a means of differential diagnosis but also because one or more of the venereal disorders frequently coexist.

Treatment. Treatment with streptomycin, tetracycline, or chloramphenicol has proved reasonably effective. Streptomycin is the only specific therapy that has proved at all successful in clearing up moderately advanced lesions. It is usually administered in a dosage of 4 gm daily for two to four weeks. For lesions that fail to respond to antibiotic therapy, resection by electrosurgical excision with wide margins and coagulation of the underlying base has given good results. The laser may be employed for such resections.

Condyloma Acuminatum

Condyloma acuminatum, an infection of viral origin that was mentioned briefly in Chapter 14, results in multiple papillary proliferations on the vulva, vagina, and less frequently the cervix. It is also probably subject to sexual transmission. There is usually an associated profuse, irritating vaginal discharge and secondary vulvitis. The lesions multiply rapidly over an ever-increasing area of the vulva, perineum, and perianal region.

Diagnosis. The diagnosis is usually obvious on clinical grounds, the typical narrow-based, pedunculated growths being readily distinguished from the more sessile, broad-based, flat condyloma latum of syphilis or from other benign tumors. However, a biopsy specimen should always be submitted for histologic confirmation; routine cultures, gonococcal cultures, and dark-field examination of the accompanying discharge should be done to exclude the presence or coexistence of other venereal diseases whenever any doubt exists.

Treatment. The most effective treatment for externally situated condylomas, provided they are small and not too numerous, has been the application of a solution of 25% podophyllum in tincture of benzoin directly to each individual growth, coating the surrounding normal skin with petrolatum. For large, coalescing lesions, surgical excision or, more often, electrocoagulation followed by curettage is usually preferable. Laser vaporization of the lesions on the vulva and the cervix offer the advantage of vaporizing the viral particles in the cell and is currently preferred over electrocoagulation whenever the laser is available. It is prudent not to use the laser on vaginal wall lesions because of postoperative vaginal scarring, adhesions, or even stenosis. For recalcitrant lesions and lesions in the vaginal wall, topical applications of 5% 5-fluorouracil in a cream base (Efudex) should be used. Cryosurgical therapy is effective but should be reserved for lesions on the cervix, especially those discovered only at colposcopy, or cervical cytology showing koilocytosis.

Immunotherapy employing interferon has been used successfully for treatment of condyloma acuminatum. Interferon is reserved for use in cases of extensive condyloma where other therapeutic methods have failed or there are persistent recurrences. Interferon is effective for both men and women with genital warts (condyloma acuminatum). The therapy is under clinical trials at the time of writing.

Herpesvirus Type 2 Infections (Herpes Progenitalis, Herpes Genitalis, Herpes Preputialis)

Type 2 herpesvirus hominis is closely related to herpes labialis (type 1 herpes simplex). It causes herpetic lesions on the cervix, vagina, and external genitalia and is considered to be the result of venereal transmission. Symptoms generally appear within three to seven days, although occasionally within less than 24 hours. Most of the patients afflicted are teenagers or young unmarried adults. For a number of reasons, herpetic infections of the genital tract occasionally involve the type 1 virus (in 5 to 10 percent), and herpesvirus type 2 is the occasional etiologic agent for lesions about the mouth (5 to 10 percent).

The herpes lesion characteristically appears on the vulva as a group of multiple vesicles surrounded by a diffuse area of inflammation and edema; the lesions are usually located on the clitoral prepuce, labia minora, and medial aspects of the labia majora. There is usually intense itching and an associated burning sensation (often preceding the appearance of the vesicles). Erosion and secondary infection of the vesicles by scratching is common and may create diagnostic difficulties. There may also be multiple small superficial ulcers, with or without vesicles, on the vulva, vagina, or cervix. Although the symptoms of herpes vulvovaginitis are usually more dramatic, cervical involve-

ment is more common and is present in 75 percent of cases. The cervix may be diffusely edematous and inflamed, bleeding easily when touched; there may be a large punched-out ulceration, or there may be a granulomatous-appearing tumor-like mass covered with gray exudate. There is often a profuse, watery discharge. However, a significant number of patients with the primary herpetic infection are completely asymptomatic, and a previous type 1 infection elsewhere in the body probably modifies the subsequent type 2 genital tract infection and minimizes its signs and symptoms. Herpes genitalis is frequently associated with *Hemophilus vaginalis* or *Trichomonas vaginalis* infections, or both, as well as with gonorrhea and condyloma acuminatum. Therefore it is important to look for all these possibilities in each patient.

The possible significance of type 2 herpesvirus infection in the etiology of cervical cancer is discussed in Chapter 26. During pregnancy herpes genitalis poses a special problem, because in early pregnancy it is responsible for an increased incidence of spontaneous abortion. Late in pregnancy, especially at delivery, there is the danger of transmitting the infection to the infant, with significant fetal morbidity and mortality.

With the initial or primary herpes infection there may be a prodromal period of several days with constitutional symptoms such as fever, malaise, and headache. The disease tends to be recurrent and unaccompanied by systemic reaction in 75 percent of cases, however, and some patients have repeated flare-ups for years, often related to the menses. These recurrent attacks probably represent reactivation of the initial, now latent viral infection. Local symptoms of vaginal and cervical involvement include leukorrhea, abnormal bleeding, vaginal pain, dysuria (sometimes so painful as to lead to urinary retention), and dyspareunia.

Diagnosis. The differential diagnosis includes any of the other venereal diseases, other types of vaginitis and cervicitis, herpes zoster, condyloma latum, and erythema multiforme; the cervical lesions even suggest carcinoma at times. A specific diagnosis can often be made on cytologic smear by recognition of the typical viral inclusion bodies. Furthermore, special cultures can be prepared from vulvar, vaginal, or cervical lesions and the herpesvirus infection easily and quickly identified. Serologic tests for type 1 and type 2 antibodies are also available.

Treatment. Symptomatic management with drying and antipruritic agents and topical anesthetic agents has been used to relieve the local discomfort while the lesions are specifically treated. Acyclovir (Zovirax) is a specific antiviral chemotherapeutic agent. It affects the viral replication by inhibiting it. Acyclovir can be applied as an ointment over lesions on the vulva followed with oral acyclovir tablets. For lesions involving the vagina and cervix, the medication is given orally. Cervical lesions of herpes can also be treated by cryosurgery or, preferably, laser vaporization.

Herpesvirus can be eradicated from the vulvar skin and mucous membranes by the local application of one of several tricyclic dyes (e.g., 1% aqueous solution of neutral red or 0.1% proflavine), followed in a few minutes by exposure of the painted area to incandescent (150 watts) or fluorescent (20 to 30 watts) light for 10 to 15 minutes at a distance of 6 to 8 inches. The same exposure to incandescent or fluorescent light is repeated by the patient 6 to 8 hours later and again 24 hours later. There is prompt relief of symptoms, often within 24 hours, and the lesions are usually completely healed within seven days. These photodynamic dyes are incorporated into the virus during replication, so that subsequent exposure to light results in inactivation of the virus. Symptomatic relief is universal, when such treatment is used during the primary phase of the infection, though the course of the disease is little altered. In the case of the recurrent form of the infection, the lesions disappear promptly along with the symptoms. The possibility has been raised that inactivating the virus may potentiate its oncogenic properties, but this issue remains highly debatable and unsettled, though many authorities believe the risk to be slight or nonexistent. This form of therapy has been superseded by treatment with acyclovir.

Acquired Immunodeficiency Syndrome

Acquired immunodeficiency syndrome (AIDS) is a disease caused by the human immunodeficiency virus (HIV-1), a retrovirus, and can be sexually transmitted. The virus is transmitted through intravenous drug use with contaminated needles; transfusion of infected blood products; direct viral contact of skin with impaired integrity; or contact of rectal, vaginal or oral mucosa with infected body fluids during intercourse. Acquired immunodeficiency syndrome is prevalent among sexually active male homosexuals, and the highest incidence continues to be in such individuals. Nevertheless, other groups, including children, get AIDS through transfusion with infected blood products or use of contaminated needles. Venereal transmission or acquisition of the virus can occur in heterosexuals who have infected partners. In the United States, women account for 7 percent of AIDS cases, and there were more than 3,000 cases of AIDS in women in 1988. Most of the women were in the reproductive age group, 79 percent between 13 and 39 years of age. The women were also significantly younger than the men with the disease. The proportion of women acquiring AIDS through heterosexual transmission has been increasing since 1982, probably because (1) women are more likely to have an infected partner since there are more HIV-infected men than women, (2) semen is a good transmission medium for HIV and AIDS has been transmitted even during artificial insemination, and (3) perhaps women may be having intercourse with partners at risk for HIV infection without knowing it.

Primary infection begins when HIV gains access to cells that are susceptible because they have the specific glycoprotein antigen CD_4 and therefore are susceptible to the virus. These cells include helper-inducer T lymphocytes, B-cells, monocytes, macrophages, endothelial cells, Langerhans' cells, astrocytes, oligodendrogliocytes, neuroretinal cells, and neurons. HIV behaves as a retrovirus and induces reverse transcriptase, allowing transcription of its RNA genome into a DNA copy in the host cell genome and leading to synthesis of viral proteins. Viral proteins are assembled on the cell surface and virions begin to bud with the glycoprotein gp 120 on the viral surface, inducing cell-to-cell fusion, which results in multinucleated giant cell (syncytium) formation, swelling or "ballooning" of the cytoplasm, and cell death. Since the T and B-cell lymphocytes are susceptible to the viral attack, HIV can cripple and paralyze the immune system with secondary infection setting in. Thus there is a high incidence of *Pneumocystis carinii* pneumonia when the macrophages are infected by the virus.

Once exposure to HIV has occurred, the infection may express itself in one of three ways:

1. Asymptomatic (incubation)—patient is contagious but has no symptoms and can remain so for up to 5 years
2. AIDS-related complex (ARC)—generalized lymphadenopathy, systemic symptoms (malaise, fever, night sweat, diarrhea, and weight loss), unusual recurrent infections (oral candidiasis, herpes zoster), and occurs at variable time intervals (4 years or more)
3. Full-blown AIDS—opportunistic infections, unusual malignancies (Kaposi's sarcoma, primary lymphoma of the brain) and wasting syndrome

Not all HIV-infected asymptomatic carriers will develop ARC or full-blown AIDS. For every 50 to 100 HIV carriers, there are only three to five cases of ARC and only one case of full-blown AIDS. Nevertheless, at any time HIV carriers can progress to the other two stages of HIV infection. The number of HIV-infected carriers as well as AIDS patients is increasing, and it is estimated that the United States may have one to two million cases of AIDS in the future.

Most HIV-infected women are in the reproductive age group, and pregnancy can affect the disease. Reduction of leukocyte chemotaxis and adherence, suppression of T-cell activity, and prevention of IgG production (all of which occur in pregnancy) compromise the immune system. Certain drugs (e.g., opiates) and alcohol reduce the effectiveness of the immune system by suppressing T-lymphocyte function. Because most HIV-positive women in the United States are drug abusers, the combined effects of pregnancy, drug abuse, and malnutrition make them particularly vulnerable to immunodeficiency. Children born to HIV-positive mothers are at high risk of becoming HIV positive.

Diagnostic Laboratory Test. The screening test for HIV infection is detection of HIV-specific antibodies in the blood of the infected person. The test is an enzyme-linked immunosorbent assay (ELISA) using beads or microtiter wells coated with antigens from HIV to which the patient's serum is added. If the patient has antibody against HIV, an antigen-antibody complex forms, which in turn is bound to the enzyme-linked antihuman IgG, thus allowing the enzyme to act on a substrate and induce a color change measured colorimetrically. The test becomes positive within 2 to 8 weeks after exposure but may not become positive for up to 6 months. A positive test is highly indicative of antibodies against HIV and therefore HIV infection, albeit still in the asymptomatic stage.

Because false-positive HIV tests can occur, positive test results should be confirmed with the more definitive Western blot assay. This test is used to detect antibodies to both the viral membrane proteins (gp 41 and gp 160) and viral core proteins (p 24 and p 31), which migrate at different rates on gel electrophoresis. The presence of antibodies to gp 41 is more reliable since they are present at all stages of the disease, whereas the antibodies to p 24 disappear during progression of the disease (therefore, they can be used to monitor disease progression).

Other tests such as tests that examine the immune status (T- and B-cell function, IgA, IgM, and IgG levels) are not specific for HIV or for AIDS but may be employed to evaluate the status of the patient.

Cultures for other sexually transmitted diseases such as gonorrhea, syphilis, and herpes genitalis should be done. Coinfection or secondary infection should also be ruled out.

Management and Treatment. There is no known cure or effective treatment for HIV at the time of this writing. Vaccines are being tested, but none is available yet. Zidovudine (zidothymidine or AZT), a thymidine analogue that inhibits replication of retroviruses will reduce the risk of opportunistic infections and is FDA approved for clinical use. Side effects include granulocytopenia, anemia, severe headaches, and sometimes neurologic changes. Other antiviral agents such as suramin, ribavirin, forscarnet sodium and inosine, pranobex are less effective. Measures should be taken to reduce the risk of acquiring opportunistic secondary infection.

Current attempts at prevention are directed at public health campaigns for better understanding of the disease transmission, changing high-risk sexual behavior to a low-risk or safer behavior, use of clean, new disposable needles in intravenous drug abusers, screening and quarantine of semen specimens from donors prior to use, and counseling on stopping drug abuse. Condom use has been widely touted as a method of "safe sex" to combat the risk of HIV transmission, but it should be emphasized that it is only a measure and is not a guarantee for "safe sex" against HIV. The only way to avoid HIV transmission through sex is to refrain from sex or to have monogamous sexual activity.

During pregnancy, HIV-infected patients should be advised to stop all drug, alcohol, and tobacco use, to attend to proper nutrition and rest, to use condoms and spermicides or abstain from sex, and to refrain from oral and anal sex. They should also be counseled on risk of transmission to the fetus and offered sterilization. Pregnancy termination is recommended by many centers if the patient is in early pregnancy. Support groups for HIV-positive patients are also available in many centers. The risk for developing tuberculosis, *Pneumocystis carinii* infection, toxoplasmosis, and candidiasis should be remembered, and measures should be taken to avoid such risk. Patients should be tested for these infections and promptly treated. Increased risk for preterm labor, premature rupture of membrane and intrauterine growth retardation have been reported in HIV-positive pregnant women. Appropriate measures should be adopted to reduce these risks.

SELECTED READINGS

Brunham, R. C., Maclean, I. W., Binns, B., et al. *Chlamydia trachomatis:* Its role in tubal infertility. *J. Infect. Dis.* 152:1275, 1985.

Dawood, M. Y., and Birnbaum, S. J. Unilateral tubo-ovarian abscess and intrauterine contraceptive device. *Obstet. Gynecol.* 46:429, 1975.

Friedman-Kien, A. E., and Eron, L. J., Conant, M., et al. Natural interferon alfa for treatment of condyloma acuminata. *J.A.M.A.* 259:533, 1988.

Guinan, M. E., and Hardy, A. Epidemiology of AIDS in women in the United States. *J.A.M.A.* 257:2039, 1987.

Hadgu, A., Westrom, L., Brooks, C. A., et al. Predicting acute pelvic inflammatory disease: A multivariate analysis. *Am. J. Obstet. Gynecol.* 155:954, 1986.

Ho, D. D., Pomerantz, R. J., and Kaplan, J. C. Pathogenesis of infection with human immunodeficiency virus. *N. Engl. J. Med.* 317:278, 1987.

McGregor, J. A. Chlamydia infection in women. *Obstet. Gynecol. Clinics North Am.* 16:565, 1989.

McNeeley, S. G. Gonococcal infections in women. *Obstet. Gynecol. Clinics North Am.* 16:467, 1989.

Minkoff, H. L. Care of pregnant women infected with human immunodeficiency virus. *J.A.M.A.* 258:2714, 1987.

Pastorek, J. G., II. Pelvic inflammatory disease and tubo-ovarian abscess. *Obstet. Gynecol. Clinics North Am.* 16:347, 1989.

Reichman, R. C., Badger, G. J., Mertz, G. J., et al. Treatment of recurrent genital herpes simplex infections with oral acyclovir: A controlled trial. *J.A.M.A.* 251:2103, 1984.

16

Spontaneous Abortion, Induced Abortion, and Ectopic Pregnancy

Most practicing physicians, but particularly gynecologists, are called on at least as often as the obstetrician to establish if a patient is pregnant. Moreover, the gynecologist or general surgeon is perhaps the physician most frequently consulted regarding the various complications of early pregnancy. The most common and important of these complications—spontaneous abortion (threatened, incomplete, complete), therapeutic abortion, and ectopic pregnancy—are discussed in this chapter. The rarer trophoblastic tumors (i.e., hydatidiform mole, chorioadenoma destruens, and choriocarcinoma) are discussed in Chapter 30. The subject of septic abortion received detailed consideration in Chapter 15, and certain aspects of habitual abortion are taken up in Chapter 8.

DIAGNOSIS OF EARLY PREGNANCY

Various clinical tests and laboratory procedures help to establish a definite diagnosis of early pregnancy and are sometimes useful for differentiating between disorders of early pregnancy and other gynecologic diseases that have similar symptoms and findings. These procedures are reviewed in detail in Chapter 2.

In addition to the history of the missed period in a woman whose cycles are invariably regular and the subjective and hence only suggestive symptoms of breast fullness and tenderness, morning nausea, urinary frequency, vomiting, and tiredness that may appear within a few weeks after conception, there are certain objective anatomic physical findings that are fairly reliable guides to a correct diagnosis. They include the typical softening of the lower uterine segment, which is usually detectable at about six weeks after the last period (Hegar's sign), and the visible bluish hue taken on by the vagina and introitus, which

usually appears near the end of the second month of pregnancy (Chadwick's sign). By this time the uterine fundus is usually one and one-half to two times enlarged and is soft and globular; and the breasts are visibly full and turgid, with heavily pigmented areolae and erect nipples from which colostrum can often be expressed. Thus the diagnosis is now fairly definite on clinical grounds alone.

When the diagnosis of pregnancy is first established, the expected time of delivery can be estimated with some accuracy as being 280 days (plus or minus two or three days) following the first day of the last period. The expected date of confinement can thus be rapidly calculated by counting ahead one year, subtracting three months and adding seven days, or by counting ahead nine months and adding seven days.

SPONTANEOUS ABORTION

Any pregnancy that terminates before 20 weeks of gestation can be called an abortion. Approximately 10 to 15 percent of all known pregnancies end in abortion. Not only does it represent immense fetal wastage, the associated maternal mortality is not insignificant, ranging from 0.1 percent to as high as 1.0 percent in various reports. Sepsis and hemorrhage are the chief causes of maternal death.

Abortions can be classified as: (1) *spontaneous abortion,* which is the result of termination of pregnancy through natural causes; or (2) *induced abortion,* which is a result of artificial means employed to terminate the pregnancy. The latter group can be further subdivided into: *criminal abortions* if the induction has been attempted or performed by the patient, unqualified individual, or another individual without legal sanction, and *therapeutic abortions* if termination of the pregnancy has been formally and openly carried out within a hospital or clinic for proper and valid medical indications and with full knowledge and medical-legal sanction of all parties concerned.

Etiology

Most simple, nonrepetitive, spontaneous abortions occur during the second or third month of gestation and are most commonly (50 to 75 percent) associated with a blighted ovum and the inevitable subsequent abnormalities of both fetal and placental development. These pregnancies were destined to fail at the outset, and the process of abortion simply represents an inevitable outcome. The primary deficiency may be maternal, paternal, or both, and may often involve improper genetic transfers during the stage of fertilization and early cell divisions within the zygote. Many studies indicate that major chromosomal abnormalities are present in a high percentage of abortuses or stillborn infants.

The maternal effects of serious acute or chronic systemic disorders (pulmonary, renal, cardiovascular, and endocrine-metabolic), certain viral infections (e.g., rubella), overwhelming bacterial infections, certain toxic drugs, and extensive local pelvic trauma of the type sometimes encountered in automobile accident victims are occasionally followed by abortion of a previously normal pregnancy, though in most such instances the resulting termination of pregnancy can hardly be considered spontaneous. Some evidence has been advanced suggesting that fertilization late in the cycle involving an "overripe" ovum may be a factor in the appearance of chromosomal aberrations, congenital malformations, and spontaneous abortions. Operations on the ovary containing the corpus luteum during the first thirty to fifty days of pregnancy such as are sometimes necessary or prompted by torsion or a vascular accident in an ovarian cyst may also result in a "spontaneous" type of abortion of an otherwise normally developing pregnancy owing to premature withdrawal of corpus luteum support before the immature placenta is capable of sustaining the gestation by adequate estrogen and progesterone production of its own.

The potential role of physical trauma (e.g., a blow to the abdomen, a fall down stairs, an automobile accident) or emotional trauma (e.g., a frightening experience, loss of a loved one) as an etiologic factor in first-trimester abortion has been questioned. Even in the presence of a history suggesting such a train of events, careful histologic study of the fetal and placental tissue obtained in instances of spontaneous abortion nearly always reveals the typical features of a blighted ovum or maldeveloped fetus and placenta, a situation that obviously antedates the apparent pre-

cipitating incident. It is usually only when direct and severe accidental injury to the uterus, the fetus within, or both has occurred that trauma per se can be incriminated as the cause of abortion of a previously normal pregnancy.

Clinical Types of Abortion

Depending on the apparent phase of abortion or impending abortion as indicated by the patient's history and findings when first seen, abortion can be classified, from a clinical standpoint, as follows.

1. *Threatened abortion.* The patient gives a typical history of early pregnancy, with a missed period or two, and then notes the onset of vaginal bleeding with or without uterine cramps. Pelvic examination reveals the cervix to be of normal length and the endocervical canal closed by an external os of normal diameter.

2. *Imminent abortion.* The patient gives the same history as that for threatened abortion but nearly always with cramps present. Examination reveals shortening and dilatation of the cervix.

3. *Inevitable abortion.* Examination discloses fetal or placental tissue or both within or protruding from the dilated, effaced cervical segment.

4. *Complete abortion.* The embryo, if present, and the entire placenta have been expelled. Obviously, diagnosis of this type of abortion depends on the physician visualizing the tissue passed. Rapid cessation of bleeding and cramps and prompt early involution of the uterus are confirmatory.

5. *Incomplete abortion.* The fetus, with or without portions of the placenta, has been expelled, but some of the products of conception (usually fragments of placenta) remain within the uterus. Inspection of the tissue passed, together with persistence of cramps, bleeding, and cervical dilatation, are usually sufficient to support this clinical diagnosis.

6. *Missed abortion.* Fetal death has occurred in utero before the twentieth week, but the pregnancy is retained for two months or longer. The presence of a missed abortion may be established before the onset

of uterine contractions if amenorrhea persists but the uterus fails to enlarge further. More frequently, the patient is first seen because of the development of vaginal bleeding and cramps (the onset of the actual abortion) and is found to have a uterus several weeks smaller than would be expected from the duration of her amenorrhea.

7. *Septic abortion.* Any abortion complicated by intrauterine infection and fever falls in this category (Chap. 15). Although secondary infection of a spontaneous abortion is theoretically possible and may rarely occur, criminal induction or therapeutic interruption must be suspected.

8. *Habitual abortion.* By definition, the syndrome of habitual abortion is said to exist when a patient has three or more successive pregnancies terminating in spontaneous abortion.

Clinical Features and Management

Threatened Abortion. Threatened abortion includes the early phases of all pregnancies that ultimately terminate in abortion, as well as episodes of vaginal bleeding in many patients with otherwise normal pregnancies but in whom bleeding occurs from marginal placental sinuses, polyps, cervical erosions, acute vaginitis, and so on. The latter situations are sometimes apparent on initial pelvic examinations, but the usual prompt cessation of bleeding and the subsequent continued normal progress of the pregnancy ultimately serve to distinguish those cases in which the initial clinical impression of threatened abortion was erroneous.

In those patients who ultimately proceed to spontaneous loss of the pregnancy, the initial bleeding and signs and symptoms of uterine irritability are the first manifestations of failing trophoblast function, the deficient hormone production resulting in the beginning of placental circulatory failure and hemorrhage into the decidua basalis. Further progression of this process leads to fetal death, placental separation, and eventually active uterine contractions. In most instances, this sequence of events, once initiated, cannot be reversed by any therapeutic maneuvers now available. The number of patients who initially present with true threatened abortion and whose pregnancies are capable of being "rescued" either by spontaneous return of normal hormonal support or by institution of bed rest or treatment with progestogens is probably small. It is estimated that, when first seen, fewer than 30 percent of patients in whom abortion is threatened have viable fetuses, and that 80 percent or more proceed to abortion regardless of management. Because it is currently impossible to differentiate by either clinical or laboratory diagnostic aids the patients who may be fortunate enough to retain their pregnancies, it is best to manage all cases of threatened abortion expectantly until the abortion becomes obvious or the signs and symptoms subside.

The possibility of the presymptomatic recognition of potential incipient threatened abortion by changes in the results of a number of laboratory tests suggestive of hormonal insufficiency has been discussed in Chapter 2. Quantitative serum chorionic gonadotropin or serum progesterone assays reflect corpus luteum or placental inadequacy and have been employed to identify patients most likely to abort. Although progesterone supplementation is widely used, there is little rational and scientific justification for such an approach except for the small percentage of abortions due to true corpus luteum inadequacy. Such women present with threatened abortion shortly after the missed period at around four to five weeks after the last menstrual period and seldom after seven weeks.

The corpus luteum is the principal source of progesterone during early pregnancy (until forty-nine days or seven weeks after the last menstrual period); thereafter, the trophoblast takes over as the major source of progesterone. Controlled studies of treating threatened abortion with progestins have shown that the outcome was no better than with placebo. At any rate, because of possible effects of the synthetic progestins on the fetus, it is best that only progesterone be employed if such therapy is warranted. Estrogens are currently not indicated for treating abortions, and certainly the experience with diethylstilbestrol used for treating abortion indicates no clear benefit but considerable risk of developing vaginal adenosis, clear cell carcinoma, and a T-shaped uterine cavity in the female fetus whose mother was treated during that pregnancy.

Imminent and Inevitable Spontaneous Abortions. In most instances of imminent and inevitable spontaneous abortion, provided blood loss does not become excessive and the patient is reasonably comfortable, continued observation for a brief period seems justified in the hope that the abortion will be spontaneously concluded and the fetus and placenta completely expelled. If this expectant program does not yield the hoped-for results within a few hours, intervention is indicated.

Spontaneous Complete Abortion. During most spontaneous complete abortions or early miscarriages the onset of labor is abrupt, and the fetus and placenta are expelled rapidly in an uncomplicated fashion with minimal cramps and bleeding, both of which cease promptly. Many such patients never visit the office or hospital; of those seen, examination even a few hours later usually reveals a firmly contracted fundus and a relatively tight cervix. If the subsequent course in such patients is uneventful, no further treatment is indicated.

It should be noted, however, that in theory no abortion or early miscarriage is actually complete because as the immature placenta separates from the uterine wall the tips of the chorionic villi invariably remain attached. Therefore some hold firmly to the belief that all abortions or early miscarriages, even though grossly "complete," should be managed by curettage to facilitate prompt convalescence and avoid post-abortal complications that often ultimately require dilatation and curettage (D&C). Certainly if any doubt exists as to whether the abortion is complete, or if cramps or bleeding persist despite the recovery of what appears to be a complete and intact placenta, curettage seems to be the wisest policy.

Spontaneous Incomplete Abortion. An incomplete abortion is the commonest disorder of early pregnancy that requires treatment, and surgical intervention is nearly always necessary. It is important to determine as promptly as possible whether an abortion is either in process (and therefore inevitable) or has already been partially completed so that definitive treatment can be instituted without undue delay, rather than pointlessly pursuing a conservative waiting pro-

gram as would be indicated in the earlier phase of threatened abortion. Ordinarily, the diagnosis of an incomplete abortion is rendered obvious by the typical history of persistent, severe uterine cramps, often accompanied by considerable bleeding and by the passage of recognizable tissue. On examination, the cervical os is found to be dilated and patulous and the cervical segment effaced. The uterine fundus is still enlarged, soft, and boggy but is ordinarily not tender or painful on motion unless one is dealing with a septic abortion.

If no obvious tissue is present in the cervix, even though the latter is dilated, and if bleeding is not excessive and there is no evidence of sepsis, the following alternatives may be elected: (1) Wait for possible spontaneous completion of abortion or (2) attempt to hasten it with intravenous infusion of oxytocin (20 units in 1 liter of normal saline) run at 10 to 12 mIU per minute. (3) If bleeding is excessive or persists, or if products of conception are visible in the cervical canal, the uterus should be promptly emptied surgically, carefully dilating the cervix further, if necessary, and then thoroughly evacuating the uterine contents. Evacuation is done by suction curettage initially when possible, employing placental forceps, and then instrumental "sharp" curettage to be certain that all placental and chorionic decidual tissues are removed. The preliminary intravenous infusion of oxytocin as above prior to curettage facilitates the latter by firmly contracting the fundus. At the conclusion of the procedure, intravenous or intramuscular injection of 0.2 mg of ergonovine helps to maintain the uterus firmly contracted and is an aid to immediate hemostasis. The suction technique has the advantages that little or no anesthesia is required, there is usually less bleeding, and in many cases the procedure can be completed in a few minutes. Occasionally, however, suction aspiration is not as effective as sharp curettage for completely removing all retained placental and decidual tissue. Once a diagnosis of incomplete abortion is definitely established, prompt curettage minimizes blood loss, reduces the chance of secondary infection, and shortens convalescence.

Occasionally, a spontaneous abortion is accompanied by a placenta accreta that resists attempts at removal and is accompanied by continued hemorrhage of serious proportions. In such cases, which are fortunately rare, emergency hysterectomy may be the only alternative and is invariably lifesaving.

Missed Abortion. The existence of missed abortion, in which fetal death in utero precedes by several weeks the onset of symptoms of the mechanical aborting process, is most often not recognized until the development of cramps and bleeding indicates that the abortion is actively under way and causes the patient to seek medical attention. In most of these patients, spontaneous delivery occurs within two to three weeks after fetal death; and under these circumstances the problem is handled in the same way as any incomplete abortion. However, the diagnosis of missed abortion occasionally becomes apparent before the onset of the aborting process, and a decision about further management must be made.

Missed abortion is suggested if cessation of fetal movements is noted by patient and physician and if the fetal heartbeat is no longer audible to the physician or found on ultrasound, or if the uterus is many weeks smaller than the duration of gestation and there is no evidence of a live conceptus. More definite evidence is the disappearance of activity on the fetal electrocardiogram or the demonstration by abdominal radiography of the subcutaneous fat layer elevated away from the fetal skull bones, the *halo sign.* If fetal death is confirmed, it appears to be perfectly safe to treat the situation expectantly for three to four weeks and await the spontaneous onset of labor, which in 90 percent of cases occurs within one month and takes place eventually in all cases.

In perhaps 25 to 35 percent of women who retain dead fetuses in utero for five weeks or longer, hypofibrinogenemia with secondary hemorrhagic phenomena develops, and alarming hemorrhage may occur from the uterus as well as at other body sites. Therefore if labor does not occur within one month of the estimated time of fetal death, weekly determinations of the serum fibrinogen concentration (normal value about 350 mg per deciliter) is a wise precautionary measure.

In any case, the uterus should probably be emptied after one month by induction of labor preferably with prostaglandin vaginal suppositories, intramuscular injections of prostaglandins or their analogs, or intravenous infusion of oxytocin (20 units oxytocin in 1 liter of normal saline), which is increased at regular intervals of no more than 30 minutes. Hypertonic saline or prostaglandins may be given intraamniotically to induce uterine contraction and abortion. Hysterotomy is occasionally required but has seldom been necessary since prostaglandins have become available. Once the cervix is dilated sufficiently to allow evacuation of the dead fetus and products of conception, evacuation should be carried out in the operating room and completed with uterine curettage. Uterine evacuation is especially indicated if the fibrinogen level falls below 150 mg per deciliter or if bleeding occurs regardless of the fibrinogen level. (The administration of fibrinogen alone, without emptying the uterus, does not effectively control the bleeding.) The ultimate labor is usually short and uncomplicated. Some patients may not want to wait once they know they have a missed abortion and may insist on evacuation of their pregnancy, which is then indicated and appropriate to perform.

Septic Abortion. The serious gynecologic emergency of septic abortion is discussed in detail in Chapter 15. It should be emphasized again that its management differs from that of a simple, spontaneous, incomplete abortion in that, unless massive hemorrhage dictates the need for earlier curettage, even with an early, uncomplicated septic abortion control of or protection against invasive sepsis is achieved first by a short (6 to 12 hours), intensive preliminary antibiotic program, together with attention to restoration of normal fluid balance and blood volume prior to surgically emptying the uterus. Prompt evacuation of the uterus shortly after institution of antibiotic therapy frequently allows removal of the septic focus before extension beyond the confines of the uterine cavity can take place. Thus spread of infection into the wall of the uterus and beyond, with the subsequent occurrence of septic and gram-negative endotoxic shock, can be prevented. Should endotoxic shock develop, the situation becomes critical, and the intensive therapeutic program presented in Chapter 15 is then of vital importance.

Habitual (Recurrent) Abortion. A patient in whom three or more consecutive pregnancies have terminated in spontaneous abortion or miscarriage before the twentieth week may be considered as having habitual abortion. However, the chance that any pregnancy will end in abortion is about 15 percent; that figure remains stable regardless of the number of abortions, although earlier reports had suggested that the risk of subsequent abortion increases with increasing number of abortions up to three. Nevertheless, there is little doubt that there is a group of women who exhibit a definite predisposition toward abortion and miscarriage, and patients in this category warrant careful study and management so that obvious causes for their inability to maintain a pregnancy normally and to carry it to term can be discovered and corrected in at least some of them.

Because the potential etiologic factors are many, and multiple causes may operate simultaneously in the same patient, the diagnostic approach should include the following: (1) an evaluation of the nutritional and general health status of both husband and wife; (2) in the woman, a search for underlying chronic diseases that may foster placental insufficiency during early pregnancy (particularly latent diabetes, thyroid disturbances, or primary ovarian dysfunction), a careful evaluation of potential, often subtle psychic factors, and finally, a thorough search for local anatomic defects that may mechanically predispose to premature termination of a pregnancy. Chronic urinary tract infections should be ruled out and antibodies to blood groups and the Coombs' test performed. There is also suggestive evidence that low grade infections of the female or male genital tracts by T-strain *Mycoplasma* organisms may be a significant cause of repeated spontaneous abortions, and that elimination of these organisms by tetracycline or doxycycline therapy can prevent subsequent fetal wastage (Chap. 13). Obviously, it is preferable to carry out the diagnostic survey before the patient conceives again, correcting any deficiencies or abnormalities prior to the next pregnancy.

The general nutritional, endocrine-metabolic, and psychosomatic aspects of the problem must be properly managed in the so-called habitual aborter during early pregnancy, including assurance of adequate dietary and vitamin intake and thyroid medication

if indicated. When an inadequate corpus luteum is demonstrable, it is desirable to give supplemental progesterone (as suppositories or as twice-weekly intramuscular injections) until eight or nine weeks' gestation. Progesterone should not be employed indiscriminately in these patients; it should be prescribed only if there is valid evidence of progesterone deficiency. Perhaps even more important is the development of a close, supportive relationship between physician and patient, the former constantly offering reassurance and encouragement at the regular prenatal visits and remaining readily available during the intervals between. It is often possible to relieve the stress and anxiety characteristically experienced by this group of patients by allowing them to relate their symptoms and verbalize their fears and apprehensions, which can then be sympathetically allayed and explained. Assuming that no local uterine abnormality or fundamental endocrinopathy exists, such a conscientious supportive program allows a substantial proportion (up to 75 to 80 percent) of these women who have habitually aborted in the past to carry to term. In nearly all reported series, no improvement in these results has been observed by adding routine progesterone medication to the regimen.

Another intriguing possibility is that in a certain percentage of women habitual spontaneous abortion may be the result of immunologic rejection of the fetus due to excessive release of fetal antigens, especially in cases where tissue antigens from the husband and those from the wife are markedly dissimilar. Accelerated rejection of skin grafts donated by the husband in a series of pregnant women who had been habitual aborters lends support to this hypothesis. Diseases such as lupus erythematosus and other autoimmune disease should be ruled out. High incidences of elevated levels of lupus anticoagulant and anticardiolipin antibodies have been reported in repeat aborters. Attempts have been made to treat such patients with immunotherapy employing blood cells (lymphocytes) from their spouse with modest success, but concerns about potential side effects have temporarily delayed further progress.

Local, mechanical causes are sometimes responsible for repeated abortion or miscarriage. The principal conditions involved here are (1) congenital anomalies of the uterus and vagina (see Chapter 8 for diagnosis and treatment), (2) submucous or intramural fibroids (Chap. 17), and (3) an incompetent cervix. Because the latter entity is of significance only in connection with habitual abortion or miscarriage, it seems appropriate to discuss it briefly here.

INCOMPETENT CERVIX AND HABITUAL ABORTION. Although most abortions occur before the twelfth week and are associated with an abnormal embryo, a significant number of patients experience repeated premature terminations of otherwise normal pregnancies during the second trimester or occasionally early in the third trimester of pregnancy (typically between the twelfth and thirty-fourth weeks). Such patients may be found to have an anatomic defect that involves the entire cervical segment and consists of abnormal cervical dilatation, particularly at the level of the internal cervical os.

This history of repeated second-trimester abortions that occur relatively rapidly and painlessly after spontaneous rupture of the membranes and usually unaccompanied by preliminary cramps or bleeding is characteristic and should be the clue that further studies are indicated to corroborate the diagnosis. If the patient first appears in the nonpregnant state, the diagnosis may be confirmed by the ease with which a No. 18 or larger cervical dilator may be introduced into the cervical canal and passed through the internal os, or by hysterosalpingography (according to standard techniques or employing a special balloon catheter or a Harris uterine injector to retain the radiopaque dye within the cervical segment), which reveals the triangularly dilated internal os and upper endocervical canal.

When, as is often the case, the patient is first seen while pregnant, the cervix is observed to undergo painless dilatation over a period of several weeks, with the fetal membranes ultimately plainly visible as they bulge through a dilated, patulous cervix (Fig. 16-1A).

Apparently, the incompetent cervix is occasionally a primary congenital condition, some patients never having carried a pregnancy beyond the second trimester. However, most patients give a history of one or more term pregnancies (often the last one was a difficult, traumatic labor and delivery) or have previously undergone what may have been a traumatic cervical D&C or cervical conization so that in most instances the defect appears to be an acquired one.

Management of the incompetent cervix during pregnancy involves surgical repair utilizing a vaginal approach and placing an encircling ligature strip of fascia, polyethylene, Mersilene (Ethicon), a synthetic polyester fiber material, or a dermal graft strip removed from the patient's lower abdominal skin. It is tied snugly about the cervix at the level of the internal os, closing the defect—so-called cervical cerclage (Fig. 16-1B and C). Often the cerclage is performed as a purse-string suture as high up the cervix as possible. This MacDonald procedure is a modification of the Shirodkar procedure and is often easier to do during pregnancy or after the cervix has dilated and the membranes are partially protruded.

With the Shirodkar operation, the bladder base must be dissected and pushed up so that the cerclage that encircles the internal os high up is not a purse-string cerclage but a complete cerclage at the level of the internal os. It is best done during the nonpregnant stage as it can produce hemorrhage during pregnancy. To obtain best results in patients with the classic history, the procedure is preferably done prophylactically, before dilatation and bulging of the membranes has occurred; however, it is wise to delay until after the twelfth week to avoid performing the procedure prematurely only to have a simple abortion due to a blighted ovum occur during the first trimester. Emergency cerclage in the face of an already dilated cervix and bulging membranes is indicated if rupture of the membranes and early labor has not begun. The membranes are gently reduced as the ligature is tied, and the procedure often successfully halts the incipient premature labor. Currently, tocolysis is carried out for 12 hours using one of the betamimetic agents, terbutaline or ritodrine, after cerclage performed during pregnancy to inhibit any impending premature uterine activity. Vaginal delivery can be accompanied by simply dividing the ligature at term and then either awaiting the spontaneous onset of labor or inducing labor in the usual manner; this regimen

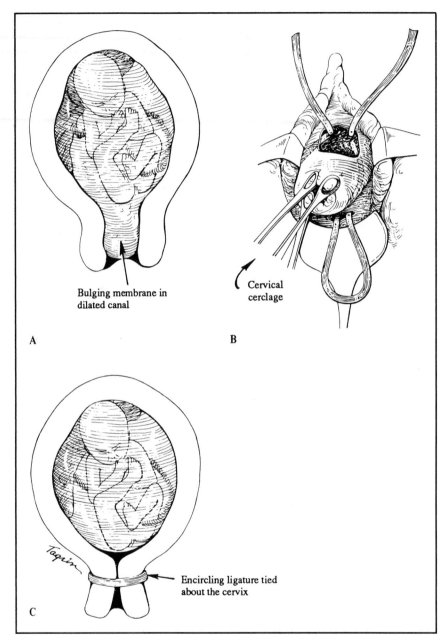

Bulging membrane in
dilated canal

A

Cervical
cerclage

B

Encircling ligature tied
about the cervix

C

Fig. 16-1. A. Cervical dilatation in midtrimester pregnancy. B. Treatment by cervical cerclage, showing
placement of the encircling ligature. C. End result of
cerclage, with restoration of adequate mechanical support of the pregnancy at the level of the internal cervical os, forestalling progressive cervical dilatation and
subsequent premature initiation of labor.

of course necessitates repeated cerclage with future pregnancies. If, on the other hand, an attempt at permanent repair is desired, cesarean section can be performed and is then mandatory with all future pregnancies as well.

If the diagnosis of cervical incompetence is established in the nonpregnant state, the alternative procedure originally devised by Lash and Lash can be utilized; it has the advantage that it permits subsequent pregnancies to be delivered vaginally without seriously jeopardizing the cervical repair. The Lash operation is also carried out vaginally and involves removal of a longitudinal segment of the anterior cervical wall approximately one-half its circumference in width, thereby reducing the previously dilated cervical canal and internal os to a normal diameter and state of competence.

THERAPEUTIC ABORTION

Medical Indications

Advances in general medicine have sharply reduced the number of valid, purely medical reasons for terminating a pregnancy that threatens the life of the mother. The mere presence of any degree of cardiac or renal disease, diabetes, tuberculosis, or other potentially chronic systemic disorder no longer warrants routine termination of pregnancy, for such diseases are now usually as amenable to therapy in the pregnant state as in the nonpregnant state. However, there remain a relatively small number of fairly generally accepted indications for considering therapeutic abortion on medical grounds alone. Chief among them are the presence of maternal disorders that pose a real threat to the health or life of the mother.

1. Severe hypertensive cardiovascular disease.
2. Severe chronic renal disease.
3. Severe rheumatic valvular heart disease with uncontrollable cardiac decompensation.
4. Serious psychiatric disorders, especially when the threat of suicide is great.
5. Carcinoma of the breast or malignant melanoma coexisting with pregnancy. Although the primary

therapy for either may remain the same, regardless of the coexisting pregnancy, there is considerable evidence that the course of either neoplasm is adversely influenced by the high levels of placental steroids, particularly estrogen, present in association with the pregnancy, and that termination of the pregnancy may improve the chances for a favorable response to treatment.
6. Carcinoma of the cervix. In this situation, which is discussed more fully in Chapter 26, proper treatment is often facilitated by the preliminary performance of a therapeutic abortion; in any case, irradiation or surgical treatment, of course, terminates the pregnancy.
7. Miscellaneous medical disorders under certain circumstances, e.g., lymphoma, ulcerative colitis, regional enteritis, multiple sclerosis, severe diabetes.

Another potential indication for therapeutic interruption of pregnancy involves situations in which it is suspected that there is a strong possibility that the fetus is abnormal. Obviously, therapeutic abortion on these grounds is a controversial, highly debatable subject; nevertheless, it is accepted as a legitimate and reasonable option under special circumstances. The classic example of such indications is found in the case of the woman who contracts rubella (German measles) during the first trimester of pregnancy. On the basis of the high incidence of defective babies born to such mothers, the poor outcome in the eyes of many women and their physicians is unacceptable. The accumulated figures from various reported series originally indicated that one-third to one-half of all such patients would either lose the baby or give birth to a stillborn or seriously defective child with fetal abnormalities such as blindness in association with cataracts, deafness, congenital heart disease, microcephaly, or severe mental retardation. Other maternal viral diseases, e.g., rubeola, mumps, chickenpox, and poliomyelitis, may also be responsible for fetal abnormalities, but the incidence of such abnormalities is considerably less.

Although based on subsequent careful prospective studies it appears that the overall risk may be more in the range of 10 to 15 percent, the problem is still a serious one. Women contracting rubella during the first trimester had a six or seven times greater chance of giving birth to defective infants than a normal control group of pregnant women. The risk is probably even greater if the disease occurs during the first two months of pregnancy, with a maximum risk of 50 to 60 percent during the first four weeks, 25 to 35 percent the next four weeks, 15 to 20 percent during the ninth to twelfth week, and 5 to 10 percent during weeks 13 to 16. Contraction of rubella during the early second trimester also increases the chance of an abnormal child or of premature delivery, but the risk is considerably less.

The safe, effective rubella vaccine now available promises to eliminate this most common infectious cause of congenital abnormalities. Because 40 percent of adult women show definite symptoms and signs of the disease following inoculation, the vaccine is best administered during childhood, none of the vaccinated children or their contacts having exhibited any clinical evidence of disease despite the successful establishment of immunity in 97 percent of those vaccinated. Administration of the vaccine during pregnancy is definitely contraindicated, however, as even attenuated viruses are potentially teratogenic. In adult women of childbearing age, the safest time to give the vaccine is immediately postpartum, with strict avoidance of another pregnancy for three months following vaccination.

Other situations in which the problem of whether therapeutic abortion is indicated include a history of serious hereditary disorders (e.g., amaurotic idiocy and hemophilia), particularly if previous offspring have exhibited these disorders, and exposure to drugs known to produce serious fetal damage (e.g., the sedative thalidomide, which produced phocomelia in a high percentage of infants born to mothers to whom it had been administered early in pregnancy). Because it is now possible to establish definitely the presence of many inherited fetal disorders by chorionic villi biopsy or amniocentesis (e.g., virtually all chromosomal abnormalities including Down syndrome, certain biochemical disorders such as Tay-Sachs disease and Hunter-Hurler's disease, and sex-linked diseases carried by females but affecting only males such as hemophilia), it is likely that there will be an increasing use of therapeutic abortion for this type of indication. Other conditions such as anencephaly, which is incompatible with extrauterine life, can be readily diagnosed by ultrasound or amniotic fluid α-fetoprotein.

Elective (Voluntary) Therapeutic Abortion for Unwanted and Unplanned Pregnancy

Changes in viewpoints toward therapeutic interruption of pregnancy among both the lay population and the medical profession have resulted not only in the adoption of more permissive legislation in most states but also in a steady increase in the number of voluntary therapeutic abortions done each year. This change in attitude has substantially reduced the number of criminal abortions performed in the United States.

Nowadays, most legal interruptions are performed because the woman does not desire to continue the pregnancy. The decision is thus a voluntary one on the part of the patient, made with the advice and consent of the physician counseling and treating her.

In most instances, voluntary abortion represents a failure to use effective contraception. Therefore there must be greater emphasis placed on improving both the quality and availability of contraceptive methods for those who need them. Contraceptive counseling should be offered to all women having abortions, as it may convince them that there are much safer approaches to fertility control.

In 1973 the United States Supreme Court ruled that the decision for or against abortion was and is the prerogative of the pregnant woman in consultation with her physician. This ruling paved the way for elective abortions during the first two trimesters to be done legally in all states. Since then, more than 1 million legal abortions have been performed annually in the United States.

First-trimester abortions are relatively simple, inexpensive, and free of significant risk of serious complications. Second-trimester abortions are much more complicated, and the potential for serious complications and an unpredictable outcome is much greater. After the second trimester, and at the time when the fetus first becomes viable (potentially capable of leading an independent life outside the mother), the safety and rights of the potential new life become a subject for legal protection by state or federal laws. Most state laws, as well as the 1973 Supreme Court ruling, therefore continue to restrict therapeutic abortions after the second trimester to those necessary to preserve the life or health of the mother. Ideally, elective (voluntary) abortions are done early in the first trimester.

Management of Therapeutic Abortion

As with any surgical procedure, informed consent must be obtained before performing an abortion. If the patient is a minor and unmarried, it is wise to obtain parental consent, if possible, although even if one or both parents refuse consent the abortion can still legally be done.

The decision to abort should be made early, preferably before the end of the first trimester, so that the pregnancy can be interrupted safely and in the simplest way—by *suction curettage* or, when necessary, formal *D&C*. A variation involving vacuum aspiration of the uterine contents (an office procedure) within 14 days of a missed menstrual period is also widely practiced and has been termed menstrual regulation or menstrual extraction. There are even fewer complications than with the preceding methods, and only 3 to 4 percent of women so managed during early pregnancy require further treatment because of method failure. Most therapeutic abortions carried out by suction curettage can be done in the operating room of a surgicenter, clinic, or hospital and require only paracervical block or a short period of general anesthesia. Although uterine perforation is rare during suction curettage, should it occur there is the possible danger that the powerful suction may draw parametrial tissues and other adjacent structures, including the uterine artery, ureter, bladder, and ileum, through the perforation in the uterine wall and into contact with the suction cannula, with resulting hematomas and traumatic lacerations. Hence suction curettage requires just as much care as regular curettage if complications are to be prevented or recognized and then treated promptly.

In addition to accidental perforation and related

trauma during D&C or suction curettage, the other common potential complication is retention of fetal or placental fragments with subsequent bleeding, intrauterine and pelvic sepsis, or both. Patients should be alerted to these possibilities and warned to report the development of cramps, abdominal pain, vaginal bleeding, or fever immediately. Such symptoms require hospitalization for a formal D&C, as well as vigorous management of pelvic infection, as discussed in Chapter 15. Long-term complications of curettage include uterine synechiae (Asherman syndrome) with oligomenorrhea or amenorrhea and infertility. Uterine synechiae are usually due to overenthusiastic curettage with or without infection.

Curettage is not a safe or feasible technique for interruption of pregnancy after the third month, especially in primigravidas. In highly trained hands, however, *dilatation and evacuation* (D&E) can be undertaken up to 14 to 15 weeks. This procedure is similar to D&C, but with D&E strong ovum forceps are used to evacuate fetal parts and the cervix is more widely dilated than for D&C. Curettage is performed after fetal parts have been evacuated and should be carried out only by trained individuals. Because of the additional cervical dilatation, a definite complication of D&E is subsequent clinical incompetence.

Alternatively, the *intraamniotic injection of hypertonic saline solution or prostaglandins* has proved to be an effective method of inducing labor after the third or fourth month, although it is not without hazard. The technique is as follows.

1. The patient's bladder is emptied, and the lower abdomen is prepared and draped using sterile techniques.
2. Under local anesthesia, a No. 16 or No. 18 needle trocar is introduced into the amniotic cavity, inserting it in the midline and well below the top of the fundus to avoid loops of bowel.
3. A total of 100 to 200 ml of amniotic fluid is removed, and then 200 to 300 ml of a 20% saline solution or prostaglandin is instilled and the needle withdrawn.

Although failures may be encountered, labor usually occurs within 8 to 20 hours, and delivery is ordinarily accomplished within a few hours. Subsequent curettage may be necessary to complete the removal of all placental and decidual tissue. If labor has not started after 12 to 24 hours, induction with an intravenous oxytocin infusion is carried out.

Aside from the dangers of introducing infection or accidental injury to adjacent viscera, the most serious complications, including several deaths, have occurred as a result of the accidental intravenous injection of the hypertonic saline solution. Cerebral convulsions, acute renal failure (the latter presumably due to hemolysis), and acute tubular necrosis have occurred, with fatal outcomes reported in several cases. Furthermore, a number of instances of disseminated intravascular coagulation and secondary maternal hemorrhage have been observed, presumably secondary to the release of tissue thromboplastin from the edematous, fragmenting placenta.

Intraamniotic instillation of the natural or synthetic prostaglandins E_2 and $F_{2\alpha}$ induces strong uterine contractions that usually result in cervical dilatation and expulsion of the fetus and placenta within 24 hours. In some clinics, in addition to the prostaglandins, *laminaria tents* are used. These plugs, made from dried seaweed, gradually swell when the substance absorbs moisture. Dilatation of the cervix is further promoted and speeded up by this mechanical means. (Laminaria tents have also been employed by some as a preliminary step prior to suction curettage, inserting one 12 hours before, especially in young nulligravidas with tight cervical canals that are otherwise difficult to dilate.) More recently, prostaglandin E_2 gel inserted vaginally into the cervix can soften the cervix in preparation for pregnancy termination. Prostaglandins appear to be safer than hypertonic saline, because their use avoids the dangers of disseminated intravascular coagulopathy and hypernatremia. However, with prostaglandin, the fetus is sometimes expelled alive; moreover, rupture of the uterus may occur posteriorly, with the fetus being expelled partially into the cul-de-sac.

The physician should be on the lookout for *psychological problems* secondary to guilt or feelings of loss over the abortion. The patient may require psychiatric consultation to help deal with her emotions. However, emotional disturbances following abortions have not been as frequent or as serious as had been anticipated; and proper preabortion counseling, together with reassurance and sympathetic support during and after the procedure, tends to minimize the emotional trauma suffered by women undergoing elective abortions.

Finally, *postabortion counseling* regarding an effective contraceptive program is of vital importance. Without a conscientious and sympathetic follow-up program, a significant number of patients who have undergone an abortion may return with another unwanted pregnancy.

If the therapeutic termination of pregnancy is performed for chronic medical or psychiatric conditions that the physician knows will be in existence at the time of any subsequent pregnancy, sterilization at the time of abortion should be seriously considered. Certainly sterilization is safer than repeated abortions or the risks of long-term contraceptive use.

ECTOPIC PREGNANCY

Failure of the fertilized ovum to migrate or to be transported to the normal site of implantation within the endometrial cavity may result in implantation at an aberrant site in the tube, broad ligament, or ovary giving rise to an ectopic gestation. The incidence of ectopic pregnancy is traditionally given as 1 in 200 live births, but it is more accurate to record it as per 1000 live births and abortions. The incidence of ectopic pregnancy is increasing. It has increased from 3.2 to 4.3 live births and therapeutic abortions in Britain and from 5.8 to 11.1 per 1000 conceptions in Sweden over a 15-year period. Similarly it has increased by 11 percent annually in the United States, from 4.8 per 1000 live births in 1970 to 19.2 per 1000 in 1983. This dramatic increase, summarized in Table 16-1, is largely due to an increase in the incidence of pelvic inflammatory disease. Other contributory factors include increased use of the intrauterine device, induced abortion, tubal surgery for infertility or sterilization, conservative management of ectopic pregnancy, delayed childbearing, and douching. Ectopic pregnancy is more frequent in blacks and nonwhites than in whites, and it is most frequent in women 35 years or older. Most such pregnancies occur in women

Table 16-1. Numbers and Rates of Ectopic Pregnancies in the United States (1970–1983)

Year	Number[a]	Rates		
		Females, ages 15 to 44+ (per 10,000)	Live births (per 1000)	Reported pregnancies[b]
1970	17,800	4.2	4.8	4.3
1971	19,300	4.4	5.4	4.8
1972	24,500	5.5	7.5	6.3
1973	25,600	5.6	8.2	6.8
1974	26,400	5.7	8.4	6.7
1975	30,500	6.5	9.8	7.6
1976	34,600	7.2	11.0	8.3
1977	40,700	8.3	12.3	9.2
1978	42,400	8.5	12.8	9.4
1979	49,900	9.9	14.3	10.4
1980	52,500	9.9	14.5	10.5
1981	68,000	12.7	18.7	13.6
1982	61,800	11.5	17.0	12.3
1983	69,600	12.6	19.2	14.0
Total	563,300	8.3	11.8	9.2

[a]Rounded to nearest 100.
[b]Rate per 1000 reported pregnancies (live births, legal induced abortions, and ectopic pregnancies).
Source: Centers for Disease Control. Ectopic pregnancy. *MMWR* 35:289, 1986.

25 to 34 years of age, but age increases the risk of ectopic pregnancy with a threefold risk at 35 to 44 years compared to that at 15 to 24 years.

Ectopic pregnancy has emerged as a leading cause of maternal mortality, although mortality from ectopic pregnancy has also declined over the years, from 3.5 deaths per 1000 ectopic pregnancies in 1970 to 0.5 deaths per 1000 in 1983. At present, 40 to 50 women die annually in the United States owing to ectopic pregnancy. It is estimated that approximately 25,000 ectopic pregnancies occur each year in the United States, the ratio of ectopic to normal intrauterine pregnancies ranging from 1:300 to as high as 1:125 in various reported studies. Although in recent years earlier recognition of this disorder with more prompt and effective treatment has brought about a reduction in deaths, ectopic pregnancy is still a significant cause

of maternal mortality. Fatalities are nearly always the result of failure to make the diagnosis, delayed or inadequate surgery, or ineffective therapy for shock in patients with tubal rupture and massive intraperitoneal hemorrhage.

Etiology

A preexisting chronic salpingitis, whether of gonococcal, mixed bacterial (postabortal or puerperal), or tuberculous origin, is commonly found in association with ectopic pregnancy. It is currently estimated that approximately 25 percent of all ectopic pregnancies occur in association with preexisting chronic salpingitis, most of which cases are of gonococcal origin. Obviously, the inflammatory disease in these cases has not resulted in complete occlusion, but the mucosal damage has been sufficient to produce luminal narrowing, distortion, and sometimes pseudodiverticulum formation, with resulting arrest and abnormal implantation of the migrating early embryo somewhere along the course of the tube, in a narrow, tortuous channel, or postinflammatory sacculation. With the advent of more effective chemotherapy for both pyogenic and tuberculous salpingitis, control of the acute phase of the disease is now more often achieved before complete tubal closure has occurred. However, some degree of mucosal damage is usually sustained, and thus it is not surprising that within recent years there has been an apparent increase in the frequency of ectopic pregnancy.

Because any pathologic condition involving the tube or the uterotubal junction results in obstruction to the normal passage of the fertilized ovum, a number of other tubal, peritubal, or uterine disorders are similarly accompanied by a high incidence of ectopic pregnancy. These disorders include congenital müllerian duct anomalies; benign tubal tumors and cysts (Chap. 18); peritubal adhesions secondary to sexually transmitted diseases such as *Chlamydia* infection, prior appendicitis, endometriosis, or a previous pelvic or abdominal operation; uterine fibroids or adenomyosis in the cornual region near the uterotubal junction; and previous tubal repair (tuboplasty) to restore patency or normal tubal pickup and transport function where these functions had been totally impaired by previous disease. The subsequent rate of occurrence of ectopic tubal pregnancies following such tubal reconstruction procedures is high, despite achieving high postoperative tubal patency rates, because tubal function may not be totally restored.

Although the probable etiology of many ectopic gestations can often be traced to one of the above specific preexisting disorders, most ectopic pregnancies (50 percent or more) occur within fallopian tubes that are apparently anatomically and histologically normal. Therefore premature arrest and ectopic implantation of the early embryo are more commonly the result of a disturbance in tubal physiology, on a hormonal or a neurogenic basis. Because of the great dependence of normal tubal physiology on adequate and properly timed ovarian hormonal stimulation of the secretory and ciliated cells of the mucosa and the smooth muscle layer of the tubal wall, minor inadequacies in corpus luteum function and hormone output in even apparently ovulatory cycles might well lead to impaired tubal transport. This situation could then result in prolonged retention of the ovum within the tube beyond the normal, approximately three-day interval required for fertilization and subsequent preliminary development of the zygote and early trophoblastic elements, as well as further conditioning of the ripening endometrium, both of which are essential if the early embryo is to be capable of implanting successfully once it has reached the endometrial cavity. In the fact of such a delay, implantation within the tube might well result.

Another plausible mechanism for delayed tubal transport of the early zygote is neuromuscular rather than hormonal in nature. Although impossible to document objectively, it seems highly likely that in some cases emotional disorders and temporary psychological disturbances could well result in interference with the normal autonomic nervous system regulation of tubal muscular activity and lead to delay in passage of the fertilized ovum in a "spastic" tube.

One other probable way in which delayed migration of the fertilized ovum is sufficient to result in ectopic implantation is suggested by the observation that in a significant percentage (in some series as high as 50 percent) of tubal pregnancies the corpus luteum of pregnancy is found in the contralateral ovary. This finding implies that either the ovum was fertilized within the free peritoneal cavity or fertilization occurred in the ampullary portion of the tube on the same side as the corpus luteum and the fertilized ovum subsequently transmigrated to the opposite tube. In either case, considerable delay would be inevitable, and the developing zygote could well enlarge sufficiently to be unable to pass through the narrow isthmic or cornual portion of the tube.

Finally, there has been interest in the possibility that delayed ovulation occurring around the twenty-first day of the cycle rather than at midcycle is the cause of ectopic pregnancy in some cases. Such a delay in ovulation and fertilization could result in an initial failure of adequate uterine implantation because of a short, inadequate luteal phase, with subsequent uprooting of the poorly implanted conceptus and its transfer to an ectopic site by tubal reflux during the menstrual flow. Retrospective histologic studies of the embryos in some series of ectopic pregnancies have verified that conception must have occurred around the twenty-first day of the cycle, and invariably the patient had experienced menstrual bleeding at the expected time, even though conception had taken place.

Contrary to the often optimistic reassurance, women who have had one ectopic pregnancy, even when the opposite tube appears grossly normal, have a seven to ten times greater chance of having another than do women who have never had such a pregnancy (about 10 percent have another ectopic pregnancy at some future time). Unfortunately, only about one-third succeed in having a live baby, although a somewhat larger number conceive only to lose their pregnancies through abortion, miscarriage, or another ectopic gestation.

Another example of tubal dysfunction leading to ectopic pregnancy is the rare occurrence of ectopic pregnancy after postcoital prevention of an unwanted conception by giving large doses of diethylstilbestrol or other estrogenic compounds (the "morning-after pill"), which alter tubal motility and transport and may lead to arrest and implantation of the embryo in the tube. On the other hand, the frequent occurrence of ectopic pregnancy in women using an intrauterine device is believed to be due to the device eliminating intrauterine pregnancies but not ectopic pregnancies, thereby contributing to the incidence of ectopic pregnancy.

Sites of Ectopic Pregnancy

Fallopian Tube. Most ectopic pregnancies (95 percent) occur within the fallopian tube, usually in the ampullary or isthmic portion (Fig. 16-2). Interstitial or cornual pregnancies are less frequent but of considerable significance, as rupture of a cornual pregnancy usually takes place earlier and is often associated with the sudden onset of such massive hemorrhage that even the slightest delay in diagnosis and treatment can prove fatal.

Bilateral tubal pregnancies occurring simultaneously are rare, although several cases have been recorded. Similarly, the simultaneous occurrence of a tubal and a normal intrauterine pregnancy is only infrequently encountered.

Ovary. Primary ovarian pregnancies comprise about 1 percent of all types of ectopic gestation (Fig. 16-2). Such pregnancies are due to the following: (1) The ovum fails to be properly extruded and is fertilized within the early corpus luteum; or (2) after fertilization within the tube or free peritoneal cavity, the ovum fails to continue on its transtubal journey, implanting instead on the surface of the ovary, where it temporarily burrows into the ovarian cortex.

Because the clinical manifestations are similar to those of an ectopic tubal pregnancy, the diagnosis of an ovarian rather than a tubal gestation can be made definitively only at laparotomy and only after the tube itself is clearly shown to be completely uninvolved in the implantation site. Not infrequently, an early ovarian pregnancy cannot be grossly distinguished from rupture or hemorrhage into a simple cyst. Only when histologic examination of the resected specimen reveals chorionic villi does the true nature of the acute ovarian process become apparent. Women using intrauterine devices have a higher rate of ovarian pregnancies than do nonusers.

Cervix. Cervical pregnancy (Fig. 16-2) appears to be the rarest type of ectopic gestation, probably because the chances are remote that a fertilized ovum that has passed completely through the uterus retains sufficient capacity to implant in the relatively unfavorable en-

Fig. 16-2. Sites of ectopic pregnancy.

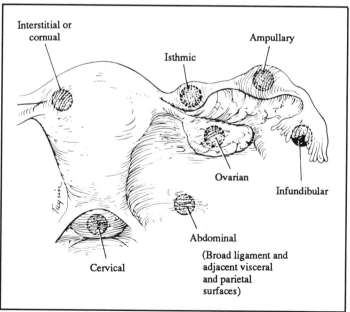

vironment afforded by the cervical endothelium and glands.

Abdominal Sites. Tubal, ovarian, and cervical pregnancies rarely survive more than two to three months and never reach the state of fetal viability. One type of ectopic gestation that occasionally approaches term with the development of a viable fetus is the *abdominal* pregnancy. The balance of evidence suggests that nearly all abdominal pregnancies begin initially as tubal gestations. The latter are then "aborted" from the tube relatively early in their development and implant on the neighboring broad ligaments and adjacent uterus, bowel, and parietal peritoneum, the sites of placental development in an abdominal pregnancy. The availability of an adequate blood supply in these areas makes further growth of the pregnancy possible. Thus prior pelvic inflammatory disease, known to be associated with an increased incidence of tubal pregnancy, is also considered to be the most important etiologic factor in the occurrence of abdominal pregnancy. Partial tubal obstruction leads to temporary tubal implantation, which later may be converted to an abdominal pregnancy if tubal abortion occurs while the early pregnancy is still capable of reimplantation. The incidence of abdominal pregnancy in a general population is about 1 per 15,000 live births, but it appears to be higher in blacks, possibly because of the greater frequency of chronic salpingitis in black women.

Migration of what was initially an intrauterine pregnancy via rupture of a previous cesarean section scar has been shown to be another mechanism by which an abdominal pregnancy can develop. (There is usually a demonstrable uteroplacental fistula in these cases.) Finally, initial implantation of a fertilized ovum on abdominal peritoneal surfaces with a resulting primary abdominal pregnancy has been fairly well documented in an occasional case, but it is exceedingly rare.

Diagnosis and Management

The patient frequently experiences mild abdominal pain and transient vaginal bleeding approximately six weeks after the last menstrual period (coincident with "tubal abortion"), and she then may be relatively asymptomatic for several weeks or months, presenting with what appears to be a normal intrauterine pregnancy. As the pregnancy enlarges, abdominal pain and gastrointestinal or urinary tract disturbances develop. On physical examination, clues such as easily palpable superficial fetal parts, excessively loud fetal heart tones, or a fetal mass that feels separate from the uterus may be detected.

The finding of an abdominal fetal position (transverse lie or breech) with the presenting part high above the pelvic inlet should always raise the suspicion of abdominal pregnancy, as such fetal malpositions are inevitable in and characteristic of this condition. Sonography, pelvic roentgenography utilizing soft-tissue techniques, and occasionally hysterography may be employed to confirm the diagnosis.

There are many recorded instances in which an abdominal pregnancy has been spontaneously and indefinitely retained without benefit of medical attention, with subsequent partial or complete resorption, skeletonization or lithopedion formation, or the development of a pelvic abscess or a fistulous tract involving the vagina, abdominal wall, bladder, or rectum through which fetal parts are extruded. Deliberate conservative medical management carries a high mortality and is not recommended. Once abdominal pregnancy is definitely diagnosed, prompt laparotomy is indicated, regardless of the stage of gestation, to avoid dangerous complications—in particular, massive, spontaneous intraabdominal hemorrhage or serious pelvic sepsis. The fetus should be removed, ligating the umbilical cord close to the placenta; if the stage of viability has been reached, a live baby that survives and is relatively normal is obtained in approximately 20 percent of cases.

The principal problem confronting the surgeon dealing with an abdominal pregnancy is management of the placenta at laparotomy. If the blood supply of the placental attachments can be readily identified and completely and safely ligated (i.e., when essentially all of it is derived from the uterine vessels, ovarian vessels, or both), the placenta should usually be ligated and removed, as the risk of later hemorrhage is remote. Furthermore, the subsequent convalescence is greatly simplified by eliminating the need for spontaneous resorption of the placenta, which in some instances is accompanied by sepsis, hemorrhage, and intestinal obstruction or fistula formation. On the other hand, if the placental attachment is broad or its blood supply diffuse and not readily identified or available for safe and complete ligation, the placenta should be left completely undisturbed after removal of the fetus and the abdomen closed without drainage, accepting the possibility of a more prolonged and complicated convalescence and even the occasional need for reoperation. Any attempt to define the placental site and its vascular supply further in such cases—and particularly any ill-advised efforts at partial or total removal—are definitely contraindicated, as alarming and often fatal hemorrhage may result, either immediately or during the early postoperative period.

Tubal Pregnancy

Pathologic Features. The tubal environment is not a favorable one, and even though implantation occurs the embryo often fails to develop or is malformed. The wall of the tube becomes edematous, and there is vascular engorgement. Although chorionic villi usually undergo early development, there is little if any decidual response on the part of the tubal mucosa and no hypertrophy of the tubal musculature. Accordingly, the tubal wall remains thin as the tube becomes increasingly distended; and if tubal abortion does not occur first, as is frequently the case (such an event may go totally unrecognized or be accompanied by minimal symptoms and spontaneous resolution and recovery), rupture or penetration of the wall of the tube is inevitable, usually within six to eight weeks of onset.

If functional activity of the chorionic villi is adequate during the early stages of a tubal pregnancy, the uterus undergoes enlargement, occasionally attaining the size of a three-month pregnancy, and there is a definite decidual change in the normal endometrium. With the onset of tubal abortion or often well in advance of impending rupture of the ectopic gestation, and as a result of a rapid decline in human chorionic gonadotropin secretion, sloughing and hemorrhage from the uterine decidua (now deprived of its hor-

monal support) result in the onset of the abdominal vaginal bleeding frequently seen in patients with tubal pregnancies. Occasionally, this sequence of events results in the passage of a decidual cast, which should further alert the physician to the possibility of ectopic pregnancy.

Diagnosis

SIGNS AND SYMPTOMS. Only a few patients with tubal pregnancy, perhaps 15 percent, present the classic history: initial amenorrhea with one or two missed periods, accompanied by symptoms suggestive of early pregnancy. This phase is followed by the appearance of vaginal bleeding, signifying the impending termination of the pregnancy. Then, after a variable interval of hours or days, abdominal pain suddenly develops, indicating rupture of the tubal pregnancy and the onset of intraperitoneal bleeding. At first the pain is unilateral and pelvic in location but shortly becomes generalized throughout the abdomen. It is often associated with shoulder pain as the hemoperitoneum increases and blood accumulates under the diaphragm. Thereafter, there is rapid progression to an obvious acute surgical abdominal emergency, with generalized abdominal tenderness and spasm, marked vaginal vault tenderness, and characteristically exquisite pain on motion of the cervix (cervical motion tenderness). A tender adnexal mass is usually palpable, although this finding may be obscured if sufficient blood and clots are present in the pelvis. Cullen's sign (bluish discoloration of the umbilicus) and a cul-de-sac that feels doughy and may have a bluish color are sometimes present and further indicate massive hemiperitoneum. The classic picture is completed by the obvious associated surgical shock, often with syncope, that promptly ensues as a result of the continuous, steady or abrupt massive hemorrhage.

On the other hand, most patients (85 percent) exhibit subacute and atypical manifestations. Although some irregularity of the recent menstrual pattern has usually occurred, 25 to 40 percent of patients experience no interval of amenorrhea whatsoever. It is important to ascertain not only the last menstrual period but also the period prior to that, as well as the nature, duration, and amount of flow. This information assists in deciding which is likely to have been the last menstrual period. Morning nausea, breast soreness and fullness, and other symptoms commonly associated with early pregnancy are often absent or minimal. When abdominal or pelvic discomfort (present in 90 percent of cases) does appear, it is frequently mild, sometimes poorly localized, and intermittent at first; the distress is often associated with similarly vague and inconstant symptoms of bowel or bladder irritability. Typically, the early pain is crampy or colicky in nature and generally is referred to one of the lower abdominal quadrants. Only when bleeding or rupture occurs does the pain become severe and steady. Abnormal vaginal bleeding, a manifestation that occurs only slightly less frequently than abdominal pain and that is present in 80 percent of patients, is also often mild, intermittent, and frequently of considerable duration before the patient seeks medical advice. The patient is often more concerned about her pain than her other symptoms, and the physician frequently must elicit specifically the information concerning the irregular flow. Finally, the findings on physical examination are often unremarkable or equivocal; there may or may not be significant pelvic or abdominal tenderness, and in 50 to 75 percent of the cases no definite adnexal mass is palpable. Secondary uterine enlargement is also a highly variable feature. Occasionally, the temperature is slightly elevated, but most of the patients are afebrile.

Thus it is the clinical picture in most patients with subacute signs and symptoms that makes tubal pregnancy "the disease of diagnostic surprises" and the "great masquerader." Only by maintaining a high index of suspicion of the possibility of its presence in any woman of childbearing age who complains of abdominal pain and irregular bleeding can this disorder be consistently recognized, particularly in its early stages. Ectopic pregnancy represents a constant diagnostic challenge, not only because of its own frequently vague manifestations but also because a wide variety of other pelvic and abdominal disorders are accompanied by similar signs and symptoms.

DIFFERENTIAL DIAGNOSIS. The differential diagnosis of tubal pregnancy should include the following.

1. Early normal intrauterine pregnancy, with some other cause of abdominal and/or pelvic pain and with or without a tender adnexal mass, e.g., ruptured, bleeding corpus luteum of pregnancy; painful, tender, normal corpus luteum; painful stretching of the round ligaments; torsion of the ovary containing the corpus luteum or twisted ovarian cyst; spontaneous torsion of the fallopian tube during pregnancy; torsion or degeneration of a pedunculated fibroid; appendicitis; ureteral colic

2. Intrauterine pregnancy with simple implantation bleeding or with "threatened," missed, or incomplete spontaneous abortion

3. Pregnancy or hematometrium in a rudimentary uterine horn

4. Anovulatory cycles with a painful, tender follicle cyst and irregular bleeding
   a. Dysfunctional
   b. In association with acute and chronic pelvic inflammatory disease
   c. In association with polycystic ovarian disease

5. Complications of endometriosis, pelvic inflammatory disease, ovarian tumors, pedunculated fibroids (torsion, rupture, hemorrhage into or from), or ovarian cysts (hemorrhage into and rupture or further bleeding from a corpus luteum cyst being a common entity simulating ectopic pregnancy)

DIAGNOSTIC PLAN. *It cannot be overemphasized that prompt and accurate diagnosis is facilitated by constantly including ectopic pregnancy among the diagnostic possibilities in women of childbearing age who are suffering from abdominal pain and menstrual irregularities.*

In patients with a "classic history" who are in shock with obvious internal bleeding, the diagnosis is nearly always apparent from the history and examination alone. Confirmation by recovery of blood on culde-sac aspiration may also be sought but is often unnecessary. Operative treatment (laparotomy) should proceed forthwith, following a brief period of preparation with transfusions to relieve shock and restore a satisfactory blood volume for safe anesthesia and surgery.

In patients with the more usual, atypical, subacute clinical picture, a period of observation in the hospital or even on an ambulatory basis may be needed, during which time the findings on repeated pelvic examinations, the results of serum hCG titers (see below), blood counts, vital signs, and the further clinical course of the illness are utilized to arrive at a correct diagnosis. A falling hemoglobin or hematocrit may be helpful; the white blood cell count may be normal or moderately elevated and is of no diagnostic value; the temperature usually remains normal or only slightly elevated.

Serum hCG titer measured by specific radioimmunoassay using antibodies against the β-subunit of hCG (see Chapter 2) in combination with ultrasonography (see Chapter 3) has proved to be a valuable adjunct in the early diagnosis of ectopic pregnancy. Early diagnosis reduces morbidity and mortality, allows prompt laparoscopy and definitive surgical or medical therapy, and enables salvation of the affected tube in tubal pregnancy. Almost all patients suspected of having an ectopic pregnancy have a positive serum hCG by the specific radioimmunoassay, usually with low titers, while those who are not pregnant have a negative hCG level. A subnormal or low serum hCG titer is suggestive of a nonviable pregnancy that can be either a threatened (or missed) abortion or an ectopic pregnancy and less commonly a trophoblastic disease. A slow rise in serum hCG titer also suggests an ectopic pregnancy or a nonviable pregnancy (serum hCG titers double every two to three days in early normal intrauterine pregnancy). Serum hCG titers of 6,000 mU/ml are usually reflective of normal intrauterine pregnancy, and a pregnancy sac is readily seen on transabdominal pelvic sonography. With transvaginal pelvic sonography, an intrauterine pregnancy sac is visible much earlier at hCG titers of 1,000 to 1,600 mU/ml, usually about 5 weeks and certainly by 6 weeks from the last menstrual period. Thus, if an intrauterine pregnancy is seen and/or the serum hCG titers are consistent with the early stages of pregnancy as described, expectant management of a suspected ectopic is permissible; if the serum hCG titer doubles every two to three days, ectopic pregnancy is unlikely.

Cul-de-sac aspiration (culdocentesis) has frequently been employed as a guide to whether prompt surgery is indicated. Although often helpful, too great reliance on this maneuver can prove misleading because with early, unruptured ectopic pregnancy no blood is obtained, whereas with many of the acute disorders simulating ectopic pregnancy blood may well be obtained on culdocentesis.

The most effective and satisfactory diagnostic procedure is laparoscopy. It should be performed almost immediately on all patients suspected of harboring an ectopic pregnancy (excluding the obvious cases, of course) because visualization of the tubes is the only way the diagnosis can truly be established or excluded in most patients. Prompt laparoscopy completely eliminates the need for a prolonged, somewhat hazardous, and often expensive observation period and the various frequently inconclusive or even misleading laboratory studies and diagnostic maneuvers. It avoids unnecessary laparotomy for diagnosis only when conditions not requiring surgical treatment are responsible for the symptoms and findings. When no ectopic pregnancy is found, laparoscopy has the added advantage in most cases of accurately identifying some other cause for the symptoms, which is information that may be important in itself for further management of the patient.

Finally, if curettage has been done because a diagnosis of incomplete abortion was mistakenly entertained, a pathologist's report of an atypical, decidual type of endometrium in the absence of chorionic villi should immediately alert the physician to the possible existence of an ectopic pregnancy.

A specific histologic picture in the endometrium, the *Arias-Stella phenomenon,* is often seen in the presence of a bleeding tubal pregnancy, although it may be observed in aborting intrauterine pregnancies as well. It consists in marked secretory and proliferative activity (often within the same endometrial glands), piling up of cells within the gland lumens to form syncytial masses, and tall "bizarre" cells with foamy cytoplasm and hyperchromatic nuclei.

Operative Treatment. Obviously, the sooner the diagnosis is established, the more likely it is that a relatively conservative surgical procedure can be done. Depending on its size and the extent of local tubal damage produced by the ectopic gestation, several maneuvers may be considered.

1. Simple, manual extrusion by "milking" the ec-

topic pregnancy from the tube may be possible in the case of abortion with minimal bleeding of an early tubal pregnancy located in the ampullary region. This procedure can be performed laparoscopically or at laparotomy, but the milking must be gentle to reduce tissue trauma.

2. Resection of the involved segment of the tube and end-to-end anastomosis or resection, and tubal reimplantation if the ectopic pregnancy is in the isthmic or cornual region, can be done for early ectopic pregnancy with localized tubal damage when the remaining portion of the tube is normal. The repair or reanastomosis of the tube can be undertaken at the same time as resection of the ectopic pregnancy, or definitive tubal repair or reconstruction can be performed a few months later as an interval procedure. The advantages of the latter are that less-vascular tissues are encountered in the nonpregnant state and there is better surgical preparation when done as an elective procedure. Microsurgical technique must be employed.

3. Salpingectomy is indicated when dealing with advanced lesions, where hemorrhage and rupture have produced extensive damage to the tube and mesosalpinx or when there is uncontrollable bleeding if conservative repair of the tube is attempted. Although ipsilateral oophorectomy was previously advocated with salpingectomy on the questionable assumption that it enhances conception by guaranteeing ovulation in the remaining ovary with a tube, current availability of in vitro fertilization and newer reproductive technologies make preservation of both ovaries desirable.

4. Salpingostomy may be done. Favorable experiences have been reported when fairly large ectopic pregnancies were managed by incision of the distended tube with evacuation of the ectopic pregnancy, control of all bleeding points with microcauterization, and preservation of the tube if it is still viable. Although there is much claimed about high subsequent tubal patency rates, there are neither sufficient data on subsequent pregnancy rates, repeat ectopic pregnancies, and permanent tubal occlusion nor comparisons with resection of the ectopic pregnancies followed by reanastomosis at a later date. However, salpingostomy should be seriously considered if the opposite tube has previously been removed. The salpingos-

tomy can be performed using needle microcautery or a laser and is best left open after evacuating the ectopic pregnancy.

5. Laparoscopic surgery may be appropriate. Several of the above procedures, including resection of the ectopic pregnancy, salpingostomy, and milking of the tube, can be undertaken through the laparoscope if there is adequate equipment for translaparoscopic surgery, the surgeon is trained for it, and the ectopic pregnancy is unruptured.

Regardless of the operative approach employed, all gross blood and clots should be removed, as it is easier and quicker to give patients transfusions or iron therapy than to await resorption of peritoneal blood. Moreover, fewer intraperitoneal adhesions that might interfere with subsequent fertility result.

Postoperatively, if the patient is Rh-negative and does not already have an anti-D antibody, she should promptly receive RhoGAM, a purified human anti-Rh gamma globulin preparation. RhoGAM should be used to prevent sensitization whenever an Rh-negative woman may have received Rh-positive blood cells. Therefore this measure is indicated when such a patient has suffered an ectopic pregnancy, has undergone a spontaneous or therapeutic abortion, or has delivered an Rh-positive baby. RhoGAM appears to act by destroying Rh-positive blood cells before the recipient's immune system recognizes that an antigen is present (1 ml of RhoGAM destroys approximately 10 ml of Rh-positive blood cells).

Nonsurgical Management. Because some unruptured tubal ectopic pregnancies undergo spontaneous resorption, tubal abortion, and spontaneous resolution, attempts have been made to develop a system of conservative nonsurgical management for selected patients. Methotrexate, a folic acid antagonist, has been used with promising success in several small studies to induce repression of the ectopic pregnancy with subsequent tubal patency and viable pregnancies.

First, laparoscopy is necessary to establish that the ectopic pregnancy is unruptured and is less than 3 cm in size. Methotrexate is then given intravenously followed by citrovorum factor (folinic acid) the next day to overcome the toxic side effects of methotrexate.

This regimen is repeated for a total of eight days, i.e., four days of methotrexate and four days of citrovorum factor. Thus far it has been found that the smaller the ectopic pregnancy, the more likely is the therapy to be successful. Surgery may still be necessary if the ectopic pregnancy ruptures or bleeds during the chemotherapy. Although chemotherapy offers an interesting alternative and advantage over conservative surgery, the success rates and selection of suitable cases must be better established.

Another type of nonsurgical treatment of ectopic pregnancy is direct injection of methotrexate or prostaglandin $F_{2\alpha}$ into the pregnancy. Direct injection of methotrexate into a cervical pregnancy has been successfully carried out with good outcome and avoiding surgical removal of the ectopic pregnancy. Direct injection of prostaglandin $F_{2\alpha}$ into unruptured tubal pregnancies has also been performed in a series of patients with good outcome. With better image definition of transvaginal sonography, the prostaglandin could be injected with ultrasound guidance.

SELECTED READINGS

Atrash, H. K., Friede, A., and Hogue, C. J. R. Ectopic pregnancy mortality in the United States 1970–1983. *Obstet. Gynecol.* 70:817, 1987.

Atrash, H. K., et al. Legal abortion mortality in the United States: 1972 to 1982. *Am. J. Obstet. Gynecol.* 156:605, 1987.

Couzinet, B., et al. Termination of early pregnancy by the progesterone antagonist RU 486 (Mifepristone). *N. Engl. J. Med.* 315:1565, 1986.

DeCherney, A. H. Tubal ectopic pregnancy. In S. J. Behrman, R. W. Kistner, and G. W. Patton (Eds.), *Progress in Infertility* (3rd ed.), Boston: Little, Brown, 1988. Pp. 181–194.

Lindblom, B., et al. Local prostaglandin $F_{2\alpha}$ injection for treatment of ectopic pregnancy. *Lancet* 1:776, 1987.

Morris, N. D., McCallum, G. I., and Hammond, L. Preoperative cervical dilatation: A trial of laminaria tents and prostaglandin $F_{2\alpha}$ gel. *Aust. NZ. J. Obstet. Gynecol.* 26:36, 1986.

Nyberg, D. A., et al. Endovaginal sonographic evaluation of ectopic pregnancy: A prospective study. *A. J. R.* 149:1181, 1987.

Ory, S. J., et al. Conservative treatment of ectopic pregnancy with methotrexate. *Am. J. Obstet. Gynecol.* 154:1299, 1986.

Pouly, J. L., et al. Conservative laparoscopic treatment of 321 ectopic pregnancies. *Fertil. Steril.* 46:1093, 1986.

Romero, R., et al. The value of serial human chorionic gonadotropin testing as a diagnostic tool in ectopic pregnancy. *Am. J. Obstet. Gynecol.* 155:392, 1986.

Stray-Pedersen, B., and Stray-Pedersen, S. Etiologic factors and subsequent reproductive performance in 195 couples with a prior history of habitual abortion. *Am. J. Obstet. Gynecol.* 148:140, 1984.

17

Benign Diseases of the Uterus: Leiomyomas, Adenomyosis, Hyperplasia, and Polyps

Benign conditions of the uterus are the most frequent indications for hysterectomy. Performed for the proper indications this operation provides relief of many gynecologic symptoms, including abnormal and heavy bleeding (menorrhagia, menometrorrhagia), pain (dysmenorrhea), and pelvic pressure. Some of these conditions can be easily diagnosed, whereas the diagnosis of others may be elusive and not established until the pathologist has studied the histology. The differential diagnosis of these conditions, especially in women after age 35, must always include the possibility of a malignancy (endometrial adenocarcinoma, uterine sarcoma, ovarian cancer, or cervical carcinoma).

LEIOMYOMAS

Popularly known as fibroids, leiomyomas are sometimes also called *myomas* or *fibromyomas*. In actuality, they are benign tumors of smooth muscle cell origin. It is only after atrophic and degenerative changes have occurred that the grossly and histologically obvious element of fibrosis is introduced. Leiomyomas may develop in any structure or viscus that contains smooth muscle cells. For example, they occur occasionally throughout the gastrointestinal tract, arising in the muscular layer of the esophageal, gastric, or intestinal wall and usually project within the lumen as an intramural, extramucosal tumor. Leiomyomas are far more frequent in the reproductive tract and represent the most common pelvic tumor. Sites for their occurrence include not only the uterus itself but also the fallopian tubes, cervix, vagina, vulva, and round and uterosacral ligaments. Although brief reference in the appropriate chapters is made to their appearance and varying manifestations at extra-

uterine sites, most leiomyomas develop within the uterus, a fact that is undoubtedly related to the various relatively poorly understood etiologic and developmental factors that influence their initial formation as well as their subsequent rate and pattern of growth. It is estimated that uterine leiomyomas develop in at least 20 to 30 percent of all women. Many of these lesions remain completely asymptomatic and relatively insignificant in size and so represent incidental findings.

Histologically, a leiomyoma in its initial stages is a localized proliferation of smooth muscle cells. It is not clear why leiomyomas develop in some women and not in others. It is apparent, however, that black women are far more likely to have leiomyomas than are white women (the incidence is perhaps 50 percent or more in black women but only about 20 percent in white women). Moreover, clinically significant fibroids develop in black women at a considerably younger age, and the growth rate of their leiomyomas appears to be more rapid.

The growth-promoting effects of estrogen with respect to leiomyomas are well known. This fact is clinically apparent in the sudden increase in the growth rate of uterine fibroids frequently noted in association with pregnancy (although much of the enlargement noted during pregnancy may be due to edema superimposed on the actual increase in proliferation of smooth muscle cells), the invariable cessation of growth following menopause, and the resumption of growth and occasionally dramatic increase in size of known fibroids in postmenopausal women to whom estrogens are given. There is no evidence that an endocrine imbalance is present prior to the genesis of a leiomyoma, and fibroids develop in vast numbers of women who by all clinical and laboratory criteria have perfectly normal ovarian function.

Pathologic Anatomy

Leiomyomas may be solitary in the uterus but most frequently are multiple and are found in a variety of locations in the uterus. Grossly, the uterus may appear symmetrically enlarged; more often, however, multiple fibroids give the uterus an irregular, "knobby" shape. The cut surface of the leiomyoma is lighter in color than the normal myometrium and appears as a white, whorled configuration. The original areas of smooth muscle cell proliferation appear within the myometrial layer; if the leiomyoma maintains this same relative position within the wall of the uterus as it enlarges, it is termed an *interstitial (intramural) fibroid* (Fig. 17-1). It is probably most likely to occur if the area of smooth muscle proliferation arose initially in the central portion of the myometrium. Because intramural fibroids are thus surrounded on all sides by approximately equal thicknesses of myometrium, they tend to remain spherical.

The surrounding muscular wall of the uterus is in a perpetual state of intermittent contraction about these initially small interstitial tumors, so there is also a considerable tendency for them to be pushed either inward toward the endometrial cavity or outward toward the peritoneal surface of the uterus, particularly if they originally arose in the inner or outer portions of the myometrium. When this change occurs, leiomyomas tend to lose their original spherical shape and develop varying degrees of asymmetry. Furthermore, as they become more or less extruded from the muscle layer, the thin connective-tissue attachment, with its contained relatively sparse vascular and lymphatic channels, invariably becomes increasingly attenuated, and the fibroid may assume the form of a pedunculated tumor with a narrow pedicle. When the leiomyoma protrudes into the cavity of the uterus, it is termed a *submucosal (intracavitary) fibroid;* when it bulges through the outer surface of the uterine wall it is termed a *subserosal fibroid* (see Fig. 17-1). In either case, such fibroid tumors often ultimately become markedly *pedunculated.*

If the original leiomyoma is so situated that on its subsequent outward extrusion it appears and continues its growth between the leaves of the broad ligament, it is termed an *intraligamentous (or broad-ligament) fibroid.* Leiomyomas in this location are of considerable significance for two reasons: (1) Their later location sometimes makes it difficult or impossible to be certain they are uterine fibroids and not ovarian tumors (true also of any laterally placed pedunculated subserosal fibroid), and (2) the distortion of the uterine blood supply and the displacement of the ureter from its normal course through the broad

ligament produced by the intraligamentous fibroid often makes hysterectomy technically more difficult than usual and exposes the ureter to a greater risk of accidental injury if the operation is carelessly or improperly carried out.

Occasionally in pedunculated fibroids of considerable age, the pedicle and the accompanying vascular channels become progressively smaller, while at the same time adherence to adjacent tissues (e.g., the neighboring broad ligament or, less often, the omentum) may result in the development of an accessory blood supply that grows in from such a secondary, external source. If under these circumstances the blood supply of the true pedicle eventually becomes inadequate, thrombosis and infarction of the pedicle alone may occur, with the fibroid completely separating from the uterus and maintaining its viability through its now well established accessory vascular channels. Although they are encountered only rarely, such "wandering" leiomyomas of the broad ligament or omentum are termed *parasitic fibroids.*

Finally, although most fibroids develop in the wall of the uterine fundus, perhaps 5 to 10 percent appear in the muscular wall of the cervix (*cervical fibroids*). Here there is a universal tendency for them to protrude into the endocervical canal as they grow larger, the surrounding rim of normal cervix becoming progressively dilated and thinned. Superficial ulceration, necrosis, secondary infection, and hemorrhage are common in cervical fibroids; and as they become pedunculated, they often come to lie within the vaginal canal and can be easily removed surgically by transvaginal resection. A considerable number retain their endocervical location, however; and large cervical fibroids in this position pose the same potential technical problems during hysterectomy as do broad-ligament fibroids because their size often makes adequate exposure of the uterine vessels and adjacent ureter difficult.

From a histologic standpoint, the original pure collection of proliferating smooth muscle cells soon begins to undergo a chronic process of atrophy and hyaline degeneration. It is particularly obvious within the central portion of the growing tumor because the blood supply of a leiomyoma is relatively sparse at best, and with continued growth it becomes increas-

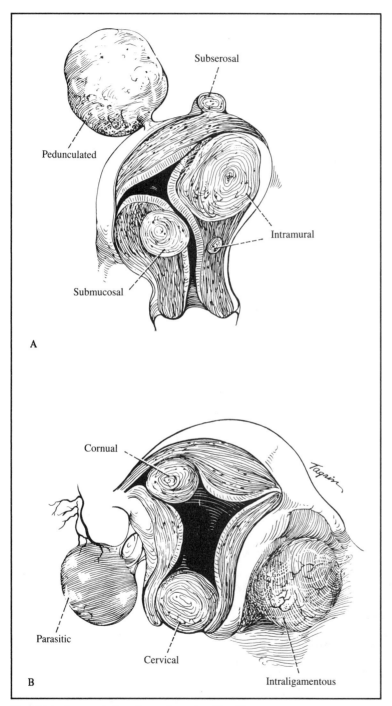

Fig. 17-1. Anatomic locations of uterine fibroids.
A. Types. B. Locations.

ingly limited in areas farthest removed from the capsular vascular channels. Areas in which atrophy and degeneration have occurred are most often replaced by fibrous tissue, which gives the usual fibroid its typical firm consistency, particularly noticeable in the hard central core.

At the periphery, a pseudocapsule is permanently maintained, and there is usually a distinct line of cleavage between the leiomyoma and the surrounding normal myometrium. As a result, local removal of the fibroid (myomectomy) is readily accomplished by incising the overlying muscular wall down to the surface of the pseudocapsule of the fibroid itself, which can then be easily shelled out.

As the smooth muscle atrophy, fibroblast replacement, and progressive impairment of blood supply proceed, further chronic degenerative changes, particularly apt to occur in large tumors, may result in a myxomatous type of degeneration with diffuse edema and a soft, gelatinous consistency. In some instances this process progresses to cystic change within the softer areas of the fibroid. More often, fatty necrosis

and ultimately calcification take place. Calcification of fibroids (Fig. 17-2) is commonly seen in postmenopausal women in whom the fibroids have obviously been undergoing degenerative change over a period of many years.

Acute degenerative change caused by a sudden infarction of all or a large portion of a leiomyoma may also take place. This change is particularly prone to occur in pedunculated fibroids, when, as a result of torsion or spontaneous thrombosis of the narrow pedicle, the blood supply is suddenly cut off. A specific form of acute degenerative change of this type, termed *red degeneration* or *carneous degeneration,* is most commonly seen during pregnancy. In this situation the increased growth of the fibroid, stimulated by the extremely high and rising estrogen levels, leads to an equally rapid outstripping of the precarious blood supply. The situation is further aggravated by the

Fig. 17-2. Typical radiographic appearance of calcified fibroids. The patient was a 70-year-old woman with asymptomatic pedunculated fibroids. The pessary ring she wore for an associated uterine prolapse is visible on the radiograph.

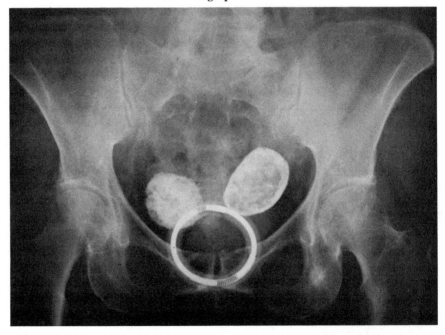

often marked edema of the fibroid as well as by the pressure of the enlarging pregnant uterus. At some point, whether due primarily to arterial or venous insufficiency or to a combination of the two, sudden vascular impairment develops, often in the nature of acute venous thrombosis, and may or may not proceed to total infarction. On cut section, a leiomyoma that has undergone acute carneous degeneration looks like raw, red meat; and on microscopic examination marked edema, pronounced vascular engorgement with evidence of extravasation of blood into tissue spaces, and varying degrees of hyaline degeneration are seen.

From a clinical standpoint, this acute vascular accident poses obvious problems in the differential diagnosis as well as in management in both the pregnant and the nonpregnant patient. During pregnancy the resulting increased uterine irritability predisposes to abortion, miscarriage, or premature delivery. In general, because the acute process often subsides without the development of infarct necrosis, a conservative program of observation and supportive therapy is usually indicated initially in the pregnant patient. Increasing evidence of ischemic necrosis and deterioration of the patient's general condition may ultimately make surgical exploration necessary, however, and the risk that myomectomy may further increase the likelihood of loss of the pregnancy must be accepted. In the nonpregnant patient the process is usually less acute and dramatic, but persistence of symptoms for more than a day or two or a steady increase in their severity is usually sufficient indication for exploration and myomectomy or hysterectomy, depending on the circumstances.

A rare complication is the development of an abscess within a degenerated leiomyoma. Organisms such as the coliforms, streptococci, or anaerobes enter the degenerated fibroid directly from the uterine cavity or via hematogenous or lymphatic spread, producing suppuration and gas formation; the latter is readily demonstrated on a plain abdominal radiograph. If this gas abscess is unrecognized and untreated, rupture into the peritoneal cavity, with resulting generalized peritonitis, or perforation into the bowel or bladder may occur. Occasionally there is spontaneous drainage into the uterine cavity. Although the radiographic picture is fairly characteristic, the possibility of gas formation accompanying either a tuboovarian or a pelvic abscess developing on some other basis (e.g., diverticulitis) must also be considered.

The older literature has suggested that leiomyomas may undergo change to a highly malignant sarcoma. Whether a true sarcomatous change can take place in what was originally a completely benign leiomyoma is a somewhat controversial issue. Obviously, such a malignant transformation is difficult to prove in most instances, although suggestive evidence is at hand in some cases in which a leiomyosarcoma is found growing in a local area within the capsule of what appears grossly to be a simple fibroid, all other areas of which are histologically benign. Circumstantial clinical evidence of the possibility of sudden change in the character of a leiomyoma is also present in some patients who, having been followed for many years with clinically benign "fibroids" that have not increased in size, abruptly show evidence of rapid growth of their tumors, which after excision are found to be leiomyosarcomas. On the other hand, this association of sarcomas and leiomyomas is likely supported coincidentally by the evidence that leiomyomas are frequent whereas sarcomas are rare. Conversely, most sarcomas are not associated with leiomyomas. The simultaneous occurrence of a leiomyoma and sarcoma is reported to be 0.1 to 0.5 percent.

Intravenous Leiomyomatosis and Leiomyomatosis Peritonealis Disseminata

Intravenous leiomyomatosis and leiomyomatosis peritonealis disseminata are benign forms of leiomyomatous tissue spread that may simulate malignancy and thus be erroneously considered manifestations of leiomyosarcoma. Both are rare and usually occur in patients who have ordinary uterine fibroids as well. With intravenous leiomyomatosis, smooth muscle cells enter and grow within vascular spaces and venous channels, sometimes implanting in the vena cava, heart, and lungs. However, the clinical course in these patients is relatively benign and usually prolonged. The microscopic appearance of the leiomyomatous tissue remains benign, with no cellular atypia and few mitotic figures.

Similarly, with leiomyomatosis peritonealis disseminata, a patient who appears to have simple uterine fibroids is found at the time of planned hysterectomy or myomectomy to have numerous intraperitoneal nodules of varying size, superficially resembling implants of metastatic carcinoma and involving omentum as well as visceral and parietal peritoneal surfaces. On close inspection of these nodules, however, even their gross appearance is seen to be that of small, benign leiomyomas, which is confirmed by detailed microscopic examination of both the uterine leiomyomas and the "metastatic implants." In extreme cases the patient may have had signs and symptoms of an advanced malignancy with masses throughout the peritoneal cavity. As with leiomyomas, leiomyomatosis peritonealis disseminata appears to be stimulated by high levels of estrogen, as occurs during pregnancy. All the "metastatic" leiomyomas that are technically easy to remove should be resected and hysterectomy or myomectomy carried out as planned. The patient is unlikely to have any further manifestations of this unusual form of spread of a benign leiomyoma.

Secondary Pathologic Changes in the Fibroid Uterus

The wall of the uterus surrounding a leiomyoma may thin out as a result of the pressure atrophy produced by the enlarging fibroid; or, on the other hand, the myometrium surrounding multiple fibroids may hypertrophy as a result of the stimulus to increased contractility produced by their presence, the result being a large, thick-walled uterus. Endometrial polyps are also commonly found in association with uterine fibroids. The development of polyps may be the result of interference with the blood supply to the endometrium overlying the fibroids, with a consequent disturbance in the endometrial growth pattern, leading to local hyperplastic change and eventual polyp formation. There is good evidence that both endometrial polyp formation and an increased rate of growth of fibroids are often secondary to a relative preponderance of estrogen, so ovarian hormone imbalance may also be a factor in their frequent coexistence.

Symptoms and Clinical Manifestations

Although probably most uterine fibroids remain small and clinically insignificant, symptoms sufficiently severe to require treatment develop in a large number of women with these tumors. Subserosal fibroids, even those attaining considerable size, are most likely to remain asymptomatic, whereas submucosal (intracavitary) and intramural fibroids are more likely to cause difficulty and may do so even when relatively small. The symptomatic manifestations produced by fibroids vary considerably, depending primarily on their size, number, and location. The chief symptoms are described in the sections that follow.

Pain. Approximately one-third of patients with leiomyomas experience pain. Pain is usually crampy in nature and secondary to the presence of submucous and intramural fibroids. Most typically pain occurs at the time of menstruation (dysmenorrhea); less often it occurs intermenstrually. Acute pain may be caused by infarction due to sudden degeneration or torsion of a pedunculated subserosal or intracavity fibroid. The uterus may attempt to expel a pedunculated submucosal fibroid, and symptoms may be similar to the cyclic contractions of normal labor until the fibroid is "delivered" through the cervix.

Pressure Symptoms. Pressure symptoms are due to the enlarging uterine mass and include pressure effects on the bladder (frequency, urgency, incontinence), colon (constipation, rectal pain, difficult defecation), and small bowel (abdominal cramps); there may also be pelvic and lower abdominal discomfort or increased abdominal girth. Pressure on the ureter, usually at the pelvic brim, may lead to obstruction (hydroureter), pyelonephritis, and ultimately chronic renal injury.

Other situations warranting surgical intervention include rapid growth of apparent fibroids (particularly at or after menopause), which may suggest the possibility that a uterine sarcoma or ovarian neoplasm is present, and an inability to differentiate between a lateral fibroid and an ovarian tumor. In the latter instance, laparoscopy may be adequate for diagnosis in patients in whom the fibroids are asymptomatic and who otherwise require no treatment once the possibility of an ovarian tumor is excluded. Leiomyomas may cause dystocia during labor and delivery, especially if located in the cervix or filling the sacral hollow, thus obstructing the birth canal. Delivery by cesarean section is necessary, but myomectomy should be delayed until the increased vascularity of pregnancy has resolved.

Abnormal Bleeding. Abnormal bleeding is reported in 30 percent of patients and takes the form of menorrhagia, with increased amount and duration of flow. It ordinarily occurs only in association with submucous or multiple intramural fibroids. The etiology of this bleeding may be the following.

1. Pressure necrosis and ulceration of the endometrium often with heavy bleeding, an event particularly likely to occur in the presence of submucous fibroids
2. Impaired normal endometrial vascular reactions and hormonal responses by interference with the normal blood supply, particularly in the endometrium directly overlying the fibroids (despite normal ovarian hormonal production and balance)
3. Interference with the normal myometrial contraction about the spiral uterine arterioles, normally an important auxiliary hemostatic mechanism

The increasingly excessive chronic blood loss over the course of months or years often occasioned by the presence of uterine fibroids may not be obvious to the patient, who gradually becomes accustomed to the heavier flow. However, a severe simple iron deficiency anemia frequently develops in this way, and it is not uncommon to find the hemoglobin levels in the range of 4 to 5 gm per deciliter in women whose menorrhagia is due to fibroids.

Irregular menstrual cycles or intermenstrual bleeding are rarely due to the presence of fibroids alone, and some other cause for this type of abnormal menstrual function should be sought, even though fibroids may be present. In fact, it is important to point out that in many patients with abnormal uterine bleeding coexisting fibroids are unrelated to the source of the abnormal flow, which is most often due to hormonal imbalance and occasionally to endometrial hyperplasia or polyps or to carcinoma of the cervix or fundus. Hence before deciding that the bleeding is related to the presence of fibroids, one must take into account their number, size, and location and exclude bleeding from hormonal imbalance or other neoplastic processes.

Infertility. Less often, fibroids may cause infertility due to interference with the normal tuboovarian pickup and transport mechanisms by intramural or multiple large subserosal fibroids, particularly if they are located in the cornual regions. Infertility also may be secondary to abnormal early implantations and habitual abortion in the presence of submucous or multiple intramural fibroids. Obviously, before concluding that a known uterine fibroid is playing a significant role in a couple's failure to conceive, both the wife and husband should undergo a complete infertility investigation to be certain that other, often far more important factors are not overlooked. Only when all other possible causes have been excluded or corrected and pregnancy still fails to occur should myomectomy be considered. When such a thorough preliminary investigation has been done, however, the results following myomectomy in the management of the otherwise normal infertile woman with uterine fibroids are often highly successful and gratifying with respect to subsequent fertility and pregnancies carried to term.

Diagnosis

The clinical diagnosis of leiomyoma(s) usually is based on the findings of a careful abdominal, vaginal, and rectal examination. The clinician often notes an enlarged uterus or a mass that moves with the uterus, most often irregular in shape. Often discreet leiomyomas may be palpated in the pelvis. The uterine size may vary from only a slight, irregular enlargement to a mass filling the entire pelvis and abdomen. It is the larger masses (those extending above the pelvic brim, or of 12 weeks' gestational size) that are difficult to distinguish clinically from other pelvic pathology such as an ovarian neoplasm. It is obviously of great importance to be certain that the lesion in question is indeed simply a fibroid and not an adnexal mass—particularly not an ovarian tumor—even if it is asymptomatic. When symptoms are present, as already emphasized, one must not be too quick to assume that they are due to fibroids, as the latter frequently coexist with other, more significant pelvic disease.

Laparoscopy may be of value in questionable cases, as previously mentioned, for differentiating a laterally situated uterine fibroid from an ovarian mass. Occasionally, the presence of a submucous fibroid can be demonstrated or confirmed by hysterosalpingography or curettage. Frequently, the typical pattern of concentric calcification in older, degenerated fibroids is noted on abdominal radiographs, and the radiographic appearance is usually sufficiently characteristic to be diagnostic of a leiomyoma. Pelvic, ultrasound, computed tomography (CT) scan, or magnetic resonance imaging also may be of value for distinguishing and locating leiomyomas in the uterus.

Treatment

Although surgical removal is the definitive treatment for leiomyomas, in most of these women conservative management is possible. It is wise to evaluate the pelvic findings every six months to avoid any possibility of a mistake in diagnosis and to obtain a general impression of the rate of growth of the fibroids. At these checkups the patient should also be evaluated for new symptoms such as bleeding, pain, or pressure. Because the growth rate of leiomyomas is usually slow, most patients can be carried through to menopause if when originally seen they are asymptomatic or have only minimal symptoms. Growth of a fibroid during menopause is abnormal and warrants immediate surgical intervention. In most cases this growth represents another neoplasm such as a sarcoma or ovarian neoplasm. Mild pain and pressure symptoms may be controlled by intermittent use of analgesics or nonsteroidal antiinflammatory agents. More recently, gonadotropin-releasing hormone (GnRH) analogs have

been found to diminish the size of fibroids; however, when the GnRH is discontinued the fibroids appear to regrow.

If symptoms are sufficient to warrant treatment (removal), whether myomectomy or hysterectomy is done is determined largely by whether the individual circumstances make preservation of childbearing function desirable and important. The general indications of surgical intervention are listed in Table 17-1.

Myomectomy. Myomectomy, the removal of leiomyomas with preservation of the uterus, is invariably possible, regardless of the size, location, or number of fibroids. Large submucous fibroids may require that the uterus be opened (hysterotomy), but the leiomyomas can then be dealt with and removed in the usual manner. A helpful technical maneuver that minimizes blood loss during myomectomy involves local intrauterine injection of vasopressin solution and may be combined with the use of noncrushing clamps or tourniquets to the uterine or ovarian vessels. It is important to resuture the wall of the uterus carefully in layers to obliterate all deadspace and create a strong, solid scar. Properly closed myomectomy incisions in the nonpregnant uterus heal well, and cesarean section is thus not mandatory if the patient subsequently becomes pregnant. The exception is the myomectomy

Table 17-1. Indications for Surgical Removal of Leiomyomas

Persistent abnormal uterine bleeding, especially causing anemia (other pathology has been excluded)
Pain or pressure symptoms not relieved by medical management
Rapidly enlarging pelvic mass
Pelvic mass of more than 12 to 14 weeks' gestational size
Increase in size after menopause
Obstruction or compression of ureter or bowel
Infertility with no other cause
Habitual abortion
Uncontrolled pain in pregnancy
Infection of infarcted necrotic fibroid
Fibroid located in adnexa (usually pedunculated) that cannot be clinically distinguished from an adnexal mass of more severe pathology

that requires entry to the endometrial cavity. In this circumstance, as after classic cesarean section, the risk of uterine rupture during labor is increased; therefore planned cesarean section before the onset of labor is advised.

Undoubtedly, depending largely on the patient's age and the care and completeness with which the fibroids are removed, the recurrence rate after myomectomy (the subsequent development of new leiomyomas) has been in the vicinity of 30 percent in most large reported series, with 10 to 20 percent of these women eventually requiring hysterectomy. However, the subsequent uncomplicated term pregnancy rate following myomectomy has been satisfactory, approaching that for normal women of comparable age. The results in women undergoing myomectomy because of infertility (after a thorough infertility investigation has excluded other significant factors) have been particularly gratifying in many instances, with 40 to 50 percent of the women conceiving successfully. In view of these results, the risk of recurrence, which should be known and accepted by both patient and physician, seems well worth taking in younger women who have been infertile or who desire additional children.

Hysterectomy. In the woman who has completed her family and who has multiple, symptomatic leiomyomas, it is usually wiser to perform a hysterectomy, preserving the ovaries when possible and indicated. Ordinarily, the presence of fibroids poses no special problems during hysterectomy. However, as previously noted, in the case of broad-ligament or cervical fibroids, it is particularly important to bear in mind the course and location of the ureters and bladder, to mobilize the fibroid, and to dissect and display carefully the displaced ureters and uterine vessels before beginning removal of the uterus.

ADENOMYOSIS

Adenomyosis is a condition resulting from the ingrowth and pinching off, within the muscular wall of the uterus, of islands of normal endometrial glands and stroma derived from the endometrial cavity proper.

It has been termed *internal endometriosis;* but as emphasized in Chapter 12, this term should probably be discarded, as the lesion appears to be unrelated in nature and etiology to true or "external" endometriosis, even though the histologic appearances of the two are essentially identical. Adenomyosis and endometriosis are found to coexist in only 20 percent of cases. The endometrial islands of adenomyosis are situated within the myometrium, interspersed between the smooth muscle bundles. They frequently retain a direct anatomic connection, however tortuous and hidden, with the surface endometrium lining the uterine cavity. Thus the pathogenesis of adenomyosis is entirely different from that of endometriosis. This difference in etiology is also reflected in the fact that adenomyosis is essentially a disease of multiparous women in their late thirties and forties, whereas endometriosis is characteristically seen in the young, relatively infertile woman. It therefore seems likely that the myometrial dispersion of islands of normal endometrium found with adenomyosis may be secondary to the traumatic and disruptive effects on the uterine wall produced by repeated pregnancy, delivery, and postpartum involution. A less common causative factor in some cases may be an unduly deep and vigorous curettage. Finally, because adenomyosis is frequently (in 35 to 50 percent of cases) accompanied by varying degrees of cystic and adenomatous hyperplasia of the endometrial islands within the myometrium, it seems possible that a hormone imbalance with a preponderance of estrogen may favor the persistence, growth, and activity of the aberrant endometrial islands within the myometrium. Such an ancillary causative mechanism might also account for the somewhat increased incidence of fibroids, endometrial polyps, and even endometrial carcinoma that has been noted in association with adenomyosis.

Pathologic Features

Grossly, adenomyosis exhibits two forms. Most frequently it consists in a diffuse, uniform involvement of the entire uterine wall, the myometrium presenting a characteristic trabeculated appearance on cut section, with occasional blood-filled cystic spaces also visible. The myometrium itself invariably undergoes hypertrophy, and in most cases the uterus becomes symmetrically enlarged to two to three times normal size. In such cases the underlying pathology may be mistaken clinically as leiomyomas. Less often the process is more focal and produces an adenomyoma, a localized tumor that is clinically indistinguishable from a leiomyoma. However, in either case, the process is in the nature of an infiltration of the surrounding myometrium, and there is no tendency to encapsulation. Thus although a local adenomyoma can be resected, it cannot be "shelled out" like a leiomyoma because no capsule is present. Adenomyosis is most often found in the posterior wall of the fundus, less commonly on the anterior wall, and only infrequently in the cornual or cervical segments. Rarely, a focal adenomyoma may become pedunculated and behave like a submucous fibroid.

From a histologic standpoint, the endometrial tissue in areas of adenomyosis consists of both glands and stroma and is often immature or atrophic. Evidence of normal cyclic changes (occasionally, decidual transformation in the presence of pregnancy) is found in only 25 percent of cases. This situation is likely explained by the finding of low levels of estrogen and progesterone receptors in the adenomyosis tissue compared with those in the coexisting normal endometrium. It also explains why adenomyosis is unsuccessfully treated with hormone manipulation. Hemosiderin deposits within phagocytes are often observed in the myometrium adjacent to areas of adenomyosis. Not infrequently the aberrant endometrial glands show cystic hyperplasia, and occasionally even glandular atypicalities are seen; true malignant change, however, rarely if ever occurs.

This picture is in sharp contrast to the situation encountered with the entity known as *endolymphatic stromal myosis of the uterus,* which cannot properly be considered a variant of adenomyosis despite the fact that it too involves infiltration of the myometrium by endometrial elements (stromal cells unaccompanied by glands). Although this stromatosis of the uterine wall sometimes exhibits a benign microscopic appearance and benign clinical behavior, the evidence suggests that it is a true neoplastic process and that it is most frequently encountered in its highly malignant form (endometrial stromal sarcoma).

Clinical Manifestations and Diagnosis

Although the frequent coexistence of other uterine and pelvic disease and the nonspecific nature of its symptomatology frequently tend to obscure the manifestations of adenomyosis and render a definite preoperative diagnosis difficult, there is a tendency to certain characteristic and progressive symptoms and signs that should enable it to be recognized in many instances. It is a more common disorder than has generally been appreciated, with an estimated incidence in the range of 15 to 25 percent of all women and in up to 60 percent of women 40 to 50 years of age. As already noted, it is encountered more frequently in older women, with a peak incidence during the fifth decade. The patients in whom it is found are invariably multiparas. In many women it remains minimal and asymptomatic and is either never discovered or is detected as an incidental finding in a hysterectomy specimen removed for other reasons.

The classic symptom complex accompanying adenomyosis and the one most often encountered is the following triad: (1) increasing menorrhagia, the menstrual flow becoming both heavier and of longer duration; (2) an acquired type of dysmenorrhea that becomes progressively more severe; and (3) a steadily enlarging uterus that is usually symmetric, firm and globular, and typically tender to palpation, especially around the time of the menses. Occasionally, the uterus is somewhat irregularly nodular to palpation ("nutmeg uterus"), and not infrequently pelvic findings mistakenly suggest the presence of uterine fibroids; in the case of a localized adenomyoma, differentiation from a leiomyoma may be impossible. Other symptoms often present include metrorrhagia, dyspareunia, a sense of pelvic pressure or diffuse pelvic and lower abdominal pain, secondary bladder or bowel irritability, and a "pelvic congestion" type of premenstrual syndrome produced by the appreciable increased vascular supply to the uterus that uniformly develops if the adenomyosis is extensive.

Although the presence of associated disease may

well be responsible for some or all the symptoms in many cases, adenomyosis per se can and does produce this characteristic complex of symptoms and signs in the absence of other lesions. Its presence alone can seriously interfere with the usual endometrial and myometrial hemostatic mechanisms and produce menorrhagia; and the marked distention of the uterine wall honeycombed with the highly vascular, swollen areas of adenomyosis readily accounts for the severe dysmenorrhea, dyspareunia, and painful, tender uterine enlargement.

Treatment

As previously noted, adenomyosis does not cycle with the menstrual cycle and is associated with low numbers of estrogen and progesterone receptors. Hormone therapy with oral contraceptives or cyclic estrogen or progesterone therefore does not alleviate the symptoms. In fact, estrogens given alone during the second half of the menstrual cycle definitely increase the menorrhagia. For the older woman with symptoms severe enough to warrant definitive treatment, total hysterectomy is usually the treatment of choice. Preservation of the ovaries may be considered in young women. Resection of localized areas of adenomyosis with preservation of the uterus, especially in cases of true adenomyoma formation, is often feasible and is occasionally indicated in women in their late twenties or thirties, particularly if they have not yet had all the children they desire.

ENDOMETRIAL HYPERPLASIA

Hyperplasia of the endometrial glands and stroma is most often recognized in the perimenopausal or postmenopausal woman presenting with abnormal uterine bleeding. Hyperplasia usually results from the noncyclic influence of estrogens on the endometrium with inadequate or no progestin withdrawal. This effect may be caused by the prolonged use of unopposed exogenous estrogen therapy for the treatment of menopausal symptoms or the unopposed estrogen stimulation by the anovulatory ovary during the perimenopausal years. Polycystic ovarian disease and

obesity may also lead to higher levels of endogenous estrogen without the normal cyclic progesterone influence, thereby producing hyperplasia in young women. Finally, estrogen-producing tumors (e.g., granulosa theca cell tumors) may lead to abnormal endometrial proliferation.

Endometrial hyperplasia, as previously noted, is usually recognized when the patient presents with abnormal uterine bleeding. There is no typical bleeding pattern associated with endometrial hyperplasias, except that the bleeding is usually not cyclic. In premenopausal women who are anovulatory, this pattern may be characterized by lengthy episodes of amenorrhea (several months) followed by excessively heavy bleeding for many days or weeks. It may also be recognized as intermenstrual spotting or bleeding. Any postmenopausal patient with uterine bleeding may have endometrial hyperplasia. Examination of cytology specimens obtained from the cervix or the endometrial cavity rarely reveals or suggests endometrial hyperplasia. It is therefore imperative that histologic study of the endometrium be performed. The most straightforward and frequently used method to evaluate the endometrium is an outpatient endometrial biopsy, or aspiration biopsy. Should an outpatient biopsy be inconclusive or not easily obtained (e.g., secondary to cervical stenosis or patient intolerance), fractional dilatation and curettage (D&C) under adequate anesthesia must be performed. In most patients, however, outpatient biopsy is adequate to establish a diagnosis of hyperplasia and to exclude the possibility of endometrial cancer.

The classification of endometrial hyperplasias is important in that *atypical adenomatous hyperplasia* carries a modest risk of malignant transformation, whereas other hyperplasias do not. The malignant potential of endometrial hyperplasia has been confused in the past by lack of uniform terminology and has probably led to the aggressive surgical therapy of many patients who did not have a premalignant neoplasm. Most endometrial hyperplasia can be managed medically, and it is important to follow a standard histologic classification. Endometrial hyperplasia therefore should be subdivided into three groups: (1) cystic hyperplasia; (2) adenomatous hyperplasia (simple and complex); and (3) atypical adenomatous hyperplasia. It is the atypical adenomatous hyperplasia that carries significant potential to become an adenocarcinoma of the endometrium if left untreated.

Histologically, *cystic hyperplasia* is characterized by dilated endometrial glands lined by a single layer of columnar epithelium. These dilated glands have a characteristic "Swiss-cheese" microscopic pattern. *Adenomatous hyperplasia,* both simple and complex, is typified by an increased number of endometrial glands crowding each other but maintaining a single layer of columnar epithelium in each gland. The intervening stroma between these glands in the more complex cases may be sparse, but there is no cytologic or nuclear atypia.

Atypical adenomatous hyperplasia takes on an even more complex and more densely crowded glandular pattern, with minimal or no intervening stroma and heaping-up of the glandular epithelium with budding into the gland lumen. The cytologic atypia confirms the diagnosis of atypical adenomatous hyperplasia. No invasion is noted in this situation. The criteria for diagnosis of atypical adenomatous hyperplasia may vary from one pathologist to another, and some pathologists interpret it as a well differentiated adenocarcinoma. In other classifications, the severely atypical adenomatous hyperplasia has been called adenocarcinoma in situ. Squamous metaplasia may be noted within any of the hyperplasias, but it has no clinical significance. Furthermore, hyperplasias may be noted to be focal in the endometrium but more commonly are diffuse. Hyperplasias may also be noted in endometrial polyps.

The malignant potential of the three subtypes of endometrial hyperplasia has been debated over the past several decades. It appears at the present time that in the absence of cellular atypia hyperplasia should not be considered premalignant. Therefore therapy for cystic hyperplasia and adenomatous hyperplasia may be medical in many cases. In long-term follow-up studies of patients diagnosed as having cystic hyperplasia, progression to invasive cancer has been noted infrequently (approximately 1 percent of the time). Adenomatous hyperplasia likewise has an infrequent potential to become invasive, and during long-term follow-up of untreated patients the progression to invasive cancer is noted in approximately 3 percent of the patients. On the other hand, atypical adenomatous hyperplasia appears to be at significant risk of becoming endometrial carcinoma and has been found to progress to invasive adenocarcinoma in approximately 30 percent of patients. In nearly all instances, the adenocarcinoma found after the diagnosis of atypical adenomatous hyperplasia is a well differentiated adenocarcinoma with an excellent prognosis.

The treatment of endometrial hyperplasias should consider the reproductive status of the patient as well as the severity of the hyperplasia. In premenopausal women who have cystic or adenomatous hyperplasia, elimination of the unopposed estrogen stimulation of the endometrium may be sufficient therapy. Cyclic withdrawal of the endometrium with progestins reverts the hyperplastic endometrium to a benign-appearing resting endometrium more than 90 percent of the time. If the unopposed estrogen cannot be eliminated (as in patients with morbid obesity), continued cycling with progestins may be necessary to keep the endometrium from reverting back to a hyperplastic pattern. On the other hand, patients in whom high levels of unopposed estrogen are eliminated (after removal of a granulosa cell tumor or resolution of polycystic ovarian disease) may not require lifelong progestins.

In general, atypical adenomatous hyperplasia should be treated by total hysterectomy. The exception to this admonition is the young patient who desires fertility or the older patient who is medically unsuited to undergo a major surgical procedure. In the young patient who wishes to become pregnant, the endometrium should be withdrawn using oral progestins followed by the pursuance of cyclic ovulation induction. In the older, medically inoperable patient, progestin therapy may be used in a cyclic fashion with expectant follow-up by serial biopsies of the endometrium to confirm that the hyperplasia has been eliminated. Progestin therapy in patients with atypical adenomatous hyperplasia may be successful in causing regression of the disease in more than half of these patients. Nonetheless, the patients remain at high risk for recurrence of atypical adenomatous hyperplasia or cancer. There-

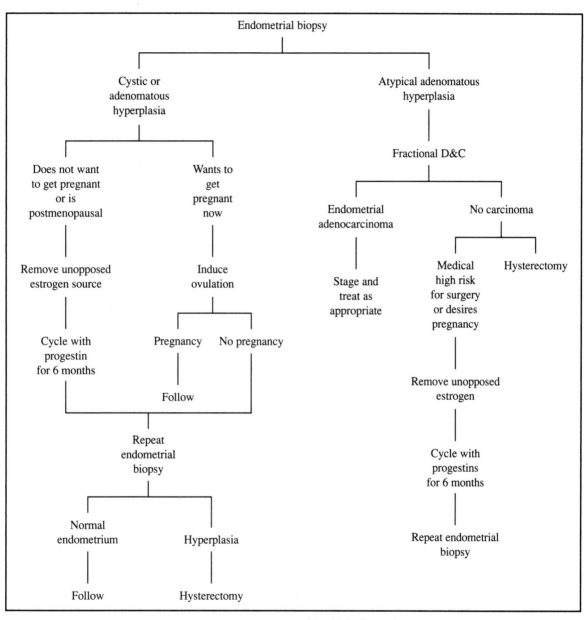

Fig. 17-3. General management plan for endometrial hyperplasias.

fore, if there is no contraindication to surgical therapy, hysterectomy is advisable in this setting. A general management schema for the evaluation and treatment of patients with endometrial hyperplasia is shown in Figure 17-3.

POLYPS

The frequently encountered *endometrial polyp*, together with the common *cervical* and *endocervical polyps* discussed in Chapter 14, make up another large group of benign uterine tumors. Whereas cervical polyps usually arise on an inflammatory basis in connection with chronic cervicitis, endometrial polyps must often develop in association with endometrial hyperplasia, each being due to a hormonal imbalance. Prolonged stimulation by estrogen in relative excess leads to diffuse cystic or adenomatous endometrial hyperplasia as well as to focal areas of gross mucosal hypertrophy that ultimately become polypoid in structure. Although they may occur at any age, endometrial polyps are most commonly seen in premenopausal or postmenopausal women, at a time when ovarian endocrine dysfunction is also almost universal. Endometrial polyps occur in approximately 10 percent of women and are usually asymptomatic. When symptomatic, their principle manifestation is intermenstrual or postmenopausal bleeding. Polyps range in size from a few millimeters to several centimeters. Large polyps may dilate the cervix and protrude into the vagina. Although they may be seen by hysteroscopy or hysterosalpingography, D&C is required for definite diagnosis. Diagnostic curettage is also indicated to rule out the possibility of cancer of the fundus or endocervix. When polyps are found, they are readily removed by a combination of curettage and careful exploration of the uterine cavity with curved polyp forceps.

Malignant change in an endometrial polyp (adenocarcinoma) is rare, and when it does occur it is usually superficial and of low histologic grade. Malignant mixed müllerian tumors may also appear grossly as an endometrial polyp (Chap. 27). Histologically, an endometrial polyp is composed of a vascular core covered by endometrium and endometrial stroma. The endometrium may be hyperplastic (usually cystic) and may be ulcerated at the tip. Treatment of polyps is surgical removal (D&C). Polyps rarely respond to hormonal therapy.

One additional type of benign polypoid lesion is the so-called *placental polyp*. Here again, a localized area of mucosal proliferation and heaping-up of a somewhat hyperplastic endometrial lining takes place about a fragment of retained decidual tissue, the constant uterine contractions about the area gradually leading to polypoid transformation. Except for the fact that it follows pregnancy and hence occurs in a relatively younger age group, the symptoms are essentially identical with those produced by a simple endometrial polyp; it should be noted, however, that the interval between the antecedent pregnancy and the appearance of a symptomatic placental polyp may be lengthy, sometimes amounting to several years.

PYOMETRA

A pyometra is defined as the development of a collection of "pus" (sterile in 40 to 50 percent of cases) within the cavity of the uterine fundus as a result of interference with the normal dependent drainage of the uterus. Invariably, the obstruction occurs within the cervical canal (usually within the endocervix), but it occasionally is secondary to obliteration of the external os. Although carcinoma of the cervix or endometrium is sometimes the cause of the condition (in 15 to 20 percent of cases), benign cervical stenosis due to atrophic changes similar to those affecting the vagina postmenopausally or to old inflammatory changes or old obstetric trauma with secondary scarring and fibrosis is a more common cause, accounting for roughly 40 percent of cases. Prior irradiation for cervical cancer and previous cervical surgical procedures (including D&C, cauterization, and cone biopsy) are other frequent causes and account for the remaining 40 percent of cases.

Pyometra usually occurs in postmenopausal women, with a peak incidence in the age range 55 to 70. The most common presenting symptom is an abnormal vaginal discharge, usually yellowish-brown, or vaginal bleeding; less often, the patient complains of lower abdominal pain due to the uncomfortable uterine distention from backed-up secretions and old blood. Roughly one-fourth of patients are asymptomatic, although an enlarged, soft, "cystic-feeling" uterus is noted on routine pelvic examination. Pelvic ultrasound or CT scan may be helpful for determining the nature of such a pelvic mass. It is rare for the condition to be associated with fever, leukocytosis, or other signs or symptoms of a true infection.

A pyometra should be managed by careful cervical dilatation and then meticulous fractional curettage of the endometrial cavity and endocervix to confirm or rule out the possibility of cervical or endometrial carcinoma. (Occasionally, the curettage must be delayed until the cavity has been allowed to drain for a week or two, permitting the uterine wall to involute and regain its normal thickness.) If either cervical or endometrial cancer is detected, drainage of the uterine fundus for several weeks with a rubber T-tube (such as that employed for drainage of the common bile duct) anchored by a suture to the cervix is indicated before radiotherapy is begun or radical surgery contemplated. If only a benign stricture is present, simple T-tube drainage for one month after completion of the D&C should suffice to correct the condition, with follow-up cervical dilations in the office as indicated. Postoperative antibiotics are usually not necessary unless there is some suspicion that uterine perforation has occurred during the procedure.

MISCELLANEOUS BENIGN UTERINE DISORDERS

Fibromas and Cysts

Fibromas, or true benign connective-tissue tumors, occasionally arise in the wall of the fundus or cervix, but they are relatively rare in comparison with the ubiquitous leiomyoma. Cystic lesions of the uterus are also uncommon; most are pseudocysts that result from areas of degeneration and cystic change within what were originally leiomyomas or adenomyomas. However, in rare instances, a true cyst, congenital in origin and derived from mesonephric duct remnants or cell rests, may be encountered. (These lesions are thus related in nature and etiology to parovarian cysts and to Gartner's duct cysts of the vagina.)

Idiopathic Uterine Hypertrophy

An entity termed idiopathic uterine hypertrophy, myometrial hypertrophy, or diffuse myometrial sclerosis (also sometimes called fibrosis uteri or chronic sub-

involution) is occasionally encountered. The uterus is symmetrically enlarged, and the patient is prone to excessive bleeding for which there is often no other explanation, as the process is frequently unaccompanied by any other pathologic process in the uterus or ovaries. The patient is invariably a multipara and frequently complains of dysmenorrhea, low backache, and a constant sense of pelvic pressure. Thus symptomatically and on pelvic examination, myometrial hypertrophy may simulate either adenomyosis or a solitary, large, centrally located submucous or intramural fibroid.

The uterine enlargement and considerably thickened uterine wall are due in part to hypertrophy of smooth muscle fibers, which in turn may be secondary to progressively increasing subinvolution of the uterus after multiple pregnancies. There is also a marked increase in the amount of fibrous tissue between the smooth muscle fibers, which is most responsible for the sometimes dramatic increase in the volume of the uterine fundus. The tendency to excessive bleeding may well be the result of impaired myometrial contractility at the time of the menstrual flow. However, in many patients there is associated uterine disease (leiomyomas or adenomyosis), which could equally well be the cause of the pain and excessive flow.

Most of the hypertrophied uteri are either asymptomatic or cause minimal difficulty. However, when symptoms are severe and menorrhagia is marked, hysterectomy may be required for relief.

SELECTED READINGS

Berkeley, A. S. Abdominal myomectomy and subsequent fertility. *Surg. Gynecol. Obstet.* 156:319, 1983.

Buttram, V. C., Jr. Uterine leiomyomata: etiology, symptomatology, and management. *Fertil. Steril.* 36:433, 1981.

Coulam, C. B., Annegers, J. F., and Kranz, J. S. Chronic anovulation syndrome and associated neoplasia. *Obstet. Gynecol.* 61:403, 1983.

Filicori, M. A conservative approach to the management of uterine leiomyomata: pituitary desensitization by a luteinizing hormone releasing hormone analogue. *Am. J. Obstet. Gynecol.* 147:726, 1983.

Fox, H. The endometrial hyperplasias. *Obstet. Gynecol. Annu.* 13:197, 1984.

Gal, D. Long-term effect of megestrol acetate in the treatment of endometrial hyperplasia. *Am. J. Obstet. Gynecol.* 146:316, 1983.

Gross, B. H. Sonographic features of leiomyomas: analysis of 41 proven cases. *J. Ultrasound. Med.* 2:401, 1983.

Koss, L. G. Detection of endometrial carcinoma and hyperplasia in asymptomatic women. *Obstet. Gynecol.* 64:1, 1984.

Kurman, R. J., Kaminski, P. T., and Norris, H. J. The behavior of endometrial hyperplasia: a long-term study of "untreated" hyperplasia in 170 patients. *Cancer* 56:403, 1985.

Tada, S. Computed tomographic features of uterine myoma. *J. Comput. Assist. Tomogr.* 5:866, 1981.

Winer-Muram, H. T. Uterine myomas in pregnancy. *Can. Med. Assoc. J.* 128:949, 1983.

18

Evaluation of Pelvic Masses and Management of Benign Neoplasms of the Ovaries and Fallopian Tubes

The discovery of a pelvic mass in a woman, no matter what the age, confronts the gynecologist with many challenges during evaluation and treatment. Any mass raises the specter of possible malignancy and the need for extensive surgery. Most masses, however, are benign; and some do not require surgery at all. With the myriad possible diagnoses and the variety of surgical procedures that might be used for definitive treatment, it is imperative that the patient be fully evaluated with due consideration of all possibilities prior to suggesting recommendations for therapy.

When developing a differential diagnosis, the gynecologist not only must focus on the reproductive system but should consider all organs in the pelvis that might create a mass. Therefore the differential diagnosis of a pelvic mass must include the gastrointestinal and genitourinary systems, as well as neoplasms arising in the retroperitoneal space from lymphatics, blood vessels, bone, and neural tissue. In most cases the differential diagnosis can be narrowed considerably by careful history and astute physical examination. Thereafter, the selection of laboratory and radiographic tests might be narrowed to a few studies that should clarify the clinician's impression. Although this process requires careful thought and clinical skills, it should not be a lengthy procedure requiring weeks of studies. The clinician who must obtain every test and radiograph in the book clearly is throwing clinical judgment and acumen to the wind and thereby does a disservice to the patient, especially when it means that definitive treatment is unduly delayed.

EVALUATION OF THE PELVIC MASS

Once a mass is discovered or suspected, initial evaluation should proceed with a complete history and physical examination.

Symptoms

Although symptoms are not specifically diagnostic, they may be of significance for pointing the clinician to particular questions or laboratory investigations and may provide a strong clue about the etiology of the mass. One of the current problems in the treatment of ovarian cancer is the delay in diagnosis, which is partly due to the fact that the disease is relatively *asymptomatic*. Other benign pelvic masses may also be asymptomatic for long periods and be discovered only on routine gynecologic examination.

Pain is a frequent presenting symptom of a pelvic mass. The pain may be described as acute in onset and severe, suggesting an accident such as ovarian torsion, infarction, or hemorrhage. Cyclic, premenstrual and menstrual pain, on the other hand, that is chronic in nature is more likely to suggest endometriosis or adenomyosis. Chronic pelvic pain with acute exacerbations may raise a suspicion of chronic pelvic inflammatory disease.

Another common presenting symptom is *pelvic pressure*. It is often surprising, however, to find a mass extending above the umbilicus and filling the entire pelvis that creates minimal signs and symptoms of pressure on the adjacent gastrointestinal or genitourinary tract. Nonetheless, because the pelvis is a closed space laterally, pressure symptoms as the mass reaches the pelvic brim or impinges on the bladder or rectum are infrequently reported.

Pressure or invasion of the gastrointestinal tract may cause other problems, such as nausea and vomiting, diarrhea, constipation, blood or pus in the stool, rectal pain, or abdominal distention. These *gastrointestinal symptoms* may be secondary to extrinsic involvement of the gastrointestinal tract or may represent primary gastrointestinal disease. One must recall, for example, that colorectal carcinoma is significantly more frequent than ovarian carcinoma in women in the United States.

Genitourinary tract symptoms may also be a presenting or coexisting complaint. Most frequently noted is pressure on the bladder, causing urinary frequency and nocturia. Partial or complete obstruction of the ureter may cause flank pain and pyelonephritis secondary to urinary stasis. Again, genitourinary tract symptoms may be due to extrinsic compression or involvement of a nongenitourinary tract tumor, or they may represent a primary neoplasm of the urologic system such as a pelvic kidney.

Vaginal bleeding may be an early symptom of a pelvic mass, although it raises many other possibilities as well, including disorders of pregnancy, carcinoma of the vagina, cervix, uterus, or ovary, or other uterine neoplasms such as a leiomyoma.

Although none of these symptoms is necessarily specific, and many may be vague in nature, the patient should be questioned about them even when they are not voluntarily presented.

Medical History

The age of the patient should be considered when evaluating the pelvic mass. Logically there are three groups of women: those in childhood and early adolescence who are premenarchal; women during their menstrual and reproductive years; and postmenopausal women. Certain causes of pelvic masses are more likely or less likely to occur in a particular age group. For example, colonic carcinoma is unlikely to be the cause of a pelvic mass in a child or a woman younger than age 30. On the other hand, functional ovarian cysts are frequent in the menstrual age group but unheard of in the premenarchal or postmenopausal woman. Consideration of the patient's age combined with physical examination findings and symptoms often assists in eliminating several possibilities from the differential diagnosis and focuses the laboratory and radiographic investigations more appropriately.

The patient's medical history may point to possible causes of the pelvic mass. A complete *gynecologic history* should be obtained including inquiry as to menstrual history, age at menarche, and recent menstrual periods. A seven-year-old who has had vaginal bleeding may likely have an ovarian tumor stimulating the endometrium prematurely. Pregnancy also may be mistaken as a pelvic mass, or the pelvic mass may be secondary to an ectopic pregnancy, which might be suggested by an aberration of recent menstrual periods in the woman of reproductive age.

The contraceptive history should be complete. It is especially helpful for determining if a moderate-size adnexal cyst is due to corpus luteum, which might be expected to resolve spontaneously. For example, a woman taking oral contraceptives correctly should not develop a corpus luteum cyst; and therefore a delay in further investigation of this patient and definitive therapy is inappropriate.

A history of pelvic inflammatory disease might increase the likelihood of the adnexal mass being a tuboovarian abscess, hydrosalpinx, or pyosalpinx. A history of uterine leiomyoma(s) or of a benign ovarian neoplasm may increase the likelihood of either of these processes recurring. The patient with a history of a dermoid cyst or an ectopic pregnancy is known to carry a 10 to 15 percent chance of recurrence of these processes in the contralateral ovary or fallopian tube, respectively.

Other organ systems should be reviewed for significant history. In the *gastrointestinal system,* a history of Crohn's disease (regional enteritis), ulcerative colitis, or colonic carcinoma should be sought. Likewise, a history of diverticulitis or symptoms of appendicitis should be carefully reviewed. With a definite history of any of these conditions a recurrence of these problems should be strongly considered and appropriate further tests performed to include or exclude these processes in the differential diagnosis. Obviously, a history of appendectomy reasonably excludes the possibility of an appendiceal abscess as the cause of a patient's right pelvic mass with associated fever and leukocytosis.

In a similar fashion, the *urologic system* history should be reviewed for the possibility of known urologic disease such as a pelvic kidney or ureterocele. Spinal cord injuries and other conditions causing neurogenic bladder (including the history of radical hysterectomy or posterior exenteration) may explain the pelvic mass that resolves when the urinary bladder is catheterized.

A history of treatment for some carcinomas may increase the possibility that the adnexal mass is a metastasis (recurrence) to the ovary. Carcinomas known to metastasize with some frequency to the ovary include colon cancer, breast cancer, endometrial carcinoma, and gastric carcinoma. A history of abdominal and pelvic surgery should be sought, as further clues may be obtained regarding preexisting conditions that may cause new onset of a pelvic mass.

Physical Examination

Physical examination often improves the diagnostic accuracy and eliminates a significant number of problems from the differential diagnosis. A thorough and complete physical examination should be performed in all patients with a pelvic mass, searching for abnormalities not confined to the pelvis.

Palpation of *lymph nodes,* including supraclavicular, axillary, and inguinal nodes, may identify significant adenopathy and suggest the possibility of large pelvic sidewall nodes as the source of a pelvic mass more consistent with lymphoma or Hodgkin's disease. Adenopathy might also suggest widespread metastases from other carcinomas.

Examination of the *chest* may reveal a pleural effusion that may be either malignant or benign (Meigs' syndrome). Diagnostic thoracentesis may assist in the further evaluation of this particular patient.

Breast examinations, searching for a mass, or recognizing a patient who previously had breast cancer surgery may raise the specter of recurrence in the pelvis. On the other hand, it is highly unlikely that an occult breast carcinoma that cannot be detected on breast examination would present as a metastasis in the ovary.

A thorough examination of the *abdomen* may be helpful for determining the character of the mass and any other related abnormalities. Prior to abdominal and pelvic examination, the bladder and rectum should be emptied so the examiner does not confuse an overdistended bladder or colonic contents with an intraabdominal or pelvic mass. Observation and palpation should seek to determine the size of normal organs (liver and spleen) as well as any indication of an

omental "cake." Ascites should be sought by percussion, looking for shifting dullness or a fluid wave. Most masses in a normal-size person are palpated above the pubis if they reach 12 weeks' gestational size or more. Other factors to consider include bowel sounds and evidence of hyperactivity, tenderness to palpation, and local or diffuse rebound tenderness. Palpation of a mass in the periumbilical region may be suggestive of a "Sister Mary–Joseph nodule," seen when carcinoma metastasizes to the lymphatics in the periumbilical region.

Thorough *pelvic examination,* as described in Chapter 1, should be performed in all patients with a known or suspected pelvic mass. Particular attention should be given to the identification of any other lesion in the vulva, vagina, or cervix that might represent a primary or metastatic site of malignancy. Mobility of the cervix and tenderness to cervical motion should be noted, as it is suggestive of pelvic inflammatory disease. The size and consistency of the cervix might suggest an endocervical carcinoma. Palpation of the uterus should determine its size and location and if it is separated from the mass. The examiner must always consider that the pelvic mass might be an enlarged uterus or a pedunculated fibroid arising from the uterus, but feeling separate on clinical examination. The size and consistency of the mass may be described as doughy, cystic, solid, or nodular. Its mobility should be noted when bimanual examination is performed.

Rectovaginal examination should search for extension of the mass into the rectum or cul-de-sac and nodularity in the cul-de-sac or uterosacral ligaments. The stool should be checked for occult blood.

The complex of physical examination findings often leads the clinician to correctly rank order a differential diagnosis. For example, a patient with an epigastric mass, ascites, and a nodular pelvic mass most likely has an ovarian neoplasm. On the other hand, a 30-year-old woman with dysmenorrhea, dyspareunia, and a somewhat tender mass with nodularity of the uterosacral ligaments most likely has advanced endometriosis. A smooth cystic mass that is mobile and often anterior to the uterus in a 30-year-old woman is often found to be a dermoid cyst.

Laboratory Evaluation

After the history and physical examination, selective use of laboratory evaluation may further define the nature of the mass and direct appropriate therapy. The use of laboratory tests, however, should be selective and based on sound clinical judgment. The "shotgun" approach—obtaining every potential test listed in this section—is condemned as unnecessary health care expenditure and points to the physician's lack of clinical experience and judgment. In many instances, surgical intervention is required for ultimate diagnosis and treatment, and so to delay surgery for days or weeks of testing is usually unnecessary.

The first temptation of many clinicians is to perform some sort of imaging of the pelvic mass. Technology available today includes abdominal radiography, ultrasonography, computed tomography (CT scanning), and magnetic resonance imaging (MRI). In most instances, the performance of one or more of these tests is of little ultimate value. In menopausal women or in children (with the exception of a follicular cyst of the newborn) all ovarian masses are abnormal and should be removed surgically for histologic diagnosis and treatment. Therefore to perform radiographic imaging in these two age groups to determine whether the mass is solid or cystic or associated with ascites or upper abdominal metastases or masses is rarely of assistance.

In the menstrual age woman with a mass of less than 8 cm, it is possible that the mass is a functional cyst that will resolve spontaneously. If the pelvic examination is equivocal or the nature (solid or cystic) of the mass cannot be determined, ultrasound might be helpful. If a solid mass is found despite the fact that it is less than 8 cm, surgery should be expedited. On the other hand, if the mass is a simple uncomplicated cyst (no septa or solid areas), the presumptive diagnosis of a functional cyst might be made, and conservative management with observation over a period of six weeks can certainly be considered. If the origin of the mass is not clear (i.e., it might be arising from the uterus, colon, urologic system, or retroperitoneal space in the pelvis), imaging might assist when planning surgery and having the appropriate

surgical consultation available in the operating room.

For distinguishing a uterine from an adnexal mass, ultrasonography, a CT scan, or MRI is often helpful. However, an ovarian neoplasm (especially if it is solid) that is adherent to the uterus may be mistaken as a uterine neoplasm by the radiologist.

Search for a gastrointestinal cause of the mass should be carried out especially if the patient has gastrointestinal symptoms or a history of them. Barium enema and upper gastrointestinal series are the most helpful tests in this regard and may be augmented by proctosigmoidoscopy or colonoscopy.

Involvement of the urologic system by a pelvic mass or the urologic system as the cause of the pelvic mass should be considered. CT scan with contrast or an intravenous urogram is often the most helpful test in this regard. The exclusion of a pelvic or a horseshoe kidney (although rare) should be considered. Probably more importantly, the pelvic mass may involve the urologic system, especially the distal ureter, which may be obstructed by extrinsic compression or encroached on by a neoplasm invading the retroperitoneal space. The course of the ureter and exclusion of a duplicate or an absent ureter should be considered prior to undertaking pelvic surgery. This condition is best identified with an intravenous urogram. More specific bladder symptoms or an abnormal urinalysis might prompt investigation with cystoscopy.

Blood work obtained during the evaluation of a pelvic mass should also be selective. Overall, blood laboratory tests are often of limited value when evaluating the pelvic mass. On the other hand, many laboratory tests are part of the standard medical evaluation of patients prior to undertaking major surgery. Such tests are helpful only for the diagnosis of pelvic neoplasms, which may produce a particular hormone or antigen that might be detected in the serum. Germ cell tumors of the ovary (usually occurring in children and young women) may produce human chorionic gonadotropin (hCG) or α-fetoprotein or lactate dehydrogenase (LDH). Therefore patients with an adnexal mass in the age group where one might consider germ cell ovarian tumors as a reasonable possibility should undergo these tests preoperatively.

More recently, serum antigens have been detected

and associated with epithelial ovarian carcinoma. One antigen, CA-125, appears to be present in the serum of approximately 80 percent of patients with epithelial ovarian carcinoma. The CA-125 level is also elevated in some patients with benign gynecologic disease (e.g., endometriosis, pelvic inflammatory disease, and leiomyoma uteri) as well as in those with other nongynecologic malignancies. Therefore the serum CA-125 assay is not absolutely sensitive or specific for the detection and diagnosis of epithelial ovarian carcinoma.

Carcinoembryonic antigen (CEA) is often present in the serum of patients with recurrent metastatic colorectal carcinoma. Therefore, if a patient has a history of colorectal cancer, the CEA assay should be done if a pelvic mass is detected.

Abnormal liver function tests might suggest liver metastases and should be done in patients in whom a malignancy is suspected. Patients with possible pelvic inflammatory disease should have a white blood cell count obtained. As mentioned, many other blood tests including complete blood count, renal function and liver function tests, and serum chemistries are usually performed in patients prior to undertaking surgery but are reasonably nonspecific in terms of pointing to a diagnosis or the etiology of the pelvic mass.

A chest radiograph is usually obtained preoperatively but is of little assistance in the diagnosis of a pelvic mass. Nonetheless, if one finds evidence of pulmonary metastases or a pleural effusion, the surgical approach or technique might be altered by such information. One must always remember that in the patient with ascites and pleural effusion, Meigs' syndrome may be the etiology (see later in this chapter).

A flat plate radiograph of the abdomen may strongly suggest the presence of a dermoid cyst, especially if teeth or a portion of bone is located in the region of the pelvic mass. Other microcalcifications might suggest psammoma bodies. These calcified areas in an ovarian neoplasm are not necessarily associated with malignancy.

Differential Diagnosis

After the history, physical examination, and selective laboratory work, the physician should develop a dif-

Table 18-1. Common Nongynecologic Causes of a Pelvic Mass

Bowel
    Sigmoid or cecum filled with stool or gas
    Diverticulitis abscess
    Regional enteritis (Crohn's disease)
    Colon cancer
    Appendicitis abscess
Urinary tract
    Distended bladder
    Horseshoe kidney
    Wilms' tumor
    Pelvic kidney
    Ureterocele
Other retroperitoneal structures
    Retroperitoneal sarcoma
    Lymphoma–Hodgkin's disease
    Retroperitoneal fibrosis
    Anterior sacral meningocele

ferential diagnosis of the pelvic mass to expedite appropriate management. For the purposes of discussion of this gynecologic textbook, we do not delve into the nongynecologic causes of a pelvic mass at length. Nonetheless, the astute physician should always consider the possibility of gastrointestinal, urologic, and retroperitoneal sources as the cause of a pelvic mass. These masses are usually outside the purview or surgical training of the gynecologist and should be referred to the proper surgeon or clinician for definitive treatment. The differential diagnoses of nongynecologic pelvic masses are listed in Table 18-1 and are often suggested by the complete history and physical examination.

The true adnexal mass is any mass arising in the adnexal structures adjacent to the uterus: fallopian tube, ovary, mesosalpinx, round ligament, and broad ligament. The exact location of an adnexal mass is difficult to determine on clinical examination or radiographic studies. Therefore any mass arising in the adnexal region detected by pelvic examination must be considered to have arisen from any one or more of these structures. The most common adnexal masses are ovarian neoplasms and functional cysts, followed in frequency by tubal and paratubal cysts or neoplasms and then the rare tumors of the broad ligament or round ligament. On occasion, a pedunculated uterine myoma is mistaken clinically and radiographically as an adnexal mass (Chap. 17).

Ovarian neoplasms may arise from any of the tissues in the ovary, and it is therefore useful to consider these tissues in order to understand the breadth and variation of ovarian neoplasms. Most ovarian tissue can produce both benign and malignant neoplasms from the same cell type. For purposes of convenient classification, ovarian neoplasms may be divided according to their cell line of origin: epithelial neoplasms, neoplasms arising from germ cells, neoplasms of stromal and sex cord origin, and malignancies metastatic to the ovary. Of critical importance in the differential diagnosis of an ovarian neoplasm is the age of the patient. The female reproductive years may be conveniently divided into (1) children and adolescents, (2) menstrual-age women, and (3) postmenopausal women. Almost any neoplasm may arise in any age group, although certain lesions are seen most commonly at a particular age (Table 18-2).

The remainder of this chapter discusses the benign neoplasms of the adnexa. Malignancies of the ovary and fallopian tube are discussed in Chapter 28.

BENIGN OVARIAN CYSTS AND NEOPLASMS

Physiologic Ovarian Cysts

In the menstrual age group of women, physiologic ovarian cysts are the adnexal masses most often detected. In most cases the cysts resolve spontaneously and do not require surgical intervention or more than conservative management. The two most common cysts that arise in this age group of women are the follicle cyst and the corpus luteum cyst. Both are normal components of the ovarian cycle and occur each month on a subclinical basis. On occasion, however, these cysts enlarge enough to cause symptoms or be detected on bimanual pelvic examination.

The normal follicle, prior to ovulation, usually is less than 3 cm in diameter. Enlargement of this follicle, for whatever reason, to more than 3 cm may lead to its detection on pelvic examination. Enlarged *follicle cysts* are usually asymptomatic but may be associated with menstrual irregularity. Pain from torsion of the cyst or dyspareunia may also be reported. Should the cyst rupture, intraperitoneal bleeding may cause increasing pain or some abdominal distention, although it is rarely serious. In general, follicle cysts

Table 18-2. Most Common Ovarian Neoplasms in Different Age Groups

Age	Benign	Malignant
Infancy and childhood	Cystic teratoma (dermoid) Serous cystadenoma Follicle cyst	Dysgerminoma
Menstrual/reproductive years	Follicle cyst/corpus luteum Serous cystadenoma Cystic teratoma (dermoid) Mucinous cystadenoma Fibroma-thecoma	Epithelial ovarian carcinoma Germ cell tumors
Postmenopausal years	Serous cystadenoma Cystic teratoma (dermoid) Mucinous cystadenoma Fibroma-thecoma	Epithelial ovarian carcinoma Stromal-sex cord tumors

are less than 8 cm in diameter and are relatively asymptomatic. The recognition on clinical examination of such a cyst requires appropriate clinical judgment and management. Because they are physiologic cysts, most resolve with time. Management of these cysts requires reassuring the patient and repeat evaluation after a menstrual cycle. Most of the cysts resolve within four to six weeks of recognition and require no therapy. The cyst that persists after four to six weeks of observation, that enlarges, or that is initially larger than 8 cm requires more definitive diagnosis by surgical removal and histologic evaluation.

Corpus luteum cysts are likewise physiologic cysts but are less common than follicle cysts. In contrast to the frequently asymptomatic follicle cyst, corpus luteum cysts are often associated with pain, delayed menses, or intermenstrual spotting. Because of these symptoms and an associated adnexal mass, the differential diagnosis of threatened abortion (Chap. 16) or ectopic pregnancy is frequently entertained. Both of these complications of pregnancy can usually be excluded by performing a serum hCG assay. Like follicle cysts, corpus luteum cysts are almost always unilateral and mobile, and are seldom larger than 10 cm in diameter. Cysts less than 8 cm in diameter should be managed similarly to follicle cysts, with conservative observation for four to six weeks. Cysts larger than 8 cm or those that do not resolve require surgical intervention. Some investigators have suggested that in patients in whom a functional ovarian cyst is considered a one- to two-month course of oral contraceptives might aid in the differential diagnosis. It is suggested that oral contraceptives eliminate the gonadotropins that stimulate the ovary, thereby allowing regression of a physiologic cyst. The cyst, however, usually regresses without the need for oral contraceptive suppression. Furthermore, should the cyst not resolve, the use of oral contraceptives increases the patient risk for surgical complications.

Another benign ovarian mass is the slightly enlarged ovary, often associated with *polycystic ovarian disease* (Chap. 13). These ovaries may reach two to three times normal size and are usually suspected in the clinical constellation of a patient with polycystic ovarian disease. Surgical intervention for the diagnosis or management of the slightly enlarged polycystic ovary is not necessary.

Theca Lutein Cysts

Theca lutein cysts are physiologic cysts arising secondary to high hCG levels. These high levels of hCG, especially associated with hydatidiform mole and gestational trophoblastic disease (but sometimes seen with normal or complicated pregnancies), lead to excessive luteinization of the ovarian stroma. Additionally, use of gonadotropins or clomiphene citrate for the treatment of infertility may cause similar cysts. The cysts are most often bilateral and may achieve a size of up to 25 cm in diameter. Maternal virilization has been recognized in some patients with theca lutein cysts, although fetal virilization is not generally noted.

Because the cysts are responsive to hCG, evacuation of the hydatidiform mole leads to reduction in the size of the cyst, which ultimately regresses to a normal-sized ovary. It is perfectly safe and advisable to simply follow a patient who has a theca lutein cyst rather than submit her to surgical exploration and removal of the cyst. Although the cyst may undergo torsion, rupture, or hemorrhage, which would require surgical intervention for an acute abdomen, in most patients the cyst regresses spontaneously.

Pregnancy Luteoma

Another physiologic ovarian mass associated with pregnancy is the pregnancy luteoma. In contrast to the theca lutein cyst, pregnancy luteomas are usually solid, nodular masses that are often not recognized unless the patient is studied by ultrasonography or the mass is discovered at the time of cesarean section. The pregnancy luteoma is often bilateral and multinodular, and it may achieve a size of 20 cm. Histologically, ovarian lutein cells display nodular hyperplasia. Virilization of the mother is noted in 10 to 15 percent of cases, and virilization of the female fetus may be noted in 50 percent of newborns. Because the mass is solid and multinodular, concern about some other solid ovarian neoplasm is usually entertained, and therefore excision of a single nodule for histologic evaluation is recommended. However, complete excision or oophorectomy is not recommended and, in fact, is contraindicated as the luteoma will regress postpartum.

Hyperthecosis

Hyperthecosis is usually noted and found in women in the menstrual age group. In many ways, it is similar to the ovary of polycystic ovarian disease in that the ovary is usually two to three times normal size and multicystic. Hyperplasia of the ovarian stroma leads to excessive androgen production, and virilization of the patient is often more extreme than that noted with polycystic ovarian disease. The serum testosterone level here is usually higher than that noted with polycystic ovarian disease. The use of clomiphene citrate for ovulation induction in patients with hyperthecosis is reported to be less successful than in women with polycystic ovaries, and this condition seems to be more resistant than polycystic ovarian disease to medical management in general. Ultimately, bilateral salpingo-oophorectomy may be necessary to control androgen excess.

Massive Ovarian Edema

Massive ovarian edema is most often found in women in their early twenties. The etiology of the edema is unclear, although it is thought to be associated with intermittent ovarian torsion leading to vascular occlusion and subsequent edema. The most frequent presenting symptom of massive ovarian edema is lower abdominal pain, but there may also be menstrual aberrations. Androgen excess noted clinically is found in approximately 10 percent of the patients. Because the diagnosis of ovarian edema is difficult to establish clinically, and because it is often associated with significant pain due to torsion, exploratory surgery is usually required. At exploratory laparotomy, 50 percent of patients have torsion of the ovary that may require oophorectomy. The ovary is usually moderately enlarged (8 to 10 cm); and because of its soft consistency does not resemble other physiologic tumors. In addition, a conclusive diagnosis of massive ovarian edema on frozen section is difficult. Nonetheless, this

rare diagnosis should be entertained in the differential diagnosis of a patient in this age group so that oophorectomy is not performed unnecessarily. In fact, ascites and hydrothorax have been reported to be associated with massive ovarian edema (pseudo-Meigs' syndrome). The diagnosis of ovarian edema may not be established until final permanent sections of the ovarian wedge biopsy are interpreted by a skilled pathologist. The treatment for massive ovarian edema is suspension or fixation of the ovary so that it does not twist.

BENIGN OVARIAN NEOPLASMS

Epithelial Ovarian Neoplasms

Approximately two-thirds of ovarian neoplasms arise from the coelomic epithelium that invests the surface of the ovary. This epithelium, which is in continuity with the remainder of the peritoneum, has the potential to give rise to a variety of cystadenomas and cystadenocarcinomas. In fact, 85 percent of all ovarian cancers are epithelial in origin.

Whether benign or malignant, epithelial neoplasms may differentiate histologically along several cell lines, mimicking other epithelium of the female reproductive tract. The most frequent lesions are serous ovarian neoplasms that differentiate into a fallopian tube-like epithelium with ciliated columnar cells predominating. Mucinous ovarian neoplasms histologically resemble the mucin glands of the endocervix or, in some cases, colonic intestinal epithelium. Endometrioid epithelial neoplasms are rare and appear similar to the glandular epithelium of the endometrium. These tumors must be distinguished from an ovarian endometrioma, which arises from ovarian involvement with endometriosis (Chap. 12). The Brenner tumor, a rare epithelial ovarian neoplasm, is usually a solid tumor that is similar to the transitional epithelium of the urinary bladder.

The presentations of epithelial ovarian neoplasms are not necessarily characteristic, and these lesions cannot be differentiated based on symptoms or physical examination findings. Both serous and mucinous cystadenomas are in general cystic and may be multiloculated with septa identified radiographically. Calcification of these cysts due to psammoma bodies is noted in as many as 25 percent of cases. The Brenner tumor is characteristically a solid tumor and usually reasonably small compared to the serous, mucinous, and endometrioid cysts. The symptoms of an epithelial ovarian neoplasm tend to parallel the size of the tumor, with pain, pressure, and abdominal distention being frequent presenting signs. In the smaller size range (up to 12 cm) the cyst is often mobile and smooth. When it achieves a larger size it tends to become less movable on abdominal and pelvic examination. These cysts may be associated with minimal amounts of ascites, which should be studied cytologically.

The potential for all of these epithelial neoplasms to be either benign or malignant or to fall into a category of tumors of borderline malignant potential must be emphasized. The characteristics and management of benign epithelial ovarian neoplasms are discussed later in this chapter. The management of borderline and frankly invasive ovarian carcinomas is discussed in Chapter 28.

Serous Cystadenoma. The most common of the benign epithelial ovarian neoplasms is the serous cystadenoma. These cysts usually arise in the menstrual or postmenopausal age group of women and account for 25 to 30 percent of all benign ovarian neoplasms. The cysts may vary in size and become reasonably large, although the truly massive ovarian cysts are usually mucinous in origin. Nonetheless, serous cystadenomas may range from several centimeters to 20 cm in size. The gross characteristics of a serous cystadenoma at the time of surgery are those of a smooth cyst that may transluminate or have a dense, white capsule. These cysts are often loculated into several compartments, and on cut section an occasional papillary projection may be noted in the interior wall of the cyst. Any evidence of papillary excrescences into the cyst or on the surface of the cyst raise the specter of malignancy and require careful histologic study. However, not all papillary projections are malignant, and most contain only benign epithelium. Histologic study may also identify psammoma bodies (calcified granules in

the epithelium) in up to 25 percent of cases. These psammoma bodies, if dense, may be seen on a plain flat plate radiograph of the abdomen preoperatively. Psammoma bodies may also be identified in the malignant counterpart of serous cystadenomas. Ten to fifteen percent of serous cystadenomas are bilateral.

Treatment of the serous cystadenoma is surgical removal, usually requiring oophorectomy. In the young patient in whom some identifiable normal ovarian tissue is present at the base of the cyst, an ovarian cystectomy may be performed. Most cases should be studied immediately by frozen section to screen or exclude the possibility of obvious ovarian carcinoma. Ovarian carcinoma tends to occur more frequently in the older woman who does not desire preservation of reproductive function. Therefore oophorectomy is the logical choice of definitive therapy.

Mucinous Cystadenomas. Mucinous cystadenomas account for approximately 15 percent of ovarian neoplasms. Five percent of the time, bilateral mucinous cystadenomas are recognized at the time of surgery. Of the ovarian neoplasms, mucinous cystadenomas tend to be the largest, with cases reported of mucinous cysts weighing 100 to 200 pounds (Fig. 18-1). The mucinous cystadenoma tends to have a smooth capsule that may be septated or loculated. The contents of the mucinous cystadenoma tend to be mucinous, with a sticky gelatinous material noted in most instances. Mucinous cystadenomas occasionally appear to arise from a benign ovarian teratoma (dermoid). In other instances, histology may show a mixture of other epithelial elements, such as serous or endometrioid epithelium.

Treatment of mucinous cystadenoma requires surgical resection, usually oophorectomy and rarely ovarian cystectomy in the young reproductive age woman. Rupture of the mucinous cystadenoma is thought to increase the patient's risk of developing pseudomyxoma peritonei.

Pseudomyxoma peritonei is a benign condition in which mucinous cells implant throughout the peritoneal cavity, secreting the gelatinous mucin material usually found in mucinous cystadenoma. This mucinous material ultimately fills the peritoneal cavity,

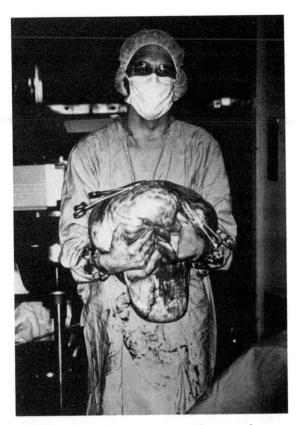

Fig. 18-1. Mucinous cystadenoma. A large mucinous cystadenoma was removed from a 35-year-old woman who had noted increasing abdominal girth over a two-year period.

causing a scirrhous reaction of the peritoneum leading to multiple loculations. As the mucinous material progressively accumulates, abdominal distention, early satiety, and intestinal obstruction result.

This process tends to be a slowly progressive one with no successful treatment available today. In most instances, multiple surgical procedures are required to drain this thick mucin material and thereby relieve intestinal obstruction. Although the histology of the mucinous glands implanted in the peritoneal cavity may remain benign or of low malignant potential, most patients ultimately succumb to intestinal obstruction over a course of years. Because mucinous cystadenomas and pseudomyxoma peritonei are asso-

ciated with mucocele of the appendix, the appendix should be routinely removed at the same operation. In a setting where mucinous cystadenoma of the ovary is ruptured intraoperatively or preoperatively, implantation is therefore possible although probably infrequent. Extensive irrigation of the peritoneal cavity at the time of surgery may dilute or eliminate the mucinous cells, which might ultimately implant on peritoneal surfaces. In large series the five-year survival for patients with pseudomyxoma peritonei is approximately 45 percent. Many clinicians therefore have attempted aggressive therapy such as chemotherapy, radiation therapy, or intraperitoneal radioisotopes. To date there is no known effective treatment for pseudomyxoma peritonei except for surgical relief of intestinal obstruction and removal of the collected mucin. Because of the thick, tenacious nature of the mucin, less-interventional procedures such as paracentesis are usually futile.

Endometrioid Cystadenoma. An endometrioid cystadenoma of the ovary is generally similar but much rarer than the serous cystadenoma. The multiloculated cyst is usually lined with a simple layer of epithelium appearing similar to endometrial tissue. In contrast to endometriomas arising from endometrial implants, endometrioid cystadenomas do not tend to be hemorrhagic or contain "chocolate" material. Endometrioid cysts tend not to be large and are much rarer than the other previously mentioned epithelial ovarian tumors. Endometriomas are considered and discussed in the context of endometriosis in Chapter 12.

Brenner Tumors. Brenner tumors are the rarest of the epithelial ovarian neoplasms and account for less than 1 percent of all ovarian tumors. Grossly, the Brenner tumor is small and often found only at the time of exploratory laparotomy. Most are less than 5 cm in diameter. The Brenner tumor, in contrast to other epithelial tumors, is usually solid or contains only microcysts. On gross examination, a small tumor is noted on the ovary that is smooth and solid in nature. On cut section, it is grayish-white and is similar in consistency to an ovarian fibroma. Brenner tumors are bilateral in approximately 5 to 10 percent of cases and are associated with mucinous cystadenomas in approximately 20 percent. About one-half of women with Brenner tumors are postmenopausal. On pathologic evaluation, the solid tumor shows a pattern of transitional epithelium (similar to that of the bladder) embedded in an abundant stroma. Only 1 to 2 percent of Brenner tumors develop into a malignant neoplasm.

In the reproductive age group, Brenner tumors may be managed by simple excision or oophorectomy. The contralateral ovary should be inspected carefully because of the potential for bilaterality. Ovarian function in one ovary can usually be preserved, however. In the menopausal woman bilateral salpingo-oophorectomy should be performed as definitive treatment.

Adenofibromas and Cystadenofibromas. Adenofibromas and cystadenofibromas are solid or solid and cystic tumors composed of epithelium and connective tissue. Adenofibromas appear solid and are nearly impossible to distinguish grossly from an ovarian fibroma. On microscopic examination, small microcysts of benign epithelium (usually serous) are noted. A cystadenofibroma is grossly a mixed solid and cystic tumor. These tumors usually arise during menopause and may reach 15 cm in diameter. Twenty percent are bilateral, and some have papillae on the surface of the ovary raising some concern as to the potential for malignancy. Careful pathologic evaluation is therefore required.

Germ Cell Ovarian Tumors

A number of tumors can arise from the ovarian germ cells, the most frequent of which is benign cystic teratoma (dermoid). Although the dermoid is a common benign ovarian neoplasm, the other germ cell neoplasms of the ovary are highly malignant and are discussed in Chapter 28. Dermoids are the most common ovarian tumor in children, adolescents, and teenagers. Other germ cell neoplasms of the ovary include the immature teratoma, endodermal sinus tumor, dysgerminoma, ovarian choriocarcinoma, and embryonal tumors.

The term *dermoid,* implying a cyst or tumor of der-

mal origin and content, is actually a misnomer; although dermal elements (e.g., cutaneous epithelium and its appendages, sebaceous fluid, hair, and teeth) predominate in most dermoid cysts, careful histologic study reveals tissues derived from all three germ cell layers, which confirms the true teratomatous nature of the cyst. Dermoid cysts must be distinguished from immature teratomas, which are malignant tumors composed of immature germ cell elements, most frequently neural tissue (Chap. 28). It is well established that dermoid cysts are parthenogenic tumors that arise from a single germ cell after the first meiotic division but before the second. They represent about 20 to 25 percent of all ovarian neoplasms and constitute 33 percent of all benign ovarian tumors (excluding follicular and corpus luteum cysts).

Benign cystic teratoma (dermoid) is the most common ovarian tumor of childhood; and although it may occur at any age, it usually appears during active reproductive life. These lesions are also frequently multiple, with several developing in the same ovary and with bilateral ovarian involvement in 25 percent of cases. Nonovarian teratomas may arise in any midline structure where germ cells resided during embryonic life.

Grossly, the cystic teratoma usually attains only moderate size (80 percent are less than 10 cm in diameter) and presents as a thick-walled, grayish-white, well encapsulated, globular cyst projecting from the surface of the ovary or attached to it by a pedicle. The bulk of the cyst contents are usually composed of a fatty, semisolid sebaceous material, which gives these cysts their characteristic doughy consistency. Collections of matted hair are also commonly found. Well formed teeth, often arising from a rudimentary jaw, are present in 50 percent of cases and are visible on radiographs of the abdomen and pelvis (Fig. 18-2). Most of the solid components are found arising from one localized area of thickening within the cyst wall (tubercle of Rokitansky). The lining of the dermoid cyst is otherwise smooth and composed essentially of skin. Microscopically, various types and combinations of tissue representative of all three germ cell layers may be found: skin, hair, sebaceous glands, teeth, and even fingernails and rudimentary portions of

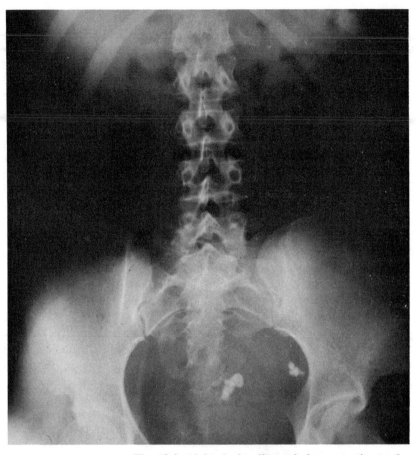

Fig. 18-2. Abdominal radiograph demonstrating teeth in a large dermoid cyst (mature teratoma).

the eye and the central nervous system (ectodermal); bone, cartilage, muscle, fat, and connective tissue (mesodermal); and gastrointestinal tract mucosa, respiratory epithelium, and thyroid tissue (entodermal).

Aside from their obvious presence as an ovarian mass, the most common clinical manifestation of dermoid cysts is acute pelvic and lower abdominal pain secondary to torsion, sometimes with infarction, to which their smooth free-lying nature predisposes them. Acute or chronic discomfort due to acute rupture or to intermittent leakage of the highly irritating cyst contents into the peritoneal cavity is also noted with some frequency. Malignant change, usually squamous cell carcinoma, developing in one of the epidermal elements of the cyst, is rare, occurring in 1 to 3 percent of cases and invariably in women well past menopause. The development of adenocarcinomas and carcinoid tumors in dermoid cysts has also been reported, but these cases are rare. Struma ovarii is a rare variation of cystic teratoma in which a preponderance of thyroid tissue is found. About 5 percent of struma ovarii have enough production of thyroid hormone to cause thyrotoxicosis. A dozen cases have been reported in which benign cystic teratoma has been accompanied by severe autoimmune hemolytic anemia, with the hemolysis and anemia disappearing completely when the ovarian tumor was removed. The factors underlying this rare association are not clear.

Because cystic teratomas arise with reasonable frequency in children and young women wishing to retain reproductive potential, conservative management should be carefully considered. In most cases, the cyst is well encapsulated and unilateral. In these circumstances, incising the cyst wall and simply "shelling out" the cyst may be accomplished with the remainder of the ovarian tissue reconstructed and preserved. The latter may be accomplished even when bilateral ovarian cystic teratomas are encountered. On rare occasion, oophorectomy must be performed, with the contralateral ovary being preserved. In the past, the general advice was to bivalve the contralateral ovary to be certain that a bilateral dermoid cyst was not present. It has now been clearly shown that bivalving a grossly normal-appearing ovary is unnecessary, as the yield for detecting an occult cystic teratoma is infrequent. On the other hand, bivalving a normal ovary increases the risk of hemorrhage into the ovary with its subsequent loss or the creation of adhesions from the fallopian tube to the ovary with subsequent infertility. Although the contralateral ovary should be inspected carefully, our advice today is not to bivalve the ovary in a woman desiring subsequent fertility.

Stromal–Sex Cord Tumors

Tumors arising from the ovarian stroma and sex cord cells account for only 5 percent of ovarian tumors. In general, these neoplasms are benign and are therefore discussed in this chapter. Their rare malignant counterparts are discussed in Chapter 28.

The stromal sex cord tumors are often considered "functioning" ovarian tumors because they produce steroid hormones, thus causing end-organ manifestations such as precocious puberty, endometrial hyperplasia, postmenopausal bleeding, and hirsutism. Fifteen percent of sex cord tumors are hormonally inert. It should be recognized when discussing functioning ovarian tumors that any ovarian neoplasm (including metastatic carcinoma to the ovary) may stimulate the ovarian stroma to produce steroids.

Embryologically, the gonad is sexually bipotential,

and therefore ovarian stromal tumors often parallel testicular tumors. The granulosa cell tumor of the ovary is histologically identical to Sertoli cells in the male testes, and theca cells of the ovary are similar to Leydig cells in the testicle. Therefore these tumors may produce either female or male hormones. Ovarian sex cord tumors and stromal tumors are classified according to their differentiation toward ovarian follicles, testicular tubules, Leydig cells, or adrenocortical cells.

Ovarian Fibroma. The ovarian fibroma is the most common benign solid neoplasm found in the ovary. This tumor, arising from the fibrous stroma of the ovary, may vary in size from small nodules on the ovary to huge ovarian masses weighing up to 20 kg. The average size of an ovarian fibroma is 6 cm. These tumors are often palpated on pelvic examination as a firm smooth or nodular mass. Because of their consistency, which is similar to that of leiomyomas, they may be mistaken for a uterine fibroid on pelvic examination. Like leiomyomas of the uterus, 10 percent of ovarian fibromas are calcified. On cut section, the ovarian tumor is solid with a grayish-white appearance. Ten percent are bilateral. Because these solid ovarian tumors are most often found in perimenopausal and postmenopausal women, they may be managed by simple oophorectomy. Careful histologic study is required to exclude the possibility of a malignancy such as a fibrosarcoma or a malignant Brenner tumor.

Ovarian fibromas may also cause other signs and symptoms associated with malignancy, especially ascites or a pleural effusion. The constellation of ascites, pleural effusion, and a pelvic mass that is ultimately found to be an ovarian fibroma is called *Meigs' syndrome.* The ascites and pleural effusion disappear completely and permanently following removal of the ovarian fibroma (Fig. 18-3). Approximately 40 percent of fibromas larger than 6 cm in diameter are accompanied by ascites, but fewer than 5 percent of all fibromas give rise to Meigs' syndrome. Meigs' syndrome is also encountered occasionally in the presence of thecomas and other fibroma-like benign tumors. It should be emphasized that Meigs' syndrome does not include the development of ascites and pleural effusions secondary to metastasis from ovarian or other abdominal carcinomas, although it may simulate this situation, including a malignant-appearing cachexia. Occasionally, other tumors and cysts of the ovary and, rarely, even large uterine fibroids may be accompanied by ascites and a hydrothorax, a condition referred to as *pseudo-Meigs' syndrome.*

The formation of ascites depends on fluid formation (a transudate of extracellular fluid) and leakage through the thin capsule surrounding the myxoid tissue of the usually markedly edematous fibroma (the most widely accepted explanation). Alternatively, ascites may result from fluid formation secondary to local peritoneal irritation or even to some more generalized response of the peritoneal cavity. Hydrothorax presumably results from the passage of excessive abdominal fluid through the lymphatics of the diaphragm. Although pleural effusions may be noted bilaterally on the chest radiograph, the right thorax is more often involved.

It is important to be aware of Meigs' syndrome, as it is often highly suggestive of advanced, hopeless cancer; many patients have not been treated in the past, thus dying of a benign, easily curable condition. The need to establish a definite histologic diagnosis in any patient with an ovarian tumor, ascites, and hydrothorax is obvious.

Thecomas. The ovarian thecoma is another solid ovarian tumor that grossly appears similar to an ovarian fibroma. In fact, many tumors arising from the ovarian stroma may be of mixed composition, containing both theca cells and connective tissue of fibromas; they are classified according to their predominant element. Thecomas occur in approximately the same age group as do ovarian fibromas and are bilateral only about 10 percent of the time.

Thecomas frequently have estrogenic activity, causing postmenopausal bleeding or menometrorrhagia in the menstrual age woman. Because of the estrogenic activity and its effect on the endometrium, 50 percent of patients with ovarian thecomas have endometrial hyperplasia, 20 percent have endometrial polyps, and 10 percent have well differentiated endometrial adenocarcinoma.

Management of the ovarian thecoma requires sur-

Fig. 18-3. Meigs' syndrome. Chest radiograph demonstrates a right hydrothorax (left) and diffuse ascites (center) in a patient who had a 15-cm ovarian fibroma. After removal of the ovarian fibroma, the ascites and hydrothorax resolved spontaneously, as demonstrated in a chest radiograph obtained two months later (right).

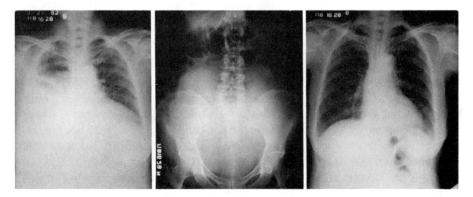

gical removal. In the perimenopausal and postmenopausal woman, assessment of the endometrium is also mandatory because of the noted propensity for endometrial hyperplasia and neoplasia. In the postmenopausal woman, hysterectomy is usually advised as part of the treatment plan for ovarian thecoma to remove the possibility of an occult carcinoma. Ovarian thecomas are rarely malignant.

Granulosa Cell Tumors. In many textbooks granulosa cell tumors are considered in the section on malignant ovarian neoplasms. However, most granulosa cell tumors are benign in nature, and even when they are malignant they carry an excellent prognosis especially when diagnosed at an early stage. In addition, granulosa cell tumors may occur at any point in the woman's life-span from the prepubertal years to postmenopausal age. Most granulosa cell tumors, however, occur in postmenopausal women, with fewer than 5 percent in children. Because the granulosa cells are responsible for production of estrogen, these tumors also frequently produce estrogen, causing isosexual precocious puberty in children, menorrhagia and irregular bleeding in the menstrual age woman, and postmenopausal bleeding and breast fullness in the postmenopausal woman. The stimulation of the endometrium by this unopposed endogenous production of estrogen often leads to endometrial hyperplasia; and endometrial adenocarcinoma is found to coexist in approximately 10 percent of patients with granulosa cell tumors.

The granulosa cell tumor is usually solid with some cystic components. Often hemorrhage into the tumor is noted. Characteristically, the solid tumor is small and not suspected unless there is abnormal bleeding; or it may be large and ultimately rupture, causing bleeding and signs and symptoms of an acute abdomen. Eighty-five percent of granulosa cell tumors are found to be confined to the ovary. For these Stage I tumors, a more than 95 percent five-year survival rate is reported. On the other hand, granulosa cell tumors found to have spread beyond the ovary are malignant and so are discussed in more detail in Chapter 28. Histologic study of the Stage I tumors is important, especially noting cellular atypia and evaluating

mitotic activity. The size of the ovarian tumor is associated with the long-term outcome, with an excellent prognosis found in tumors measuring less than 5 cm in diameter.

Juvenile granulosa cell tumors account for 85 percent of granulosa cell tumors in children. Seventy percent of these children manifest precocious puberty, and the tumor itself is usually palpable on abdominal or rectal examination. Rarely (less than 5 percent of the time), these tumors are bilateral or have spread beyond the ovary. Histologically, the nuclei of juvenile granulosa cell tumors appear less mature than those in the adult granulosa cell tumor.

Granulosa cell tumors occurring in children and in women wishing to preserve reproductive function may usually be managed by unilateral salpingo-oophorectomy. Careful histologic study is advised to identify those tumors with a higher malignant potential. Nonetheless, the overall outcome of women with Stage I tumors following surgical resection is excellent. In the postmenopausal patient or the menstrual age woman, endometrial sampling is advised because of the high association with hyperplasia and adenocarcinoma of the endometrium. In the postmenopausal patient, resection of both ovaries and the uterus is advised and should serve as definitive therapy.

Sertoli-Leydig Cell Tumors (Androblastomas). Sex cord tumors that differentiate toward testicular structures are histologically identified as Sertoli-Leydig cell tumors. Although some may differentiate as pure cell lines of Sertoli or Leydig cells, most are of dual cell origin and therefore termed androblastomas. These rare tumors (comprising fewer than 1 percent of ovarian tumors) are generally benign. More than 60 percent are associated with virilization, which may be slow in onset. Other androblastomas may produce estrogen or progesterone, and 15 percent have no clinically obvious hormonal activity. Most patients with Sertoli-Leydig cell tumors are in the menstrual age group, with a median age of 25 to 30 years. In addition to virilization (including clitoromegaly, hirsutism, acne, hoarseness, increased libido, temporal balding, and rarely an increase in muscle mass), some patients present with oligomenorrhea or genital or breast atrophy. Many of these tumors are not palpable on abdominal or pelvic examination, and therefore the clinical signs and symptoms of virilization should lead the clinician to further investigate the specific etiology, including consideration of a virilizing ovarian tumor (see Chapter 18 for further evaluation and discussion of virilism). The malignant potential of androblastomas is low and is most frequently seen in tumors that are histologically poorly differentiated or those with heterologous elements, especially skeletal muscle or cartilage.

Pure Sertoli cell tumors are rare and frequently manifest excessive production of unopposed estrogen, leading to menorrhagia. Pure tumors composed of Leydig cells or hilus cells are usually small and unilateral, may produce testosterone, and occur in a slightly older age group (average age 50 years). Gynandroblastoma has a mixture of elements, including granulosa cells, plus tubules and Leydig cells. These tumors may produce estrogen, androgens, or both.

The management of stromal and sex cord tumors is usually directed toward local excision. In the perimenopausal and menopausal age group, bilateral salpingo-oophorectomy and abdominal hysterectomy should be performed, as fertility is no longer a consideration. Preservation of the contralateral ovary and uterus in the older woman allows the patient to retain genital organs that might later develop another ovarian neoplasm, secondary endometrial hyperplasia, or adenocarcinoma. In the child and menstrual age woman in whom fertility preservation is strongly considered, local excision of the tumor (usually oophorectomy) should suffice as adequate therapy. The tissue should be carefully evaluated histologically for malignant elements, but the usual additional staging biopsies and lymph node dissection advised for other ovarian malignancies need not be carried out in most instances. As a general rule, in the woman wishing to preserve fertility, conservative surgical resection should be performed with careful intraperitoneal exploration, followed by careful histologic evaluation and consultation. If in the final analysis the tumor is found to be malignant, repeat operation may be necessary for further staging and resection. On the other hand, it is inappropriate to remove both tubes and ovaries as well as the uterus in a young woman without a clear-cut diagnosis of malignancy. The management of advanced and malignant stromal and sex cord tumors is discussed in Chapter 28.

Parovarian Cysts

Cystic structures may arise from the broad ligament and mesosalpinx that are clinically indistinguishable from an adnexal mass and ovarian cyst. Radiographic studies, including ultrasonography, CT scan, and MRI, are rarely helpful for distinguishing the origin of the adnexal cyst, and therefore surgical exploration is necessary in most cases. It is often only at surgery that the cyst is determined to be of parovarian origin rather than from the ovary itself. Parovarian cysts arise in the broad ligament from either the embryonic müllerian remnants or embryonic mesonephric (wolffian duct) remnants, or as a peritoneal inclusion cyst. Most of these cysts are noted in the reproductive age group, and most are asymptomatic.

Although the cysts may be tense on pelvic examination, many are less firm, with a softer, mushy consistency on bimanual examination. Symptoms associated with parovarian cysts are usually due to torsion, which may be intermittent or acute and persistent. Torsion and infarction of a right parovarian cyst may mimic appendicitis in the young woman. Surgical removal of these cysts is usually easily accomplished; and in the setting where fertility is to be maintained, the surgeon should take care to avoid excessive tissue trauma or the use of reactive suture material, which might ultimately lead to adhesions and tubal obstruction.

NEOPLASMS OF THE FALLOPIAN TUBE

True neoplasms of the fallopian tube are rare and are usually discovered as incidental findings during pelvic surgery or only after resection of the fallopian tube in combination with the uterus and ovary. Most clinically detected masses arising from the fallopian tube are associated with inflammatory processes. A tubo-ovarian abscess is often an adherent mass of infected fallopian tube and mesosalpinx joined by adherent ovary, small bowel, and broad ligament. Later in the course of pelvic inflammatory disease the chronic adhesion formation around the fallopian tube and ovary may result in a palpable mass. Hydrosalpinx may occur following tubal infection and pyosalpinx or tubal ligation. Ectopic pregnancy may also cause clinically detected enlargement of the fallopian tube, which is indistinguishable from other adnexal structures on pelvic examination. The diagnosis and management of pelvic inflammatory disease, tuboovarian abscess, hydrosalpinx, and ecotopic pregnancy are discussed in Chapters 15 and 16, respectively.

Adenomatoid Tumors of the Fallopian Tube

Adenomatoid tumors are the most common benign neoplasms arising from the fallopian tube. Although usually small and asymptomatic, they are of some importance because their histologic appearance has sometimes led to an erroneous diagnosis of a low grade adenocarcinoma of the fallopian tube. In gross appearance, adenomatoid tumors are firm, discrete nodules, grayish-white or yellow, lying within the muscle layer of the tube and rarely exceeding 3 cm in diameter. The distinctive histologic picture is one of solid cords and gland-like spaces lined by cells that may be flattened, resembling endothelial cells, or large and vacuolated suggesting either epithelial or mesothelial cells—hence the occasional confusion with low grade adenocarcinoma in the past.

Benign Tubal Tumors with Clinical Significance

Occasionally, leiomyomas, fibromas, and cystic or solid teratomas, by virtue of their size or an associated vascular or inflammatory complication, produce either acute or chronic symptoms. They also may simply present as a palpable adnexal mass of unknown nature. Ultimately they require surgical exploration and removal.

True leiomyomas are usually small, solitary, and asymptomatic; and probably many are never reported. When large, they occasionally produce acute tubal torsions; more rarely they have been implicated as a cause of ectopic pregnancy. Leiomyomas of the fallopian tube are subject to the same degenerative changes that occur with uterine fibroids, and acute or chronic

symptoms may likewise result. The disparity between the low incidence of leiomyomas of the fallopian tube and their frequent occurrence in the uterus is surprising, as both are of müllerian duct origin, but it may be partly related to the relative unresponsiveness of the tubal smooth muscle to estrogens compared to the responsiveness of the myometrium.

Teratomas of the fallopian tube are of the dermoid cyst variety in most instances, although solid teratomas have been encountered. Many of these tumors are small and asymptomatic and are incidental findings, usually arising by a thin interluminal pedicle from the mucosa of the distal portion of the fallopian tube. However, large teratomas frequently cause a palpable mass and chronic symptoms either because of their increasing size and pressure on adjacent viscera or because of a secondary inflammatory reaction. Recurrent bouts of abdominal pain and fever may simulate chronic pelvic inflammatory disease. Acute or chronic intermittent torsion may also occur. The etiology of teratomas in the fallopian tube appears to be primordial germ cells whose migration to the ovary has been arrested, with subsequent neoplastic changes leading to the histology commonly found in ovarian mature cystic teratomas.

Finally, the commonest of all noninflammatory benign tubal lesions are the *hydatid cysts of Morgagni* (Fig. 18-4). Hydatid cysts of Morgagni are usually small and asymptomatic, occurring as pedunculated cystic structures near the fimbriated end of the fallopian tube. Most are asymptomatic and are recognized only at the time of pelvic surgery. Most achieve the size of a centimeter or so and are not usually palpable on pelvic examination. Rarely, intermittent torsion or infarction of hydatid cysts of Morgagni causes unexplained intermittent or acute pelvic and lower abdominal pain that is usually unilateral and colicky; it may be associated with nausea, vomiting, and signs of peritoneal irritation, a tender adnexal mass, and low grade fever. If symptoms are severe enough and especially if torsion of the entire adnexa has been precipitated by the twisting hydatid cyst, laparotomy may be indicated. Most hydatid cysts of Morgagni are easily removed surgically with preservation of the remainder of the fallopian tube.

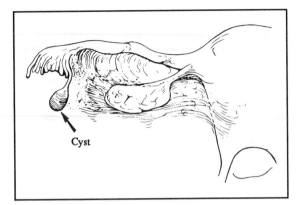

Cyst

Fig. 18-4. Hydatid cyst of Morgagni.

GENERAL MANAGEMENT OF THE ADNEXAL MASS

Whereas a pelvic mass may be of gastrointestinal, urologic, or retroperitoneal origin, this chapter has focused on the adnexal mass arising from gynecologic organs. Astute clinical judgment combined with appropriate use of laboratory and radiographic testing can usually exclude or identify patients with a mass caused by disease of another organ system. In those cases, appropriate referral should be made immediately.

We must therefore consider management of the adnexal mass of gynecologic origin in a comprehensive discussion. The implications of an adnexal mass obviously raise the concern of ovarian cancer. In addition, concerns about preservation of fertility are raised in the child or young woman. Because of the variation and type of adnexal masses occurring in different age groups, a logical treatment schema may be devised dividing women into three categories: (1) infants and children prior to menarche; (2) menstrual age women desiring preservation of fertility; and (3) perimenopausal and menopausal age women.

Adnexal Mass in Children

Aside from the adnexal mass occurring in the neonate—often a follicular cyst secondary to maternal hormone stimulation of the fetal ovaries—there are no normal adnexal masses. In the neonate, a cystic structure in the pelvis or abdomen should be observed

over the ensuing few weeks after delivery and can be noted to regress if it is truly a follicular cyst. On the other hand, a persistent mass in the neonate, or an abdominal or pelvic mass in children or adolescents, is abnormal and requires thorough evaluation and surgical exploration.

Nongynecologic causes of an abdominal and pelvic mass in children include Wilms' tumor, neuroblastoma, tumors of the gastrointestinal tract, lymphomas, and mesenteric or omental cysts. Most true ovarian neoplasms of childhood are benign, many being dermoid cysts. Functional cysts (follicular or corpus luteum cysts) are the second most common cause of an adnexal mass during childhood. Of ovarian cancers, dysgerminoma is most frequently diagnosed, and other germ cell tumors are less frequent. Epithelial ovarian tumors and stromal sex cord neoplasms are rarer still.

At surgical exploration of the child with a persistent adnexal mass, primary consideration should be given to the preservation of fertility and of the uninvolved ovary. In most instances, dermoid cysts and cystadenomas may be removed by cystectomy, thereby preserving the normal ovarian tissue at the base of the cyst. The remaining ovarian tissue should be reconstructed with low inflammatory suture material and care taken to minimize tissue trauma, which might induce peritubal adhesions. Solid tumors of the ovary (e.g., dysgerminoma or granulosa cell tumor) are difficult to remove, leaving residual ovarian tissue behind. In most instances, oophorectomy is required. All neoplasms of the ovary have a small potential to be bilateral. The contralateral ovary therefore should be carefully inspected. However, because of the risk of injury to the contralateral ovary, which would cause loss of the normal ovary or excessive adhesion formation, the practice of bivalving the other ovary in search of an occult neoplasm should be condemned.

Adnexal Mass in Menstrual Age Women

Management of the adnexal mass in the menstrual age group provides the gynecologist with an enormous clinical challenge, on occasion requiring considerable judgment both preoperatively and intraoperatively. Because many adnexal masses in the menstrual age woman may be functional cysts (follicle or corpus luteum cysts), which usually regress spontaneously, there is a significant role for conservative management.

In general, if the adnexal mass appears to be cystic on pelvic or ultrasound examination and less than 8 cm in diameter, observation of the mass through a menstrual cycle or for up to six weeks is advised. During this six weeks of observation, most corpus luteum or follicle cysts regress and require no surgical intervention. On the other hand, if the cyst is still present after six weeks of follow-up, the strong possibility of a persistent ovarian neoplasm should be entertained and surgical exploration with removal of the mass undertaken.

In all cases of a solid adnexal mass, or one that shows solid and cystic structures on ultrasonography, the patient should undergo immediate surgical exploration. Most of these masses are benign. The patient's desire for preservation of fertility should be clarified prior to undertaking surgery.

In most instances, dermoid cysts may be removed by cystectomy, thereby preserving both ovaries. Epithelial ovarian cysts are more difficult to remove by cystectomy, although it should be attempted if possible.

Solid ovarian neoplasms such as a granulosa cell tumor or fibroma are more difficult to excise, and usually unilateral oophoretomy is required. Large or rapidly growing adnexal masses, especially in adolescents or teenagers should raise the possibility of an ovarian germ cell malignancy and be managed as discussed in Chapter 28.

Selecting an incision to explore a patient with an adnexal mass during the menstrual years may be difficult. Clearly, a large mass reaching to the umbilicus or above requires a midline or paramedian incision to allow adequate exposure for surgical removal. On the other hand, an 8 cm mass in the pelvis may be explored through a transverse incision (e.g., Pfannenstiel or Maylard incision). Because most of these masses are not malignant, this incision allows adequate exposure to perform surgical resection necessary to manage the benign neoplasm. If a patient at exploration is found to have an ovarian malignancy, the transverse incision must be modified to allow adequate, complete exploration for surgical staging and tumor debulking as discussed in Chapter 28.

At the time of exploratory laparotomy, several gross characteristics of the mass and associated findings suggest whether it is benign or malignant (Table 18-3). The pelvis and abdominal cavity are carefully explored in all patients; and in cases where the diagnosis is not clear, peritoneal washings or free peritoneal fluid should be submitted for cytopathologic evaluation. Frozen section of the adnexal mass usually defines the benign or malignant nature of the lesion. Management of the patient with an adnexal

Table 18-3. Clinical Characteristics of Benign and Malignant Adnexal Masses*

Status of mass	Characteristics	Associated findings
Benign	Smooth capsule	No ascites
	Cystic	Smooth peritoneal surface
	Unilateral	Stable weight
	Capsule intact	
	Mobile	
	Smooth inner wall of cyst capsule	
Malignant	Excrescence on capsule	Ascites
	Solid	Peritoneal nodularity/excrescences
	Bilateral	Weight loss
	Ruptured capsule	
	Adherent/fixed to adjacent organs	
	Excrescences into cyst	

*None is definitely diagnostic.

mass that is not clearly defined as benign or malignant, based on frozen section, should be conservative until the final pathology report is available. Occasionally, on further study a "benign" ovarian neoplasm is found to be malignant and further surgery is required to completely stage and debulk the ovarian malignancy. Because these circumstances occur infrequently, the pelvic surgeon is encouraged to be conservative in women with a unilateral adnexal mass who wish to preserve fertility.

Laparoscopy may prove useful when there is only the suspicion of ovarian enlargement or when it is a matter of definitely identifying a lateral, pedunculated fibroid for which no treatment is necessary once the possibility of an ovarian lesion has been excluded. The use of laparoscopy today has no role in the management of other adnexal masses, as surgical excision is required and should not be performed through the laparoscope for fear of rupturing the occasional early stage ovarian cancer. The use of laparoscopy, therefore, in cases of suspected ovarian enlargement that cannot be confirmed by other noninvasive studies, or when the diagnosis of a pedunculated uterine fibroid is entertained, avoids a number of unnecessary laparotomies for diagnosis only.

Adnexal Mass in Menopausal Women

Any adnexal mass during menopause must be considered abnormal, raising a more significant specter: the possibility of ovarian carcinoma. In fact, because of atrophy of the ovary during menopause, any enlarged ovary found on routine gynecologic examination in the menopausal woman must be considered abnormal even though it does not reach 5 to 8 cm in diameter and may well be asymptomatic. Likewise, because of the higher probability of ovarian cancer, the menopausal woman should undergo exploration through a midline or paramedian incision. It seems foolhardy to explore a postmenopausal patient through a Pfannenstiel incision for an adnexal mass that is then found to be malignant. Likewise, in the setting of a benign adnexal mass, most postmenopausal patients should undergo total abdominal hysterectomy with bilateral salpingo-oophorectomy. Preservation of a senescent ovary is of little or no benefit and simply allows

the patient to retain an organ that may subsequently develop a neoplasm, requiring further surgery.

In all instances, the surgeon or gynecologist undertaking exploration of a woman with an adnexal mass should be prepared for the worst possible findings. That is, the surgeon must be prepared mentally and have the surgical skills to adequately manage the patient should ovarian carcinoma be found. As discussed in detail in Chapter 28, it should include a thorough knowledge of and the capability to perform surgical staging as well as aggressive tumor debulking for advanced ovarian carcinoma. The skills required include the ability to operate in the retroperitoneal space and to perform lymphadenectomy, omentectomy, and intestinal surgery. If the surgeon does not have these capabilities for managing the patient intraoperatively, he or she should seriously consider referring the patient to a surgeon who has these capabilities and resources.

SELECTED READINGS

Barber, H. R. K., and Graber, E. A. The PMPO syndrome (postmenopausal palpable ovary syndrome). *Obstet. Gynecol.* 38:921, 1971.

Chaitin, B. A., Gershenson, D. M., and Evans, H. L. Mucinous tumors of the ovary: a clinicopathologic study of 70 cases. *Cancer* 55:1958, 1985.

Dockerty, M. B., and Masson, J. C. Ovarian fibroma: a clinical and pathological study of 283 cases. *Am. J. Obstet. Gynecol.* 47:741, 1944.

Doss, N., Forney, P., Vellios, F., et al. Covert bilaterality of mature ovarian teratomas. *Obstet. Gynecol.* 50:651, 1977.

Dunnihoo, D. R, and Wolff, J. Bilateral torsion of the adnexa: a case report and review of the world literature. *Obstet. Gynecol.* 64:55S, 1984.

Hallatt, J. G., Steele, C. M., and Snyder, M. Ruptured corpus luteum with hemoperitoneum: a study of 173 surgical cases. *Am. J. Obstet. Gynecol.* 149:5, 1984.

Hibbard, H. Adnexal torsion. *Am. J. Obstet. Gynecol.* 152:456, 1985.

Hunter, D. J. S. Management of a massive ovarian cyst. *Obstet. Gynecol.* 56:254, 1980.

Killackey, M. A., and Neuwirth, R. S. Evaluation and management of the pelvic mass: a review of 540 cases. *Obstet. Gynecol.* 71:319, 1988.

Laing, F. C., Van Dalsem, V. F., Marks, W. M., et al. Dermoid cysts of the ovary: their ultrasonographic appearances. *Obstet. Gynecol.* 57:99, 1981.

Meigs, J. V. Fibroma of the ovary with ascites and hydrothorax—Meigs' syndrome. *Am. J. Obstet. Gynecol.* 67:962, 1954.

Ong, H. C., and Chan, W. F. Mucinous cystadenoma, serous cystadenoma and benign cystic teratoma of the ovary. *Cancer* 41:1538, 1978.

Peters, W. A., Thiagaraja, S., and Thornton, W. N. Ovarian hemorrhage in patients receiving anticoagulant therapy. *J. Reprod. Med.* 22:82, 1979.

Spanos, W. J. Preoperative hormonal therapy of cystic adnexal masses. *Am. J. Obstet. Gynecol.* 116:551, 1973.

Voss, S. C. Ultrasound and the pelvic mass. *J. Reprod. Med.* 28:833, 1983.

19

Disorders of Pelvic Support and Urinary Incontinence

L. Lewis Wall

Support of the pelvic viscera and intraabdominal contents presents a significant anatomic engineering problem. The pelvic floor, composed primarily of muscles, connective tissue ("fascia"), and ligaments, not only must be able to support the pelvic and abdominal contents (which are focused on this area in the upright position) but must also allow correct function of the urinary, reproductive, and gastrointestinal "canals," which penetrate and exit through this floor. Voluntary control of bladder and bowel function (after toilet training) is usually taken for granted.

There are many forces and events during a woman's lifetime that may diminish the support function of the pelvic floor. Most notable is the vaginal delivery of a child, the process of which tremendously dilates the vaginal canal and pelvic floor muscles and fascia. The tone and strength of the pelvic floor after pregnancy and delivery are rarely fully retained. Repeated deliveries further reduce support mechanisms. Pressure on and relaxation of the pelvic floor are increased with age and aging of tissues. Loss of estrogen stimulation of lower reproductive tract tissues causes further stretching of the vaginal wall and supporting fascia.

This chapter addresses the mechanisms of normal pelvic support, the causes and anatomic defects caused by loss of support, and the corrective measures that may be offered. Because stress urinary incontinence is a major problem resulting from loss of support of the base of the bladder and urethra, it is discussed in detail, but within the broader context of urinary incontinence.

DISORDERS OF PELVIC SUPPORT

Support of the Uterus

The uterus may occupy a number of positions within the female pelvis. They may be simple anatomic variations of normal, not implying pathology or loss of normal anatomic support; or they may be the result of progressive relaxation of the normal supporting structures of the pelvic floor and perineum. The former, which may be called *simple displacements,* are usually both asymptomatic and insignificant in terms of normal function.

Simple Displacements. A number of terms are used to describe the position of the uterus within the pelvis. *Anteversion* and *anteflexion* refer to a uterus that is tipped forward toward the anterior abdominal wall. A *military* or *midplane* uterus lies fully extended in the pelvis with its long axis in a straight line. A *retroverted* or *retroflexed* uterus lies tipped backward toward the bottom of the pelvic basin and the vaginal canal. The uterus may also be described as deviating to the left or right side in its position in the pelvis. These positions are usually easily determined by bimanual and rectovaginal-pelvic examination. The most frequent position occupied by the uterus is in the midpelvis and moderately anteverted, but other positions are not significant so long as the uterus is freely mobile and nontender to palpation: They are merely anatomic variations of normal and are of no functional significance. However, because historically retroversion of the uterus was thought to be abnormal and because it may be associated with pelvic pathology, it is worth brief consideration.

RETROVERSION OF THE UTERUS. Simple retroversion of the uterus is found in 20 percent or more of otherwise normal asymptomatic women. It represents an anatomic variation of normal consisting of a somewhat shorter anterior vaginal wall in combination with more relaxed or attenuated uterosacral ligaments. This positioning allows the cervix to swing more anteriorly and permits the uterine fundus to fall back into the cul-de-sac. As a normal anatomic variation it is essentially asymptomatic and, by itself, is innocent of the list of charges ascribed to it in the past: dysmenorrhea, dyspareunia, backache, infertility, menorrhagia, and complications of pregnancy.

The normal retroverted uterus is invariably freely movable and can usually be displaced anteriorly during a pelvic examination. It may fall forward spontaneously if the patient assumes the knee-chest position. The retroverted uterus can be held anteriorly with a Smith-Hodge pessary, but simple correction of uterine position in the absence of pelvic pathology is of no clinical utility.

A *fixed retroversion* of the uterus, however, may develop secondary to pelvic pathology (e.g., endometriosis or pelvic inflammatory disease) that produces adhesions between the uterus, adnexal structures, and posterior pelvis. Large uterine fibroids or ovarian tumors may also cause the uterus to fall backward into the pelvis. Conservative surgery for these diseases aiming to preserve and improve fertility, e.g., conservative resection of endometriosis, myomectomy, lysis of pelvic adhesions, or tubal reconstruction (Chap. 13) may require mobilization of the uterus and adnexal structures and suspension to reposition them anteriorly away from potential areas of adhesion formation. This problem is the most valid indication for performing a uterine suspension operation in contemporary gynecologic practice.

A variety of surgical procedures for uterine suspension have been developed. The most satisfactory operations involve either anterior (Coffey suspension) or posterior (Baldy-Webster) plication of the round ligaments. Plication of the uterosacral ligaments may also achieve the same end. Operations for uterine suspension must avoid creating any fenestrations, bands, or cul-de-sacs that could lead to small bowel obstruction. If fertility is an issue, the uterine fundus must be left free to expand and enlarge with any subsequent pregnancy.

Anatomy of Pelvic Support

To understand the pathologic anatomy of pelvic relaxation and the general principles involved in surgical correction of its various manifestations, it is necessary to consider the basic structures that provide normal support for the pelvic viscera.

Bony Pelvis. As a result of the exaggerated lumbar spinal curve and accompanying downward tilt of the bony pelvis in humans, the anterior part of the bony pelvis (the pubic symphysis and adjacent rami) rests underneath the anteriorly situated pelvic viscera (especially the bladder) and helps support them. The widening and marked forward curve of the sacrum and coccyx (sacrococcygeal bony basin) that has evolved in the human female has placed these bony structures directly underneath parts of the more posteriorly situated pelvic organs (especially the rectum), where they also serve as a rigid, unyielding support. Unless severely traumatized, the bony pelvis does not lose its supportive function and does not require correction as part of a plan to correct loss of support. Rather, it is through the intervening space (the "floor" of the pelvis) that most anatomic defects resulting in loss of support develop.

Muscular Pelvic Floor. In the central pelvis between the peripheral anterior and posterior bony segments and lateral pelvic walls, the fan-shaped levator muscles provide support for the structures directly over the pelvic outlet (Fig. 19-1). The components of the levator complex (ischiococcygeus, iliococcygeus, puborectalis, and pubococcygeus muscles) are essentially fused on each side and blend together in the midline, where they surround and support the three canals in the pelvic floor where the urinary, reproductive, and gastrointestinal tracts exit. This "levator sling" of thick striated muscle is admirably suited for this purpose, as it fulfills the requirements of adequate long-term support and yet allows considerable temporary expansion to meet the functional demands of vaginal delivery and defecation. It is obvious that congenital deficiency or acquired weakness of this muscular supporting framework, with relaxation and widening of the outlets, leads to inadequate support and ultimately to herniation of the pelvic viscera through the pelvic floor (See Fig. 19-1).

Perineal Musculature. The superficial muscles of the perineum (ischiocavernosus, bulbocavernosus, and superficial and deep transverse perineal muscles) together with the external anal sphincter and the mus-

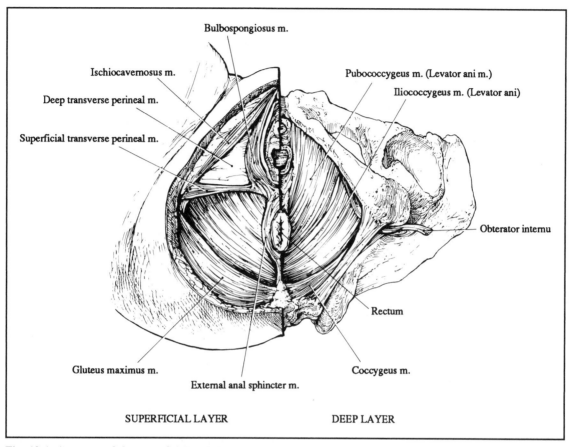

Bulbospongiosus m.

Ischiocavernosus m.

Deep transverse perineal m.

Superficial transverse perineal m.

Pubococcygeus m. (Levator ani m.)

Iliococcygeus m. (Levator ani)

Obterator internu

Rectum

Gluteus maximus m.

External anal sphincter m.

Coccygeus m.

SUPERFICIAL LAYER   DEEP LAYER

Fig. 19-1. Anatomy of the superficial and deep components of the pelvic diaphragm.

culofascial tissues of the urogenital diaphragm form a second supporting mechanism that is less important for pelvic support than the levator sling. This second line of defense against the forces tending to produce pelvic descent is considerably less effective and rarely if ever prevents eventual herniation of the uterus, bladder, or rectum once the supports of the levator complex have been seriously weakened.

Uterine Ligaments and Endopelvic Fascia. Two pairs of intrinsic uterine ligaments (uterosacral and round ligaments) normally help support the uterus, although they do not actually hold the uterus up against the forces that tend to push it down. They function, rather,

to keep the uterus in proper alignment with the vaginal canal, which passes obliquely through the muscular pelvic floor. The uterosacral ligaments are the most important factor here, as they hold the cervix firmly posteriorly, with the result that the uterus remains perpendicular to the axis of the vaginal canal and positioned over the thick muscular plate of the levator sling. This muscular plate can therefore oppose the forces tending to drive the uterus down and out of the pelvis through the weak spot of the vaginal canal and its surrounding muscular outlet. The round ligaments make a slight contribution to this mechanism by pulling the uterus forward into optimal position, but they are so elastic and easily stretched (as during pregnancy) that they play a relatively minor role. If the uterosacral ligaments are weak and attenuated, either congenitally or through acquired injuries, downward forces cause the cervix to ride forward and the axis of the uterus comes to rest directly over the vaginal canal. The uterus then acts like a piston or wedge when downward forces come into play and gradually further dilates the aperture of what is usually by now an already stretched and weakened levator sling. Uterine prolapse and other forms of pelvic relaxation then begin to develop. The broad ligaments play no real supporting role and are not true ligaments in the generally accepted sense of the word.

The "cardinal ligaments" are actually composed of blood vessels and lymphatic channels traveling between the pelvic walls and the uterus at the level of the cervix. They gain their supportive strength (which is often considerable) by virtue of the condensation of areolar and fibrous tissue around them, the "endopelvic fascia," which is reflected from the pelvic walls medially along all the vascular, muscular, and peritoneal tissue planes running toward the central pelvic viscera. (The term "fascia" is used rather loosely, as nowhere in the pelvis is there grossly or histologically any fascia in the true sense of the word, except in the case of the true muscle fascia, which covers the striated muscles of the pelvic floor.) The cardinal ligaments are actually only the thickest, strongest, and most anterior sections of wider vascular "webs" that bring the blood and lymphatic supply from the main vessels along each pelvic sidewall and run medially to the central pelvic organs. They may maintain support for the uterine fundus for a time even in the face of a markedly weakened levator sling. (In this situation the cervix, which is poorly supported below the level of the cardinal ligaments, often becomes markedly elongated.) Ultimately, however, the cardinal ligaments also give way, with the development of a prolapse of the uterine fundus as well once the fundamental support of the levator sling has been impaired.

Pelvic Relaxation and Abnormalities of Visceral Support

The following forms of pelvic relaxation may develop largely as the result of weight-bearing during pregnancy and the trauma of delivery through the pelvic floor (levator sling and the perineal musculature). The normal weight-bearing of abdominal contents and the stress of increased intraabdominal pressure (lifting, coughing, laughing) also stretches the pelvic support over time. Finally, withdrawal of estrogen, as during menopause, causes weakened pelvic tissues. Each form of pelvic relaxation is a recognizable entity, but several may, and often do, exist together in one patient and may require simultaneous correction. Impaired pelvic support is uncommon in nulliparous women, although a combination of congenitally weak musculature, menopause, and subsequent atrophy may produce a simple prolapse or cystocele even in a virginal woman.

Uterine Prolapse. Prolapse of the uterus through the pelvic floor and vaginal outlet is traditionally rated in three degrees (Fig. 19-2).

First degree prolapse: the cervix descends to the introitus
Second degree prolapse: the cervix protrudes through the introitus
Third degree prolapse (total procidentia): the entire uterus protrudes through the vaginal outlet

Symptoms are due to mechanical discomfort and inconvenience as well as to the irritation of the exposed cervix and vaginal walls. In its early stages prolapse sometimes consists almost entirely of a markedly elongated cervix: It may be 5 to 10 cm in length, in contrast to the normal length of 3 cm. The protruding cervix and vaginal walls may become eroded owing to chronic abrasion leading to vaginal discharge and bleeding. Prolapse is frequently accompanied by marked perineal relaxation, cystocele, rectocele, and often enterocele as well (Fig. 19-3).

Although the ideal treatment of uterine prolapse is surgical, conservative management (as with a pessary) is indicated in certain patients (Fig. 19-4). The various forms of treatment are listed in general order of preference. Details of the operative procedures are discussed in the references listed at the end of the chapter.

SURGICAL TREATMENT. The most effective and reliable method of correcting the problem of uterine prolapse and the frequently coexisting problems of cysto-

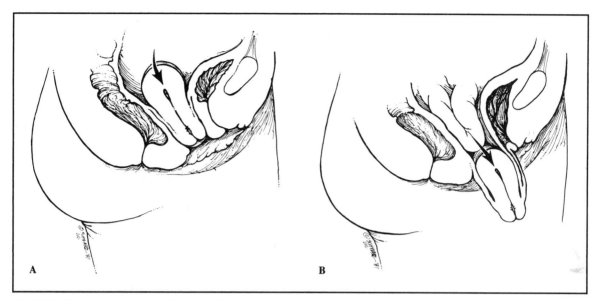

Fig. 19-2. Uterine prolapse. A. Descent of the uterus and cervix to the introitus is designated first degree prolapse. B. Complete prolapse of the cervix and uterus beyond the introitus is third degree prolapse.

cele, rectocele, and weakness of the levator sling and perineum is *vaginal hysterectomy with simultaneous anterior and posterior colporrhaphy.* After hysterectomy, skillful "reconstruction" of lost pelvic support by obliterating the posterior cul-de-sac, incorporating the uterosacral and cardinal ligaments into the vaginal cuff, and plicating the stretched endopelvic fascia and the levator and perineal muscles usually yields excellent results in terms of restoration of normal anatomic support. It also allows preservation (and sometimes improvement) of normal vaginal function and provides relief from secondary bowel or bladder dysfunction.

Two other operations are discussed briefly for historical completeness, although they are rarely performed today. Their main advantage was shortened operating time during an era of less adequate anesthesia and postoperative medical management.

The *Manchester (Fothergill) operation* involves amputation of the cervix with combined anterior and posterior colporrhaphy. Although originally designed during the nineteenth century as an operation that would preserve childbearing ability, the damage done to reproductive function by cervical amputation is

enormous. The main indication for this procedure appears to have been rapid operation in a patient unable to tolerate more prolonged surgery.

The *LeFort operation* (partial vaginal closure) is one of the most rapidly performed operations for the cure of prolapse. It involves removing a long rectangular strip of mucosa from the anterior and posterior vaginal walls with subsequent closure of the exposed submucosal and muscular tissues. This technique has the effect of elevating the prolapsed cervix back up into the vagina and burying it behind the vaginal mucosa. Good short-term results can be obtained with this procedure, which should be performed only in patients for whom the operative risk of hysterectomy is great. It can be performed only on postmenopausal women (because it precludes the flow of menstrual blood); moreover, because it results in marked closure of the vagina, it should not be performed on a sexually active woman without an extensive discussion of its coital consequences. It has the further disadvantage of burying the uterus behind an obliterated vaginal canal, which creates serious problems should a uterine malignancy develop in the future. Performance of this operation should be preceded by obtaining adequate cervical material for cytologic study and samples of the endometrium to rule out the possibility of malignant disease.

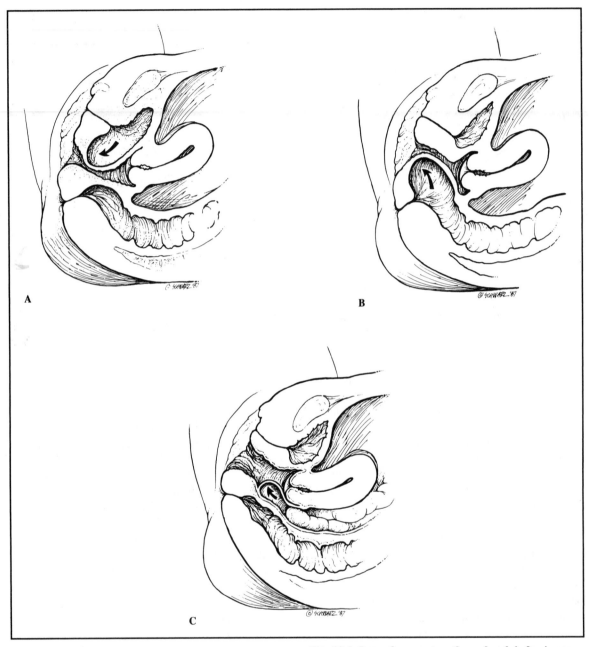

A

B

C

Fig. 19-3. Loss of support on the endopelvic fascia may
result in a cystocele (A), rectocele (B), or enterocele (C).

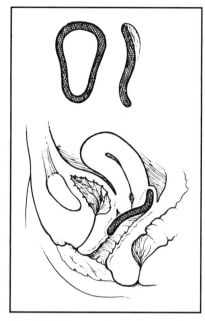

Fig. 19-4. Pessary. Pessaries may be used to relieve symptoms of uterine prolapse, cystocele, or rectocele.

Abdominal uterine suspension procedures for prolapse are mentioned here only to point out their shortcomings and to condemn their use in any but the most exceptional circumstances. None of the uterine suspension operations provides any but the most temporary support, as they do not correct the fundamental weaknesses in the pelvic floor that have led to the problem in the first place. The attempt to use highly elastic structures such as the round ligaments to provide support is doomed to failure, as they rapidly stretch into uselessness and the problem promptly recurs. Even if ventral fixation of the uterine fundus to the anterior abdominal wall is performed, the uterus simply elongates over time owing to lack of support from below, and ultimately the cervix again prolapses through the introitus within a few years. Uterine suspension also does not correct concurrent relaxations such as a cystocele or rectocele.

CONSERVATIVE THERAPY WITH A PESSARY. The use of pessaries in older patients at high risk for complications of surgery is probably preferable to either the LeFort or the Manchester operation. A pessary is fit-

ted into the vagina and usually held in place by its position behind the pubis and the levator plate. The pessary then elevates the cervix and uterus (Fig. 19-4). A pessary is not always effective as it may not be retained if the pelvic floor and perineum are too badly damaged. Neither is a pessary always well tolerated, as discomfort, discharge, and vaginal erosion with bleeding may prevent its continued use. A variety of pessaries are available, and today they are largely constructed of plastic materials that are far superior to the more irritating rubber that was used in the past.

Cystocele. When the normal striated muscular support of the vaginal canal and levator sling is damaged by the widening and stretching that often accompanies repeated childbirth, the vaginal walls and endopelvic fascia also tend to bulge and stretch in response to the constant force of gravity and the increased intermittent stresses of coughing, lifting, straining, defecating, and so on. Marked descent of the anterior vaginal wall and the base of the bladder may ultimately occur, creating a *cystocele* (Fig. 19-3A). If the urethra is also involved in this prolapse, it is termed a *cystourethrocele* (isolated urethroceles are rare).

The chief symptoms associated with a cystocele are the result of mechanical inconvenience, with a sense of insecurity and an uncomfortable bearing-down sensation. Furthermore, poor bladder emptying with residual urine often produces urinary frequency and urgency and may create a stagnant pool of urine in the bladder that becomes a focus of chronic and recurrent urinary tract infection. Stress incontinence of urine may also occur but is *not* a symptom of cystocele alone and may occur in the absence of a cystocele. (Stress incontinence is discussed later in this chapter.)

The primary treatment for cystocele is anterior colporrhaphy combined with posterior colpoperineorrhaphy if indicated for other concurrent relaxations. Occasionally only a pessary is indicated in an elderly high-risk patient who would not tolerate surgery.

Rectocele and Relaxed Perineum. The posterior vaginal wall and underlying rectum also commonly tend to bulge forward and eventually protrude through the vaginal introitus when the pelvic floor and perineal musculature have been weakened and stretched. This condition is called a *rectocele* (Fig. 19-3B). The chief symptoms result from the uncomfortable protrusion of the rectocele and the frequently associated difficulty when emptying the bowel. With a large rectocele, stool accumulates in the hernia and is not funneled down toward the anus as it should be. This situation results in chronic "constipation," incomplete emptying, and prolonged straining during defecation, which serves only to exaggerate the rectocele instead of helping to empty the bowel. Patients may be forced to disimpact their bowels manually or to reduce the rectocele by placing a finger in the vagina to complete a bowel movement.

The treatment of a rectocele and relaxed perineum consists in posterior colporrhaphy and careful repair of the perineum (perineorrhaphy). Special attention must be paid to rebuilding the injured perineal body, which serves as an anchor for the surrounding perineal tissues. Because perineal relaxation is usually marked, conservative treatment with a pessary is rarely successful. If the anal sphincter has been damaged by obstetric trauma, it may be necessary to reconstruct it at the same time.

Enterocele. An *enterocele* is a true hernia occurring in the area between the uterosacral ligaments just posterior to the cervix (Fig. 19-3C). The hernial sac usually contains small bowel, particularly when the patient is standing. The enterocele dissects down through the rectovaginal septum. This hernia may be congenital (a thin-walled, narrow-necked peritoneal sac found in a nullipara) or, more often, acquired through delivery trauma. In the latter case, a large but short, blunt sac is often present. Frequently the hernia remains occult until it is exaggerated by the pelvic-floor injuries of childbirth. It often goes unrecognized owing to failure to consider it as a possibility, and it may be overlooked in the presence of a more obvious uterine prolapse or rectocele. An enterocele may be more obvious after a vaginal operation to cure a rectocele or uterine prolapse when the physician and patient both become aware that a problem is still present. Careful examination of the patient both before and during surgery should prevent this embarrassing situation. The examiner should place a finger in the rectum and thumb in the vagina. The patient then strains (valsalva maneuver), preferably in the standing position. The enterocele, if present, descends into the rectovaginal septum and can be readily felt between the two examining fingers.

Surgical evaluation may also detect an enterocele. The hernial weakness of the enterocele and its accompanying sac can be readily sought at the appropriate site during laparotomy and should be obvious. From the vaginal side the enterocele sac, which lies anterior to the rectum, should be felt during any rectocele or perineal repair. When the peritoneum is first opened during vaginal hysterectomy, the area between the uterosacral ligaments and the anterior wall of the cul-de-sac should be palpated to identify any existing enterocele, which may then be repaired.

The repair of an enterocele follows the same basic principles used for repairing any hernia: careful, complete dissection of the sac; closure of the sac at its neck and amputation of any excess peritoneum; and reinforcement of the closure by approximating available soft tissues surrounding it. It can be accomplished by the abdominal or the vaginal route. Vaginal repair of a huge enterocele may require additional reinforcement by a combined abdominal approach at the same operation.

Total Prolapse of the Vagina. Total vaginal prolapse is a relatively uncommon (but distressing) sequel to progressively increasing uterine prolapse, but more often it is a complication of a previous vaginal hysterectomy. It is almost invariably accompanied by enterocele and often by cystocele.

A number of surgical operations exist for treatment of this unfortunate condition. *Colpocleisis,* or total vaginal obliteration and surgical closure, is an effective, reliable procedure for patients in whom preservation of coital function is not an issue, such as the elderly debilitated patient. Preservation of a functioning (or potentially functioning) vagina, however, may be of importance even to nonsexually active patients; and such wishes should be respected and surgical plans made accordingly, if possible.

There are several operations that can correct vaginal vault prolapse and still preserve sexual functioning. Abdominal *sacral-colpopexy* is a surgical technique whereby the apex of the vagina is suspended to the sacral promontory by use of a fascial or synthetic (e.g., Mersilene mesh) strip. Alternatively, the apex of the vagina may be suspended to either the right or the left sacrospinous ligament using a vaginal approach. The *Zacharin procedure* utilizes a combined vaginal and abdominal approach to plicate the levator muscles, closing the widened levator hiatus and then suturing the apex of the vagina to the reconstructed pelvic diaphragm. All of these procedures have good success rates and have greatly improved the lives of many women suffering from vaginal inversion following a hysterectomy.

URINARY INCONTINENCE

Incontinence is defined as a condition in which involuntary loss of urine is a social or hygienic problem and is objectively demonstrable. Urinary incontinence is frequently, but not invariably, associated with various other forms of pelvic relaxation. The most common type of female urinary incontinence is stress incontinence; but because the differential diagnosis, diagnostic evaluation, and choice of therapy are more complex than for other disorders of pelvic support, it is discussed here in some detail.

The term *stress incontinence* refers to three entities that must be clearly distinguished from one another: a symptom, a sign found at physical examination, and a definitive diagnosis. As a *symptom,* stress incontinence refers only to the patient's statement that she loses urine when undertaking activities that increase intraabdominal pressure (e.g., coughing, sneezing, laughing, lifting, exercising). The *sign* of stress incontinence refers to the objective observation of urine loss from the urethra immediately on such an increase in intraabdominal pressure. As a *diagnosis,* however, "genuine stress incontinence" refers to urine loss due to urethral sphincter incompetence without demonstrable contraction of the bladder detrusor muscle. Making the diagnosis of genuine stress incontinence presupposes that other causes of urinary incontinence have been investigated and excluded.

Because urinary incontinence may arise from different causes that require different treatments, it follows that the incontinence must be meticulously evaluated before embarking on a course of therapy and particularly before performing a major surgical operation to correct it. To understand how urinary incontinence may occur, it is first necessary to understand how urinary continence is maintained.

Mechanism of Urinary Continence

As an involuntary organ under voluntary control, the bladder is one of the most complex and least understood organs in the human body. It has two essential functions: (1) It dilates passively and stores urine, which is continually received from the kidneys via the ureters; and then (2) on command and not before, it expels urine voluntarily at a socially acceptable time and place. Performing this function successfully requires a complex interaction of anatomic, mechanical, and neurologic functions.

At its most rudimentary level, urinary continence is a matter of basic physics. When the pressure in the urethra exceeds the pressure in the bladder, no urine is lost and continence is maintained. When the balance of pressure is greater in the bladder than in the urethra, urine is lost. When loss occurs involuntarily, incontinence results. Numerous factors enter this pressure equation and influence the relative increase or decrease of urethral closure or bladder pressure. The amount of urine the bladder can hold is influenced by the viscoelasticity of the bladder wall. The detrusor muscle, which contracts to empty the bladder upon micturition, must be suppressed during filling and contract only on voluntary command. Bladder sensation must be normal and appropriate for the amount of urine contained in the bladder. The anatomic supports of the bladder neck and urethra must be intact and properly aligned. All of these components must respond appropriately to increased stress to maintain continence, and they must respond appropriately to initiate spontaneous voiding, with relaxation of the urethra, opening of the bladder neck, and adequate sustained contraction of the detrusor to empty the bladder completely.

The bladder neck and urethra are suspended by ligaments attached to the pubic bone and by the levator fascia, which serve to keep them suspended within the abdominal cavity. If these supports become loose or relaxed (as with the strain and trauma of pregnancy and childbirth), the bladder neck may drop below the pelvic floor. Under normal circumstances increases in intraabdominal pressure are transmitted equally to the bladder, bladder neck, and proximal urethra, as all of these structures normally lie within the abdominal cavity. This equal distribution allows the urethral closure pressure to rise as bladder pressure rises, maintaining continence by maintaining the pressure gradient in favor of the urethra. However, if significant damage to the supporting mechanism of these structures has occurred, intraabdominal pressure increases (e.g., coughing, sneezing, lifting) may be transmitted unequally, allowing bladder pressures to exceed the urethral closure pressure with consequent urine loss (Fig. 19-5).

Classification of Urinary Incontinence

Urinary incontinence may occur via two principal pathways: extraurethrally or urethrally. Each must be carefully considered during the evaluation of patients who present with urine loss.

Extraurethral urine loss is found infrequently and often presents as continuous urinary leakage. It occurs through an abnormal opening from the urinary tract to the outside and may be congenital (e.g., bladder extrophy, ectopic ureter) or an acquired fistula (e.g., vesicovaginal fistula, ureterovaginal fistula).

Involuntary loss of urine through the urethra may be due to one of several causes. It is most commonly due to urethral sphincter incompetence (genuine stress incontinence), but it frequently is caused by instability of the detrusor muscle, which can contract involuntarily to cause urinary leakage. The latter may be due to an underlying neuropathy (detrusor hyperreflexia) or can occur on an idiopathic basis in an otherwise neurologically intact patient. Urine loss may occur because of chronic urinary retention with resultant overflow, a urethral diverticulum that stores urine and allows it to drain unexpectedly, congenital lesions (e.g., epispadias), or drug effects on the lower urinary tract. Urinary tract infections can cause marked temporary urgency, frequency, dysuria, and urge incontinence, as can idiopathic disorders of urinary sensation (e.g., "urethral syndrome"). Finally, there are occasional patients who seem to suffer from urinary incontinence due to what can only be described as functional or psychosomatic reasons.

Evaluation of the Incontinent Patient

Clinical Assessment. Urinary incontinence is not a life-threatening condition, and not all incontinence requires major intervention. Most women lose urine occasionally, and it may not be anything more than a passing inconvenience for them. Loss of an occasional drop of urine while playing tennis, for example, is a far different thing than the continued social embarrassment and gradual social isolation that results from repetitive daily urine loss requiring frequent changes of clothing and continuous bathing to remove the smell of stagnant drying urine. To be significant, urinary incontinence must present a social or hygienic problem, or both.

Evaluation of the incontinent woman should begin with a careful history. The exact nature of her com-

Fig. 19-5. Urinary continence and incontinence are related to the transmission of intraabdominal pressure (*arrows*) to the bladder and urethra. A. Urinary continence is maintained by the equal transmission of abdominal pressure to the bladder (V) and the urethra (U) when they are in their proper anatomic locations. B. When the urethra is found underneath the pelvic floor, however, abdominal pressure is transmitted only to the bladder, which can cause a pressure rise that exceeds urethral closure pressure with subsequent urine loss.

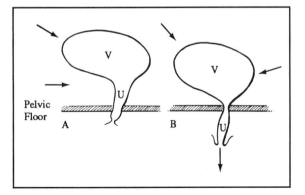

plaint should be carefully detailed and the degree of incapacity it gives her noted. The circumstances surrounding urine loss should be investigated: Does it occur with standing? Is there marked urgency to urinate preceding urine loss? Is urination painful? The frequency of voids should be noted (more than seven times during the day and more than twice at night is considered abnormal). Having the patient keep a "frequency/volume chart" may be especially useful in this regard. Over the period of a few days the patient records all voids and the amounts of urine passed, episodes of urine loss with subjective evaluation of the amount (e.g., "a few drops," "soaked underwear") and a notation of the circumstances under which urine loss occurred (e.g., sneezing, picking up a laundry basket, running tap water at the sink). This method allows objective evaluation of fluid intake, frequency, nocturia, and the pattern of urinary leakage.

Patients with marked urgency, frequency, and urge incontinence are more likely to have detrusor instability than those complaining only of the symptom of stress incontinence, but this statement is only broadly true. Many patients with detrusor instability have uncontrollable bladder contractions triggered by coughing, sneezing, or other stimuli. Careful prospective studies have shown a wide overlap in the presenting symptoms of patients with genuine stress incontinence and incontinence due to detrusor instability.

The obstetric, general medical, and past surgical histories should also be carefully reviewed, with particular attention paid to neurologic disorders, diabetes, psychiatric history, and any previous urologic or gynecologic surgery for correction of urinary incontinence. Any current medications should be carefully detailed, as the number of drugs with side effects on the urinary tract is enormous.

Following the history, a careful general physical examination should be performed, with special attention to the neurologic examination. Although the number of patients with an occult neurologic disorder are few, patients presenting with urinary tract symptoms do have a higher incidence of neuropathy than the general population. Particular attention should be paid to the examination of the lower extremities and the sacral dermatomes involving the anus, buttocks, and posterior thighs. A thorough pelvic examination

should be performed with careful attention paid to the urethra and bladder neck. The bladder should be palpated to check for a large residual urine volume and any evidence of pelvic relaxation that might need simultaneous correction if surgical treatment of incontinence is contemplated. Above all, objective confirmation of urine loss under conditions of stress must be obtained. No woman should undergo incontinence surgery on the basis of her history alone. In addition, all patients should have a urinalysis and urine culture to exclude a urinary tract infection, which should be treated before any further studies or therapy are undertaken.

Specialized Studies. With the history, physical examination, and urine culture completed, patients must undergo specialized studies depending on their clinical picture and presentation. Many investigators have consistently demonstrated that the history alone is an unreliable guide to obtaining the final diagnosis, and some form of objective evaluation of the lower urinary tract is mandatory. Mention has already been made, for example, of the use of *frequency/volume charts* to document urinary frequency and incontinence. A wide variety of special technical studies are available for investigation of the urinary tract. A full review of all of them is beyond the scope of this chapter; however, some discussion of the main procedures available is in order.

Cystoscopy and urethroscopy are important in some patients to exclude intrinsic bladder or urethral pathology as the cause of their disorders. Bladder stones, bladder tumors, interstitial cystitis, and urethral diverticula can be excluded by these studies. Radiographic plain films of the lower abdomen can help evaluate the presence of bladder stones or occult spina bifida as a cause of urinary dysfunction. An *intravenous pyelogram* can be used to help exclude ectopic ureters or damage to the upper urinary tract. All patients with complete uterine procidentia should undergo preoperative intravenous pyelography for this purpose, as pronounced uterine prolapse may pull the bladder down to such a degree that the ureters become kinked bilaterally, with subsequent degeneration of the upper urinary tract. Lateral *bead-chin cystourethrograms* may be of use for evaluating the descent of the bladder neck with stress and the alignment of the urethra and bladder neck to the symphysis pubis. However, previous concepts of the importance of the posterior urethrovesical angle have diminished as our understanding of dynamic bladder physiology has increased. The role of *ultrasonography* in the evaluation of the bladder neck is also currently being explored. *Urethral pressure profilometry* aids in evaluating the integrity of the urethral closure mechanism, and *voiding cystourethrography* under fluoroscopy can provide a dynamic evaluation of the bladder neck, as well as give valuable information on such parameters as ureteric reflux and urethral or bladder diverticula.

CYSTOMETROGRAPHY. The procedure of greatest utility for investigating the urinary tract is *cystometrography.* The cystometrogram is a simple means of evaluating the two principal functions of the bladder: urine storage and urine expulsion. Evaluation of the filling and voiding phases of the bladder cycle provides much information about the integrity of the nervous system and its control of bladder functions. Cystometrography is the only way to definitively diagnose detrusor instability.

A *cystometrogram* is essentially a careful study of the pressure-volume relation that exists in the bladder. As such, the technique necessitates measuring bladder volume and the components that contribute to bladder pressure. Bladder volume is measured by emptying the bladder and filling it at a constant rate with a fluid, usually sterile water. Measuring pressure is more complicated. What is of real interest, physiologically, is knowing the amount of pressure generated within the bladder by the contraction of the detrusor muscle. Because the bladder is an intraabdominal organ, however, another component of bladder pressure is contributed by the surrounding intraabdominal pressure. To differentiate these two components, the pressure in the bladder is measured by a fine bladder catheter and the surrounding abdominal pressure is subtracted to obtain the true detrusor pressure. The abdominal pressure is approximated by measuring rectal pressure with another fine catheter.

TECHNIQUE. Cystometrography is performed in the following manner. The patient first voids and empties her bladder, which may be done on a urine flowmeter to obtain a urine flow rate. A catheter is then passed into the bladder, and the residual urine (if any) is measured. At the same time, another smaller line for measuring intravesical pressure is also passed. A second line is placed in the rectum to measure intraabdominal pressure (Fig. 19-6). The patient's bladder is then filled with sterile water, usually at a rate of 100 ml per minute (patients with a known neuropathy may require a slower filling rate of 10 ml per minute or less). Filling is usually done in a supine or sitting position. The patient is asked to tell the clinician when she feels the first desire to void, and the volume at which it occurs is noted. Bladder filling is then continued until bladder capacity is reached and the patient has her maximum desire to void. She should be comfortably full at this point, not in pain, and the bladder should not be overdistended. The response of the detrusor muscle and the presence or absence of urinary leakage is noted throughout filling.

Provocative tests such as coughing or running tap water in the background may be done and the response of the detrusor noted. At full bladder capacity the patient is asked to stand, and any change in detrusor activity is noted. She is asked to cough once, and the presence or absence of urinary leakage is noted. If no leakage occurs, she is asked to cough vigorously six times and is again observed for urinary leakage or uninhibited detrusor contractions. Other provocative tests such as walking, heel-bouncing, or running tap water may also be undertaken.

After these tests are completed, the patient is asked to sit on a commode attached to a urine flowmeter and is told to void (Fig. 19-7). The flow rate, maximum detrusor pressure, and voiding pattern are recorded, as are the intravesical and rectal pressures. During voiding the patient is asked to stop her urine stream, and the isometric detrustor pressure that results is measured; she then voids to completion, and the residual urine volume is calculated. These studies may be performed using radiographic contrast under fluoroscopic guidance to produce a filling and voiding cystometrogram combined with a radiographic picture of the bladder, bladder neck, and urethra. Normal cystometric findings are given in Table 19-1.

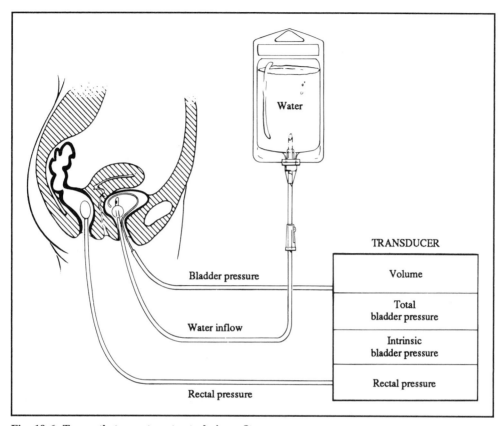

Fig. 19-6. Two-catheter cystometry technique. It records total bladder pressure, rectal pressure, and intrinsic bladder pressure.

Obviously, a great deal of information about normal and abnormal bladder function can be obtained from a cystometrogram. It is beyond the scope of this chapter to discuss this subject in detail. Suffice it to say that the diagnosis of genuine stress incontinence is made when objective evidence of urinary loss is obtained in the absence of detrusor contractions. *Detrusor instability* is diagnosed when the detrusor is shown objectively to contract, either spontaneously or on provocation, during the filling phase while the patient is attempting to inhibit micturition.

INDICATIONS. The principal indication for a cystometrogram (or other urodynamic studies) is to confirm clinical diagnosis using objective measurable data. It is useful when diagnosing the cause of incontinence and is the only test that reliably establishes the presence of detrusor instability (Fig. 19-8). It helps detect potential voiding difficulties in otherwise asymptomatic patients preoperatively and allows the objective assessment of bladder function in patients with known neuropathies. A cystometrogram allows a baseline determination of bladder function to be made prior to radical pelvic surgery or radiation therapy (both of which may adversely affect bladder physiology), and it should routinely be performed as part of the initial evaluation of urinary incontinence prior to corrective surgery—as much, unfortunately, for legal as for medical purposes. The evaluation of bladder function by cystometry is also important for the evaluation of drugs acting on the lower urinary tract and is especially helpful for following the progress of patients being treated pharmacologically for detrusor instabil-

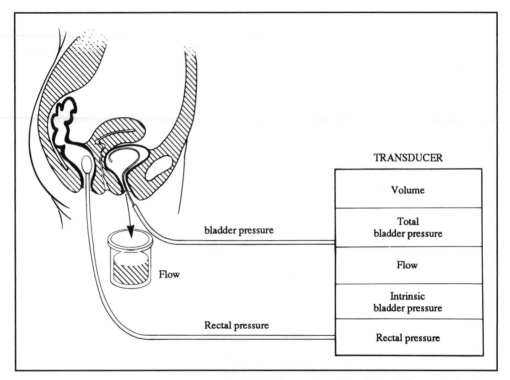

TRANSDUCER

Volume
Total bladder pressure
Flow
Intrinsic bladder pressure
Rectal pressure

bladder pressure

Flow

Rectal pressure

Fig. 19-7. Flow cystometry. Water inflow catheter is removed, and the total bladder pressure, rectal pressure, and flow rate are recorded simultaneously.

Table 19-1. Normal Cystometric Findings

First bladder sensation: 150–200 ml
Bladder capacity: 400–500 ml
Detrusor pressure rise on filling: <15 cm H_2O
No incontinence seen on coughing, straining, etc.
Urine flow rate: >15 ml/second with a minimum volume
  of 150 ml
Detrusor pressure on voiding: >70 cm H_2O
Residual urine: <50 ml
Patient can interrupt urine stream on command

ity. In some cases it is a useful tool for teaching bio-feedback techniques to patients with lower urinary tract symptomatology.

**Surgical Correction of
Genuine Stress Incontinence**

Once the diagnosis of genuine stress incontinence has been made (which presupposes that urinary leakage has been objectively demonstrated and other causes of urinary incontinence, e.g., detrusor instability, have been effectively ruled out), consideration can be given to surgical correction. Because urinary incontinence is not a life-threatening condition, corrective surgery is not always indicated. The decision to perform surgery depends on the patient's general state of health and the degree of social disruption she experiences as a result of her incontinence. If it is decided to proceed with surgical repair, the surgeon must then choose the operation appropriate for the patient.

Perhaps 100 operative procedures have been devised for the correction of urinary incontinence due to urethral sphincter incompetence. It is beyond the scope of this chapter to describe all of them or to provide detailed descriptions of how they are performed; however, a brief survey of the principal operations

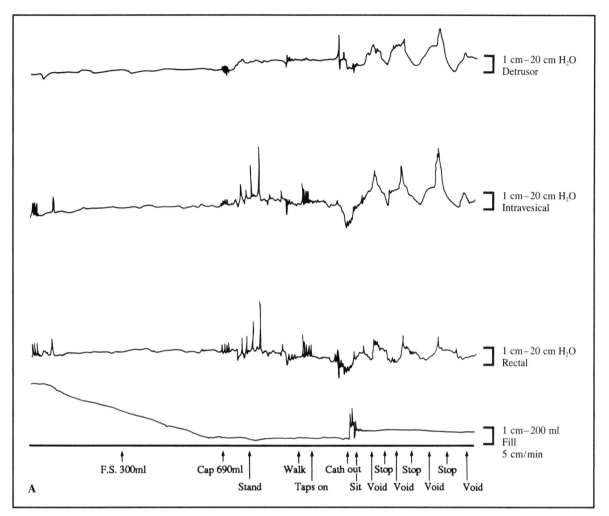

Fig. 19-8. A. Normal twin-channel subtracted systometric tracing.

now in use is appropriate. For more information the interested reader is referred to the Selected Readings at the end of the chapter.

Anterior Colporrhaphy. Anterior colporrhaphy is primarily an operation for the correction of cystocele. It is often used, however, to correct genuine stress incontinence, particularly in patients undergoing vaginal hysterectomy with posterior colporrhaphy for other, associated forms of pelvic relaxation. The op-

eration involves careful dissection of the pubocervical and endopelvic fascia from the anterior vaginal wall, which is then carefully reapproximated in the midline to buttress and elevate the bladder neck. The redundant vaginal mucosa is then excised and closed.

Many surgeons view the use of anterior colporrhaphy for treatment of stress incontinence as controversial. There is a consensus that if all patients were operated on from a retropubic (rather than a vaginal) approach the overall cure rate for stress incontinence would be much higher. However, many surgeons have had excellent results using anterior repair, undoubt-

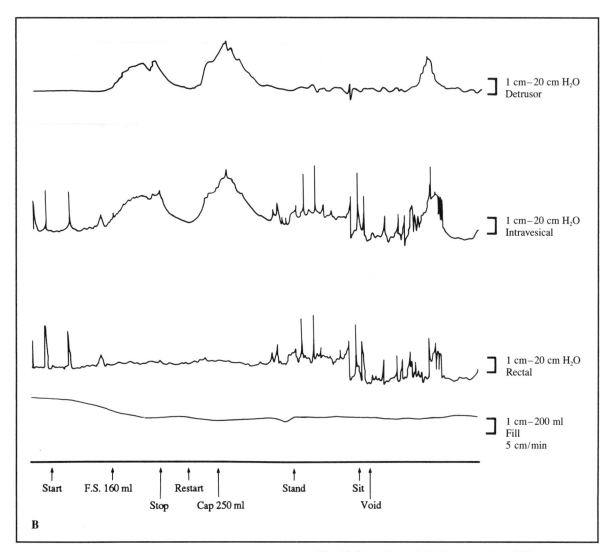

1 cm–20 cm H$_2$O
Detrusor

1 cm–20 cm H$_2$O
Intravesical

1 cm–20 cm H$_2$O
Rectal

1 cm–200 ml
Fill
5 cm/min

↑ Start   ↑ F.S. 160 ml   ↑ Stop   ↑ Restart   ↑ Cap 250 ml   ↑ Stand   ↑↑ Sit Void

B

Fig. 19-8 (continued). B. Detrusor instability is demonstrated on this twin-channel subtracted cystometric tracing.

edly reflecting both careful patient selection and the skill of the operating surgeon. If anterior colporrhaphy is contemplated, there is little doubt that it should be performed as a primary operation only on patients with mild to moderate symptomatology—not on those who have already had a previous anterior repair or a previously unsuccessful operation for incontinence.

Retropubic Operations. An alternative to surgical repair via the vagina is to approach the bladder neck and urethra from above, through retropubic dissection into

the space of Retzius. Retropubic operations for stress incontinence attempt to elevate the bladder neck and proximal urethra by hoisting these structures up and attaching them to or suspending them from more solid anatomic structures, such as the symphysis pubis. These procedures offer stronger structural foundations for repair than anterior colporrhaphy, which attempts to push the bladder neck up from below by plication of the pubocervical and endopelvic fascia,

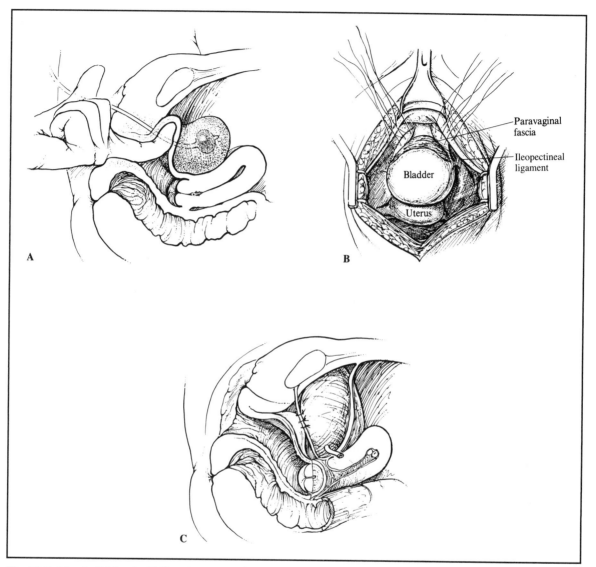

Fig. 19-9. Marshall-Marchetti-Krantz cystourethropexy. A. Note the elevation of the anterior vaginal wall lateral to the urethra and base of the bladder. B. Sutures are placed in the paravaginal fascia and il- **iopectineal ligament but are not yet tied. C. With the sutures tied, the bladder neck and bladder base are elevated on a shelf of paravaginal tissue, thereby restoring the urethrovesicle angle and urinary continence.**

which is subject to recurrent weakening and relaxation. Several varieties of retropubic suspensory operations have been described.

The *Marshall-Marchetti-Krantz cystourethropexy* (Fig. 19-9) is an effective operation for correction of

genuine stress incontinence. It involves dissection into the space of Retzius from above to expose the bladder neck, urethra, and endopelvic fascia overlying the anterior vagina. Sutures are then placed on either side of the proximal urethra through the endopelvic fascia and passed through the periosteum of the pubic symphysis to elevate the urethra and urethrovesical junction. A high success rate (around 80 percent) can be achieved with this operation, but it cannot effectively correct a coexistent cystocele. In addition, osteitis pubis from the sutures placed in the pubic symphysis complicate approximately 5 percent of cases.

The *colposuspension operation* first described by Burch and subsequently modified by others has become the most widespread and best studied operation for genuine stress incontinence. Like the Marshall-Marchetti-Krantz operation, it involves careful dissection of the space of Retzius underneath the pubic symphysis to expose the bladder neck, urethra, and paravaginal endopelvic fascia. With this operation, however, the sutures are placed through the paravaginal tissues along the lateral edges of the bladder down to the bladder neck and then sutured to the iliopectineal ligaments (Cooper's ligaments) along the back of the pubic symphysis. When tied down, these sutures elevate the lateral vaginal fornices to create a "hammock" for the bladder neck and urethra in a high position behind the pubic arch. The long-term success rate for this operation is in excess of 80 percent. This operation has the further advantage that it can correct a coexistent cystocele.

Surgeons undertaking colposuspension should ensure that the patient's vagina possesses adequate capacity and mobility to allow approximation of the lateral vaginal fornices to Cooper's ligaments. This requirement can be assessed preoperatively by a vaginal examination in which the examining fingers are spread laterally and elevated toward the iliopectineal line on either side. Because marked elevation of the anterior vaginal wall occurs with the colposuspension operation, any concurrent rectocele or enterocele should be repaired simultaneously, as it may otherwise worsen under the increased anterior tension created by vaginal elevation.

A variety of procedures combined with endoscopic observation have also been developed for elevating the bladder neck. With these procedures incisions are made in the abdomen and anterior vaginal wall, and needles carrying permanent suture are passed through the tissues on each side of the bladder neck. A small

buttress of either Dacron or Silastic is threaded on the suture, which is then passed back through the tissues lateral to the bladder neck. When the sutures are tied to the rectus fascia, the bladder neck is elevated to restore continence. The patient is cystoscoped to ensure that no sutures have been passed through the bladder. The main difficulties of the operation are the avoidance of penetrating the bladder with the long needles (multiple passes may be necessary to ensure correct placement) and knowing how tight to tie the sutures.

Sling Procedure. Nothing is more discouraging for the surgeon and the patient than the development of recurrent urinary incontinence after an attempt at surgical repair. Whereas an anterior colporrhaphy should not be attempted after a previous failed operation, a Marshall-Marchetti-Krantz operation or a colposuspension may be successful.

A more complicated but highly effective operation, particularly for recurrent incontinence, is a *urethrovesical sling procedure.* Many variations of this operation have been developed, but the underlying principle is the same—to provide a sling of artificial or natural material to support the urethra and bladder neck in the face of pronounced pelvic floor weakness. Many materials have been used: pyramidalis muscle, round ligament, rectus fascia, fascia lata obtained from the thigh, Mersilene, or Silastic. The procedures involve creating a tunnel under the bladder neck and then passing the sling material through this tunnel and attaching it to the rectus fascia or iliopectineal ligaments to provide the necessary elevation and support (Fig. 19-10). These operations are often complex and frequently require a combined abdominal and vaginal surgical approach. The most difficult aspect of a sling operation is determining how much tension to place on the sling, and as yet there is no objective way of determining the tension; it remains part of the art of gynecologic surgery.

Patients with genuine stress incontinence who have undergone multiple unsuccessful surgeries to correct their problem may end up with a scarred and functionless "drainpipe" urethra that leaks nearly continuously. These patients may be best served by surgery to occlude the urethra and drain the bladder with a permanent indwelling suprapubic catheter, by continent

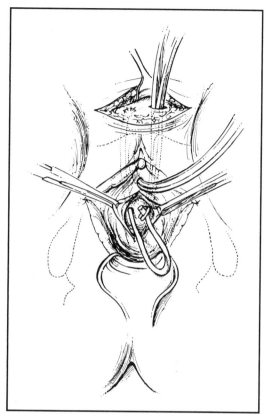

Fig. 19-10. Fascia lata sling cystourethropexy. The fascia lata strap is passed underneath the urethra and then retropubically. The strap has been anchored to the rectus fascia on the patient's right side. After the strap is drawn under the urethra and up to the left side, the tension is adjusted and the strap sutured to the left side.

urinary diversion such as an ileal conduit, or, more attractively, by implantation of an artificial urinary sphincter. Developments in prosthetic materials and implantation technology have made such implants an excellent therapeutic option in selected, severely incontinent patients.

Nonsurgical Treatment of Urinary Incontinence

Because urinary incontinence is not a life-threatening condition and the degree of incapacitation varies greatly from patient to patient, not all women need or desire surgery to improve their condition. Special exercises of the pubococcygeal muscles (*Kegel exercises*) help restore tone to the levator complex and may be the only therapy necessary in mild cases of genuine stress incontinence. Other exercises are also available, including the use of progressively weighted vaginal cones to build up muscle tone. Mild stress incontinence may be helped by sympathomimetic drugs that increase urinary sphincter resistance, such as ephedrine or phenylpropanolamine (α-adrenergic agonists); and estrogen cream helps restore tissue integrity in postmenopausal women with severe vaginal and urethral atrophy. A variety of electric stimulating devices are available that can increase the tone of the muscle groups important for maintaining urinary continence. In elderly women, stress incontinence and cystocele occasionally are managed with the use of a vaginal pessary. In all cases the fundamental guiding principles remain the same: a careful history to ascertain the nature of the patient's complaint and the extent to which it incapacitates her followed by a thorough and objective evaluation of her physical condition and bladder function. Only when these steps have been accomplished can the appropriate therapy be prescribed for the patient's individual needs.

SELECTED READINGS

Abrams, P., Feneley, R., and Torrens, M. *Urodynamics.* New York: Springer-Verlag, 1983.

Addison, W. A., Livengood, C. H., III, Sutton, G. P., and Parker, R. T. Abdominal sacral colpopexy using Mersilene mesh in the retroperitoneal position in the management of posthysterectomy vaginal vault prolapse and enterocele. *Am. J. Obstet. Gynecol.* 59:140, 1985.

Bates, C. P., Loose, H, and Stanton, S. L. The objective study of incontinence after repair operations. *Surg. Gynecol. Obstet.* 136:17, 1973.

Beck, R. P., and McCormick, S., Treatment of urinary stress incontinence with anterior colporrhaphy. *Obstet. Gynecol.* 59:269, 1982.

Beecham, C. T. Classification of vaginal relaxation. *Am. J. Obstet. Gynecol.* 136:957, 1980.

Burch, J. Urethrovaginal fixation to Cooper's ligament for correction of stress incontinence, cystocele and prolapse. *Am. J. Obstet. Gynecol.* 81:281, 1961.

Cardozo, L., and Stanton, S. L. Genuine stress incontinence and detrusor instability: a review of 200 patients. *Br. J. Obstet. Gynaecol.* 87:184, 1980.

DeLancey, J. O. L. Correlative study of paraurethral anatomy. *Obstet. Gynecol.* 68:91, 1986.

Donovan, M. G., Barrett, D. M., and Furlow, W. L. Use of the artificial urinary sphincter in the management of severe incontinence in females. *Surg. Gynecol. Obstet.* 161:17, 1985.

Enhorning, G. Simultaneous recording of intravesical and intra-urethral pressure: a study on urethreal closure in normal and stress incontinent women. *Acta Chir. Scand.* [*Suppl.*] 276:4, 1961.

Green, T. H., Jr. Urinary stress incontinence: differential diagnosis, pathophysiology and management. *Am. J. Obstet. Gynecol.* 122:368, 1975.

Marshall, V. F., Marchetti, A. A., and Krantz, K. E. The correction of stress incontinence by simple vesicourethral suspension. *Surg. Gynecol. Obstet.* 88:509, 1949.

Nichols, D. H. Sacrospinous fixation for massive eversion of the vagina. *Am. J. Obstet. Gynecol.* 142:901, 1982.

Parker, R. T., Addison, W. A., and Wilson, C. J. Fascia lata urethrovesical suspension for recurrent stress urinary incontinence. *Am. J. Obstet. Gynecol.* 135:843, 1979.

Porges, R. F. Changing indications for vaginal hysterectomy. *Am. J. Obstet. Gynecol.* 136:153, 1980.

Ridley, J. H. Evaluation of the colpocleisis operation: a report of fifty-eight cases. *Am. J. Obstet. Gynecol.* 113:1114, 1972.

Stamey, T. A. Endoscopic suspension of the vesical neck for urinary incontinence. *Surg. Gynecol. Obstet.* 136:547, 1973.

Stanton, S. L. (ed.), *Clinical Gynecologic Urology.* St. Louis: Mosby, 1984.

Stanton, S. L. Stress incontinence: why and how operations work. *Urol. Clin. North Am.* 12:279, 1985.

Stanton, S. L., and Cardozo, L. A comparison of vaginal and suprapubic surgery in the correction of incontinence due to urethral sphincter incompetence. *Br. J. Urol.* 51:497, 1979.

Stanton, S. L., and Tanagho, E. A. (eds.), *Surgery of Female Incontinence* (2nd ed.). New York: Springer-Verlag, 1986.

Ulfelder, H. The mechanism of pelvic support in women: deductions from a study of the comparative anatomy and physiology of the structures involved. *Am. J. Obstet. Gynecol.* 72:856, 1956.

Zacharin, R. F. Pulsion enterocele: review of functional anatomy of the pelvic floor. *Obstet. Gynecol.* 55:135, 1980.

Zacharin, R. F., and Hamilton, N. T. Pulsion enterocele: long-term results of an abdominoperineal technique. *Obstet. Gynecol.* 55:141, 1980.

20

Sexual Assault and Rape

Charles R. B. Beckmann

Sexual assault is the nonconsensual performance by one person upon another of acts that in a consensual setting would be sexual or that involve genital structures in such a manner that the victim perceives a sexual intrusion. Threatened or actual violence is always an important part of the assault and is coupled with a sense of loss of control. This lack of control is the most serious immediate emotional problem faced by the victim of sexual assault. Although life-threatening trauma is uncommon, minor trauma is seen in perhaps one-fourth of victims. Pregnancy ensues in about 5 percent of fertile female victims.

A sexual assault occurs every 1 to 10 minutes in the United States. One in every four women and children and an unknown number of men are victims of sexual assault. Because of the stigmas associated with sexual assault, it is believed that only one in every ten victims seeks help from anyone. Those victims who do seek help often find themselves as traumatized by those from whom they seek help as from those who assaulted them.

ADULT VICTIMS

Initial Treatment

Because neither physicians, nurses, social workers, nor any other professionals have all the skills and knowledge needed to provide the total care required by a victim of sexual assault, a multidisciplinary team approach that involves the use of prepared care protocols is the best organization for care. At the time of initial treatment, three tasks are especially important: *caring for the victim's emotional needs, medical evaluation and treatment, and collection of forensic specimens.*

On arrival at the hospital or other health care setting, the victim is taken to a private area where a supportive member of the health care team remains with her. Using a supportive, nonjudgmental manner, this person encourages the patient to talk about the assault and her feelings, thus starting the patient's emotional care as well as the history-taking that is needed. If the patient sustained life-threatening trauma, appropriate emergency treatment is instituted. If such emergency care is required, it is important to tell the patient why there is a rush and to obtain as much of a consent as is practical or possible. Even in life-threatening situations, any sense of "control" that can be given the patient is helpful. Obtaining consent for treatment initially and at pivotal times during her care (e.g., before the pelvic examination or prior to taking the history of the assault) is important. Returning this particular control to the patient is the key to starting the patient's returning sense of control. For adults, it includes deciding whether to cooperate with the police. Patients are often reticent to do so but should be gently encouraged to work with the police, as such cooperation is clearly associated with improved emotional outcomes for victims. This initial police contact should usually be limited, with a more detailed discussion after the victim has completed her initial medical care.

History

History-taking is difficult in cases of sexual assault, for both the victim and the members of the care team who obtain and record the information. The process should not, however, be an additional trauma. Instead, it is both a necessary activity to gain medical and forensic information and an important therapeutic activity.

By recalling the details of the assault in the warm, supportive environment of the care setting, the victim begins to understand what has happened, that she can deal with the events, and, importantly, that others do not shun her because she is the victim of a violent crime. Victims of sexual assault characteristically perceive themselves as guilty of causing the assault, especially in situations where they have used poor judgment, e.g., hitch hiking. To say that the activity was acceptable when it was poor judgment is a lie that destroys the patient's ultimate trust and the care provider's credibility. Instead, it is well to remind the patient that "poor judgment is not a rapable offense," which helps the patient to start to place blame where it truly belongs.

All care team members obtaining information should record their findings in a concise and legible manner, signing and dating every page of the record on which they work. It is controversial whether this information should be recorded as a summary of the victim's statements and a professional evaluation of the victim's feelings or as a series of direct quotations from the patient. Professional summaries may be viewed as valid and useful or as "colored" with the professional's interpretations. It is unclear which approach is best, although this author recommends professional summaries. Table 20-1 reviews the information that should be obtained and some specific interventions based on positive responses to specific questions.

Table 20-1. History: Information To Be Obtained and Kept in the Patient's Record

1. **General information.**
   a. Date and time of assault.
   b. Place where assault occurred (e.g., at home, at work).
   c. Identity, sex, race, and relationship to patient of assailant(s) if known.
   d. How did the patient present for care? How did patient arrive? Was patient accompanied? If so, by whom? What is their relationship to the patient? How much time elapsed from the incident to her presentation for care?
   e. Does the patient wish anyone called? If so, it should be done. If not, the patient should be gently encouraged to select someone to call so she does not leave alone.
   f. Does the patient have any immediate concerns about someone else's welfare (e.g., family, children)? If so, these concerns should be communicated to appropriate authorities and documented in the record.
2. **Specific information about the assault.** *A description of what happened before, during, and after the assault must be elicited in as much detail as possible.* Specific questions should be asked to help the patient talk about the assault and to remember what happened. Such questions include the following.
   a. Was she hit, strangled or choked, abused with a foreign object (if so, what and how?)? Bound? Forced to take drugs or alcohol?
   b. Where did the assailant make contact with the victim and with what? Questions must be asked about each anatomic area of the victim.
   c. Since the assault, has she washed her face, hands, body, or genitals, including douching? Has she applied makeup or changed clothes since the assault?
   d. Has she been unconscious—during or after the assault? Did she use any drugs, medications, or alcohol before the assault or afterward?
3. **Medical and sexual history.** A medical and sexual history must be obtained, including the following information.
   a. *Medical history,* including allergies, major medical problems, current medications, history of previous sexually transmitted disease, and previous hospitalizations and surgery. *Obstetric and gynecologic history,* including menarche, LMP and PMP, number of pregnancies, abortions, or miscarriages. If the patient thinks she is pregnant, her EGA should be calculated. A contraceptive history should be taken if appropriate.
   b. The *sexual history* is taken to provide specific information needed for her medical management and for forensic purposes. It is important to explain these reasons to the patient so she does not make assumptions about a pejorative intent in the questions. Information that should be obtained includes the following.
      (1) If the victim had been sexually active within one week before the assault or afterward.
      (2) If the patient had been a victim before, and if so when and how.
      (3) If the patient has frequented prostitutes or been prostituted.
      (4) If any of the victim's sexual contacts belong to groups identified as at high risk for HIV (AIDS) virus infection (drug users, those who have required multiple blood product transfusions, those of Haitian or African background, male or female prostitutes, gay or lesbian life style).

Physical Examination

A complete physical examination, including pelvic examination, collection of forensic specimens, and culturing for sexually transmitted diseases, is required. It has been suggested that a female physician is preferable for this examination, but in fact the sex of the physician is unimportant compared to the requirement that the physician be warm and empathetic. It may be argued, in fact, that an empathetic male physician is of benefit to help the patient regain control of her interpersonal skills with a nonthreatening, supportive man. Table 20-2 lists the procedures that should be performed and those that may be performed if clinically indicated.

Testing for the HIV virus is a difficult issue. Although single-coitus transmission of the AIDS virus is known to be possible, the risk of acquiring the virus during sexual assault is unknown. Until sufficient data are collected to address this question, it is assumed that AIDS can be transmitted during sexual assault just as any other sexually transmitted disease. The risk of transmission of the AIDS virus in this situation, however, should be low compared to the situation of multiple exposures during sequential consensual coital events.

The collection of *forensic specimens* and the "legal entanglements" that may follow are usually a concern to physicians, nurses, and other care team members. It is important to remember that the responsibilities of the care team are primarily good medical and emotional care. Doing these tasks well, following the di-

Table 20-2. Physical Examination and Laboratory Evaluation

1. *General description* of the patient's overall appearance and emotional state.
2. *Physical examination,* including a thorough general physical examination as well as abdominopelvic examinations. Using full-figure front and back diagrams of the body and genital area, draw any lacerations or abrasions and indicate their size. Photographs are especially helpful for forensic purposes if the means to take them are available.
3. The following *laboratory studies* and *forensic specimens* SHOULD be obtained.
   a. Cytopathology smear (Papanicolaou smear) fixed in the usual fashion and not air-dried.
   b. Cultures (*Neisseria gonorrhoeae, Chlamydia, Mycoplasma*) from cervix/vagina and rectum and from oropharynx if clinically indicated.
   c. Wet (saline) preparations may show motile sperm up to 72 hours following an assault, and nonmotile sperm may be seen for several days thereafter. This examination is useful only if correlated with a history of consensual or nonconsensual sexual activity (or both) during the week preceding the assault. The examination is of little value from a forensic standpoint after 72 hours have elapsed from the time of the assault.
   d. Acid phosphatase is present in ejaculate but not normal vaginal fluid. Its presence may be especially useful in the case of an assailant who has had a vasectomy.
   e. RPR.
   f. Pregnancy test for *all* menstrual-age females regardless of contraceptive status, including having had a tubal ligation.
   g. Blood type/Rh.
   h. Gross specimens of blood, dried fluids, and so forth should be saved in labeled bags. If they are on clothes the victim wore at the time of the assault, the clothes should be sent to the laboratory undisturbed.
4. The following *laboratory studies* and *forensic specimens* MAY be obtained where clinically indicated.
   a. CBC.
   b. Hepatitis antigen.
   c. HIV antibody titer.
   d. Urinalysis or urine culture and sensitivity.
   e. Drug and toxicology screen.
   f. Fingernail scrapings.
   g. Pubic hair combings and sample. A sample of the assailant's hair may be caught in the victim's pubic hair and compared to samples of the pubic hair from the assailant and the victim.
   h. Herpes virus cultures.

rections on the forensic specimens kit used in each locality, and carefully documenting their activities fulfills the professionals' social and legal responsibilities. It is important that these specimens be kept in a "chain of evidence," which simply means that the specimens must be kept in someone's possession or control, free of the opportunity for tampering or confusion with another sample, until turned over to a forensic officer.

Medical Management

All adult victims should be offered *antibiotic prophylaxis* after an explanation of the risks and benefits of treatment and withholding treatment while awaiting cultures or clinical signs of infection. Oral tetracycline (500 mg four times a day) or oral doxycycline (100 mg twice daily) for seven days is recommended. For pregnant women or victims allergic to tetracyclines, oral amoxicillin (3 gm in a single dose) plus probenecid (1 gm as a single oral dose), followed by oral erythromycin base (500 mg four times a day for seven days is recommended). In areas with a prevalence rate that is higher than 1 percent for antibiotic-resistant strains of *Neisseria gonorrhoeae,* ceftriaxone (250 mg IM for one dose) followed by doxycycline (100 mg PO b.i.d. for 7 days) is recommended. All victims should be treated for any identified sexually transmitted disease in either the victim or the assailant.

Diethylstilbestrol (DES; 25 mg orally twice a day for five days) or ethinyl estradiol (5 mg orally twice a day for five days) with compazine (10 mg orally every 8 hours) may be given as a *postcoital contraceptive medication.* Because neither is Food and Drug Administration (FDA)-approved for this purpose despite long-standing use, the victim should be told that there is an estimated 5 percent chance of pregnancy for a fertile woman after an assault and a 1 percent failure rate for the postcoital medications that are recommended. Furthermore, these medications are teratogenic, so that a therapeutic abortion is recommended if pregnancy ensues after their use. Some victims choose to take such postcoital medication, whereas others may choose to wait and have an abortion or carry the pregnancy if pregnancy ensues.

Tetanus toxoid is administered if indicated. Of course, any trauma is treated according to the location and severity of the lesions.

Emotional Treatment

Emotional treatment depends on an understanding of the rape trauma syndrome. The reactions to sexual assault, collectively called the *rape trauma syndrome,* begin during the assault at the moment when the victim believes that she cannot escape the situation and has lost control. The syndrome is comprised of three phases.

The *acute phase* of rape trauma syndrome occurs immediately after the disclosure of sexual assault or immediately after the sexual assault itself. In this emotionally volatile state the victim may appear calm or may be tearful and agitated. She may move from one extreme to another, especially if she experiences flashbacks of the assault. Cognitive dysfunction, an inability to think about issues clearly, is a particularly distressing aspect of the acute reaction for victims. She may have difficulties remembering her own medical history and is at times inconsistent in her descriptions. Sensitive, nonjudgmental persistance can assist the victim to reestablish cognitive control. Prior to seeking care, the victim may have performed routine tasks such as shopping or going to the bank. This retreat to routine activities represents an attempt to regain control and should not be misinterpreted as an indication of the severity of the assault. Safety and regaining control over her life are the victim's main emotional needs during this time. The patient should be reassured about her immediate safety and offered as much control over events as is reasonable for her clinical situation. Paradoxically, discussing the sexual assault within a supportive health care environment facilitates a sense of control. Helping the victim with pragmatic concerns such as how to get home (or where to go if home is not an appropriate place) and who to call after she leaves if she has problems or questions are also important.

The "readjustment," or *middle phase,* is a transition time when to outward appearance the patient seems to resolve most issues about the assault. In fact, this resolution usually means a rationalization that she could or should have prevented the assault and unrealistic plans to avoid another assault. This pseudo-resolution eventually breaks down during the *late (re-organization) phase,* which may last a long time as the victim begins to deal with the reality of her victimization. This period is a difficult, painful time, often characterized by drastic changes in lifestyle, friends, and work. Victims benefit from ongoing counseling throughout this period.

Follow-up Treatment

Victims of sexual assault should have some contact, usually a telephone call but sometimes an office visit, *within 24 to 48 hours of their initial treatment.* Immediate physical or emotional problems can be dealt with at this time and the plans for initial follow-up visits reenforced. Gentle questioning by the caller can also evaluate for potentially serious problems the victim may either not recognize or be unable to verbalize because of fear or continued cognitive dysfunction, e.g., suicidal ideation, issues of safety, and vaginal or rectal bleeding.

Victims should be seen *one week* after their initial treatment. At this time their physical and emotional progress is evaluated, and further plans are made. Physical examination is not necessary unless new symptoms are present or laboratory results from the initial evaluation are noted that require reexamination. The next "required" visit is at *six weeks,* when a complete evaluation, including physical examination, repeated cultures for sexually transmitted diseases, and a repeat rapid plasma reagin test (RPR) for syphilis is needed. If the victim is at risk for HIV virus exposure, another visit at 12 to 18 weeks may be indicated for repeat HIV virus titers, although our present understanding of HIV virus infection does not allow an estimate of the risk of exposure of sexual assault victims, nor do we know the best interval for follow-up testing.

Each victim should receive as much counseling and support as is necessary. If no long-term care program is available at the site of initial care, referral should be made to an appropriate local resource, which may in-clude a rape trauma organization, a local mental health agency, or an individual social worker, psychologist, psychiatrist, or gynecologist with special expertise in the psychosocial issues involving sexual assault.

CHILD VICTIMS

When a child is the victim of sexual assault or abuse, special problems arise, not the least of which are the various definitions of childhood and the disparity between these factors and the medical and emotional realities. The National Center for Child Abuse and Neglect defines *anyone under 18 years of age as a child,* yet state and local laws may differ, especially when the child is pregnant and thereby in most localities legally an "adult." Furthermore, it is common to consider a female child as an adult with respect to "gynecologic" matters after menarche. Emotionally, individuals between menarche and 18 years of age vary greatly in their emotional maturity, whereas those under 13 are more often immature in a manner roughly appropriate to their chronologic age.

Matters are further complicated by the dependence of children on their parents and the love they have (or want) from them versus the fact that more than *90 percent of the traumatized children are abused by persons known to the family, most often parents or close relatives.* The abuser has usually offered the child a combination of threats ("Mommy will leave Daddy if you tell, and she will hate you") and enticements ("Doesn't what we do feel good? You don't want it to stop, do you?") leaving them in a conflicted situation.

To deal with this situation and to get to the truth about events, *child victims should always be interviewed apart from parents and family—if possible by interviewers skilled in child interview techniques.* Several interviews are often needed to ascertain what has happened. Although such interviewing and the interpretation of information gained is difficult, one general rule is that a child who displays a knowledge of sexual matters, anatomy, or function beyond that expected for his or her years is likely a victim of sexual abuse. During the interim, it is the responsibility of the care team to determine if the child may safely return home or if the risk of ongoing abuse requires foster home placement or hospitalization. Because *suspected child sexual abuse must be reported to police and child welfare authorities,* they may help in this decision, although responsibility rests with the care team at the time of the initial disclosure.

Physical Examination

The physical examination of adolescent victims is usually little different from that of adults. The examination of younger children is much different, with small children unable to allow much of the examination, especially pelvic and rectal examination. If the history or those physical findings that can be atraumatically obtained indicate the medical need for a complete examination, the examination should be done in the operating room under general anesthesia. Heavy sedation in the outpatient area is dangerous and rarely allows proper examination. Such a determination should be made by an experienced pediatrician in consultation with a gynecologist.

Treatment

Child victims should undergo *antibiotic treatment* if there are signs or symptoms of infection, the assault was by a stranger, or there is evidence the assailant is infected. In addition, the author recommends consideration of treatment of all child victims given the risks of infection on the patient's reproductive future. Such treatment is, of course, preceded by a full explanation of the risks and benefits of treatment and refusing treatment.

For most patients, oral amoxicillin (50 mg per kilogram of body weight as a one-time dose) plus oral probenecid (25 mg per kilogram of body weight to a maximum dose of 1 gm) is adequate therapy. Intramuscular spectinomycin (40 mg per kilogram of body weight) or intramuscular ceftraxone (125 mg as a one time dose) followed by either oral tetracycline or erythromycin (50 mg per kilogram of body weight for seven days) is used for children allergic to penicillin or in geographic areas with a high prevalence of penicillinase-producing or resistant gonococci. Children under eight years of age should not be given tetracycline. Menstrual age children should be offered postcoital medication if they do not have an effective method of contraception (in the same manner as adults). The other medical treatment of children is similar to that of adults.

SELECTED READINGS

Abarbanel, G. Helping victims of rape. *Social Work* 21:478, 1976.

Beckmann, C. R. B. Taking better care of sexual assault victims: a challenge for health professionals. *J. Urban Health* 1298:35, 1983.

Burgess, A., Holstron, G., and Lytle, L. Rape trauma syndrome. *Am. J. Psychiatry* 131:981, 1974.

Finklehor, D. *Child Sexual Abuse: New Theory and Research.* New York: Free Press, 1984.

Fox, S., and Scherl, D. Crisis intervention with victims of rape. *Social Work* 21:27, 1972.

Glaser, J., Hammerschlag, M., and McCormack, W. Sexually transmitted diseases in victims of sexual assault. *N. Engl. J. Med.* 315:625, 1986.

McCombie, S. *The Rape Crisis Intervention Handbook.* New York: Plenum Press, 1980.

Sutherland, S., and Schrel, D. Patterns of response among victims of rape. *Am. J. Orthopsychiatry* 40:503, 1970.

Sgroi, S. *Handbook of Clinical Intervention in Child Sexual Abuse.* Lexington, MA: Lexington Books, 1985.

21

Sexual Function and Dysfunction

John F. Steege

Approximately 40 percent of happily married couples experience some significant sexual dissatisfaction or sexual dysfunction at some point in time. Appropriate gynecologic care can do much to improve this picture, especially when intervention takes place early in the course of a sexual problem. This chapter reviews basic sexual physiology with special emphasis on how it is affected by gynecologic disease processes; also discussed are sexual dysfunctions, how to take a sex history, and office counseling.

SEXUAL PHYSIOLOGY AND DYSFUNCTIONS

Following the historic precedent of Kinsey, Pomeroy, and Martin, William H. Masters and Virginia E. Johnson expanded our understanding of human sexual physiology by their direct observations of sexual response in the laboratory. They described sexual response as consisting of (1) changes in muscle tension and (2) changes in blood flow. The subjective sense of sexual arousal ordinarily follows the same time course as the muscular and vascular changes. These investigators divided the sexual response cycle into four phases: excitement, plateau, orgasm, and resolution.

Helen S. Kaplan added to their work by emphasizing the importance of the desire phase, preceding the physiologic response phase as described by Masters and Johnson. She collapsed the excitement and plateau phases into a single phase (Fig. 21-1). Figures 21-2 and 21-3 describe these phases in sequence. There are no time units on each graph, indicating that the duration of sexual response varies dramatically among individuals, even among different instances in the same

individual, and over the course of a person's lifetime. These phases describe a continuum with indistinct boundaries, but they provide a framework for discussion and a useful scheme for taking a sex history and making clinical decisions about treatment of sexual problems.

Dysfunction can occur during each of the phases of the sexual response cycle. As a rough generalization, the earlier in the response cycle that dysfunction takes place, the more complex may be the personal and relationship factors and the more difficult the dysfunction is to treat. The practicing gynecologist or other physician can often successfully treat problems that appear late in the response cycle; however, the more complex difficulties are usually the province of the mental health specialist.

Desire Phase

"Inhibited sexual desire" refers to the persistent and pervasive absence of fantasy, absence of initiating behaviors, or absence of physiologic arousal in the presence of adequate sexual stimulation. The condition is frequent in both men and women, affecting approximately 40 percent of couples seeking help from sex therapists. Kaplan's work revealed that many individuals in fact do not have totally absent sexual desire; rather, they "turn off" early in the process in response to negative feelings associated with sexual activity, such as fears of intimacy or commitment or specific negative feelings about the partner. In an unfortunately large percentage of cases, such problems stem from long-standing difficulties with relationships in general; or it may be the sequela of experiencing sexual abuse during childhood or sexual assault during adult life.

Careful questioning is needed to distinguish the person who truly has no desire from the person who has somewhat shut off or ignored her own sexual feelings after disappointing or uncomfortable sexual experiences, e.g., dyspareunia or vaginismus. The former problem (disappointment) is more difficult to treat and is almost always best handled by the mental health professional; the latter can be treated by the primary care physician under the right circumstances.

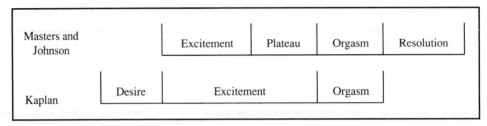

Fig. 21-1. Comparison of the models of sexual response proposed by William H. Masters and Virginia E. Johnson, and by Helen S. Kaplan.

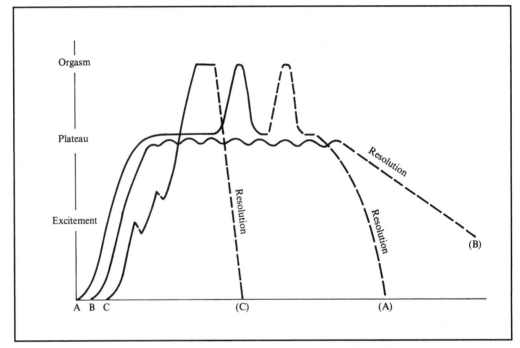

Fig. 21-2. Female sexual response cycle. Patterns A, B, and C may occur at different times in the same individual. Pattern A illustrates the possibility of multiple orgasms. The rapid response of pattern C is more typical with direct clitoral stimulation by self or partner.

Excitement Phase

Vaginal lubrication begins within 20 to 30 seconds of effective stimulation. The moisture produced is a transudate of the vaginal wall, not the product of cervical or introital glands. The rate of lubrication slows somewhat with age, even before menopause, as does the speed of penile erection. As a parasympathetically medicated function, it may be adversely affected by any drug with parasympatholytic side effects. Estrogen is vital to maintaining the vascularity, elasticity, and lubricating capacity of the vagina. Hence women in hypoestrogenic states (breast feeding, menopause, or use of low-estrogen oral contraceptives) complain of vaginal dryness during sexual intercourse (coitus). Some women who cannot (e.g., breast cancer victims) or will not use estrogen replacement ther-

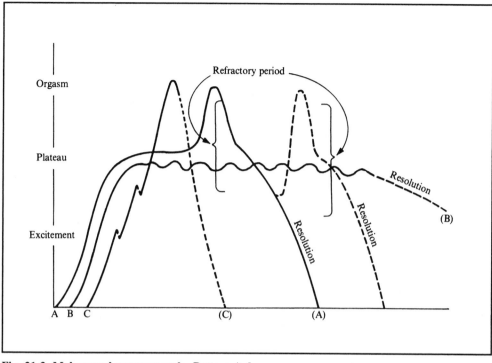

Fig. 21-3. Male sexual response cycle. Pattern A demonstrates the refractory period that must pass before a complete sex response cycle can again occur after orgasm.

apy after menopause maintain a healthy and responsive vaginal lining by means of frequent coitus alone.

Inhibited sexual excitement is marked by the partial or complete failure to attain or maintain the lubrication–swelling response of sexual excitement while engaging in sexual activity that is judged to be adequate in focus, intensity, and duration. Assuming an adequate level of sexual desire, relatively few cases of nonarousal of sexual excitement on a psychogenic basis have been reported in women. Most cases appear due to estrogen deficiency, although any gynecologic condition that causes vaginal or deep pelvic pain can cause inhibition of lubrication despite adequate sexual desire. In some instances, the continued experience of pain can cause the sexual process to be arrested even earlier, during the desire phase.

Orgasm Phase

The subjective sense of reaching a sexual peak, or *orgasm,* is accompanied by wave-like rhythmic contractions beginning at the fundus of the uterus and proceeding caudad. Vaginal and peroneal muscles, as well as the external rectal sphincter, may also contract, all starting 0.8 seconds apart at first, with longer intervals thereafter. Muscle contractions of course occur in skeletal muscle groups in a more variable pattern.

As humans have evolved, personality, culture, and emotions have risen to a position of importance at least equal to that of anatomy and endocrinology in determining sexual response. The capacity for orgasm is enigmatic; it is frustratingly elusive for some, whereas others continue to experience it despite extensive gynecologic surgery, including removal of the entire clitoris and large portions of the upper vagina. An especially sensitive area in the midportion of the anterior vaginal wall along the urethra has been labeled the *Grafenberg spot,* or "G-spot." Although the existence of the sensitive area is becoming less controversial, the anatomic basis for it is disputed. The effect of gynecologic surgical procedures, such as anterior colporrhaphy, on this sensitivity has not been investigated.

The hormonal substrate needed for orgasm is also highly variable. Many women note a decline in the ease of attaining orgasm and a decrease in its intensity with age alone and after menopause. Some with positive sexual experiences and attitudes remain fully responsive despite oophorectomy and in the absence of estrogen replacement therapy. For the average person, however, a certain level of estrogen supply is needed to maintain vaginal elasticity and lubricating capacity, as well as ready orgasmic response. These effects are probably mediated by the ability of estrogen to maintain the vascularity of receptive tissues, as well as its role in maintaining neurologic sensitivity. For the female, dysfunction in this phase is defined as recurrent and persistent inhibition of orgasm following a normal sexual excitement phase during sexual activity that is judged to be adequate in focus, intensity, and duration. This situation means that female sexual functioning is not defined in terms of male events, i.e., the timing of climax relative to the male partner's climax. Many loving and caring women report an enjoyable sexual relationship even though an orgasm is difficult or impossible to achieve. An even larger number may experience orgasm through manual or oral vaginal and clitoral stimulation but are unable to experience it during intercourse in the absence of additional clitoral stimulation. Although behavioral techniques and counseling may facilitate improvement in sexual response, the clinician must always be careful about labeling any particular response pattern as abnormal.

Women who develop difficulty reaching orgasm after years of experiencing a more intense response often are experiencing relationship or marital difficulties that contribute to the inhibition. No particular personality variable has been shown to be related to this difficulty, except for marital "happiness." Paradoxically, women who have never experienced orgasm by any means can, given sufficient motivation, learn to experience it by clitoral stimulation a high percentage of the time. Transferring this response to coitus is a bit more difficult and requires a comfortable emotional relationship with an understanding and cooperative partner.

Functional Vaginismus

The diagnostic label *functional vaginismus* is applied when there is a history of recurrent and persistent involuntary spasm of the muscles of the outer third of the vagina that interferes with intercourse. The condition may be situation-specific: for example, it may be present during sexual activity but not during pelvic examination or vice versa. Vaginismus includes a continuum of symptoms that may range in severity from unconsummated marriage to intercourse that is possible but painful. In an occasional instance, a woman may even experience orgasmic response but still describe painful involuntary introital tightening. This reaction is usually present throughout attempted coitus, although milder versions may be present initially and then disappear as lubrication increases and sexual arousal progresses.

Upon experiencing pain with attempted intercourse, many women become concerned that they may be "built small," i.e., have a congenitally anomalous small vaginal opening. It is important for the clinician to not directly or indirectly support this idea through verbal or nonverbal cues during the interview and examination. True anatomic anomalies of this type occur but are rare. On average, the vaginal tissues are enormously elastic: Witness the ability to deliver an infant's head, often without significant tissue damage. Surgery to enlarge a "small" vaginal opening is therefore to be condemned.

With time, the earliest portions of the sexual response cycle may diminish in the face of continued negative experiences, leading the woman to present as an apparent desire phase problem, even though the problem began with pain. Psychosocial factors associated with vaginismus include negative childhood conditioning to sexual activity and a history of physically or psychologically painful sexual experiences. With the growing recognition of the high prevalence of sexual abuse during childhood, we should expect to obtain this history from a large number of women who have had long-term introital dyspareunia.

Functional Dyspareunia

Functional dyspareunia is defined as recurrent and persistent deep pelvic pain that cannot be attributed to a physical disorder, lack of lubrication, or functional vaginismus. The use of this label obviously implies that a thorough evaluation, usually including diagnostic laparoscopy, has been carried out. A sense of deep pelvic discomfort often described as "bumping" may take place when the cervix or uterus is struck by the erect penis. It is clearly more uncomfortable when the cervix is inflamed (cervicitis, vaginitis) but may also persist as a conditioned pain response even when such inflammatory processes have been appropriately treated and resolved. Sexual response is often inhibited in this instance, diminishing the degree of vaginal expansion and uterine elevation that normally take place during the arousal phase (Fig. 21-4).

Fig. 21-4. Vaginal elongation and transverse expansion during the later excitement (plateau) phase.

DIAGNOSING A SEXUAL PROBLEM

With some practice, a clinically useful history of sexual dysfunction can be obtained in a relatively short period of time. The process is helped by having a format in mind to organize the data (Fig. 21-5). The purpose of taking a sex history varies with the clinical setting. Often there is hesitation to ask about sexual matters for fear that material will be discovered that cannot be adequately dealt with in the time available. Although this premise is often true, obtaining the history can help direct the patient to appropriate medical or counseling help and at the same time can legitimize the patient's concerns as worthy of thoughtful review. We should not underestimate the value of respectful and interested listening.

Introductory Questions

The questions in Table 21-1 may be used to introduce the subject either in the course of a general history if

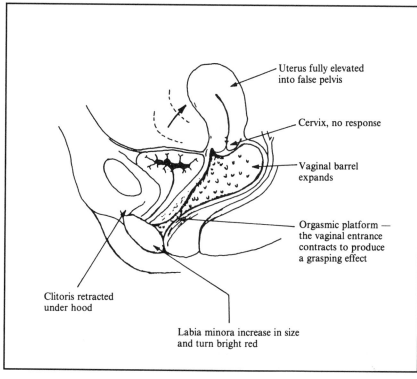

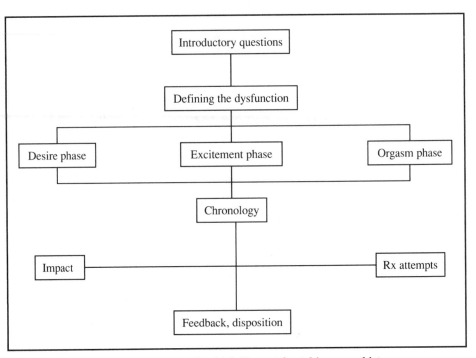

Fig. 21-5. Format for taking a sex history.

Table 21-1. Sex History: Introductory Questions

How are things at home?

How are things sexually? Any discomfort? Any questions or concerns?

How often do you have sex? Is that satisfactory for you?

Is there any way you would like your sexual life to be different (physically or emotionally)?

sexual dysfunction is pertinent to the chief complaint or present illness (e.g., diabetes, heart disease, pelvic surgery) or during a review of systems. The questions are designed to be nonintrusive and open-ended, allowing the opportunity for the patient to share these personal concerns if he or she wishes. If such questions are routinely asked during regular office care, the patient soon understands that the physician regards sexuality as a legitimate part of overall health.

Individuals who want to talk about sexual difficulties offer valuable information in response to these beginning questions. When sorting out the data, the interviewer should try to: (1) define where in the sex-

ual response cycle the process is interrupted; (2) whether the dysfunction has been present throughout a person's lifetime (primary sexual dysfunction) or it began after a period of satisfactory functioning (secondary sexual dysfunction); and (3) whether the dysfunction is constant (present in all situations and with all partners) or situational (present in some instances or with only some partners). Dysfunctions that are of more recent onset are generally more easily treated. Obviously, dysfunctions that are situational are more often psychologically based than organically based. Knowing where in the sexual response cycle progress is interrupted has important meaning when deciding what kind of help is necessary. Specific questions help to define the exact difficulty.

Nonorgasmic Response. The inquiry might begin with a broad question such as: "How do you feel about your own responses during sex?" Or, to be more precise, "Are you able to reach climax?" "How regularly does it occur?" If there is a problem with orgasmic response, it is useful to understand to what factors a woman attributes this difficulty. The next question, then, is "What do you think most influences your response?" Often answers include concerns about the menstrual cycle, emotional factors, pain during intercourse, or simply the timing of sexual encounters.

Female Excitement Phase. If a person is generally nonorgasmic, she should be asked about earlier sexual responses, perhaps: "Do you have positive sexual feelings?" "Can you identify vaginal wetness or lubrication during sex?" "Does the lubrication appear early and disappear, or does it take awhile to appear?"

If lubrication difficulties are clearly present, one must inquire about possible complicating medical factors such as recurrent vaginal or bladder infections and medications such as antidepressants, antibiotics, diuretics, vaginal medications with irritative effects, and vaginal douches. Women who douche frequently find that it relieves an uncomfortable discharge temporarily. However, the vaginal lining often responds with an inflammatory response to the douching compound, leading to a rapidly recurring discharge. Continued vaginal pain and irritation can be present when a woman responds to this pattern by increasing douche frequency.

Finally an open-ended question again is usually productive: "What do you think most influences your sexual arousal?"

Desire Phase. If organic factors inhibiting vaginal lubrication are absent and yet no sexual response is experienced physiologically or subjectively, one must begin to suspect difficulty with the desire phase of sexual response. Questions are then directed as to whether a person currently experiences positive sexual feelings. If such feelings were experienced in the past, an account of when the feelings changed can most often shed light on the intrapersonal or relationship issues causing the problem.

Chronology

As mentioned, the duration of a sexual difficulty has great impact on how difficult it is to solve. Clearly, the person who notices a change and seeks help fairly promptly is often comfortable confronting sexual is-

sues. Complicating relationship difficulties such as accumulated resentment and anger are less of a problem when the dysfunction is of short duration. For example, it has been found that problems of erectile dysfunction, if they have lasted more than five years, are difficult to solve no matter what the relative contributions of the organic and psychological etiologies might be.

Questions that fill in the chronology might include the following: "Is this problem a change from the past, or have things always been this way?" "Does this problem occur all the time or just some of the time?"

When sexual difficulties are sufficient to prompt a person to ask for assistance, the possibility of extramarital affairs has almost always occurred to the patient. It is therefore perfectly appropriate to ask these questions: "Have you considered having sex with someone else to see if it were any different?" "Have you worried that your husband/partner might find someone else?" These questions must be asked in a manner that does not imply you are suggesting a solution but, rather, recognizing that such thoughts and actions are common and would certainly present difficulties that might make a solution more elusive.

Finally, sexual difficulties are rarely the same all of the time. You might therefore ask these questions: "Have there been better times along the way?" "What do you think caused those better times?" "Were there any particular stresses or changes in your life that occurred around the time that things turned for the worse (or better)?" Such life events might include childbirth, illness of one or the other partner, an accident, a job change, death of a family member, or moving. It is useful to know how individuals and couples have coped with such stressful events; in particular, the level of constructive problem-solving and intimacy they demonstrate in these efforts may have direct bearing on their sexual interactions.

Impact

It is obviously useful to know if the sexual difficulty is a matter of mild concern or if it is seen as a serious threat to a person's relationship. One might therefore ask these questions: "How do you think this problem has affected you in general?" "What effect has it had on your relationship?" "How has this effect showed up (fighting, distance, decreased signs of affection in general, anxiety, etc.)?" Finally, the "what if" question is useful: "What do you think will happen to you and to your relationship if this problem cannot be solved?"

EFFORTS AT SOLUTION

Having understood the basic parameters of the problem, it is then useful to know what efforts have been made to fix it. After asking in precise and direct terms what happens sexually between a couple, one might then ask other questions: "What happens when things don't go well for the two of you sexually?" "How do the two of you talk about this problem with each other?" "Have you tried any different sexual techniques to solve the problem?" "Have you read any books or seen any films together that might help?" These questions again should not be asked in a way that implies a specific bias in what *ought* to be done but, rather, as a way of determining the acceptable level of discussion for this particular individual or couple.

There is a final crucial question the primary care physician should ask: "Have you discussed seeing someone about counseling?" Often counseling has been considered by one or the other partner but has not been discussed by the couple because of apprehension about the other person's response. It is often easier to have the idea introduced by a health professional; and the response is often remarkably positive. Even if this notion is not immediately acceptable, opening the discussion at least legitimizes the idea, perhaps allowing appropriate referral in the future.

What to Do Now

It is often said that physicians evaluating emotional problems should not open areas of discussion with which they cannot deal. However, when tactfully and respectfully carried out, it is doubtful that defining the problem as described above can do any damage. Rather, if done in the right way, the patient can be provided with perhaps her first experience at talking about important sexual concerns in a way that respects her feelings and legitimizes their importance. In essence, it can be seen as a "free sample" of what counseling might be like. Even if no immediate solutions appear in the discussion, this comfortable talk with her physician may make it easier for her to seek further help.

At this point in the discussion, a summary of what has been discussed so far may be helpful, with some comforting comments about the ubiquity of sexual difficulties and some fair and legitimate statistics about chances of cure. For example, women with vaginismus can be reassured that with appropriate treatment this disorder can be cured about 80 to 90 percent of the time. Similar statistics might be cited for premature ejaculation, and approximately 70 percent of men with secondary erectile dysfunction can be helped. Men with lifelong (primary) erectile dysfunction have a lower cure rate, about 40 to 50 percent, similar to that seen with even the best care for major desire phase dysfunctions. Female orgasmic response can be learned about 80 to 90 percent of the time, especially by those who have simply never experienced an orgasm by any means. Perhaps ironically, those who have been regularly orgasmic but have lost this response in the context of a particular relationship have a lower cure rate, as relationship factors themselves are most often involved. Of the women who learn to experience orgasm by manual, oral, or other means of stimulation, about half are able to transfer this learned response to intercourse.

At this point in the discussion it is useful then to ask these questions: "Would you like to have the opportunity to talk more about this problem?" "Would you like to talk to someone together with your partner?" "Do you think that some reading material might be of some use to you?" Extensive self-help literature is available and is often useful for problem-solving or at least for promoting appropriate help-seeking.

Office Counseling for Sexual Dysfunctioning

Most physicians learn relatively little about office counseling in the course of their medical school and residency training. The major reason is the frequent rotation among subspecialties during medical school and among different clinical services during a residency training program. However, when the opportunity exists for continuity of care, clinicians are often struck with how often sexual concerns emerge.

A few simple guidelines help the clinician choose individuals who might profit from short-term office counseling. First, individuals should have only a single sexual dysfunction. For example, couples for whom both premature ejaculation and vaginismus are a problem most often require the skills of a qualified mental health professional. Second, dysfunction should have been present for one year or less. Third, careful questioning should reveal that the marriage is relatively stable and that no significant discord has been present. Fourth, the specific dysfunctions of premature ejaculation, female nonorgasmic response, vaginismus, and functional dyspareunia seem to be conditions that lend themselves most readily to office counseling. Conversely, any disorder of long duration, any disorder present in a highly dysfunctional marriage, and any disorder involving a significant desire phase component are far less likely to respond positively to brief office counseling.

The structure of office counseling is of paramount importance. Time limits for office visits should be clearly defined, usually 20 to 30 minutes. The number of visits should be limited, often to three to six visits, and they should occur at regularly scheduled intervals, rather than simply making a new appointment if it appears to be needed at the end of each session. It is important to not allow pelvic examinations to take up part of the counseling time; and finally, the office staff not allow interruptions such as phone calls during the sessions. Although the time intervals seem short, often a remarkable amount can be accomplished when that time is clearly protected.

TREATMENT OF SPECIFIC DISORDERS

Before embarking on counseling, the history, as outlined earlier in the chapter, should be carefully carried out to screen for interfering illnesses and medications that may need treatment or adjustment as well as for affective or other psychiatric disorders that might block progress.

Arousal Phase

Lubrication difficulties may be due to hypoestrogenism, vaginal bacterial imbalance, overgrowth or infection with particular pathogens (e.g., *Trichomonas*), or anxiety. Hypoestrogenic states, e.g., the postpartum period or after menopause, are often associated with vulnerability to vaginal infection as well as diminished intrinsic vaginal lubrication to sexual stimulation. Specific infections should be treated as described in this volume. Vaginal pH often shifts toward neutral from its normal acidic level of approximately pH 4.5 after menopause and in women on oral contraceptives. Restoring vaginal acidity with acidifying vaginal gel often helps maintain bacteriologic homeostasis. Such medications can be used as needed but often can be diminished to once every week or two after an initial, more intense dose schedule. Supplemental lubrication is often useful when dryness is a problem. Water-soluble lubricants such as K-Y Jelly are time-honored but have the liability of drying out when exposed to air for more than a few minutes. This drawback presents problems when couples are finding that they need to take their time to allow significant arousal to occur. In this case, lubrication with an ordinary vegetable oil often works better.

When sexual arousal is slow to occur, couples also often find themselves "waiting" for sufficient lubrication to appear. When it finally does, they frequently shift to either the female-superior or male-superior intercourse position immediately. Psychologically, this move often signals an increased level of demand, which then creates anxiety and shuts off lubrication. The position shown in Figure 21-6 may allow an easier and less anxiety-provoking transition to coitus. The female partner lifts the leg closest to her partner and allows him to take her opposite leg between his two legs. This move allows each partner to rest comfortably, the woman on her back and the man on his side, and allows continued manual clitoral stimulation if it is desired. The degree and depth of vaginal penetration can be controlled by the woman with her legs if verbal cues are not comfortable. At the same time the angle of penile insertion can be controlled by the tilt of the man's body. This position often allows the couple to avoid uncomfortable pressure on an irritated

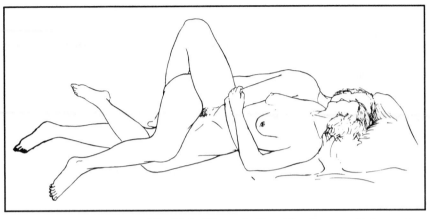

Fig. 21-6. "Crosswise" position for sexual intercourse.

bladder or on tender areas deep inside the pelvis (in the case of a severely retroverted uterus, pelvic inflammatory disease, or endometriosis). The position is also useful during pregnancy and in postoperative women when pressure on the abdomen might be uncomfortable.

During the course of office counseling, one must ask not only what behavioral responses have occurred following these suggestions but also what feelings were present in each partner and how they were shared. When communication seems to be progressing and physiologic improvement is also happening, counseling may legitimately continue. When significant blocks occur in emotional communication, the clinician must then judge if they are within his or her capabilities to handle or if referral should be made. The office counseling process therefore attempts to be therapeutic. However, when it is not, it can at least be diagnostic and pave the way for further work.

Orgasm Phase

The complaint of not being able to experience orgasm during intercourse is a common one for women. Although it happens at least some of the time to perhaps at least half of all women, it is a more pervasive difficulty for approximately 15 percent of women. Those who require additional manual stimulation to have orgasm as part of their intercourse experience can be firmly reassured that it is normal. If they have difficulty dealing with feelings of inhibition or guilt about

incorporating clitoral stimulation, the crosswise position previously described may be helpful by allowing partner stimulation to be added.

If orgasm cannot be experienced under any circumstances, the most effective method of treatment is a program of learning about one's own sexual response through self-stimulation. Self-stimulation to orgasm (masturbation) is routinely practiced by approximately 50 to 75 percent of women, according to various surveys. It is therefore by no means abnormal, although it is difficult for some women to accept. Excellent self-help literature is available if a woman believes this approach is acceptable, and it has been shown to be as effective as group therapy; the latter discusses sexual concerns in a group and assigns self-stimulation practice sessions in the privacy of the home. If self-stimulation is not acceptable, orgasmic response can be learned with a partner. However, this method often requires the skills of a mental health professional, as complex interchanges of feelings are usually involved.

Vaginismus

Treatment of involuntary vaginal introital spasm is well within the capacity of the interested family practitioner, internist, or gynecologist. Again, dysfunctions of a relatively mild or moderate level and of brief duration are readily approached, whereas long-standing vaginismus in the setting of a highly conflicted relationship is best left for the sex therapist.

Therapy begins with an educational pelvic examination. Offer the patient a hand mirror to hold so that she may see the external genitalia and hear the explanation of normal anatomy. During this review, the woman may see for herself the involuntary vaginal introital spasm. The physician then places an index finger in the vagina as comfortably as possible and asks for voluntary contraction and relaxation. This maneuver helps to identify the site of the problem as well as to provide instruction for vaginal relaxation exercises to be prescribed later.

At a psychological level, the most important part of treating vaginismus is to establish a "no pain" contract with the patient, wherein she does not allow pain to occur during examinations and certainly not during any attempts at sexual contact that she may have. The woman is given total control of vaginal events, this control being reinforced as constructive and the only way to resolve the problem. Simply allowing the pain to decrease enough to the point where she can "put up with it" aggravates the problem by reinforcing the conditioned muscular contraction. If the patient, her partner, and her physician are comfortable with this approach, it is often useful to have the male partner present during the examination to visualize the involuntary contraction for himself. It helps him to recognize the problem as something outside the woman's conscious control and therefore not a specific rejection of him as a man or as a partner.

When the examination is completed, instructions may be given for vaginal relaxation exercises to be done at home. To begin, the woman should seek the most comfortable setting for her, which usually means being alone. Perhaps while relaxing in a warm bath or just prior to going to sleep, she should gently place one index finger in the opening of the vagina to a point that is comfortable. She should then voluntarily try to contract and relax the vaginal introital muscles, using the index finger as "feedback" on how well she is able to do it. This muscular skill is often learned fairly quickly, although it may take awhile in an apprehensive patient. Regular daily practice is most productive, but the frequency and duration of the practice sessions should be also completely under the woman's control. She needs to go at her own speed.

When voluntary control is achieved, she can then proceed through a series of steps toward intercourse.

This phase might first involve having her partner present in the room while she does the exercises, then including him in the exercises by having him place his index finger in the vagina, gradually proceeding to intercourse. Intercourse is best approached by her assuming the female superior position or in the crosswise position, which allows her to have control over the depth of penetration. Even at this point, she must remain in control, and the "no pain" contract must be adhered to. Increasing coital motion may then take place only as is comfortable.

In this setting, especially with the female partner being given total control, about 15 percent of men have transient erectile difficulties. Such problems usually resolve spontaneously or with simple reassurance. Obviously, a positive alliance with the office counselor helps a great deal and hence the utility of including the partner in the counseling sessions as much as possible.

Throughout these efforts, it of course remains important to ask not only about the events that are occurring but also about the feelings of both partners concerning those events. When progress is halted or feelings become difficult to manage, appropriate referral should be made. Careful judgment must be used to accomplish this referral, and it should be done before the patient and her partner become too discouraged and see the entire effort as yet another failure.

Deep Dyspareunia

Women often note diminished sex response when sex is painful owing to organic conditions such as cervicitis, endometriosis, or pelvic inflammatory disease. In such cases, vaginal expansion (Fig. 21-4) fails to occur, and tender areas are closer to the vaginal introitus and hence more likely to be painfully stimulated. A vicious cycle of pain—less response—more pain becomes established.

This situation can often be ameliorated by: (1) explaining the phenomenon to the patient and the partner; (2) instructing them in the cross-wise position (Fig. 21-6); and (3) establishing a "no pain" contract between patient and partner. When this contract can be trusted, the sex response may resume and a better adjustment achieved, albeit with some limitations, e.g., shallow vaginal entry in extreme cases of pelvic pathology.

IMPACT OF GYNECOLOGIC SURGERY ON SEXUALITY

Much has been said and written about the effects of removing gynecologic organs on the sexual response. Although the subject remains controversial, there is growing agreement that it may not be fair to offer blanket reassurance to the woman facing hysterectomy. Many gynecologists with an interest in sexual counseling have learned that when a woman identifies uterine contractions as her cue that orgasm has occurred, or if she regards uterine contractions as a major part of the physical response she experiences, that sensation will certainly change when the uterus is removed. Preoperative counseling should explore these issues and should suggest that a woman intentionally focus on other aspects of her orgasmic response as part of her own preparation for surgery. It has traditionally been thought that the uterus and cervix should always be removed when it is surgically necessary to remove both ovaries. However, because the sexual impact of removing the uterus remains debated, this question should be the focus of further research.

Women experience depression more often after hysterectomy than after other abdominal surgery. Decreased libido is often one of the symptoms. Depressed affect may begin soon after surgery, but many times onset is delayed until physical healing has occurred. Unless it becomes sufficiently severe to require medication, the surgeon is often unaware of it as it may start after the usual six-week postoperative examination. Similarly, deep dyspareunia may be present during initial coital attempts owing to tenderness of freshly healed tissues. If vaginal expansion fails to occur because of residual pelvic disease, postoperative scarring, or insufficient sex response, a cycle may begin: pain—poor sex response (absent vaginal expansion)—more pain. Both depression and sex response changes are more likely to occur in women who had no pathologic findings at surgery, have misunderstandings about sexual response, have unsupportive or uninformed partners and families, or who have had previous psychiatric problems with depression or severe anxiety. Appropriate preoperative education and counseling can help alleviate these problems.

SUMMARY

Sexuality is an important part of life and sexual health an important part of health care. Office counseling for sexual difficulties draws on the clinician's best interpersonal skills and sensitivity as well as his or her medical knowledge. Beginning clinicians/counselors should intentionally choose the easiest cases to work with and should not allow patients' intrapersonal or financial pressures to influence them to begin counseling in cases for which they are not qualified. It is an area of health care that will improve with practice and experience, and it can be a rewarding part of clinical practice.

SELECTED READINGS

Andersen, B. L. Primary orgasmic dysfunction: diagnostic considerations and review of treatment. *Psychol. Bull.* 93(1):105, 1983.

Duncan, E. H., and Taylor, H. C. A psychosomatic study of pelvic congestion. *Am. J. Obstet. Gynecol.* 64:1, 1952.

Fordney, D. S. Dyspareunia and vaginismus. *Clin. Obstet. Gynecol.* 21(1):205, 1978.

Kaplan, H. S. *Disorders of Sexual Desire.* New York: Brunner-Mazel, 1979.

Lamont, J. Vaginismus. *Am. J. Obstet. Gynecol.* 131:632, 1978.

Masters, W., and Johnson, V. *Human Sexual Response.* Boston: Little, Brown, 1966.

Masters, W., and Johnson, V. *Human Sexual Inadequacy.* Boston: Little, Brown, 1970.

Sarrel, P. M., Steege, J. F., Maltzer, M., et al. Pain during sex response due to occlusion of the Bartholin's gland duct. *Obstet. Gynecol.* 62:261, 1983.

Steege, J. F. Dyspareunia and vaginismus. *Clin. Obstet. Gynecol.* 27:750, 1984.

22

Contraception

Birth control and population control have been practiced since ancient times. Over the years, a number of methods of varying degrees of effectiveness and acceptance have evolved, including abstinence for long intervals, withdrawal (coitus interruptus), the rhythm method ("safe period"), the condom, special vaginal tampons, immediate postcoital douches, cervical caps, intrauterine stem pessaries, intrauterine rings, vaginal spermicidal jellies, creams, or suppositories, the vaginal diaphragm, and most recently ovulation-inhibiting agents. Some of the older methods that are known to be ineffective and potentially harmful physically and psychologically continue to be used, particularly among underprivileged populations.

Continuing interest in curbing global population growth as well as the need to have both highly effective agents and those that are side effect free or acceptable have produced significant advances in our understanding of the regulation of male as well as female reproductive physiology. Such progress has contributed to the development of new forms of contraception, refinements of current forms of contraception, and treatment of infertility. Additionally, the medical profession is better equipped to provide the best possible advice and methods for planning and restricting family size. Such capability represents an important facet in the overall role that today's physician plays in improving the stability and happiness of marriage and family life among patients.

Fear of unwanted pregnancy or the stresses imposed by the attempt to rear and educate a larger number of children than had been desired or planned for may be the basis for serious marital discord and may result in unhappy, insecure families. The unfortunate end results are all too frequently seen in terms of dis-

abling psychosomatic or emotional disorders and are reflected in the rising incidence of abortion, divorce, and juvenile delinquency.

Information about contraception (including abstinence) should be made readily available to sexually active individuals or those about to embark on their sexual activities, as prevention of unwanted pregnancy is desirable and can reduce the current epidemic of teenage pregnancies as well as the use of abortion. There are considerable variations in acceptance of the methods of contraception by different religious groups, and it is imperative that the physician not impose his or her own religious convictions on medical advice, which should be predicated on scientific foundations. The various options available and their advantages and disadvantages for the particular couple should be freely discussed with them. Birth control has been employed to curb rapid population growth among lesser developed countries and low socioeconomic groups of certain populations allegedly to permit socioeconomic development, but it is important that physicians are not unintentionally swayed into pressuring patients to use a particular form of contraception against their wish.

METHODS OF CONCEPTION CONTROL

In most instances, it is the female partner who seeks contraceptive advice. Because she is fundamentally the one most concerned and the one most likely to carry it out properly and faithfully, the female partner has in the past been made responsible for the couple's contraceptive practice. Today this one-sided approach is slowly giving way to counseling that involves the couple, and many men are undergoing vasectomy. As more advances are made in male contraception, the male partners will have to participate more actively and responsibly in the couple's contraceptive program.

Before prescribing any one method, the couple or the patient should be offered a brief outline of the techniques available, with their advantages and disadvantages and their potential side effects. By supplying this information and answering the patient's questions, the physician can make it easier for the patient to select the program most acceptable to her and her partner. The following sections outline the principal methods currently in use, together with the essential details of their application.

Condoms

Use of the condom by the man is probably the usual method employed, being used by 10 to 20 percent of couples practicing birth control in the United States many of whom never sought advice from a physician or clinic. Simple for the untutored to use, its effectiveness is highly variable (70 to 90 percent protection). If properly used, the effectiveness of condoms should be much higher, closer to 100 percent. Many of the failures are due to careless use, intermittent use, careless removal of the condom containing the ejaculation upon withdrawal, late withdrawal (after penile flaccidity sets in), or having intercourse first and withdrawing, following by completion of the coitus using a condom. In practice, condom use can be physically unsatisfactory or aesthetically unacceptable to many couples. Use of the condom requires motivation on the part of the male partner.

There has been reemphasis and growth in the use of condoms, largely due to the increased incidence of acquired immune deficiency syndrome, which is due to the virus being transmitted through body fluids, most often semen. Attention has been redirected to the protective benefit of condoms and similar barrier contraceptives against acquisition of sexually transmitted diseases. Condoms are available in lubricated and nonlubricated forms. The lubricated condom often has a spermicidal agent in the lubricant. The effectiveness of condoms for preventing pregnancy is further increased when they are used in combination with a spermicidal jelly inserted into the female vagina prior to intercourse.

Rhythm Method

Prevention of pregnancy is possible by avoiding coitus during the ovulatory phase of each monthly cycle. Difficulty achieving complete conception control by the biologic or rhythm method stems from the fact that the exact day of ovulation is not only impossible to pinpoint but may vary considerably even in women whose cycles are consistently of the same length. Furthermore, the cycle length in 70 to 80 percent of women varies five or more days, and in some the variation is as much as eight or nine days. Hence to achieve any degree of reliability with respect to protection against pregnancy, the potential fertile period during which intercourse is to be avoided may necessarily be lengthy and the corresponding "safe" period relatively short.

The most reliable formula for determining the fertile time and the "safe period" is the schedule, proposed by Ogino, which assumes that ovulation usually occurs 12 to 16 days premenstrually, that the ovum may survive about 24 hours, and that sperm capable of ovum impregnation may survive in the female genital tract for about three days. Properly employed, this schedule provides roughly a 95 percent chance of avoiding pregnancy. The patient can effectively use the rhythm method of conception control in accordance with this formula if she carefully follows the regimen prescribed.

1. The patient keeps a precise record of her menstrual dates (day and hour of the onset of menstruation) for at least one year, calculating the length of each menstrual cycle and thus determining the length of the shortest and the longest cycles. This information is of paramount importance inasmuch as it is impossible to predict the length of any current cycle and all calculations of the potential fertile period must be based on the known variations in cycle length in the recent past (ovulation occurs relatively early in short cycles and late in longer cycles). Because the extent of variation in cycle length may change over the years, it is probably wise to have the patient continue to keep a careful record to be certain that all her cycles continue to fall within the initially calculated range or to make any necessary corrections should the cycles become longer or shorter.

2. The beginning of the potential fertile period, or the first unsafe day, is determined by subtracting 18 days from the shortest cycle length. The last unsafe day, or end of the fertile phase, is found by subtracting 10 days from the longest cycle length. There can never be fewer than nine unsafe days by this formula,

regardless of cycle length or variation. [Even in a woman whose cycle length is constant, these nine days of potential fertility are accounted for by the five-day interval during which ovulation is most likely (twelfth through sixteenth premenstrual days) plus one day of potential ovum survival, plus three days of potential sperm survival.]

For example: For a woman whose menstrual cycles vary between 25 and 31 days, the fertile period is calculated as extending from day 7 (25 minus 18) to day 21 (31 minus 10). The safe intervals, during which intercourse is highly unlikely to result in conception, include the days immediately following menstruation through day 6 (the last preovulatory safe day) of the cycle and the interval from day 22 (the first postovulatory safe day) through the onset of the next menstrual period.

Although there are a number of printed calendar devices on the market that allegedly simplify the task of calculating the safe period, nearly all are unduly complicated and expensive, and none is necessary. The woman's careful and continuing record of her cycles and the routine arithmetic previously described are all that are required if she has been properly instructed and understands the simple basic facts about ovulation and the menstrual cycle itself. It cannot be overemphasized, however, that her calculations must be based on prior data of cycle length and variations thereof collected over a period of at least a year (13 cycles) if she is to achieve the 95 percent protection potentially offered by the Ogino formula. The risk of conception is roughly only 0.001 per cycle under these conditions, whereas it is twice as great if computations are based on a study of nine cycles, and three to seven times as great if they are based on data obtained from only six cycles.

The safe period or rhythm method of birth control can be further refined by incorporating daily urinary luteinizing hormone (LH) determinations close to the time of ovulation until ovulation can be carried out by the woman using home kits such as the Ovustick Kit, First Response, and so forth (Chap. 13). This method enables expansion of the period or window for the safe period and introduces greater reliability to this contraceptive method. However, the home kits for

urinary LH are not only costly and therefore not easily affordable by many patients but they can have interpretation difficulties and so require motivation and some level of skill on the part of the woman. Alternatively, tests using urine or even saliva to determine critical hormone changes or enzyme changes in the cervical mucus are being developed that could be deployed to enhance the accuracy and reliability of the safe period. Other than abstinence, this technique is the only method of contraception thus far sanctioned by the Catholic church.

Vaginal Diaphragms

Use of the vaginal diaphragm continues to be one of the frequent methods selected by couples wishing to practice contraception. A number of pharmaceutical or medical supply houses manufacture reliable diaphragms. Although there are minor variations in style and construction, all the devices consist basically of a thin, slightly cup-shaped diaphragm of latex rubber or similar material mounted on and covering a completely flexible circular coiled spring or a flat or arching simple watch-type spring. The external diameter of the commercially available contraceptive diaphragms varies from 50 to 105 mm in gradations of 5 mm, so that an appropriate size may be chosen for each user. (The most commonly required size is 75.) A set of fitting diaphragms for office use is readily available from any of the manufacturers.

It is important that the proper size be selected. The diaphragm should be as large as is comfortable for the patient and then extend easily over the cervix in cup-like fashion in such a way that the back rim is firmly and snugly anchored behind the cervix in the posterior fornix and the front rim similarly "locked in place" anteriorly behind the pubic symphysis (Fig. 22-1). (It is thus fitted in place in the identical way that a Smith-Hodge pessary is inserted for correcting uterine retroversion.) During intercourse the properly fitted diaphragm lies snugly applied to the anterior vaginal wall, cervix, and upper portion of the posterior fornix, effectively shielding the cervical os, without its presence being noted by either partner.

A diaphragm that is either too small or too large may become displaced during intercourse, allowing

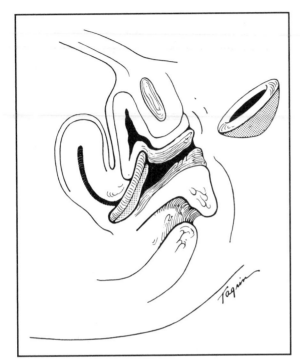

Fig. 22-1. Proper placement of the vaginal diaphragm. The diaphragm covers the cervix while holding spermicidal gel in its concave portion.

semen to gain access to the cervix. The appropriate size may change after pregnancy and delivery, so that refitting six to eight weeks postpartum is desirable if the couple wishes to resume the program of family planning. Because the area of junction between the diaphragm and the vaginal walls theoretically cannot prevent passage of an organism as minute as a spermatozoon, spermicidal jelly or cream is prescribed for use as a lubricant and protective coating on the rim of the diaphragm and is applied to it just before insertion.

A complete examination should always precede a diaphragm fitting to avoid overlooking unsuspected pelvic disease and to be certain that an anatomic variation precluding effective use of the diaphragm does not exist, e.g., severe pelvic-floor relaxation, a large cystocele, or marked congenital retroversion with an excessively short anterior vaginal wall. The proper size is determined, and a diaphragm of this size is in-

serted and checked by the physician. The patient is then helped to examine the diaphragm in place, learning the feel of the covered cervix, and particularly the feel of the front rim locked in place subpubically. The latter is her best and easiest landmark and test of proper placement. The patient should then be allowed to remove and reinsert the diaphragm herself, the physician checking once more to be sure that she has mastered the procedure. Only rarely is a patient encountered who simply cannot accomplish what is ordinarily a simple maneuver. In that event, some other means of conception control must be chosen.

The diaphragm should be coated externally with spermicidal jelly or cream, a dab of which is also placed in the center of the inner cup where it will be applied against the cervical os. It is inserted before intercourse (not more than 6 to 12 hours before, however, and preferably only shortly before) and left in place for 6 to 8 hours or more after intercourse (not more than 24 to 36 hours, however, and preferably no more than 8 to 12 hours). If a second intercourse follows while the diaphragm is still in place, an application of spermicidal jelly or cream should be inserted into the vagina before the second intercourse. When left in place for the recommended time interval following coitus, douching at the time of removal is unnecessary. Instructions for the cleaning and care of the diaphragm are provided by the manufacturer, who usually supplies kits containing diaphragm and storage container, a tube of spermicidal jelly, and an "introducer," the latter probably not employed by most users, who simply carry out insertion and removal manually. With proper care the same diaphragm suffices for as long as five to six years.

Cervical Cap

The centuries-old cervical cap (dates back to 500 BC) finally won approval by the Food and Drug Administration in 1988 for use as a contraceptive. Like the vaginal diaphragm, the cervical cap is a barrier contraceptive that blocks sperm from passing from the vagina into the uterus. The cap is a thimble-shaped device made from rubber or plastic. Measuring about 1½ inches in diameter, the cap fits snugly over the cervix and is held in place by suction. The cervical cap must be fitted by a physician or midwife and should be used with a spermicidal jelly or cream.

This method is about 85 percent effective in preventing pregnancy. Advocates of the cervical cap claim it has several advantages, including greater durability than the diaphragm and allowance of greater sexual spontaneity and gratification, as it can be worn for up to 48 hours (compared with 24 hours for the diaphragm). The cervical cap is recommended only to women with normal Papanicolaou smears, as American studies have shown that women who use cervical caps rather than diaphragms initially have a higher rate of abnormal Papanicolaou tests. Women may also find the cervical cap more difficult to insert and remove than the diaphragm.

Contraceptive Jellies, Creams, and Foams

Use of a vaginal spermicidal agent alone is a temporary alternative for the virginal woman about to be married for whom it is impossible to fit a diaphragm or for the patient in whom, for anatomic or other reasons, a diaphragm cannot be successfully inserted. These agents are available as suppositories, creams, jellies, and aerosol foams. The various manufacturers supply syringe-type applicators designed for ready filling from the tube or container of contraceptive jelly or cream and for subsequent insertion into the vagina by the patient and delivery under moderate pressure of the recommended dose (usually 5 ml) of the agent into the upper vagina. The gel should be inserted just prior to intercourse, placing the applicator well into the vagina so that the gel is deposited near the cervix. Postcoital douching is unnecessary but if desired should be delayed at least 6 hours. An aerosol foam type of spermicidal agent (e.g., Emko Vaginal Foam, Dalkon Foam) is preferred by many women; and its reliability is reputedly enhanced by virtue of the foaming action and more thorough surface dispersion of the agent. Although these agents are reasonably effective, with an average of 80 percent protection, none appears to approach the 90 to 95 percent protection afforded when used in conjunction with a diaphragm or condom.

Contraceptive Sponge

The contraceptive sponge method essentially employs a spermicide contained in a sponge placed in the vagina; it is aesthetically more pleasant than squeezing spermicidal jellies or cream into the vagina. TODAY is an example of the contraceptive sponge. TODAY is a soft polyurethane foam sponge containing the spermicide nonoxynol-9 (1 gm). TODAY is claimed to prevent pregnancy safely and reliably through three actions: (1) It continually releases an effective spermicide that kills sperms on contact; (2) it blocks the pathway of upward migration of the sperm in the vagina; and (3) it absorbs sperms.

The contraceptive sponge is moistened with water, and after squeezing out excess moisture it is folded upward and inserted deeply into the vagina. The woman is afforded immediate contraceptive protection for up to 24 hours without need to add any further spermicide. Coitus may be resumed as many times during the 24-hour period so long as the sponge is not removed. This contraceptive is not recommended for women who have experienced warning signs of or who have had toxic shock syndrome. As in the case of the diaphragm and condom, user motivation and correct use are critical for high efficacy rates of the contraceptive sponge.

Oral Contraceptive

The use of ovulation-inhibiting agents to achieve a "physiologic" type of conception control, as contrasted with the biologic (rhythm method) and mechanical (diaphragm and spermicidal jellies) approaches previously discussed, has made significant progress with the development of the new, synthetic, highly potent oral progestogens. When administered cyclically throughout most of the menstrual cycle in proper dosage, these oral progestogens in combination or in sequence with synthetic estrogens completely suppress ovulation, presumably by inhibiting the output of pituitary gonadotropins, with the result that the normal cyclic ovarian function is totally interrupted. At the same time, the periodic short interruption of drug therapy allows an interval of withdrawal bleeding to occur that simulates the normal menstrual flow and avoids the undesirable side effects of a pseudodecidual type of endometrial hyperplasia, excessive breast stimulation, and so on, which would accompany prolonged, continuous therapy.

If each pill contains both a progestogen and an estrogen, the drug is classified as a *combination* type oral contraceptive. If the initial 14 to 16 tablets in each month's package contain only estrogen, the progestogen being added to only the last 5 or 6 tablets in the treatment cycle, the product is termed a *sequential* oral contraceptive. The combination types were the first to be introduced and continue to be the most widely used. Sequential products were subsequently devised in the belief that they would be more physiologic, but there is nothing physiologic about inhibiting ovulation on a monthly basis. Use of oral contraceptives is pharmacotherapy. The sequential oral contraceptive pill is now no longer available for clinical use by patients because of concerns about the development of endometrial neoplasia associated with its use.

Combination formulations containing two or three different amounts of the same estrogen and progestin are referred to as *biphasic* or *triphasic* and are generally referred to as *multiphasic*. Each of the tablets containing one of the various dosages are taken for intervals varying from 5 to 11 days during the 21-day menstrual period. Both the combination type as well as the triphasic type of oral contraceptives are nearly 100 percent effective in preventing pregnancy.

All oral contraceptives now available in the United States, except for two daily progestin-only pills, contain varying doses of an estrogenic compound and a progestogen. The estrogenic compound is either ethinyl estradiol or mestranol, and one of five 19-nortestosterone gestagens (i.e., norethindrone, norethindrone acetate, norethynodrel, ethynodiol acetate, or norgestrel) is the progestin. Mestranol, which is the 3-methyl ether of ethinyl estradiol, has to be demethylated by the liver to ethinyl estradiol to become biologically active. The completeness of this hepatic conversion varies from individual to individual, but ethinyl estradiol has an overall potency of 1.7 times that of the same weight of mestranol. With regard to the gestagen, norethindrone acetate and ethynodiol

diacetate are metabolized in the body to norethindrone, all three of which are about equipotent for progestational activity on a weight basis. However, levonorgestrel is 10 to 20 times more potent than norethindrone.

The patient begins the oral contraceptive drug on the fifth day of the menstrual cycle, taking one tablet daily for the prescribed 20 or 21 days. Usually within 48 hours of cessation of the drug she experiences an "artificial period." On the fifth day after the onset of this withdrawal flow, she begins another 20- or 21-day treatment program. In the case of some products, the patient simply stays off the medication for seven days after completing a 21-day pill cycle and then automatically begins the next pill cycle, regardless of when, or if, her artificial withdrawal period occurs. Most manufacturers also supply 28-tablet packages that include 7 placebo tablets at the end of the 21-day active drug tablet supply in each package, thus allowing the patient to take a tablet every day during each 28-day cycle in the hope of avoiding mistakes in timing. In most instances, the artificial, drug-created menstrual cycle is regular, more so than the patient's normal, spontaneous cycle. This fact is preferably explained in advance to the patient. Patients ordinarily suffering from menstrual cramps (primary dysmenorrhea) also find relief of their dysmenorrhea.

There has been a steady trend over the years in the direction of lower doses of both the progestational agent and especially the estrogenic compound used in the commercially available oral contraceptives, with a resulting decrease in side effects without compromising the effectiveness of the product. So-called low-dose preparations have become popular but may not be satisfactory for some patients because of an increased incidence of troublesome breakthrough bleeding during each cycle. A few products containing a low dosage progestogen alone without the addition of an estrogen (the so-called mini-pill) and taken by the patient on a continuous daily basis are now on the market (Table 22-1). Observations so far have revealed a negligible pregnancy rate (Table 22-2), only slightly higher (three pregnancies per 100 woman-years) than that encountered with the standard oral contraceptives (one pregnancy per 100 woman-years). Furthermore, the absence of estrogen seems to eliminate many side effects and should reduce the more se-

Table 22-1. Oral Contraceptives Available in the United States and Their Steroid Composition

Product	Type	Progestin	Estrogen	Manufacturer
		Combination Type		
Ethinylestradiol 35 μg				
Loestrin 1/20	Comb[a]	1.0 mg Norethindrone acetate	20 μg Ethinyl estradiol	Parke-Davis
Loestrin 1.5/30	Comb	1.5 mg Norethindrone acetate	30 μg Ethinyl estradiol	Parke-Davis
Lo/Ovral	Comb	0.3 mg Norgestrel	30 μg Ethinyl estradiol	Wyeth
Nordette	Comb	0.15 mg Levonorgestrel	30 μg Ethinyl estradiol	Wyeth
Ethinylestradiol 35 μg				
Modicon	Comb	0.5 mg Norethindrone	35 μg Ethinyl estradiol	Ortho
Ortho-Novum 1/35	Comb	1.0 mg Norethindrone	35 μg Ethinyl estradiol	Ortho
Brevicon	Comb	0.5 mg Norethindrone	35 μg Ethinyl estradiol	Syntex
Norinyl 1/35	Comb	1.0 mg Norethindrone	35 μg Ethinyl estradiol	Syntex
Demulen 1/35	Comb	1.0 mg Ethynodiol diacetate	35 μg Ethinyl estradiol	Searle
Ovcon-35	Comb	0.4 mg Norethindrone	35 μg Ethinyl estradiol	Mead Johnson
Ethinylestradiol 50 μg				
Ovral	Comb	0.5 mg Norgestrel	50 μg Ethinyl estradiol	Wyeth
Ovcon-50	Comb	1.0 mg Norethindrone	50 μg Ethinyl estradiol	Mead Johnson
Norlestrin 1/50	Comb	1.0 mg Norethindrone acetate	50 μg Ethinyl estradiol	Parke-Davis
Norlestrin 2.5/50	Comb	2.5 mg Norethindrone acetate	50 μg Ethinyl estradiol	Parke-Davis
Demulen 1/50	Comb	1.0 mg Ethynodiol diacetate	50 μg Ethinyl estradiol	Searle
Mestranol-containing pill				
Norinyl 1 + 50	Comb	1.0 mg Norethindrone	50 μg Mestranol	Syntex
Norinyl 1 + 80	Comb	1.0 mg Norethindrone	80 μg Mestranol	Syntex
Norinyl 2	Comb	2.0 mg Norethindrone	100 μg Mestranol	Syntex
Ortho-Novum 1/50	Comb	1.0 mg Norethindrone	50 μg Mestranol	Ortho
Ortho-Novum 1/80	Comb	1.0 mg Norethindrone	80 μg Mestranol	Ortho
Ortho-Novum 2	Comb	2.0 mg Norethindrone	100 μg Mestranol	Ortho
Ovulen	Comb	1.0 mg Ethynodiol diacetate	100 μg Mestranol	Searle
Enovid-E	Comb	2.5 mg Norethynodrel	100 μg Mestranol	Searle
Enovid 5	Comb	5.0 mg Norethynodrel	75 μg Mestranol	Searle
Enovid 10	Comb	9.85 mg Norethynodrel	150 μg Mestranol	Searle
		Multiphasic Type		
Ortho-Novum 10/11	Comb-biphasic	0.5 mg Norethindrone	35 μg Ethinyl estradiol	Ortho
		1.0 mg Norethindrone	35 μg Ethinyl estradiol	
Ortho-Novum 7/7/7	Comb-triphasic	0.5 mg Norethindrone	35 μg Ethinyl estradiol	Ortho
		0.75 mg Norethindrone	35 μg Ethinyl estradiol	
		1.0 mg Norethindrone	35 μg Ethinyl estradiol	
Tri-Norinyl 7/9/5	Comb-triphasic	0.5 mg Norethindrone	35 μg Ethinyl estradiol	Syntex
		1.0 mg Norethindrone	35 μg Ethinyl estradiol	
		0.5 mg Norethindrone	35 μg Ethinyl estradiol	
Triphasil 6/5/10	Comb-triphasic	50 μg Levonorgestrel	30 μg Ethinyl estradiol	Wyeth
		75 μg Levonorgestrel	40 μg Ethinyl estradiol	
		125 μg Levonorgestrel	30 μg Ethinyl estradiol	
		Progesterone-only Pill		
Micronor	Prog[b]	0.35 Norethindrone		Ortho
Nor-Q.D.	Prog	0.35 Norethindrone		Syntex
Ovrette	Prog	75 μg Norgestrel		Wyeth

Note: Many generic brands of oral contraceptives identical or similar to the above are available.

[a]Combination.

[b]Progestin only.

Table 22-2. Failure Rates of Various Methods of Contraception

Method	Failure rate (per 100 woman-years)
Sterilization	
Male	0.02
Female	0.13
Oral contraception	
Estrogen 50 μg	0.27
Estrogen 50 μg	0.16
Estrogen 50 μg	0.32
Progestogen only	1.2
IUD	
Copper T	1.2
Copper 7	1.5
Dalkon Shield	2.4
Loop A	6.8
Loop B	1.8
Loop C	1.4
Loop D	1.3
Saf-T-Coil	1.3
Not known	1.8
Diaphragm	1.9
Condom	3.6
Withdrawal	6.7
Spermicides	11.9
Rhythm	15.5

Source: M. Lawless and D. Yeates. Efficacy of different contraceptive methods. *Lancet* 1:841, 1982.

rious potential complications of the conventional oral contraceptive agents that current statistical data suggest are due to the estrogenic component. The main side effect of the mini-pill is cycle irregularity and intermittent breakthrough bleeding. When these side effects become a major inconvenience to the patient, she may find use of this method unsatisfactory and unacceptable. A shift to a standard combination agent or to a different method entirely is then indicated. Because of its slightly higher pregnancy rate, the mini-pill is not recommended if prevention of pregnancy is absolutely mandatory. In addition to probable ovulation suppression, at least some of the time, the mini-pill low-dose progestogen probably acts by producing a hostile cervical mucus that impairs sperm motility and inhibits sperm penetration; it may also alter tubal function and interfere with normal endometrial maturation.

If, as occasionally occurs, the usual artificially induced menstruation does not take place within two to three days of the cessation of the current treatment cycle, the patient should be instructed to begin the next course of the drug not later than seven days after she completed the last one because despite the absence of menstruation she will usually ovulate unless the cyclic treatment is resumed within a week's time.

Side Effects. Occasionally, breakthrough bleeding indicative of inadequate endometrial hormonal support (insufficient estrogen, too much progestin, or both) may occur during the treatment cycle, often only during the first few treatment cycles. If breakthrough bleeding remains a persistent problem, a formulation containing more estrogen should be used, or the patient may elect some other contraceptive method. Erratic intake on the part of the patient should be ruled out. If abnormal bleeding persists, organic causes should be sought.

Other side effects include nausea and gastrointestinal symptoms, abdominal pain and bloating, breast soreness and tenderness, chloasma, weight gain, edema, fatigue, headaches and exacerbation of migraines, dizziness, irritability, depression, pelvic discomfort, backache, leg cramps, changes in libido, and nervousness. These symptoms resemble a combination of those encountered during early pregnancy and with the premenstrual syndrome. In most instances they are mild and tolerable, and they tend to disappear after three to four months. As Table 22-1 indicates, some of the drugs contain larger absolute or relative amounts of the estrogenic agent. Because many of the side effects are directly related to the sodium- and water-retaining effects of the estrogen, a shift to an agent with a smaller amount of estrogen may ameliorate some of these troublesome symptoms. However, in 5 to 10 percent of patients the symptoms are persistent and severe enough to force discontinuation of this method of contraception.

Occasionally, rapid growth of uterine fibroids has been observed in patients on oral contraceptive drugs that have a relatively higher estrogen than progestin composition. Therefore the known presence of fibroids may be a relative contraindication to their use. An increased incidence of candidal vulvovaginitis has also been noted, a situation not unlike that seen in pregnant women or in postmenopausal women on estrogen therapy. On occasion, the candidiasis proves so distressing and resistant to all therapy that a switch to another method of birth control becomes necessary. Finally, androgen-dominant oral contraceptives (e.g., those containing norgestrel, norethindrone, or norethindrone acetate) tend to cause or aggravate acne and occasionally result in either hirsutism or mild hair loss, whereas estrogen-dominant agents (e.g., those containing norethynodrel or ethynodiol diacetate) tend to improve the complexions of acne-prone women, as estrogens tend to suppress sebaceous gland activity.

Patients intending to use oral contraceptives often have three major concerns regarding serious potential complications with use of the birth control pill: (1) increased risk of cancer; (2) increased risk of heart attack, stroke, and thromboembolism; and (3) interference with future childbearing.

EFFECT ON TUMORS. To date, none of the studies in the United Kingdom or the United States has found an increased risk of any type of cancer, with three possible exceptions. The Oxford study found an increased risk of cervical cancer, but it was likely due to compounding factors. Oral contraceptive users were found to have a higher incidence of both cervical cancer and cervical dysplasia, but these cervical lesions are also notoriously related to early age at first sexual intercourse, multiple partners, and herpesvirus infection. Because oral contraceptive users in the study also started sexual activity earlier and with multiple partners, these factors could have been responsible for the cervical lesions, rather than the birth control pill.

Most studies examining the potential increased risk of developing breast cancer in oral contraceptive users have not been able to show such an association except for one retrospective study (the second exception), which was subsequently shown to be flawed. Concerns about the risk of breast cancer with oral contraceptive use relate to the fact that estrogens stimulate normal breast tissue. However, the progestins in the oral contraceptive counteract any stimulatory action of estrogen. In fact, women taking oral contraceptives have a lower incidence of benign breast disease and benign cystic changes of the breast.

The third exception was the Walnut Creek study, which found an increased risk of melanoma if the woman was exposed to excessive sunlight, but this finding has not been confirmed by other studies. With respect to endometrial cancer, several studies have found that oral contraceptive users were, if anything, less likely than nonusers to develop endometrial cancer. Combined estrogen-progestin pills are known to retard development of the endometrium with consequently lighter menstrual flow as well as less endometrium to shed. Progestins are antiestrogenic, inhibit the synthesis of endometrial estrogen receptors, and therefore prevent proliferative growth-promoting action of estrogen.

Users of oral contraceptives for five years or more appear to have a greater chance (1 in 30,000 to 50,000 users per year) of developing benign liver adenomas, which, however, usually decrease in size and eventually disappear after the birth control pill is stopped. The tumors do not become malignant but rarely do rupture and bleed. No reliable screening procedure is currently available for detection of liver adenoma, but palpation of the liver should be a routine part of the periodic evaluation of pill users so that the medication could be stopped if the liver is enlarged.

EFFECT ON CARDIOVASCULAR DISEASE. The first British reports indicated that approximately 5 percent of oral contraceptive users after five years of use developed hypertension. Presumably the renin-angiotensin system is stimulated (plasma angiotensinogen is increased up to eight times normal values) by the estrogen in the pill, although the dose of the progestin component was correlated with the hypertension in one study but not in another. The reduced dose of steroid in the pill has, however, led to studies that did not find any association between oral contraceptives and hypertension.

It is important to note that variables such as previous toxemia of pregnancy, previous renal disease, and unsuspected renal disease do not predict if a woman will develop hypertension on the pill. Preexisting hypertension increases the risk of thrombosis; but with medical control of the blood pressure and close follow-up, the new low dose oral contraceptives may be judiciously used for contraception. Although oral contraceptives do not significantly affect left ventricular volume or contraction, significant increases in cardiac output, systolic blood pressure, and plasma volume have been reported. Therefore caution should be exercised in patients with questionable cardiac reserve when choosing the form of contraception.

British studies have shown that the risk of deep vein thrombosis is four times greater in oral contraceptive users than nonusers. For superficial leg vein thrombosis, it is only two times greater, but varicose veins do not appear to have any influence on deep vein thrombosis associated with oral contraceptive use. With the 50-μg pill, the risk of deep vein thrombosis was 80 per 100,000 users per year, whereas it was 112 per 100,000 users per year with estrogen doses greater than 50 μg. Likewise, in Sweden it was found that the incidence of thromboembolism decreased from 25.9 to 7.2 per 100,000 users per year when the dose of estrogen in the pill was reduced from 75 μg to 50 μg and finally to 30 μg. Thus the risk of developing thromboembolism with the use of oral contraceptive is related to the dose of estrogen in the pill; therefore the low dose estrogen preparation should usually be chosen.

Although the early British studies indicated that the risk of myocardial infarction in pill users was increased by two to seven times (30 to 39 years of age) to five to seven times (40 to 44 years of age) in pill users, it became clear that the risk was increased only in those over 35 who smoke or in those of any age who have some preexisting vascular disease such as hypertension, diabetes, or hypercholesterolemia. The absolute risk of any oral contraceptive user developing myocardial infarction is low. Few nonsmoking women under age 35 have heart attacks. There is no clear evidence that nonsmokers under 45 and smokers under 35 who use oral contraceptives have any significantly increased chance of dying from a heart attack so long as there is no underlying vascular disease. Therefore a woman under 35 who is a smoker can still use oral contraceptives, but she should be counseled to quit smoking. Those between 35 and 45 who do not smoke or who do not have an underlying vascular disease may also use the oral contraceptive. Although previously believed that oral contraceptive use should be limited to no more than 5 years because of possible increased risk of dying from cardiovascular disease with longer use, this observation was not found in many other studies.

Perhaps any small potential risk of cardiovascular and thromboembolic adverse effect associated with the use of the oral contraceptive should be placed in perspective against the risk of mortality due to pregnancy (about 22.8 deaths per 100,000 pregnant women from all causes associated with pregnancy). The psychological and sociologic problems created by the constant fear of pregnancy or the need to raise an unwanted child should also not be forgotten. The risk of death from oral contraceptive is approximately 0.3 to 3.0 deaths per 100,000 woman-years compared to 3.2 deaths per 100,000 elective abortions and 27 deaths from automobile accidents per 100,000 person-years. Certainly caution should be exercised when the patient has a history of cardiovascular disorder, and oral contraceptives are probably wisely avoided under those circumstances.

EFFECTS ON FUTURE REPRODUCTION. Although oral contraceptives may produce a short period of temporary infertility in some women after stopping the pill, this infertility is usually not permanent. Fertility rates of former oral contraceptive users are similar to those of former users of other methods of contraception. The suppressive effect of oral contraceptives on the hypothalamic-pituitary-ovarian axis disappears shortly after discontinuation of the pill; only the first postcontraceptive cycle may have a variable prolongation of the follicular phase. Delay in resumption of ovulation for varying periods may make it difficult to calculate the date of confinement if a pregnancy should ensue before spontaneous menstruation resumes. Therefore it is better to defer attempts at pregnancy until at least one or even two spontaneous menses have returned and to use barrier contraception in the interval after stopping the pill. Prolonged amenorrhea, not infrequently accompanied by galactorrhea, is encountered in a small percentage of oral contraceptive users and requires complete evaluation and treatment as necessary (Chap. 11). It should be noted that in most of these patients a history of previous irregular cycles with episodes of amenorrhea or oligomenorrhea can be elicited. Because most patients coming off the pill resume spontaneous regular cycles within one to six months, detailed investigation for postpill amenorrhea can safely be postponed until after six months.

There is no increase in the spontaneous abortion rate after stopping oral contraceptives. Although it was earlier reported that the incidence of chromosomal abnormalities was higher in abortuses of women conceiving within a few months after stopping the oral contraceptive, more recent studies have found no such increase. Specifically, normal reproductive tract function and fertility are universally restored on discontinuation of the drug, and until recently no tendency to fetal anomalies had been demonstrated. However, there have now been reports from several centers suggesting a potential teratogenicity of progestogen-estrogen agents because of a small but definite increased incidence of multiple congenital anomalies of the type covered by the acronym VACTERL (vertebral and cardiac–tracheal–esophageal–renal–limb) in the offspring, especially male offspring, of women exposed to combined progestogen-estrogen compounds during early pregnancy. Such exposures have occurred by accident, early or late in an oral contraceptive program, or while under hormone therapy for one reason or another.

OTHER PILL-ASSOCIATED SIDE EFFECTS OR CHANGES. Certain neuroocular complications, including retinal thrombosis and optic neuritis, have also been encountered in patients on oral contraceptives. No absolute cause-and-effect relation has been established, but immediate withdrawal of the drug is indicated if visual disturbances develop.

Changes in liver function test results and the occasional occurrence of cholestatic jaundice have been observed in some women taking oral contraceptives. The progestogen component of the drug appears to interfere with bile secretion in these patients, thus accounting for increased Bromsulphalein retention and, less often, jaundice. Because these alterations are much more likely to occur in patients with preexisting liver disease, the latter is a contraindication to use of the pill. There also appears to be an increased tendency toward the development of gallstones in users of oral contraceptives.

Other benign alterations in blood chemistry noted in women on contraceptive drugs include an elevation in protein-bound iodine and butanol-extractable iodine (thyroid function tests) secondary to an increase of thyroxine-binding proteins (also seen during pregnancy and estrogen administration) and a decrease in glucose tolerance, the mechanism for which remains obscure. However, there is no evidence of any fundamental effect on thyroid function (patients remain euthyroid), nor does the use of oral contraceptives in diabetic patients appear to affect the diabetic state per se or complicate its management.

Oral contraceptives do lower blood levels of the B-complex vitamins and vitamin C, but these changes are not accompanied by any clinical evidence. Supplementation of these vitamins are not specifically indicated for oral contraceptive users.

Any patient embarking on an oral contraceptive program should first be given the benefits and reassurance of a careful history, complete physical examination, cytologic smear, and any other indicated laboratory studies. Unsuspected pelvic or other diseases may be discovered, and contraindications to the use of these agents should particularly be sought.

Contraindications to the use of oral contraceptives include a history of phlebitis and embolic phenomena, preexisting genital or breast cancer, sizable fibroids, preexisting liver disease or a history of jaundice, or a history of coronary or cerebral vascular disease. Furthermore, patients on such a program should have continued supervision and regular follow-up examinations (at least yearly).

Drug Interactions Affecting Oral Contraceptives. Some drugs can accelerate the biotransformation of contraceptive hormones, particularly estrogens, to their metabolites, which are biologically less active and therefore give rise to breakthrough bleeding and breakthrough ovulation. This sequence has sometimes ended in pregnancy. Drugs that are known or have been implicated to interact with contraceptive hormones include rifampicin (a semisynthetic antibiotic used for treatment of tuberculosis), phenobarbitone, phenytion, carbamazepine, and diazepam. It is postulated that these compounds induce the formation of liver microsomal enzymes, particularly hydrolases, which accelerate the biliary excretion of drugs (e.g., estrogens) metabolized by the liver. Therefore patients who require treatment with these contraceptive hormone-interfering agents should consider alternative methods of contraception.

Noncontraceptive Health Benefits of Oral Contraceptives. Far too often there is excessive attention directed toward the adverse effects of any medication and little or no attention given to the benefits derived from use of a medication other than for the primary intended purpose. In addition to being the most effective nonsurgical contraceptive method other than absolute abstinence, oral contraceptives provide the following benefits.

1. Effective relief of primary dysmenorrhea in women suffering from it
2. Reduction of menstrual blood loss to about 20 ml, with therefore less likelihood of iron-deficiency anemia
3. Reduced likelihood of developing menorrhagia, irregular menstruation or intermenstrual bleeding (demonstrated by British studies)
4. Reduction of the relative risk of developing endometrial cancer to half that of nonoral contraceptive users
5. Reduction of the incidence of benign breast disease (directly related to the amount of progestin in the formulation) as well as chronic cystic breast disease but not fibroadenomas (reduction appears only after one to two years or more of use)
6. Reduction of the incidence of benign ovarian neoplasms and functional ovarian cysts; significantly reduced risk (by one-half) of ovarian cancer with the protection persisting for at least 10 years after stopping the oral contraceptives
7. Possible protection against the risk of rheumatoid arthritis
8. Protection against pelvic inflammatory disease

(relative risk reduced by one-half in oral contraceptive users)

Ethical Issues. One of the ethical questions posed by the increasingly widespread use of oral contraceptives is whether the physician should prescribe them for unmarried adolescents and teenagers. It is well to reiterate that at the present time there is an epidemic of teenage pregnancies in the United States. A substantial proportion (20 percent or more) of all pregnancies in unwed mothers occur in girls under the age of 17. An estimated 200,000 abortions are performed annually on teenagers. Such unwanted and unintended pregnancies have a profound adverse social impact on society as well as the individual, whose schooling and education are affected. As a result, both the immature parents and any progeny resulting from this premature attempt at adult sexuality in all likelihood are emotionally and socially crippled. Therefore for many young people it is wise to try to help them learn and believe in the value of accepting responsibility for the physical and emotional well-being of themselves and others so their sexual lives can be richer and more meaningful.

Nonetheless, there are many well adjusted, thoughtful, and responsible young women, as well as those less able to cope with the circumstances of their lives, who choose in the permissive world of today not to postpone sexual activity. It therefore seems desirable to prevent unwanted and undesirable pregnancy in these young women rather than to allow them to become entrapped in the difficult problem of premarital teenage pregnancy. The latter carries with it a severely detrimental impact on their economic and educational situation, the potential for serious disruption of their emotional health and family relationships, and even today the specter of their resorting to criminal abortion with its high morbidity and mortality. Even legalized therapeutic abortion, however well justified, is an imperfect solution at best. Making an adequately supervised contraceptive program available to these young women when and if they need it, while at the same time offering them guidance in matters of overall sexuality, seems the only logical, practical, realistic way.

Intrauterine Contraceptive Devices

The use of an intrauterine device (IUD) for contraception dates back to ancient times when a small stone was inserted into the uterus of camels to prevent pregnancy during journeys into the desert. In modern times, many IUDs have been designed and used clinically in women throughout the world. In the United States IUDs have become less readily available because of the medical-legal liabilities arising from pelvic infections and other complications associated with it. Presently only the progesterone-releasing IUD (Progestasert) is available in the United States, but in 1988 the copper-containing IUD (ParaGard) was reintroduced to the market. IUDs are made of stainless steel wires, polyethylene, or some similar plastic compounds.

Some of the more commonly employed IUDs, including those used in other parts of the world, are shown in Figure 22-2. The Lippes Loop has proved to be somewhat superior with a low pregnancy rate (1.5 to 2.5 percent), a relative expulsion rate of 10 to 12 percent, and few complications requiring removal (10 to 15 percent). The Lippes Loop was widely used in the United States until the 1980s when it was removed from the market by the manufacturer because of prohibitive product liability. The spiral IUD had a lower pregnancy rate (1.8 percent) but the highest expulsion rate (22.5 percent). The IUD rings had both high pregnancy rates (7.5 percent) and high expulsion rates (18 percent) and have been virtually abandoned in most countries. The IUD bow had a low expulsion rate (2.4 percent) but a high pregnancy rate (5.7 percent); the bow also had a high perforation rate (1 in 300), eight times greater than any of the other devices and is therefore seldom used now even in other countries. Most of the devices have a polyethylene or nylon thread tail that protrudes through the cervix to permit women to check the continued presence of the IUD.

Currently, the most commonly employed IUDs throughout the world are the Saf-T-Coil, Lippes Loop, copper-bearing IUDs such as the Copper-7 (Cu-7), the copper Tatum-T (TCu-200), and the progesterone-releasing IUD (Progestasert). In the United States only the Progestasert and the copper-containing IUD (ParaGard) are currently available.

In the Cu-7 and TCu-200, 200 mm² of copper wire are wound onto the vertical arm of the device. In the ParaGard (model T380A), the polyethylene body of the device is wound with approximately 176 mg of copper wire, and each of its transverse arms carries a copper collar of about 66.5 mg of copper, giving a total exposed surface area of 380 mm² of copper. The use of copper stems from animal studies showing copper to have a specific inhibiting effect on normal implantation. Additionally, copper may have a spermicidal and sperm-immobilizing effect. Although the original recommendation was to have copper-containing IUDs replaced every 2 to 3 years, the World Health Organization stated in 1982 that the Cu-7 is safe and effective for at least four years of use. The ParaGard (T380A) can be used for up to four years when it is removed and a new one inserted. The Cu-7 and TCu-200 had acceptable expulsion rates of 8 to 13 percent, respectively.

The progesterone-containing IUD (Progestasert) releases about 65 μg of progesterone into the uterine cavity per day, enough to exert local antifertility effects but insufficient to elevate the serum progesterone level. The Progestasert contains a reservoir of progesterone that is enough for only up to 18 months, and therefore this IUD must be removed and replaced annually.

The nonmedicated IUDs do not need replacement unless bleeding occurs after the IUD has been in place for a year or more. Bleeding is caused by calcium being deposited on the device slowly, with the resultant roughness then eroding the endometrium.

The precise mechanism by which IUDs prevent pregnancy remains to be established. The following mechanisms, however, are probably responsible either partially or collectively for the contraceptive efficacy of IUDs.

1. Spermicidal effects: IUDs produce a local sterile intrauterine inflammatory reaction with subsequent tissue (particularly leukocyte) breakdown products that are toxic to sperms.
2. Blastocidal effects: Similar to item 1, with leukocyte breakdown products also toxic to the blastocyst. Apparently, in women this toxic product exerts its action even in the tubes, as cleaving ova,

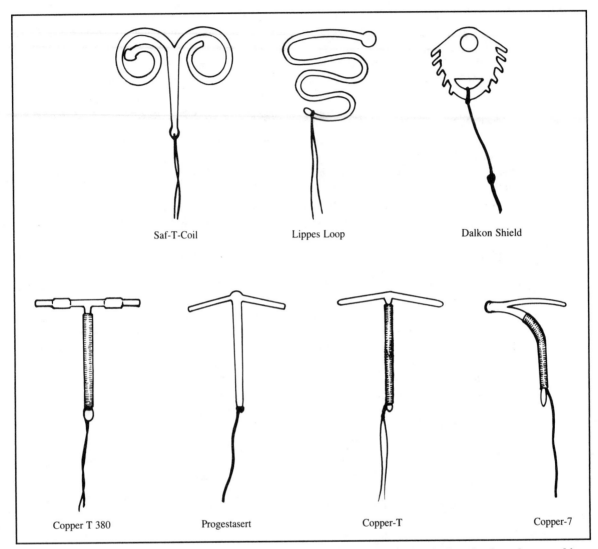

Saf-T-Coil   Lippes Loop   Dalkon Shield

Copper T 380   Progestasert   Copper-T   Copper-7

Fig. 22-2. Intrauterine devices that have been used in the United States. Many of these devices are no longer marketed in the United States but are used extensively around the world (except for the Dalkon Shield).

which can be found in tubal flushings of normal women, are absent in those of IUD users.

3. Excessive myometrial contraction: Interferes with normal implantation.
4. Excessive tubal peristalsis: Causes premature delivery of the fertilized ovum to the endometrial cavity with consequent failure of implantation.
5. Antiimplantation effect: Local, sterile intrauterine inflammatory reaction alters endometrial recep-

tivity to implantation and therefore prevents nidation (proved in rabbits).

In addition, the medicated IUDs, such as the progesterone-releasing IUD (Progestasert), releases progesterone (about 65 mg daily) within the endometrial cavity and therefore alters the development and hormonal milieu of the endometrium, making it nonconducive to implantation. The copper-bearing IUDs release small amounts of copper, which inhibits implantation. The addition of medications such as progesterone and copper enhances the contraceptive efficacy of the IUD. Thus the smaller T- and 7-shaped plastic IUDs without copper initially were associated with a much higher pregnancy rate than the larger loops and coils until copper was added, at which time their contraceptive efficacy became comparable to that of other IUDs.

The IUD can be safely inserted on any day of the cycle, but usually it is inserted during menstruation, as the cervical canal is probably widest at this time and access to it is easily gained without need for dilation. The expulsion rate for TCu-200 was lower when insertion was performed during the week after menstruation stopped, and rates of removal for bleeding and pain as well as pregnancy were higher with insertions after cycle day 18. Therefore insertion is preferably undertaken during the first 10 to 12 days of the cycle. During the postpartum period, although it is recommended that IUDs not be inserted until more than two to three months after a delivery, data indicate that copper T devices can be safely inserted at the time of routine postpartum visits. Early reports of high uterine perforation rates may be due to inadequate insertion techniques.

The flexible property of the IUD and its ability to resume its original shape render simple and painless the insertion of this device. Insertion can be carried out in the office under sterile conditions with the vagina and cervix adequately prepared. The uterus should be bimanually palpated to determine size, shape, and if it is anteverted or retroverted. The uterine cavity should be sounded to determine the length and direction of the uterine axis before inserting the IUD. Placement of the device should be as near to the fundus as possible so that expulsion is less likely. The IUD tail is then trimmed to a reasonable length so the woman can easily feel for it when she puts her fingers in the vagina but not excessively long that it could occasionally bother the male partner. Transient slight bleeding and mild discomfort are common for a short time after insertion.

The patient is instructed to check for the IUD tail regularly and after every menstrual flow. If the tail cannot be felt, she should be seen and the physician can check for it at speculum examination. Usually the check is performed after the first menstrual period with the IUD in place by the person who inserted it. Most expulsions occur within three months of insertion, usually during menstruation. Half of the women in whom the device is replaced expel it again, so that more than two or three attempts at replacement are unwarranted. Approximately 20 to 30 percent of all expulsions are not noted by the patient, and the number of pregnancies occurring in this situation add a highly significant 5 to 10 percent to the otherwise acceptable pregnancy rate of the method.

In general, IUDs are suitable only for parous women, as insertion is difficult and the expulsion and complication rates are high in nulliparas. Other contraindications to the use of an IUD include previous pelvic inflammatory disease, the presence of uterine fibroids or congenital uterine anomalies, and severe chronic cervicitis.

The main advantages of IUDs are a high level of effectiveness, lack of associated systemic metabolic effects, and the need for only a single act of motivation for long-term use. Unlike other nonpermanent forms of contraceptives, which rely on the user for effectiveness and therefore have different user-failure and method-failure rates, the IUD has similar method-failure and user-failure rates. The first year failure rates are generally 2 to 3 percent with a 10 percent expulsion and 15 percent removal rate for medical reasons (see Table 22-2). Pregnancy rates are to some degree dependent on the skill of the person inserting the IUD: Correct skillful high fundal placement of the IUD reduces the partial or complete expulsion rates, thus producing lower pregnancy rates. The accidental pregnancy rate decreases steadily after the first year of IUD use, and after several years it is similar to that of oral contraceptives. There is a steady decrease in the incidence of major adverse effects of IUDs with increasing age.

Other adverse effects of IUDs include persistent vaginal bleeding, dysmenorrhea, or diffuse pelvic pain and infection (endometritis or acute pelvic inflammatory disease). In the absence of local intrauterine anatomic pathology, persistent bleeding and dysmenorrhea have been traced to the increased endometrial prostaglandins produced as a result of the IUD-induced local sterile inflammatory reaction. Additionally, a vessel injury or defect may contribute to the bleeding. Both the dysmenorrhea and menorrhagia induced by the IUD can be effectively corrected with prostaglandin synthetase inhibitors, e.g., ibuprofen, naproxen sodium, or one of the fenamate derivatives given throughout the menstrual phase. Users of the Progestasert IUD, however, should experience no dysmenorrhea and have no increase in menstrual blood loss (their endometrial prostaglandin levels have been shown not to increase but to decrease).

Many prospective and retrospective case-controlled studies have reported a several-fold increase in the risk of developing pelvic inflammatory disease (PID). An overall relative risk of 1.9 to 5.1 has been reported in IUD users compared to nonusers; nulliparous women are at greater risk (relative risk of 1.7). The relative risk for gonococcal PID was found to be 2.8 versus 6.5 for nongonococcal PID. Although many shortcomings of these observations (including nonuniform guidelines for diagnosing PID, protective benefits of other contraceptives against PID making IUD look worse than it is, and the IUDs in such studies being the Dalkon Shield) were advanced to explain the increased incidence of PID with IUD use, a multicenter study still found that the overall risk of PID is 1.9 with IUD use, with the Dalkon Shield user having a risk of 8.3. The Dalkon Shield is of course no longer available for patient use anywhere today. The increased propensity for PID with the Dalkon Shield was attributed to breaks in the sheath around the knot attachment of the tail of the device.

The risk of developing PID is highest during the first two weeks after IUD insertion, when organisms have been found to be inoculated into the fundal area of the IUD cavity. With the Lippes Loop and Cu-7, a significantly increased risk of PID was present only during the first four months after insertion. IUD users also have an increased risk for colonizing *Actinomyces* in the upper genital tract. Therefore these organisms should be routinely sought; and if they are identified on the annual cytologic smear, the IUD should be removed. Because of the increased risk of PID

with IUD use, especially among populations at high risk (e.g., nulliparous women, those under 25 years of age, and those with multiple sexual partners), it is prudent to advise the women of these risks and the possibility of jeopardizing their fertility, and to recommend some alternative contraception. If the IUD must be employed, such patients should be taught to recognize the early symptoms of PID and to seek help early. The IUD should be avoided in nulliparous women because of increased risk of tubal causes of infertility, as reported in two studies.

If IUD users develop PID, it can usually be successfully treated with antibiotics without always having to remove the IUD until the patient becomes symptom-free. If there is evidence of a tuboovarian mass or abscess or if the Dalkon Shield is in place, the IUD should be removed as soon as therapeutic blood levels of the appropriate antibiotics have been given parenterally and there is some clinical response. Patients with a history of PID should avoid IUD use, employing some other method of contraception.

More serious complications and a few deaths have been reported as a result of perforation followed by peritonitis or intestinal obstruction. Most perforations are probably secondary to an initial, traumatic insertion, and this complication can therefore largely be avoided by proper patient selection and careful insertion. There is a ten times greater risk and higher incidence of ectopic tubal and especially ovarian pregnancies with the IUD in place. The ectopic pregnancy rate in IUD users is about 1.0 to 1.2 per 1000 woman-years. The chances of having an ectopic pregnancy is 3 to 9 percent if the patient conceives with the IUD in place compared to a regular ectopic pregnancy frequency of 0.3 to 0.7 percent of total births in similar populations. Progesterone-releasing IUDs have a higher frequency of ectopic pregnancies. Therefore ectopic pregnancy should be suspected in patients who become pregnant with an IUD in the uterus.

When pregnancy occurs with an IUD in place, it is best to remove the IUD for two reasons: First, the patient is more likely to abort if the device is left in place (50 percent chance) than if it is removed (30 percent chance). There is a high incidence of fetal wastage from all causes (abortion, ectopic pregnancy, and premature labor) if the IUD is allowed to remain.

Second—and even more important—there is a high incidence of premature rupture of the membranes complicated by serious intrauterine and intraamniotic sepsis as well as hemorrhage and septic abortion. A number of maternal deaths associated with shock and overwhelming sepsis in this situation have been reported, most of which were due to the Dalkon Shield. This increased risk of infection with the Dalkon Shield is due to the polyfilament thread acting like a wick and drawing fluid rich in bacteria from the vagina and cervix up into the uterine and amniotic cavities. Nevertheless, with any type of IUD, if a pregnancy does occur in the presence of an IUD, prompt removal is strongly recommended and the patient counseled about the risks of the IUD remaining in place versus the risks of an abortion with removal of the IUD.

The high rate of expulsions (12 to 15 percent or more), the significant pregnancy rate (if the pregnancies that occur as a result of unrecognized expulsions are included), and the significant complication rate requiring removal appear to reduce the "use effectiveness" of the method to the point where only 50 percent of women originally fitted with an IUD still have it in place two years later. For those women who experience no adverse complications or side effects, the various IUDs have proved completely satisfactory and effective.

Sterilization Procedures

Permanent sterility can, of course, be achieved by tubal ligation or hysterectomy in women or by vasectomy in men. Obviously, sterilization is not the answer for most young couples because it is irreversible in most instances. Nevertheless, these methods should certainly receive serious consideration whenever there is need in a particular patient for permanent fertility control. Voluntary sterilization is legal, and in only a few states are there restrictions regarding the indication for its performance. In countries such as India, where national population control is a particularly urgent problem, large-scale programs of voluntary sterilization have been inaugurated as a significant component of the total birth control effort.

The use of sterilization for contraception by married American women in the 15- to 44-year age group increased from 7.8 percent in 1965 to 27.5 percent in 1982. In 1982 there were nearly twice as many female sterilizations as male sterilizations. Since 1976, sterilization has become more frequent than use of either oral contraceptives or the intrauterine device.

Female Sterilization. With the increasing demand for voluntary sterilization, a number of techniques for permanent (in some cases potentially reversible) tubal occlusion or interruption have evolved, and efforts to develop simpler and safer methods continue. Tubal occlusion or interruption can be surgically carried out at present by three approaches to the tubes: (1) abdominally, through laparotomy, minilaparotomy, or laparoscopy; (2) vaginally, through culdotomy; and (3) hysteroscopically (Fig. 22-3). The most widely employed approach is via laparoscopy followed by minilaparotomy. In some parts of the developing world, the vaginal approach is preferred, where the procedure can be readily carried out from one "sterilization camp" to another with little equipment and using local anesthesia.

Laparoscopic sterilization is carried out under general anesthesia in almost all cases, but it is sometimes performed under local anesthesia or a regional block using epidural or spinal anesthesia. Currently, laparoscopic sterilization is done as a surgicenter outpatient procedure in a properly set up operating room but without need for hospitalizing the patient.

There are at least three major techniques employed for interrupting or occluding the tubes through the laparoscope: (1) electrocoagulation usually with division of the tube; (2) occlusion of the tube using the Falope ring (silicone rubber ring); and (3) occlusion of the tube using a clip (celebrated by a variety of eponyms). *Electrocoagulation* has been widely employed in the past. Whereas unipolar coagulation was previously performed, most centers currently employ bipolar coagulation to avoid thermal injury (including delayed complications). The tubes are divided after coagulation to reduce the failure rate arising from tubal recanalization after cauterization alone. To further ensure minimal failure rates after this technique of sterilization, the tubes are now usually electrocoagulated in three places adjacent to each other. Laparoscopic electrocoagulation of the fallopian tubes

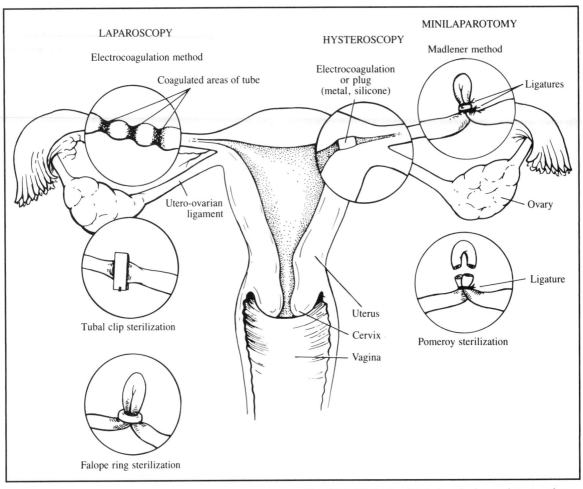

Fig. 22-3. Methods of tubal occlusion or interruption for sterilization.

carries a poor success rate for pregnancy should reversal of sterilization be requested subsequently.

The *Falope ring* is easily applied laparoscopically. To ensure good placement, a small knuckle at the proximal one-third of the tube should be lifted up and completely encircled and gripped by the Falope ring. It carries no risk of thermal injury and has a lower failure rate than electrocoagulation of the tubes. Tubal ligation with the Falope ring is easier and more successfully reversed, as tubal damage is less and adequate tubal length is often conserved. Occasionally, the Falope ring has been dislodged presumably owing to poor placement, excessive tubal activity pushing it off, or a defective ring.

Tubal *clips* have also been used through the laparoscope to occlude the tubes. Clips are composed either of metal (tantalum) or, more recently, of plastic. Unlike Falope rings, a knuckle of tube need not be lifted for occlusion, as the whole diameter of the tube is occluded at a single point, preferably in the proximal one-third of the tube. Less tube is damaged or interrupted with this procedure, but there have been high rates of the clips loosening and falling off the tubes into the pelvis. Thus the failure rates were initially high, but improvements in the design of the clips have apparently reduced the failure rates.

Laparoscopic sterilization is not without complications including occasional serious ones. Complications include hemorrhage, perforation of a viscus (bowel, bladder, stomach), perforation of large vessels including the vena cava and aorta, accidental electrical burns of the abdominal wall and bowel (occasionally with resulting perforation and peritonitis), flare-up of pelvic inflammatory disease, carbon dioxide embolism, and various anesthetic complications.

Laparotomy used to be employed for tubal ligation, but currently minilaparotomy is usually preferred. Only a small incision need be made in the lower abdomen. Minilaparotomy tubal ligation is readily carried out as a surgicenter outpatient procedure and can be performed in transient operating rooms or temporary sterilization "camps." If performed during the postpartum period, a 2- to 3-cm incision is made at the subumbilical area as for a laparoscopy and the tubal ligation performed. General, regional (epidural or spinal), or even local anesthesia can be employed for minilaparotomy postpartum tubal ligation. Several auxiliary or adjunctive steps have been introduced to elevate the uterus, thereby providing easy access and delivery of the tubes in the nonpregnant, normal-size uterus. A device called the Hulka tenaculum, which has a uterine sound as one side of the tenaculum, is used to elevate the uterus transcervically through the vagina. A loop of tube is then doubly tied with sutures, the so-called Pomeroy type of ligation. Modifications of this technique include dividing the tube between the sutures so that a piece of tube is available for histologic documentation that it was interrupted—an important consideration should the sterilization subsequently fail—and for ensuring that the round ligament was not mistaken for the tube. Various techniques have been employed for ligating or interrupting the tubes through the minilaparotomy. The Falope ring (*vide supra*) has also been used through the minilaparotomy. Fimbriectomy is rarely done unless necessary, as the chance of successful reversal is poorer than the other methods should the need arise. The failure rate of the Pomeroy type or modified Pomeroy type of tubal ligation is about 4 per 1000 women

undergoing the procedure. Linen or cotton ligatures on the tubes are avoided because the failure rate increases with such suture materials.

An alternative and equally satisfactory method uses the vaginal approach. A culdotomy (posterior colpotomy) incision is made, and tubal ligation and fimbrial resection are done (or the Pomeroy type of ligation if the patient desires a potentially reversible method) within a few minutes and under direct vision. This procedure is also feasible in the transient operating room or outpatient setting and can even be done under local anesthesia in many patients. Culdoscopy rather than culdotomy has been used by some, but the technique of ligation under direct vision is essentially the same. Culdoscopy has largely been replaced by the culdotomy technique and by laparoscopic and minilaparotomy tubal ligation.

An even simpler approach using intrauterine occlusion of the internal cornual ostia of the tubes through the hysteroscope has been explored and used for sterilization. Hysteroscopy is performed with either dextran (Hyskon) or carbon dioxide for uterine cavity distention (carbon dioxide usually being the better option). The tubes are then occluded by either electrocoagulation or local application of a sclerosing agent such as quinacrine, but either procedure must be repeated several times before complete and permanent tubal occlusion is achieved. Currently, an occlusive metal device is being evaluated for occluding the cornual ostia, but the hysteroscope requires special modification to allow flexible approach for the device applicator to reach the ostium. The use of a cornual ostium occluding device would presumably enable reversibility of the sterilization compared to chemical and thermal occlusion, which tends to be irreversible. Silicon plugs have been tried for tubal occlusion with promise of reversibility, but the success rates are not impressive and require further evaluation.

Complications with hysteroscopic sterilization include uterine and cornual perforation, thermal or chemical injury (including injury to the bowel), and higher failure rates than the Pomeroy or laparoscopic techniques for sterilization. Because of the present state of its development, safety, and efficiency, as well as the need to be trained for hysteroscopy, sterilization by this method is not widely employed. The procedure, however, can be readily carried out as an outpatient surgical procedure and should be able to be performed in transient sterilization "camps." General anesthesia can be used but is not necessary. A paracervical block may suffice.

Finally, for parous women who desire permanent sterilization and who, for example, also present signs and symptoms of pelvic support deficiencies (e.g., early prolapse, cystocele) or have persistent cervical dysplasia (both exemplify a pelvic condition that in itself is not yet necessarily a sufficient indication for surgical intervention), a case can certainly be made for vaginal hysterectomy and repair. This technique provides both permanent sterility and relief from current symptoms and future discomfort of inadequate pelvic support or protection against the progression from cervical dysplasia to carcinoma.

Male Sterilization. Permanent sterilization of men by vasectomy continues to be a simple office or transient operating room procedure, usually done under local anesthesia and with a high success rate. Ligation with division and resection of a small segment of vas followed by burying the divided ends is the usual technique. Electrofulguration or injection of sclerosing agents is used by some surgeons. After vasectomy the couple continues to employ their current contraceptive program for several months (usually three to four months) until complete azospermia is established and has been proved by several seminal analyses that show the absence of sperm.

There has been some concern about the occurrence of sperm antibody autoimmune reactions in vasectomized men. Sperm antibodies develop in 50 percent of vasectomized men and a cell-mediated immune reaction in 20 percent, but neither appears to have hazardous effects. There are no adverse hormonal changes. A study in vasectomized monkeys indicated a higher incidence of atherosclerotic disease developing than in controls, but this effect has so far not been shown in men. Possible psychological complications from or contraindications to the procedure must always be borne in mind and discussed carefully during preoperative as well as postoperative counseling.

Vasectomy can be reversed if necessary, as in the case of some forms of female tubal ligation. Reversal of vasectomy with end-to-end anastomosis is best carried out using microsurgery and by a urologist trained to do this procedure. Finally, efforts are being made to develop an easily reversible technique of male sterilization by intravas insertion of T-shaped devices with soft silicone and Dacron shuttle-stemmed microvalves within each vas; these devices would be left permanently in place, initially in the "off position" but with the possibility of readily switching them to the "on position" if desired at some future time. Thus the male partner could be literally as well as figuratively "turned on" if this experimental device should prove clinically feasible.

Postcoital Conception Control

Properly timed administration of an adequate dosage of estrogen to a woman postcoitally prevents implantation of the fertilized ovum. Although obviously not suitable for use in a routine, long-term contraceptive program, the "morning-after pill" approach is of great value in cases of rape, ruptured condom or diaphragm, or unplanned, "accidental," unprotected intercourse under a variety of circumstances.

To be effective, the estrogens must be given during the immediate postovulatory portion of the cycle, i.e., *immediately after fertilization,* real or potential, has occurred *but before the stage of implantation.* Thus if the past menstrual history indicates that exposure has occurred at or after midcycle, treatment should be started, preferably within 24 hours and not later than 72 hours. If there has been unprotected intercourse during the follicular phase, it may be wise to postpone the course of medication until just after midcycle. In either case, the patient should be warned not to have subsequent unprotected coitus in case ovulation should occur later in the cycle after the course of estrogen has been completed. Estrogen administration is not effective once implantation has occurred. Although the precise biologic mechanisms that are altered by giving large doses of estrogen are not proved (accelerated tubal transport of the ovum, abnormal endometrial maturation, and direct effects on the blastocysts are all possible factors), it is clear that failure of the implantation process is the end result.

The retroactive pill regimen consists in a five-day course of estrogen, e.g., a daily dose of 50 mg of diethylstilbestrol (DES), 30 mg of Premarin, or 5 mg of ethinyl estradiol. Transient side effects due to the excessive amount of estrogen necessary include fluid retention, breast soreness and swelling, excessive nausea, and subsequent irregular, prolonged menstrual flow. The nausea can be minimized by taking the medication with meals, together with an antiemetic drug. The patient must be warned to take all the medication despite her nausea if the regimen is to be effective. When properly administered and timed, the postcoital estrogen therapy program almost invariably prevents pregnancy. There seems to be a slightly increased incidence of ectopic pregnancy in the rare instances in which the postcoital medication program fails to prevent conception (Chap. 16). The few failures may have been associated with multiple sexual exposures, an inability to start or complete the drug program during the interval between ovulation and implantation, or inadequate estrogen dosage.

In the occasional instance of failure of the postcoital use of DES to prevent intrauterine pregnancy, therapeutic interruption is considered, both because it would best serve the interests of the patient with respect to an obviously undesired pregnancy and because of the known possibility of DES-induced adverse effects on the fetus (see detailed discussions in Chapters 8 and 16). The potential creation of the latter problem in nonexistent offspring should not be construed as a valid objection to the use of the postcoital DES regimen for preventing pregnancy when it is otherwise clearly indicated, especially as it is invariably effective in preventing pregnancy if correctly timed.

Another approach to postcoital contraception immediately after unprotected intercourse has been tried, i.e., insertion of a copper-bearing IUD. Early results suggest a high degree of protection against subsequent pregnancy. The Copper T presumably also acts by preventing nidation, and it may possess spermicidal activity. This technique is not as widely applicable

as the postcoital high dose estrogen program, but it does offer a potential and highly effective alternative for some patients.

Long-Acting Steroids

Three types of long-acting steroid formulations have been developed and have undergone clinical testing: injectable suspensions, subdermal polysiloxane capsules, and vaginal polysiloxane rings. Long-acting steroid contraception would offer a distinct advantage of infrequent administration.

Injectable Steroid Suspensions. Among the injectable steroid suspensions, the most widely used and studied is depo-medroxyprogesterone acetate (Depo-Provera) which is approved for use as a contraceptive in more than 50 countries, including Sweden and the United Kingdom. As of 1988, depo-medroxyprogesterone acetate (DMPA) is not approved for contraceptive use in the United States.

Depo-medroxyprogesterone has been used by more than 11 million women throughout the world, and there are now more than 2 million women using it. It is effective and has a failure rate of 0.0 to 1.2 per 100 woman-years—0.1 percent at the end of the first year and 0.4 percent at the end of the second year. It is given as an injection to the buttock in a dose of 150 mg at least once every three months. DMPA inhibits midcycle gonadotropin surge; the estrogen levels are low (early follicular phase levels), and progestin levels are high. Therefore the endometrium becomes low-lying and atrophic, and amenorrhea develops. In some patients breakthrough bleeding occurs 10 to 14 days per month and can be treated with low doses of estrogens on those days. Usually as the duration of DMPA use increases, the frequency of bleeding steadily declines and amenorrhea sets in. At the end of two years of treatment, 70 percent of the women are amenorrheic. Other side effects include weight gain, slight (clinically insignificant) deterioration of glucose tolerance, and delay in return of fertility. A regular cyclic menstrual pattern is established within six months of stopping DMPA in 50 percent of patients. Therefore pregnancy rates are only 50 percent at the end of a year after stopping DMPA use; that is, there is a delay of nine months in establishing similar pregnancy rates after DMPA compared to barrier contraception. DMPA has been associated with an increased incidence of mammary cancer in beagle dogs and endometrial cancer in monkeys, but up to now there is no such observation in women.

Norethindrone enanthate, an injectable progestogen given in an oily suspension, is used in Europe but not in the United States. It is given in a dose of 200 mg every 60 days for at least the first six months and no less often than once every twelve weeks thereafter. Given this way, the pregnancy rates are 0.6 percent (0.1 percent for DMPA) at the end of one year and 1.4 percent at the end of two years. Serum norethindrone levels of 4 ng per milliliter or more are reached and persist for one to two months after the injection. Norethindrone enanthate suppresses gonadotropin levels and follicular maturation. Although amenorrhea is more frequent with DMPA (55 and 62 percent at the end of one and two years, respectively) than with the norethindrone enanthate (30 and 40 percent), the total discontinuation rates are similar for the two methods (50 and 75 percent at one and two years, respectively). Moreover, less menstrual bleeding is seen, and there are fewer systemic effects with norethindrone enanthate.

Various injectable combinations of estrogen and progestogens such as dihydroxyprogesterone acetophenide with estradiol enanthate (Deladroxate) and medroxyprogesterone acetate with estradiol cypionate (Cyclo-Provera) have been tried. They have to be given monthly but produce less bleeding than the injectables. They are not used in the United States or Europe.

Subdermal Steroid Implants. The best known subdermal implant is Norplant, which is composed of polysiloxane containing levonorgestrel. Six cylindrical capsules, each 3 cm long and 2.4 mm in outer diameter, are inserted subdermally in the upper arm through a skin incision (3 mm) performed under local infiltration anesthesia. The six capsules, implanted radially, have enough norgestrel to be effective for six to seven years but are recommended for five-year use. Because the polysiloxane is not biodegradable, Norplant capsules must be removed through another incision either when the levonorgestrel has been released or when contraception is not required. Irregular bleeding episodes (spotting) are a major side effect, presumably due to the irregular estradiol levels, but total blood loss at menstruation is normal or even low normal. Norplant produces a slight decrease in serum levels of cholesterol, triglycerides, low density lipoprotein, and high density lipoprotein, but they are still within the normal range. Norplant is associated with an overall pregnancy rate of 1.5 per 100 women and an annual pregnancy rate of 0.5 percent, which is significantly lower than with oral contraceptives or IUDs. Continuation rates of use of Norplant is 80 percent at the end of one year and 50 percent at three years.

Contraceptive Vaginal Rings. Another method being evaluated for contraception is the administration of contraceptive steroids through a donut-shaped Silastic vaginal ring impregnated with a variety of progestogens. The ring (outside diameter 50 to 58 mm) is composed of an inert inner core, a concentric second layer of contraceptive steroid, and an outer ring of Silastic tubing. The ring is placed in the vagina, and the steroids are released from the ring surface to be absorbed by the vaginal epithelium. Ovulation is therefore inhibited. The ring is apparently comfortable, and neither the patient nor her partner notices its presence in the vagina. Currently the rings studied are impregnated with levonorgestrel and estradiol, releasing 300 μg and 180 μg of the respective steroids per day. The addition of estradiol to the progestogen has reduced breakthrough bleeding. There are apparently no adverse changes in the vagina. Withdrawal bleeding occurs within one to two days of removing the ring and is similar to that seen with the normal period. Multicenter studies have found pregnancy rates with the contraceptive vaginal rings to be similar to those with oral contraceptives.

Potential New Methods

Immunologic methods or approaches to fertility control raised much hope and excitement during the 1970s, but such interests are currently on a holding pattern. The principal method that was promising employed immunization to human chorionic gonadotropin (hCG) and therefore interruption of conception either at the preimplantation blastocyst stage or after implantation. Such immunizations against hCG were carried out in monkeys and women. The animal findings unfortunately produced some concern about increased abortion rates of pregnancies after discontinuation of this contraceptive method. Other approaches to immunocontraception that are or have been examined to a limited extent include development of anti-sperm antibodies in the female genital tract and antibodies against the zona of the oocytes.

Gonadotropin-releasing hormone (GnRH) and its agonists have been widely investigated as a reversible contraceptive method to be used in men. These substances down-regulate pituitary function and therefore testicular spermatogenesis. It takes three months or more to obtain satisfactory azoospermia with GnRH agonists. Moreover, the inhibition of testicular spermatogenesis inhibits testosterone secretion by the testes and results in loss of libido, which was often seen during the clinical trials in men. Attempts have been made to overcome this problem by giving testosterone supplements with the GnRH agonist administration. It takes several weeks or months for fertility to be reestablished upon discontinuing this method of contraception. GnRH or GnRH agonists have also been examined for ovarian suppression and therefore inhibition of ovulation, but the hot flushes accompanying the ovarian suppression secondary to down-regulation of pituitary gonadotropin secretion are undesirable effects. In addition, bone densitometry changes suggesting accelerated bone demineralization accompanying the hypogonadal state of GnRH agonist therapy are of concern and necessitate further investigation.

SELECTED READINGS

Alvarez, F., Guiloff, E., Brache, V., et al. New insights on the mode of action of intrauterine contraceptive devices in women. *Fertil. Steril.* 49:768, 1988.

Cagen, R. The cervical cap as a barrier contraceptive. *Contraception* 33:487, 1986.

The Cancer and Steroid Hormone Study of the Centers for Disease Control and the National Institute of Child Health and Human Development. The reduction in risk of ovarian cancer associated with oral contraceptive use. *N. Engl. J. Med.* 316:650, 1987.

Dorflinger, L. J. Relative potency of progestins used in oral contraceptives. *Contraception* 31:557, 1985.

Faich, G., Pearson, K., Fleming, D., et al. Toxic shock syndrome and the vaginal contraceptive sponge. *J.A.M.A.* 255:216, 1986.

Goldbaum, G. M., Kendrick, J. S., Hogelin, G. C., et al. The relative impact of smoking and oral contraceptive use on women in the United States. *J.A.M.A.* 258:1339, 1987.

Jones, W. R., Bradley, J., Judd, S. J., et al. Phase I clinical trial of a World Health Organization birth control vaccine. *Lancet* 1:1295, 1988.

Louik, C., Mitchell, A. A., Werler, M. M., et al. Maternal exposure to spermicides in relation to certain birth defects. *N. Engl. J. Med.* 317:474, 1987.

Massey, F. J., Bernstein, G. S., O'Fallon, W. M., et al. Vasectomy and health: Results from a large cohort study. *J.A.M.A.* 252:1023, 1984.

Phillips, J. M. Endoscopic female sterilization. A comparison of methods. Downey: American Association of Gynecologic Laparoscopists. 1983.

Svensson, L., Westrom, L., and Mardh, P.-A. Contraceptives and acute salpingitis. *J.A.M.A.* 251:2553, 1984.

Vessey, M. P., Lawless, M., and Yeates, D. Oral contraceptives and stroke: Findings in a large prospective study. *Br. Med. J.* 289:530, 1984.

23

Menopause

By definition, the term menopause is not the same as climacteric. *Climacteric* refers to the phase of the aging process of women during which they make the transition from the reproductive stage of life to the nonreproductive stage. This transition is the period of declining ovarian function, which usually becomes clinically apparent over the two to five years around menopause. The climacteric ultimately heralds menopause with manifestations of progressive tissue atrophy and aging. *Menopause* refers to the complete or permanent cessation of menstruation and is indicated by the final menstrual period, which often occurs during the climacteric. An interval of 6 to 12 months of amenorrhea is usually necessary to establish the diagnosis, but in some patients serum follicle-stimulating hormone (FSH) and luteinizing hormone (LH) levels may be necessary to differentiate this state from other causes of secondary amenorrhea.

In the United States menopause occurs between 48 and 55 years of age, with a median age of 51.4 years. Although previously suggested that the age of menopause may be increasing, data analyses indicate that it has remained unchanged for centuries. When menopause occurs at 35 years of age or less, it is classified as premature menopause (Chap. 11). Nevertheless, the clinical manifestations of menopause become apparent earlier if menopause occurs before the usual age. Therefore although the menopause that occurs at 36 years of age may not be premature by definition, the woman is nevertheless at increased risk of the same adverse effects of menopause and aging as the woman who experiences menopause at 55 years of age, only her risks begin at an earlier age. The age at which menopause occurs is influenced by several factors (Table 23-1).

The number of postmenopausal women in the United States is increasing. During the 1980s there were approximately 50 million women over 50 years of age. With a current life expectancy of 80 years, at least 30 years (or more than one-third) of her life is spent after ovarian function has failed and in a hypoestrogenic state. Furthermore, with the rising rate of pelvic inflammatory disease and its chronic sequelae, increasing numbers of young women are undergoing surgical menopause through total hysterectomy and bilateral salpingo-oophorectomy as the definitive therapy of their chronic disease. This group of young women, often in their twenties, increases both the number of menopausal women in the population and the years spent in the menopausal state. Therefore the problems of the postmenopausal period assume enormous and significant importance because of the major public health concern.

OVARIAN CHANGES

The primary basis for the progressive decrease and ultimately complete cessation of the cyclic function of the female reproductive organs at the time of menopause appears to lie in the ovary itself. Although it is commonly taught that the ovarian follicles are depleted at menopause, anatomic studies indicate that primordial follicles are still present, albeit in significantly reduced numbers. At the time the ovaries are formed in the fetus, there are approximately 6 million primordial follicles, which decrease to about 600,000 at birth, to 300,000 at menarche, and to about 10,000 or fewer near the time of menopause. Therefore progressive loss of germ cells and follicles from the ovaries is a continuous process that starts during intrauterine life and progresses throughout the reproductive years until menopause. The rate of atresia of the primordial follicles is probably determined by the intrinsic genetic program of the ovary. A few immature follicles therefore continue to undergo maturation and atresia a few years after menopause, and there are a few reports of postmenopausal ovulation. As depletion of the primordial follicles occurs, ovulation becomes irregular and steadily more infrequent, finally stopping altogether. There is an accompanying

Table 23-1. Factors Affecting the Age at Menopause

Factor	Effect on age
Menopause age of female family members	Directly related Increased if family menopausal age late Decreased if family menopausal age early
Abnormal chromosome karyotype	Early menopause (e.g., premature gonadal failure with Turner's syndrome, gonadal dysgenesis)
Obesity	Late menopause
Cigarette smoking	Early menopause
Blindness	Early menopause
Precocious puberty	Early menopause
Social class*	Late menopause with higher social class

*This factor may be more apparent than real and dependent on consequent life style, such as diet, weight, smoking, and family menopause age.

failure of progesterone production during the initial stages; and as follicle activity ceases completely, a relative lack of estrogen manifests in total cessation of menstrual function, as the amount of estrogen is insufficient to stimulate endometrial proliferation and growth. The ovary becomes smaller and fibrotic with atrophy of the ovarian cortex, which contains the primordial follicles. Thus the ovarian medulla becomes relatively more abundant with active stromal cells, which are the source of ovarian androgens. As the postmenopausal years advance, the ovaries become even more atrophic so they are eventually replaced by masses of fibrotic tissue.

ENDOCRINE CHANGES

The cessation of ovarian reproductive function gives rise to a series of endocrine changes in the hypothalamic-pituitary-gonadal axis, changes of which contribute to or are the primary basis for many of the menopausal symptoms and long-term metabolic sequelae. Several years before menopause, there is a gradual increase in circulating FSH toward the menstrual cycle, a concomitant decrease in serum estradiol values, no significant change in LH levels, and only a slight decrease in serum progesterone. These changes are still associated with follicular maturation and corpus luteum development. However, serum LH levels later become elevated but still to a lesser extent than the FSH levels. Ovulation is still recognized in some cases despite this increase in gonadotropins. Finally, at the time of menopause, gonadotropin levels are high and estrogen levels are low. Gonadotropin-releasing hormone (GnRH) levels, however, remain unchanged. Increased resistance of the remaining follicles to gonadotropins may explain the decreased estrogen production. The progressive decline in ovarian follicles gives rise to decreased inhibin levels. The combination of decreased inhibin and estradiol levels are probably responsible for the early elevation of FSH. GnRH levels have been found to remain similar to those in cycling women.

The endocrine change of widest impact during menopause is decreased estrogen production by the ovary. During the premenopausal years the ovary is a major source of estrogen; estradiol is the principal estrogen produced and is made almost entirely by the maturing follicles during each cycle. After menopause, ovarian estrogen production decreases markedly, and the principal circulating estrogen is estrone, not estradiol.

Most of the estrogen present in the circulation of the postmenopausal woman is derived from extraovarian and extraglandular production of estrone. Estrone is produced mainly in adipose tissues (in the stroma rather than the adipocytes) by aromatization of androstenedione. The amount of androstenedione converted to estrone in adipose tissue is governed by the overall amount of adipose tissue. Therefore slender postmenopausal women convert a smaller percentage (1.5 percent) of their daily androstenedione production to estrone, whereas as much as 7 percent of the daily production of androstenedione may be converted to estrone by obese postmenopausal women. The production rate of androstenedione remains similar in both slender and obese postmenopausal women, at about 3000 μg per day. Androstenedione is secreted both by the adrenal and the ovaries in the premenopausal woman. Ovarian contribution to androstenedione production decreases from 30 percent during early menopause to about 5 percent during late menopause, thus making the adrenal the source of 95 percent of the circulating androstenedione in the postmenopausal woman. The liver also converts androstenedione to estrone. The rate of conversion of androstenedione to estrone increases with age. Thus the obese postmenopausal woman who converts 7 percent of her androstenedione may be producing as much as 200 μg of extraglandular estrone per day, and the slender postmenopausal women may be producing as little as 45 μg of estrone per day. The low concentrations of estradiol present in postmenopausal women are primarily derived from extraglandular conversion of estrone and testosterone.

There is little evidence to suggest any significant alteration in adrenal hormone secretion as a result of menopause. Because of the decline in estrogen output by the postmenopausal ovary and eventually androstenedione output late in menopause, the adrenal assumes an overall important role as the principal site of androstenedione, androgen, and estrone production in postmenopausal women.

PERIMENOPAUSAL PROBLEMS

At the time of menopause and during the years immediately preceding it, the progressive and sometimes irregular decline in ovarian function often leads to functional irregularities of the menstrual cycle not unlike those seen during the early adolescent years when ovarian function began. Although the cessation of regular normal menstrual function may be abrupt and uncomplicated in some women, anovulatory cycles are common and may be manifested by (1) increasing oligomenorrhea with scanty flow or (2) irregular, often heavy and prolonged bleeding from a proliferative or hyperplastic endometrium, or both. The management of this type of dysfunctional bleeding during

the premenopausal and menopausal phases is discussed in Chapter 11.

In premenopausal and postmenopausal women with irregular vaginal bleeding, it is advisable to obtain diagnostic endometrial samples—with either suction curettage (Vabraaspiration) in the clinic or sharp curettage in the operating room—to exclude the possibility of malignancy before instituting a program of supplemental hormone therapy to control the episodes of abnormal bleeding. In many instances the curettage itself prevents recurrence of abnormal bleeding. When hormone therapy is undertaken to control dysfunctional bleeding in the premenopausal age group, estrogens may have to be employed along with progestational agents to achieve satisfactory results.

The hormonal imbalance that characteristically results from the declining ovarian activity during the premenopausal phase is nevertheless often one of a relative excess of estrogen in the presence of inadequate progesterone production. This preponderance of estrogen often leads to increased frequency of some of the other cyclic functional disorders in women approaching menopause—premenstrual tension and cystic mastitis being perhaps the most common manifestations of this tendency. The nature and management of these conditions are also discussed in Chapters 10 and 24.

POSTMENOPAUSAL PROBLEMS AND SYMPTOMS

A variety of problems or symptoms may arise at or after menopause (Fig. 23-1). Some of these problems are due exclusively to low estrogen levels or prolonged estrogen deprivation, whereas others are often aggravated or contributed to largely by the estrogen-deprived status of these women.

Psychoneuroendocrine Symptoms

Psychoneuroendocrine symptoms include headache, tiredness, lethargy, irritability, anxiety, nervousness, depression, sleep difficulties, inability to concentrate, and hot flushes. By far the commonest symptom that gets the attention of the patient and brings her to seek relief is hot flushes. As many as 85 percent of meno-

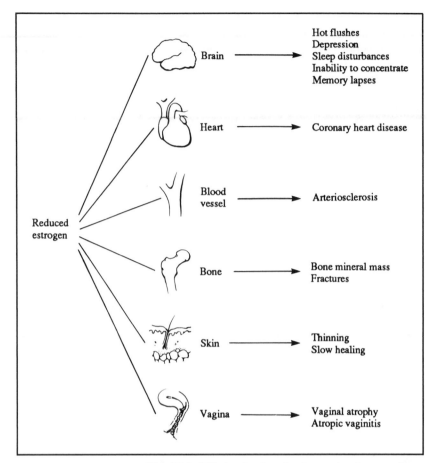

Fig. 23-1. Effects of reduced estrogen levels on various target tissues and their clinical manifestations in the postmenopausal women.

pausal women have hot flushes, and up to 45 percent of them may have hot flushes for 5 to 10 years after menopause. Hot flushes may occur months or years before the last menstrual period at menopause.

Characteristically, a hot flush begins in the head and facial areas with a typical and sudden sensation of warmth followed by facial flushing. These symptoms may radiate down the neck and other parts of the body. Each flush is followed by profuse perspiration in the same area. A hot flush is associated with an increase in temperature, increased pulse rate (average of 9 beats per minute and up to as many as 20 beats per minute), increased blood flow in the hand, and increased skin conductance, followed by a decline in temperature. Each hot flush averages 2.7 minutes. Hot flush episodes during sleep are referred to as

night sweats. The onset of each hot flush is synchronized with a luteinizing hormone (LH) pulse.

Hot flushes are the mechanism for dissipating heat through vasodilatation and perspiration in response to the thermoregulatory centers in the anterior hypothalamus around the arcuate nucleus adjusting the core temperature of the body to a new set-point. Thus a common stimulus of the arcuate nucleus or anterior hypothalamus is probably responsible for the pulsatile increase in GnRH (and therefore LH) and the hot flush.

Hot flushes are caused by a rapid estrogen withdrawal rather than a direct relation with estrogen levels. Despite high gonadotropin levels and low estrogen levels, women with ovarian failure due to gonadal dysgenesis rarely have hot flushes prior to estrogen exposure but develop them upon estrogen withdrawal after exposure. The anterior hypothalamus has estrogen and progestin receptors, and both hormones can be used effectively to treat hot flushes through binding with their respective hypothalamic receptors. Other neurotransmitters that may be involved in the pathogenesis of hot flushes include norepinephrine, an α-adrenergic agent, and endogenous opiate withdrawal. The α-adrenergic agonist clonidine effectively alleviates hot flushes through reduction of noradrenergic release, and it thereby blocks noradrenergic neuron activity associated with the rapid changes in skin temperature that occur during hot flushes and opiate withdrawal.

Sleep deprivation and interrupted sleep are reported by postmenopausal women and can contribute to nonspecific complaints such as irritability, anxiety, nervousness, fatigue, forgetfulness, and inability to concentrate. However, even if the postmenopausal woman is able to obtain an adequate amount of sleep, she usually wakes up feeling inadequately rested. In postmenopausal women not on estrogen replacement therapy, there is a decreased amount of rapid eye movement sleep and increased sleep latency interval. These two qualitative aspects of sleep are significantly improved by estrogen replacement therapy (compared to a placebo), indicating that the low estrogen levels play an important role in menopausal sleep disturbances.

Although depression and mood disturbances can certainly be triggered by the environment and changing family circumstances of the menopausal woman (e.g., children having left the home—the "empty-nest syndrome"—and the successful spouse devoting less time to his family), low estrogen levels provide the biochemical basis for development of depression. Plasma free tryptophan (the fraction not bound to serum proteins) is reduced in postmenopausal women, but total plasma tryptophan (bound and unbound fractions) remains unchanged. Trytophan is an amino acid involved in the metabolism of serotonin, alterations of which have been implicated as a mechanism for the development of endogenous depression. Plasma estrogen levels have a direct relation to plasma free tryptophan. Treatment with estrogen (but not placebo) increases plasma estrogen levels and plasma free tryptophan levels; and it is concurrently accompanied by an improvement in the depression score.

Other nonspecific menopausal complaints such as headache, tiredness, lethargy, irritability, anxiety, and nervousness may be due to family, social, and personal environmental factors of the patient. However, double-blind studies indicate that estrogen replacement significantly reduces these symptoms compared to placebo.

Cardiovascular Diseases

Based on epidemiologic data derived from deaths due to myocardial infarction, the incidence of coronary heart disease in premenopausal women is believed to be lower than in men of the same age group. After menopause, the incidence of deaths due to myocardial infarction apparently increases progressively to reach levels similar to those of men of the same age group by 70 to 80 years of age. The lower incidence of ischemic heart disease in premenopausal women compared to that in men is attributed to the protective benefits of female estrogen levels—lowering cholesterol and low density lipoprotein levels while elevating the high density lipoprotein level. The low levels of estrogen in postmenopausal women may eliminate this gender-related benefit. Alternatively, the *apparent* increase in ischemic heart disease in women after menopause may be due to an improvement in the rate of ischemic heart disease in men after 50 years of age. Most of the men with high risk ischemic heart disease have it before age 50. Nevertheless, the final verdict may not be in, as social habits such as smoking and genetic factors predisposing to hyperlipidemia have not been taken into consideration. As there are now more young women smoking than men of the same age group, the differences in incidence of ischemic heart disease between premenopausal women and men of similar age groups may narrow considerably.

Nevertheless, premature surgically induced menopause (bilateral oophorectomy) does increase the relative risk of myocardial infarction. In women less than 35 years of age the relative risk increased to 7.7 compared to 2.8 for women with natural menopause at the same age; at age 35 to 39, the relative risk of myocardial infarction from bilateral oophorectomy was 2.9 compared to 1.1 for natural menopause at this age; and after age 40, the relative risk of developing myocardial infarction with or without bilateral oophorectomy at hysterectomy remained similar. Except for two reports, studies have indicated that estrogen replacement therapy for the postmenopausal woman confers a protection against coronary heart disease and reduces the relative risk to 0.6 to 0.3.

Bone Mineral Loss and Osteoporosis

Osteoporosis is one of the most significant long-term sequelae of menopause, and it can be readily prevented or reduced through appropriate preventive management of menopause. Osteoporosis is responsible for 1.5 million fractures annually at a cost of $6 billion. By the year 2000 these numbers will have doubled, and there will be twice as many women over 65 years of age. One of every three women will have a vertebral fracture after age 65, and one in three will develop hip fracture after reaching extremely old age. Postmenopausal osteoporosis (type I osteoporosis) occurs within 15 to 20 years of menopause and is due to accelerated bone loss accompanying loss of ovarian function. The loss of bone affects predominantly trabecular bone, so that this type of bone rather than cortical bone is lost. Thus the three commonest fractures seen in postmenopausal women are fractures of the vertebra, ultradistal radius, and neck of the femur— all sites of large amounts of trabecular bone. Fracture of the neck of the femur and ultradistal radius is six times more common in postmenopausal women than in men of the same age group. Black women are slightly more protected than white women from the development of postmenopausal osteoporosis, although they are still twice as likely to develop these fractures than black men of the same age group.

Postmenopausal patients may have variable rates of bone turnover, but all of them who develop osteoporosis eventually have a level of bone resorption that is higher than the level of bone formation, so they continue to lose bone. Even if they have low bone turnover as shown by one-third of patients with vertebral fractures (one-third have normal bone turnover and one-third have high bone turnover), these patients

have had a previous period of accelerated bone loss and have therefore compromised their bone mineral mass status. The low estrogen levels of the postmenopausal woman are inadequate to antagonize the action of parathormone, the levels of which are unaffected after menopause, on bone. Therefore increased bone resorption occurs, leading to increased bone loss. The resorbed calcium from the bone is excreted in the urine so that the urinary calcium/creatinine ratio is increased in the postmenopausal woman. The urinary hydroxyproline/creatinine ratio is also increased, although serum calcium and alkaline phosphatase are not significantly altered. The reduced postmenopausal estrogen levels also may affect calcium absorption through the gut via the action of estrogen on vitamin D hydroxylation to 1,25-hydroxy vitamin D, the active form of vitamin D required for absorption of calcium. Thus estrogen replacement therapy in the postmenopausal woman reduces the urinary calcium/creatinine ratio to levels found in the premenopausal woman and promotes calcium absorption through the gut.

Menopause-related accelerated bone resorption and loss occur over an extended period (four to six years) after menopause, after which most of the loss is probably age-related. The bone loss that occurs after menopause leads to progressive shrinkage of the vertebral bodies, followed by kyphosis and loss of height. This sequence results in a postmenopausal woman who is 1 to 3 inches (as much as 8 inches) shorter than before, has a camel-like hump, a protuberant abdomen with visceroptosis, the lower ribs approximating with the iliac crest, increased transverse skin creases, and difficulty wearing her clothes although her weight may remain unchanged (Fig. 23-2).

In addition to estrogen levels, several factors appear to contribute to the development of postmenopausal osteoporosis (Table 23-2). It is obvious that a number of risk factors, e.g., smoking, high caffeine intake, high alcohol intake, inattention to a balanced diet, inadequate calcium intake, and little exercise are habits that can be readily modified. Estrogen replacement therapy has been shown to reduce hip and forearm fractures significantly as well as reduce the rate of bone mineral loss. Limited evidence suggests that progestin by itself also can reduce bone mineral mass loss.

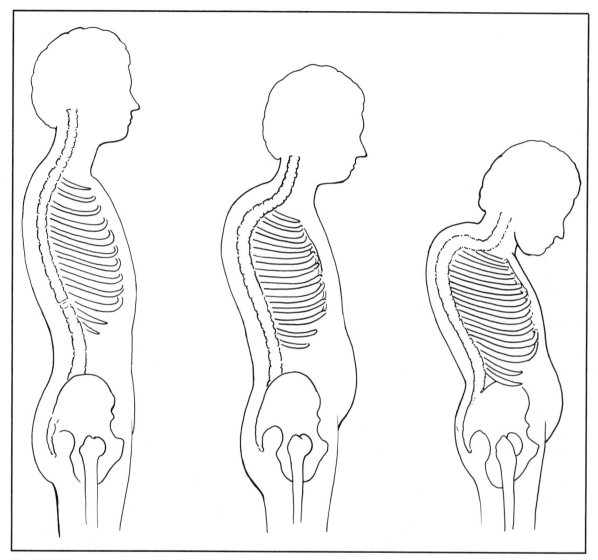

Fig. 23-2. Bone loss in the vertebral bodies in the post-menopausal woman, giving rise slowly to loss of height secondary to shrinkage of the vertebral bodies and re-alignment of their curvature. Five to ten years after menopause and without adequate treatment, the characteristic picture is that of a woman who is now several (1 to 3) inches shorter, with a camel hump on the back and a protuberant abdomen.

Epithelial Changes (Skin and Vagina)

After menopause, skin thickness is markedly decreased as a result of loss of ovarian function and decreased levels of estrogen. The loss of skin thickness is due to a significant decrease in epidermal thickness secondary to reduced epidermal cell turnover rate. When estrogen is given, epidermal cell production increases, and so epidermal thickness is restored to the levels found in premenopausal women. Postmeno-

Table 23-2. Risk Factors for Developing Postmenopausal Osteoporosis

Reduced weight for height ratio
Premature or early menopause
Family history of osteoporosis
Low calcium intake
Cigarette smoking
High caffeine intake
High alcohol intake
Low initial bone mass*
Reduced physical activity

---

*Racial and hereditary differences as well as gender differences give rise to initial bone mass.

pausal thinning of the skin results in skin that is lax, is more transparent, has more readily visible capillaries and blood vessels, and is more easily bruised. In general, healing of the skin is slowed, but the scar is less hypertrophic when union occurs.

In the vagina, the thickness of the epithelium is markedly reduced after menopause, and there is loss of vaginal rugae. The loss of vaginal epithelial thickness operates through the same mechanism as for the epidermis of the skin in other parts of the body. In addition, the vaginal epithelial cells now contain less glycogen, and the acidity of the vagina changes. Consequently, the vagina is small and atrophic, and secondary inflammation due to trauma or infection occurs much more readily. Secondary infection may occur on top of a senile atrophic vaginitis. If a uterovaginal prolapse is present in the postmenopausal woman, decubitus ulceration occurs more readily on the vagina that is already atrophic. Vaginal atrophy, atrophic vaginitis, and decubitus ulceration of an atrophic vagina can be readily treated with estrogen cream for two to three weeks, with gratifying results.

Thinning of the vaginal epithelium does not give rise to coital difficulties so long as regular coital activity is maintained. However, with severe vaginal atrophy or atrophic vaginitis, dyspareunia may occur. With prolonged interruption of coital activity, the postmenopausal vagina may undergo atrophy and narrowing so that resumption of coital activity after an extended prolonged abstinence of coitus may give rise to dyspareunia. Indeed with regular coital activity, a good proportion of postmenopausal women have reported improved sexual activity and response, as fear of pregnancy is now eliminated.

Miscellaneous Changes

The loss of ovarian function and reduced estrogen levels give rise to a number of other changes that are clinically apparent in some postmenopausal women but may not present significant medical symptoms for others. These changes include atrophic changes in the urethra and vulva, so that the external genitalia (e.g., labia majora and minora) are no longer turgid-looking and may appear crinkled. Atrophy of the ligaments supporting the uterus may give rise to uterovaginal descensus, prolapse, cystocele, and rectocele.

MANAGEMENT

The routine minimum workup for a woman entering menopause should include a complete history and physical examination followed by a Papanicolaou smear, a mammogram if one has not been done within the last year, a biopsy (Vabra curettage) of the endometrium if there is evidence of perimenopausal bleeding or irregular vaginal bleeding, and any other relevant tests as determined by the history. A Papanicolaou smear is necessary even if a hysterectomy has been done, as malignant lesions may arise in the vaginal vault. A mammogram is strongly recommended because of the increase in the incidence of breast neoplasia after age 45. Furthermore, mammograms detect lesions that are small and not readily appreciated by the examining hands. Breast cancer is a contraindication to the use of estrogen, and therefore any breast lesions or lumps require a final disposition as to their malignant or benign nature before estrogen replacement therapy can be entertained.

Management of the postmenopausal woman should be aimed at altering social habits that are adverse to the maintenance and promotion of good health, and instituting specific measures to combat the loss of ovarian function and its metabolic and endocrine sequelae. The patient should be discouraged from smoking; if she is already a smoker, she should be apprised of the risks and encouraged to stop smoking. In addition, high caffeine intake, high alcohol intake, and obesity should be reduced.

Specific measures in the management of postmenopausal woman include (1) estrogen replacement therapy, (2) attention to daily calcium intake and if necessary calcium supplements, and (3) weight-bearing exercises.

Estrogen Replacement Therapy

The benefits and potential risks of estrogen replacement therapy should be discussed with the patient prior to initiating such treatment so that a joint decision by the patient and physician is made with respect to the treatment. Certainly patients who have premature menopause, those who have high risk factors for developing osteoporosis (see above), and those with menopausal symptoms ought to be treated with the objective of overcoming some of the problems related to estrogen deficiency as discussed above. In these postmenopausal women the benefits far outweigh the risks of estrogen replacement therapy unless there are absolute medical contraindications to the use of estrogen. Such absolute contraindications include breast cancer, severe liver dysfunction, liver cirrhosis, deep vein thrombosis, pulmonary embolism, cerebrovascular accident, and myocardial infarction.

Much of the confusion surrounding the adverse effects of estrogen replacement therapy for postmenopausal women can be traced to unnecessary extrapolation of the adverse effects reported from estrogen use in the form of the birth control pill. It should be emphasized and clearly noted that many of the metabolic and cardiovascular side effects attributed to the birth control pill are related to the dose of estrogen in the pill. As the estrogen dose has been brought down—from as much as 100 μg of ethinyl estradiol initially to well below 50 μg and, in the low estrogen dose pill, even as little as 30 μg—the incidence of life-threatening side effects has been markedly reduced. Conjugated estrogens are widely prescribed in the United States for estrogen replacement therapy during menopause, and 0.625 mg of conjugated estrogens is equivalent to 5 μg of ethinyl estradiol. In clinical practice, it is rarely necessary to prescribe more than

1.25 mg of conjugated estrogens for management of the postmenopausal woman. Therefore the dose of estrogen employed in hormonal therapy of the postmenopausal woman is well below 10 μg of ethinyl estradiol, a dose considerably lower than that present in even the low dose estrogen birth control pill. The potential adverse effects of estrogen replacement therapy include endometrial hyperplasia and cancer, thromboembolism, strokes, hypertension, breast cancer, gallbladder dysfunction, and gallstones, as well as less life-threatening side effects such as nausea, vomiting, water retention, and breakthrough bleeding.

Numerous retrospective studies have indicated that prolonged unopposed estrogen therapy in the postmenopausal woman increases significantly her risk of developing endometrial hyperplasia and carcinoma of the endometrium. The increased risk is related to both the dose of estrogen used and the duration of therapy. The relative risk increases three- to fourfold with the use of unopposed estrogen and further increases to about 10-fold with 5 to 10 or more years of unopposed estrogens. The increased risk of developing endometrial hyperplasia and endometrial cancer can be eliminated by administering a progestin for 10 to 12 days each month. Indeed, the addition of a progestin for 10 to 12 days each month with estrogen replacement therapy in a menopausal woman who still has her uterus is mandatory to reduce this risk of endometrial cancer. The incidence of gallbladder disease and gallstones is increased 2.5 times with estrogen therapy. Gallstones are likely to form owing to increased cholesterol saturation in the biliary secretion. Consequently, cholecystitis and cholangitis are likely to occur secondary to the presence of the gallstones.

Although it was previously suspected that estrogen might elevate blood pressure secondary to its effect on the renin-angiotensin-aldosterone system, data based on direct observations indicate that estrogen replacement therapy in the postmenopausal woman does not induce hypertension. Mean arterial blood pressure decreases slightly with estrogen replacement therapy. Indeed, blood pressure levels in postmenopausal women with mild and moderate hypertension improve when they are put on estrogen replacement therapy. Nevertheless, it is prudent to document the blood pressure and, if it is elevated, to have a complete workup for hypertension (unles it has been done by her internist or other physician) before initiating estrogen replacement therapy. Subsequently, regular blood pressure measurements should be recorded. Postmenopausal women with severe hypertension or who have the sequelae of hypertension, e.g., thromboembolism, cerebrovascular accident, or myocardial infarction, should probably not be given estrogen replacement therapy.

With the doses of estrogen employed for postmenopausal estrogen replacement therapy (0.625 to 1.250 mg of conjugated estrogen), there is no evidence to indicate a significantly increased risk of thromboembolism, strokes, or myocardial infarction in an otherwise healthy postmenopausal woman. With higher doses of conjugated estrogens, approaching the equivalence of ethinyl estradiol dose present in birth control pills, there may be a slightly increased risk for these cardiovascular complications. However, it is rarely necessary to exceed a daily dose of 1.25 mg of conjugated estrogens for estrogen replacement therapy. There is much evidence to indicate that estrogen replacement therapy of the postmenopausal woman reduces her risk of developing coronary heart disease and myocardial infarction from a relative risk ratio of 1 to as little as 0.3.

One potential risk of estrogen replacement therapy is breast cancer. Although breast cancer, when present, can certainly be stimulated by estrogens, the balance of evidence suggests that there is no increased risk of developing breast cancer with use of postmenopausal hormone replacement therapy. In one study, an eight-year follow-up of postmenopausal women with and without estrogen replacement therapy found that estrogen as well as estrogen plus progestin given cyclically were associated with a significantly lower incidence of breast cancer than was found in women with no hormone therapy. Despite the limitations of this study, the findings are reassuring that there is no increased risk of breast cancer with postmenopausal estrogen therapy. Nevertheless, it is prudent not to give estrogen to a woman who has or had breast cancer or to a woman who has a breast lump the nature of which is not established. Additionally, mammograms should be part of the routine management of

the postmenopausal woman (see below). Other side effects of estrogen replacement therapy, e.g., nausea, vomiting, and breakthrough bleeding, can be more readily managed by adjusting the dose or formulation of estrogen used and, if necessary, performing endometrial sampling to exclude other intrauterine lesions.

In the United States estrogen replacement therapy should be given cyclically for 25 of 30 days with a five-day rest. Therefore in a woman with her uterus in place, estrogen is given for the first 25 days with a progestin added on the last 12 days (days 14 through 25) followed by five days of no medication (Figure 23-3). The usual dose of estrogen is 0.625 mg of conjugated estrogen daily or its equivalent if some other formulation is used. This dose appears to be the minimum one necessary to have a significant protective effect against osteoporosis. An alternative method is to give the estrogen continuously for 30 days of each month with progestin added on the last 12 days (days 19 through 30). This regimen is readily achieved by using a calendar month where the progestin and estrogen are given during the first 12 days and estrogen is continued for the remaining days of the month without progestin (Fig. 23-3). In the United States the most widely used progestin for hormone replacement therapy during menopause is medroxyprogesterone acetate (MPA; Provera). Although a daily dose of 10 mg of MPA has been widely recommended, there are no good objective data to substantiate the optimum minimum dose necessary. A daily dose of 10 mg MPA is usually prescribed, but this dose can be reduced to 5 mg daily if side effects of the larger dose become unacceptable to the patient. Studies are under way to determine which is the minimum dose of MPA needed.

Vaginal bleeding may occur with cyclic estrogen therapy (25 of 30 days). Although it is usually due to withdrawal bleeding, a complete uterine sampling (Vabra curettage or D&C) should be performed to rule out significant endometrial pathology when the bleeding occurs for the first time. If the endometrial histology shows normal changes, it is not necessary to perform further endometrial sampling with subsequent *scheduled* vaginal bleeding.

Although other progestins such as the 19-nor derivatives (norethindrone) can be used, MPA has been

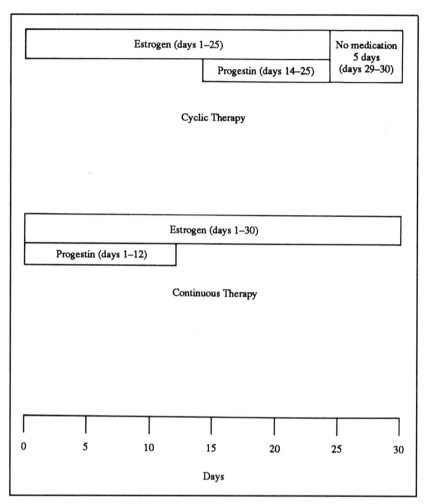

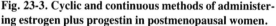

Fig. 23-3. Cyclic and continuous methods of administering estrogen plus progestin in postmenopausal women.

widely used because it causes less elevation of cholesterol and low density lipoprotein and less depression of high density lipoprotein than the 19-nor derivatives. High levels of cholesterol with increased low density lipoprotein and decreased high density lipoprotein levels have been associated with increased risk for developing coronary heart disease. Side effects of MPA include depression; breast fullness, tenderness, or soreness; a feeling of being bloated; weight gain; and premenstrual syndrome-like symptoms.

In postmenopausal women who have had a hyster-

ectomy, there is a difference of opinion as to whether progestin is needed with estrogen replacement therapy, as the risks of endometrial hyperplasia and cancer have been eliminated. Thus estrogens may be given on a continuing basis throughout the month. However, women spend half or more than half of their reproductive lives (if they have had pregnancies) in a progesterone-dominated hormonal environment. Furthermore, one study, based on an eight-year follow-up, indicated that postmenopausal women who received both estrogen and progestin for their hormone replacement therapy had a reduced incidence of breast cancer. Therefore, at present, both estrogens and progestin are given for hormone replacement therapy to postmenopausal women without uteri. The estrogens can be given continuously for 30 days each month with 12 days of progestin.

Because of cyclical bleeding or spotting occuring with the 25-day regimen of estrogen with 5 days of no medication, a regimen employing estrogen combined with a low dose of progestin (2.5 mg MPA) daily and continuously is under study. While such a combined continuous regimen eliminates the withdrawal bleeding problem, the metabolic effects of continuous progestin on lipids need to be carefully examined. This combined continuous estrogen-progestin regimen is under examination in several ongoing clinical trials.

Other Forms of Estrogen Treatment

In addition to the conjugated estrogens, several other estrogen preparations can and are used for estrogen replacement therapy: Ethinyl estradiol is widely in use in Europe; micronized estradiol is available and can be taken orally; estradiol pellets are used as subdermal implants but require placement by a physician at the time of hysterectomy or at regular intervals. To overcome the first-passage effect of estrogens on the liver and therefore on clotting factors and other liver-related metabolic effects after absorption from the gut into the circulation, alternate routes of giving estrogen have been developed.

Estrogens can be administered through the skin, and the Estraderm skin patch delivers estradiol transdermally. The Estraderm patch consists of estradiol in a reservoir with a one-way control membrane delivery system through which the hormone is released at a steady rate from the reservoir and is absorbed through the skin into the circulation. Therefore the liver does not receive a high concentration of the estradiol, as the absorbed hormone goes into the systemic circulation. The Estraderm patch has a protective liner that is peeled off to expose the adhesive surface, which can be applied to any area of the skin, bearing in mind to avoid areas that may be constantly rubbed or irritated by clothing. Estraderm patches come in two doses, 0.05 and 0.1 mg. The lower dose (0.05 mg) patch should be used first, with the higher dose reserved for use if symptoms are not adequately controlled by the lower dose. Serum levels of estradiol obtained are

comparable to those produced by daily oral administration of estradiol at about 20 times the daily transdermal dose. Therefore the dose of estradiol given is markedly reduced. Each Estraderm patch delivers estradiol for up to four days, and therefore the usual regimen is to apply one patch for three or four days, or two patches per week. An easy way to administer the Estraderm patch is to apply a new patch and remove the used one on Sundays and Wednesdays or Mondays and Thursdays every week. Progestins should still be given as with the oral estrogen regimen.

For the cyclic estrogen regimen (see above), the Estraderm patch is applied twice a week for three weeks and one patch on the fourth week, omitting the eighth patch, thus allowing an estrogen-free period of about four days. With the continuous regimen, the patch is applied twice a week throughout, and progestins are added on the third and fourth weeks for 12 days. Transdermal estrogen administration may not be suitable for all postmenopausal women. It can cause skin irritation, and some women (especially the younger ones) may not like its appearance when swimming and sunbathing. For those who do not like or cannot swallow tablets and have to remember daily medication intake, transdermal estrogen provides a convenient alternative.

Another route of giving estrogen is via a vaginal estrogen ring from which the estrogen is readily absorbed through the vagina, which has a rich blood supply. This method is not yet available for clinical use, but esthetic considerations suggest that it is unlikely to be a good alternative to the transdermal route.

Nonestrogen Therapy

For postmenopausal women who are symptomatic but in whom the use of estrogen is contraindicated, the symptoms and long-term sequelae of osteoporosis can be satisfactorily managed with alternative medications or measures. Progestins (e.g., Provera given orally or Depo-Provera given intramuscularly) and the α-adrenergic agonist clonidine are effective for relief of hot flushes. To a lesser extent, Bellergal, which contains a mixture of phenobarbital, ergotamine tartrate, and belladonna, is effective for the relief of hot flushes. If estrogen is contraindicated, progestin therapy with norethindrone can prevent bone loss and therefore postmenopausal osteoporosis. Probably other progestins would work as well. In addition, adequate calcium intake and weight-bearing exercises should further consolidate the reduction in bone loss.

Calcium

In addition to estrogen replacement therapy, attention should be focused on the intake of calcium. The median calcium intake of American men and women age 45 and above during 1971 to 1974 was 600 mg per day. The minimum calcium intake in postmenopausal women should be 1200 mg daily. If the patient is having a good intake of calcium-rich foods, it may not be necessary to supplement with calcium tablets. However, in patients who for one reason or another do not have an adequate calcium intake or absorption, supplemental calcium tablets should be prescribed or recommended. Foods rich in calcium intake include dairy products (whole milk, swiss cheese, cottage cheese, yogurt, ice cream), seafood (sardines with bones, salmon, raw oysters, shrimp), beans (soy bean or tofu), and some vegetables (broccoli, collard greens, leafy green vegetables). Patients should be encouraged to consume foods rich in calcium, but concerns for high polysaturated animal fat through dairy products can be overcome by taking low fat dairy products. It should be remembered that some foods promote the absorption of calcium from the gut: protein, lactose, carbohydrates, acids (lactic, citric) and food with a calcium/phosphate ratio of 1:1 (usually present in most dairy products). On the other hand, oxalates (leafy vegetables), phytic acid, phosphorous

Table 23-3. Calcium Content in Various Calcium Preparations

Preparation	% Calcium
Calcium carbonate	40
Calcium chloride	36
Calcium lactate	13
Calcium gluconate	9
Bone meal	31
Dolomite	22

(as in meat and soda pop), fat, and fiber tend to retard or inhibit calcium absorption. If supplementary calcium is given, it should be taken with a meal, as the fraction of calcium absorbed is then markedly enhanced. Any form of supplemental calcium, e.g., calcium carbonate, calcium citrate, calcium chloride, and other calcium preparations (Table 23-3) can be given, but the amount of elemental calcium should form the basis of the required daily intake of calcium.

Exercise

To reduce calcium and bone resorption and therefore loss of bone mineral mass, postmenopausal women should be encouraged to perform regular weight-bearing exercises. Such exercises include walking and any form of sports that include walking (e.g., golfing), jogging, tennis, aerobics, racketball, and dancing. The type of weight-bearing exercise recommended should be consistent with the life style of the woman and one that is easily carried out by her without unnecessary stress or added cost and that she might not particularly enjoy. Moderate amounts of such exercise should be enough.

POSTMENOPAUSAL BLEEDING

Postmenopausal bleeding should be regarded as a symptom of genital tract cancer until proved otherwise. Although in a large proportion of cases the apparent cause is a benign lesion, thorough sampling of the endometrium by D&C or an outpatient Vabra curettage becomes necessary. The two commonest benign causes of postmenopausal bleeding are atrophic vaginitis and cervical polyps, followed by two much less common causes: uterine fibroids and endometrial hyperplasia. Other occasional causes of postmenopausal bleeding include cervical erosion, trichomonal vaginitis, hematuria, trauma, and vaginal endometriosis. Many of these conditions are obvious and are readily diagnosed by clinical examination that includes a pelvic examination. The respective conditions should be managed as described in the various chapters, after a Papanicolaou smear and endometrial curettage have been performed to rule out cancer of the cervix and uterine body.

Atrophic vaginitis (see above) is readily visible. The vaginal walls are thin, dry, shiny, and easily abraded. The patient may complain of vaginal soreness at coitus or at other times, and often there is a thin, purulent-looking discharge that may be blood-stained. Examination of the vagina shows the walls to be red, shiny, and thin. Small bleeding spots may be obvious in more severe cases. Specific treatment of atrophic vaginitis should include administration of an estrogen cream intravaginally to improve the quality of the vaginal walls, lower the pH, and allow infection to be overcome. Cervical polyps are usually obvious and visible. The polyp needs to be avulsed and sent for histologic examination to determine whether it is benign or malignant. In addition, a search for other cervical or endometrial polyps should be undertaken, including cervical dilatation, exploration of the uterine cavity with an ovum forceps, and endometrial and endocervical curettage. Endometrial hyperplasia should be ruled out, as it may be concomitantly present with a cervical polyp.

Palpation of a fibroid in a postmenopausal woman presenting with vaginal bleeding does not necessarily mean that the fibroid is responsible for the bleeding. Although fibroids may precipitate postmenopausal bleeding, it is important to rule out carcinoma of the cervix and corpus uteri. If the fibroids are known to be increasing in size or are large enough to cause symptoms, surgery is necessary. However, treatment with gonadotropin-releasing hormone agonist is effective (Chap. 17). If adenomatous hyperplasia is found and is responsible for the postmenopausal bleeding, hysterectomy is probably indicated because adenomatous hyperplasia is a precursor of uterine carcinoma. In addition, when endometrial hyperplasia is detected in a postmenopausal woman, estrogen-secreting ovarian tumors should be ruled out. Palpable ovaries, even of normal size, in the postmenopausal woman should arouse suspicion of an ovarian tumor. If the patient is obese and the ovaries are neither palpable nor increased in volume as determined by ultrasound, the likely source of the estrogen responsible for stimulating the endometrium is the adipose tissue, where increased aromatization of androstenedione to estrone occurs. If the adenomatous hyperplasia is due to the use of unopposed estrogen for postmenopausal hormone replacement therapy, a progestogen should be given for 12 days every month. After cyclic progestogen therapy for three cycles, a repeat endometrial biopsy is performed to ensure regression of the hyperplasia. However, if the patient refuses to take a progestogen, the estrogen therapy should be discontinued if endometrial hyperplasia is present.

With more postmenopausal women taking hormonal replacement therapy, the commonest cause of postmenopausal bleeding is likely to be due to cyclic estrogen administration without progestogen. Under such circumstances, endometrial sampling is necessary only on the first occasion. If subsequently the bleeding occurs only on a scheduled basis, endometrial sampling need not be performed more frequently than once every one to two years.

SELECTED READINGS

Bergkvist, L., Adami, H.-O., Persson, I., et al. The risk of breast cancer after estrogen and estrogen-progestin replacement. *N. Engl. J. Med.* 321:293, 1989.

Christiansen, C., Christensen, M. S., Transbol, I., et al. Bone mass in postmenopausal women after withdrawal of oestrogen/gestagen replacement therapy. *Lancet* 1: 459, 1981.

Colditz, G. A., Willett, W. C., Stampfer, M. J., et al. Menopause and the risk of coronary heart disease in women. *N. Engl. J. Med.* 316:1105, 1987.

Ettinger, B., Genant, H. K., and Cann, C. E. Long-term estrogen replacement therapy prevents bone loss and fractures. *Ann. Intern. Med.* 102:319, 1985.

Gelfand, M. E., and Ferenczy, A. A prospective 1-year study of estrogen and progestin in postmenopausal women: Effects on the endometrium. *Obstet. Gynecol.* 74:398, 1989.

Hassager, C., and Christiansen, C. Blood pressure during oestrogen/progestogen substitution therapy in healthy postmenopausal women. *Maturitas* 9:315, 1988.

Laufer, L. R., DeFazio, J. L., Lu, J. K., et al. Estrogen replacement therapy by transdermal estradiol administration. *Am. J. Obstet. Gynecol.* 146:533, 1985.

Lindsay, R., Hart, D. M., and Clark, D. M. Minimum effective dose of estrogen for prevention of premenopausal bone loss. *Obstet. Gynecol.* 63:759, 1984.

Lobo, R. A. Absorption and metabolic effects of different types of estrogens and progestogens. *Obstet. Gynecol. Clinics North Am.* 14:121, 1987.

Meldrum, D. R., Defazio, J. D., Erlik, Y., et al. Pituitary hormones during the menopausal hot flash. *Obstet. Gynecol.* 64:752, 1984.

Mishell, D. R. Menopause. Physiology and pharmacology. Chicago: Yearbook, 1987.

Munk-Jensen, N., Nielsen, S. P., Obel, E. B., et al. Reversal of postmenopausal vertebral bone loss by oestrogen and progestogen: A double blind placebo controlled study. *Br. Med. J.* 296:1150, 1988.

Place, V. A., Powers, M., Darley, P. E., et al. A double-blind comparative study of Estraderm and Premarin in the amelioration of postmenopausal symptoms. *Am. J. Obstet. Gynecol.* 152:1092, 1985.

Prough, S. G., Aksel, S., Wiebe, R. H., et al. Continuous estrogen/progestin therapy in menopause. *Am. J. Obstet. Gynecol.* 157:1449, 1987.

24

Breast Disease

Evaluation of the female breast is an important part of the complete gynecologic examination. The gynecologist performs more periodic medical checkups of women today than does any other category of physician. Because they see such a large number of women for regular examinations, gynecologists need to have a thorough knowledge of the natural history, symptoms, and characteristic physical findings of the various benign and malignant breast disorders; they must also be skilled in the proper techniques of breast examination and be able to teach self-examination to their patients. It is essential, too, that they be aware of the high risk category of women especially deserving of regular surveillance. The gynecologist must be completely familiar with the screening and diagnostic modalities available, the proper indications for their use, and their limitations.

Although the screening and diagnosis of breast carcinoma is the responsibility of the primary gynecologist, the patient with breast cancer should be specifically managed by a coordinated multimodality team of oncologists with a special interest in breast cancer. Therefore the management of breast carcinoma is not included in this chapter, and the interested reader is referred to a number of current texts and references for more specifics on this subject.

EMBRYOLOGY

Breast development of the fetus begins at approximately 35 days of embryonic life. Embryologically, the epithelial ridge differentiates to form lactiferous ducts and alveoli. The functional components of the breast are complete at birth but usually lie dormant until puberty. Lactation is occasionally noted in the neonate and is due to the influence of high levels of maternal estrogen. As the systemic estrogen levels fall, lactation abates. Breast development and maturation comprise one of the landmarks of puberty. The process of breast development takes place over a three- to four-year period, ultimately resulting in an adult breast in both form and function. The various stages of development of the breast during puberty are discussed in detail in Chapter 7. The process of breast development is under the influence of estrogen, progesterone, and prolactin, ultimately resulting in the ability to lactate.

ANATOMY

The functional unit of the adult breast is composed of modified and specialized sebaceous glands. The breast parenchyma is located underneath the superficial fascial layer of the chest wall and is composed of 15 to 20 lobes, arranged in a radial fashion, which drain to the nipple via a single excretory duct (Fig. 24-1). Each lobe of the breast is composed of 30 to 40 lobules, which are the primary functional units. Each lobule is made up of 10 to 100 alveoli, which are lined by secretory cells. It is the secretory cells that form milk when under the influence of appropriate levels of prolactin. Milk is transported from the alveoli by way of 2-mm collecting ducts to lactiferous sinuses, which are approximately 5 to 8 mm in diameter. The lactiferous sinuses ultimately drain through the excretory duct and into the nipple. The ducts draining the lobules are supported by stroma composed of fibrous tissue, fat, blood vessels, lymphatics, and nerves. Whereas the lobules occupy the central portion of the breast, glandular tissue may extend toward the axilla from the upper outer quadrant (tail of Spence). The periphery of the breast is made up primarily of fat.

The breasts, which weigh 200 to 300 gm during the menstruating years, are surrounded by fascial tissue and are supported by Cooper's ligaments. These fibrous septa extend from the skin to the underlying pectoralis fascia. With stretching caused by enlargement of the breast during pregnancy and lactation, and with age, Cooper's ligaments become stretched, resulting in diminished breast support.

Lymphatic drainage of the breast is especially important with regard to the spread of breast carcinoma.

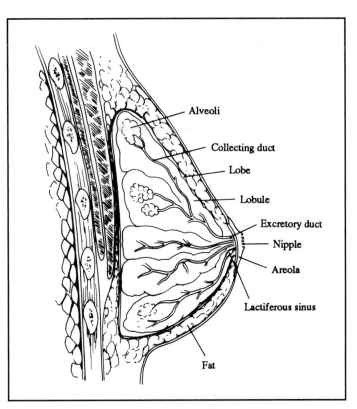

Fig. 24-1. Anatomy of the adult breast.

Ninety-seven percent of the lymphatic drainage of the breast is by way of the axillary chain of nodes. Collateral lymphatic drainage also extends along the internal mammary vessels, especially from the medial aspect of the breast. By way of the internal mammary vessels, lymphatics drain to the mediastinal, subpectoral, and subdiaphragmatic areas. It is convenient to divide lymph nodes into groups for the purpose of staging metastases of breast cancer: *Level 1 nodes* are those on the lateral border of the pectoralis minor muscle; *level 2 nodes* lie underneath the pectoralis minor muscle; and *level 3 nodes* are superior to the pectoralis minor. Interpectoral nodes are located between the pectoralis major and minor muscles. The blood supply of the breasts arises from the internal mammary arteries and the lateral thoracic arteries.

The skin supporting the breast tissue contains hair follicles, sebaceous glands, and eccrine sweat glands. Specialized pigmented skin constitutes the areola and

nipple. The pigmented areola surrounds the nipple. At the periphery of the areola are located Montgomery's glands, which are large sebaceous glands capable of secreting milk. The elevation of the duct openings are easily seen and are called Morgagni's tubercules. The nipple contains sensory nerve endings (important in the lactating reflex arc), as well as sebaceous and apocrine sweat glands.

PHYSIOLOGY

During the normal menstrual cycle, the breast undergoes cyclic changes under the influence of estrogen and progesterone. During the follicular phase, increasing levels of estrogen lead to epithelial proliferation. During the secretory phase of the menstrual cycle, under the influence of progesterone, the mammary ducts dilate and alveolar epithelial cells differentiate into secretory cells. Lipid droplets are found in the alveolar cells, and some intraluminal secretion may be noted. These responses are mediated by estrogen and progesterone receptors in the normal breast epithelium. Increased estrogen also results in increased mammary blood flow, which is most evident during the three to four days before the onset of menses. During this time, the breast volume may increase by 15 to 30 ml, and many women experience breast fullness owing to intralobular edema and ductal-acinar proliferation. With the onset of menses and the falling levels of sex steroid hormones, the secretory activity of the breast also diminishes.

Physiologic alterations of the breast are noted especially in adolescent girls, during pregnancy, and postpartum during lactation. The adolescent girl may experience several conditions that are physiologic yet disturbing. *Unilateral hypoplasia* is rare, and rarer still is congenital absence of a breast. Congenital absence is usually related to a musculoskeletal defect in the chest wall. *Premature development of the breast* is more frequent and may be present without other manifestations of sexual maturation. Functional ovarian neoplasms should be suspected in these circumstances. If no etiology for premature breast development is found, no treatment should be instituted. A common finding on physical examination of the adolescent is *asymmetric breast development*. It is not unusual to find one breast lagging behind in development, achieving equal development only over a period of months or years. Finally, *breast hypertrophy,* especially extreme cases, may be psychologically disturbing for both the young girl and her parents. Psychological counseling may be necessary, and in extreme cases reduction mammoplasty may be advised to achieve a more normal anatomic appearance.

Pregnancy causes progressive changes in breast anatomy and physiology owing to the increasing levels of estrogen, progesterone, human placental lactogen, and prolactin. During pregnancy, active growth of the breast tissue is noted with marked ductal, lobular, and alveolar growth. Increasing levels of estrogen result in the release of prolactin indirectly by reduction of the hypothalamic release of prolactin-inhibiting factor. Increasing levels of prolactin through the pregnancy result in protein synthesis by the mammary epithelium. Changes in the breast are noted as early as five

weeks after the last menstrual period. Most commonly, enlargement and fullness are noted by the woman, with the physical examination showing increased dilatation of superficial veins and increased pigmentation of the areola and nipple. As pregnancy progresses, colostrum is produced by the alveoli. By 16 weeks of gestation, the breasts are fully primed to lactate, which often occurs if pregnancy is interrupted during the second trimester. Throughout pregnancy, progressive dilatation of the alveoli, myoepithelial cell hypertrophy, and increasing fat lead to further enlargement of the breast.

Lactation is initiated after delivery of the fetus; immediate withdrawal of human placental lactogen and estrogen at the time of delivery result in an increased prolactin level, which initiates lactation in the presence of cortisol, insulin, and growth hormone. The initial secretion, during the first few days after delivery, is colostrum (a thick, sticky fluid) that gradually turns to the thin serous breast milk. Colostrum is rich in immunoglobulins and fatty acids, which may add to the immune competence of the neonate. Suckling causes and maintains prolactin release. Prolactin then causes the breast epithelial cells to have increased water transport as well as protein, milk fat, and lactose synthesis. The ejection of milk formed in the breast through the nipple to the neonate is initiated by suckling. Nerves in the areola are activated by suckling, sending messages to the hypothalamus, resulting in decreased prolactin-inhibiting factor synthesis and increased oxytocin synthesis. The oxytocin released by the posterior pituitary acts on the myoepithelial cells in the breast, which contract and eject milk from the alveoli into ducts and sinuses. This "let down reflex" may also occur after psychic stimulation, e.g., hearing the newborn cry.

EXAMINATION AND EVALUATION OF THE BREAST

Routine examination of the breast has as its primary goal the early detection and improved survival of patients with breast carcinoma. Evaluation of the breast, however, also allows recognition of more frequent, benign conditions and often affords therapy to patients who presumed that they must suffer with breast disease. Examination of the breast should therefore be part of the routine physical examination, and breast self-examination should be taught to every patient.

Breast examination should be carried out to maximize detection of breast masses and associated changes in the breast, e.g., skin or nipple retraction, subcutaneous edema, and nipple discharge. Examination in several positions optimizes detection of abnormalities (Fig. 24-2). The breast examination is usually initiated in the sitting position; the breasts are exposed, and the physician (or patient, viewing through a mirror) observes for *asymmetry of the breast*. Special attention should be paid to possible *skin or nipple retraction* or other skin changes, e.g., discoloration or edema. The patient then raises her arms over her head, and the breasts are examined with particular attention to the lower half of the breast. Elevating the arms pulls upward on Cooper's ligaments

and thereby accentuates skin retraction, especially in the lower half of the breast. The patient should then place her hands on her hips and contract the pectoralis major muscle, again attempting to accentuate skin retraction.

With the patient remaining in the sitting position, the breast is palpated. Examination using the whole hand as a unit and the pulps of the fingers rather than the fingertips affords optimal capability to detect breast lesions. The breast is palpated in an organized and systematic fashion, with additional attention to the supraclavicular areas, the neck, and the axillae. Any

Fig. 24-2. Steps of the complete breast examination. A. Inspection of the breasts in the upright position, with arms raised. B. Inspection in the upright position with hands pushing against hips. C. Palpation of the axilla and breast in the upright position. D. Palpation of the breast and axilla in the supine position.

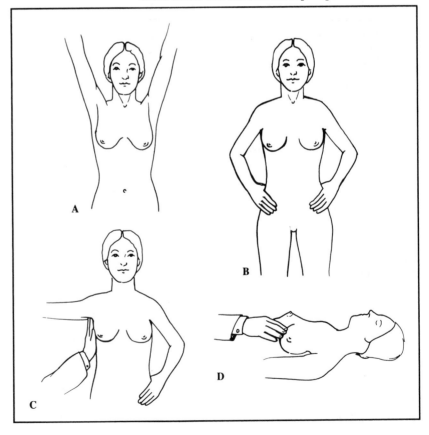

masses or nodules palpated are noted, and attention is paid to the mobility or fixation, size, and consistency of the mass(es). The patient is then asked to bend forward and, with the breast dependent, is reinspected for other skin retraction, e.g., subareolar retraction. Skin changes, especially edema of the skin (peau d'orange), suggest an underlying cancer, although fat necrosis or edema from obstructed lymph nodes may also cause these changes. Red, warm skin (erythema) suggests inflammation, mastitis, or abscess, although inflammatory carcinoma may also present as erythema and pain. The nipple is inspected with particular attention to retraction, ulceration, and discharge (see later in this chapter for the evaluation of nipple discharge).

The patient then assumes the supine position with her arms raised over the head. Palpation is repeated with attempts to spread out the breast tissue so as little as possible is palpated at any one time. Again, the breast is palpated systematically so that no areas go unexamined, with the palpation proceeding along the tail of Spence to the axilla. Assessment on palpation includes an evaluation of the background consistency of the breast. On occasion, a premenstrual patient has engorged glandular tissue that is so dense and nodular it is impossible to assess. This patient should be reexamined several days after the menstrual period. On the other hand, postmenopausal women should have no cyclic change in the breast (unless they are receiving cyclic estrogen and progesterone). Examination of the breast in the supine position includes also a search for masses or thickening. Characteristics suggestive of benign or malignant disease are listed in Table 24-1.

As the breast changes throughout a woman's lifetime, the examination also changes. As previously noted, the menstrual woman displays increased fullness of the breast along with engorgement of glandular epithelium, which makes the breast more nodular and examination of the breast more difficult. Women between 20 and 40 also tend to have an increased glandular/fat ratio and an increased incidence of fibrocystic disease. These differences through the menstrual cycle and throughout a patient's life should be taken into account when the breast is evaluated.

The physician's annual breast examination is an opportune time to teach the patient *breast self-examination*. Self-examination is to be encouraged, and it is suggested that it be performed on a monthly basis following the menstrual period. Examination in the shower when the breast is covered with soap increases tactile sensation by decreasing skin friction. The patient should also be informed that repeated examinations allow her to become familiar with her breasts, and she may therefore notice changes sooner than her examining physician. Patient teaching information—written material, videotapes, and models for practice examinations—are widely available.

MAMMOGRAPHY

The most useful imaging technique for the breast currently available is mammography. The primary value of mammography is its demonstrated role in the diagnosis of breast carcinoma before the patient develops signs or symptoms. Prospective randomized studies and demonstration projects have shown that mammography detects breast carcinoma at an early stage

Table 24-1. Findings on Breast Examination Suggesting Benign or Malignant Conditions

Condition	Mass	Nipple discharge	Skin changes
Benign	Soft Smooth Regular borders Not fixed	Clear or milky Bilateral	None
Malignant	Hard Irregular Fixed to skin or chest wall fascia	Bloody Unilateral	Skin or nipple retraction Peau d'orange changes of skin

and, with appropriate therapy, increases survival. In many instances, mammography detects lesions months or years before they are palpable. (One must realize that a clinician or patient can rarely detect a mass less than 1 cm in diameter. It is estimated that it takes breast carcinoma approximately three years to grow from a 1-mm nodule—potentially detectable by mammography—to a 1-cm nodule, which might be detectable by palpation.) Mammography is used in two situations: (1) screening for breast cancer in asymptomatic women; and (2) evaluating the breast in a patient with symptoms.

Screening Mammography

The use of mammography to screen large populations of women at risk but who are asymptomatic has demonstrated that survival from breast cancer may be increased. The most widely reported study is that of the Health Insurance Plan of New York, which performed annual mammography and has now accumulated 10 to 14 years of follow-up. In that randomized trial there was a 30 percent reduction in mortality for patients who underwent screening mammography. In the Breast Cancer Detection Demonstration Project, 42 percent of all breast cancers were detected by mammography alone. Moreover, there was a 50 percent reduction of breast cancer patients who had metastases in axillary lymph nodes. This finding is significant when one realizes that a carcinoma localized to the breast with no evidence of metastasis to the lymph nodes is associated with an approximately 85 percent survival, whereas only 53 percent of patients with metastases in lymph nodes survive. Therefore detecting breast cancer before it has metastasized to lymph nodes increases survival by about 30 percent.

To be considered an optimal screening test, mammography should be widely applicable with high sensitivity and specificity, minimal cost, and negligible risk. Although not an ideal screening test, the demonstration that mammography can reduce deaths from breast cancer certainly is compelling enough to use this test on a routine basis. Controversy arose during the 1970s regarding the radiation exposure to the breast with the potential subsequent increased incidence of breast cancer. During the 1980s, however, improvements in radiologic techniques reduced the exposure to the breast during mammography to a point where it is no longer considered a statistically significant problem. It is estimated that the routine use of screening mammography would increase the incidence of breast cancer by one new cancer among 1 million women screened. This figure is approximately the same risk of death as that encountered by driving a car 300 miles.

For optimal results, mammography equipment should be used by a properly trained and dedicated radiologist, using either xeromammographic techniques or screen film mammography. There is probably no significant difference in the accuracy of cancer detection between the two methods, and some advantages are enjoyed by each.

Xeromammography appears to be able to emphasize subtle differences in breast density and, owing to the specific technique, has improved visualization of microcalcifications and spiculations. This advantage is especially helpful for evaluating the dense or large breast.

Screen film mammography enjoys the advantage of exposing the patient to one-third to one-fifth the radiation dose that is used with xeromammography. For a two-view screen film mammogram, the breast is exposed to 0.3 cGy. Therefore screen film mammography is used most widely for breast screening. It also seems to be better at differentiating soft tissue masses from surrounding tissue (Fig. 24-3). The main disadvantage of screen film mammography is that it requires vigorous breast compression to flatten out the breast sufficiently to obtain optimal images. The patient should be informed of this discomfort prior to undergoing mammography. No matter which mammographic technique is performed, optimal results are achieved by competent technologists acquiring quality images, which are then carefully examined by a skilled, dedicated radiologist.

Current screening recommendations for asymptomatic women have been made by the American Cancer Society and supported by the American College of Obstetricians and Gynecologists. The recommended frequency of breast screening, including breast self-

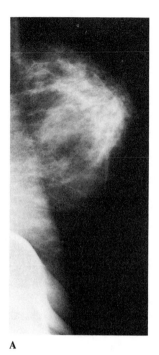 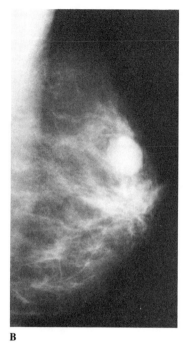 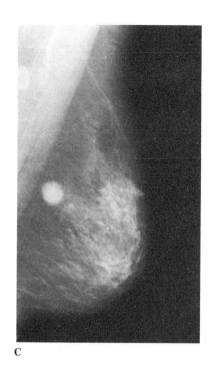

A   B   C

Fig. 24-3. A. Normal mammogram. B. Mammogram showing a typical fibroadenoma. The lesion has the same density as cancer but with a well-defined margin. Nonetheless, a biopsy is required for definitive diagnosis. C. Infiltrating ductile carcinoma in the posterior left breast. The mass is about 1.4 cm in diameter and has an ill-defined, or spiculated, margin.

examination, annual breast examination by a physician, and screening mammography, are shown in Table 24-2.

In addition to detecting subclinical breast carcinomas, mammography may also be used to localize small lesions prior to surgical biopsy: A needle is passed, under mammographic guidance, into the region of the occult lesion. Using either an injection of vital dye or a hook that holds the needle in place in the tissue of concern, the surgeon then uses the dye or hook as a guide to the tissue to be excised. Once the tissue is excised at biopsy, mammography may also be used to confirm that the suspicious lesion has truly been removed. The tissue is then evaluated histologically.

Table 24-2. Recommendations for Screening for Breast Cancer in Asymptomatic Women

Age of woman (years)	Recommendation
>21	Instructed to perform breast self-examination monthly
35–40	Annual breast examination by a physician and baseline mammogram
40–50	Annual breast examination, screening mammography at 1- to 2-year intervals
>50	Annual breast examination and annual mammographic examination

Mammography in the Symptomatic Woman

In a patient who has a palpable breast mass or other symptoms, mammography may be of additional assistance for evaluating the nature of the mass and detecting other occult disease, either in the breast of concern or the contralateral breast. All patients with a palpable breast mass or nipple discharge should undergo mammography prior to biopsy. The value of mammography lies in its ability to detect other associated breast lesions that might not be clinically recognized. In addition, mammography may give further indication as to the nature of the mass and whether it should be of concern or can simply be followed. Therefore mammography and physical examination are complementary; they do not replace each other.

Anatomic architectural changes found on mammography may lead to a greater or lesser level of suspicion for malignancy. Calcifications found on mammography are often smaller than 0.5 mm and may require magnification for detection by the radiologist. Clusters of calcifications have been associated with malignancy, but as a single finding are benign in 75 percent of cases. When calcifications are associated with a spiculated ill-defined margin of a mass, a diagnosis of cancer is confirmed in up to 90 percent of cases (Fig. 24-3C). Other subtle changes associated with breast cancers include a single dilated duct, architectural distortion, and developing density. Although these findings are clinically occult, they are associated with breast cancer in approximately 20 to 30 percent of patients. Unfortunately, the radiographic characteristics of a benign mass and malignant disease often overlap, and therefore mammography cannot entirely obviate the need for surgical biopsy. Mammography, however, easily identifies calcified fibroadenomas and radiolucent lesions such as lipomas, galactoceles, and intramammary lymph nodes.

OTHER IMAGING TECHNIQUES

Ultrasonography

The use of ultrasonography for evaluation of the breast has increased since the early 1970s with improvement in technology and resolution. Nonetheless, it is not sensitive enough to be used as a screening technique for detection of early breast cancer in asymptomatic women. Overall, ultrasonography misses approximately 50 percent of lesions less than 2 cm in diameter and therefore cannot be used in place of mammography for screening. The primary role of ultrasonography is for differentiating a mass that may be solid or cystic. In the patient in whom the breast mass cannot be aspirated based on palpation alone, ultrasonography may be used to direct a needle into the mass for aspiration, thereby avoiding surgical excision. Additionally, some nonpalpable mammogram-detected lesions that are suggested to be cysts may be aspirated by ultrasonographic guidance. Ultrasonography is less accurate than mammography for distinguishing benign masses from those that are malignant.

Transillumination

Passing light waves through the breast (*transillumination*) has been evaluated for detection of an increased blood supply to a tumor; such a condition produces greater light absorption, thereby casting a shadow. However, lesions that can be detected by transillumination must be reasonably large, and all such lesions would be diagnosed either by physical examination or mammography. To date there is no proved rationale for using transillumination to detect or diagnostically differentiate breast lesions.

Miscellaneous Techniques

The measurement of skin surface temperature (*thermography*) has been evaluated as a possible screening test for breast cancer. An advantage of this method is that it requires no radiation exposure. However, frequent false-positive and false-negative results make thermography unsuitable for detection of asymptomatic malignancies. Therefore thermography has no role in the evaluation or management of patients' breasts. *Computed tomography* (CT) and *magnetic resonance imaging* remain experimental techniques for the evaluation of the breast. CT scanning requires higher radiation exposure than mammograms, the use of intravenous contrast material, and a longer time to perform the study. The only advantage of CT scanning at the present time is for localization of a lesion that is seen by only one view of a mammogram.

EVALUATION OF A BREAST MASS

Evaluation of a breast mass is directed at confirming or excluding the possibility of breast cancer. All ap-

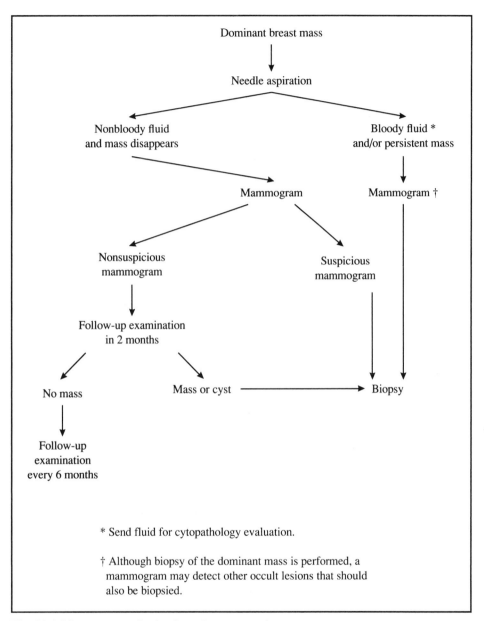

Fig. 24-4. Management of a dominant breast mass in a premenopausal woman.

propriate diagnostic modalities, including physical examination, mammography, and ultrasonography, are employed. Patients may be conveniently grouped as those of pre- and perimenopausal age and those who are postmenopausal. Because many dominant masses in premenopausal women are benign cysts, needle aspiration should be initially attempted. The schema of management of a mass in a premenopausal woman is shown in Figure 24-4. On the other hand, a dominant mass in the postmenopausal woman should be evaluated by mammography and biopsy (Fig. 24-5), as cysts are rare and malignancy is more common.

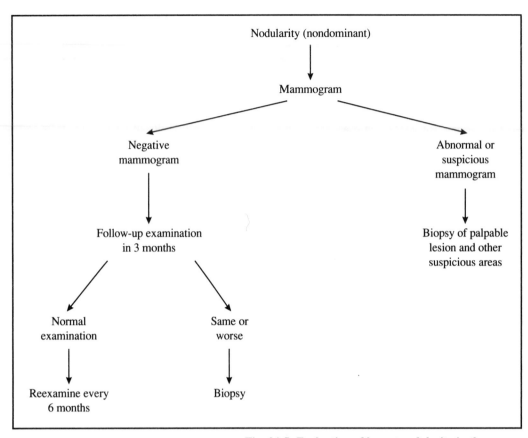

Fig. 24-5. Evaluation of breast nodularity in the postmenopausal woman.

Nodularity or thickening in the postmenopausal breast is a more difficult problem, the resolution of which may be aided by mammography (Fig. 24-6).

In pre- and perimenopausal women, a breast mass may have a reasonably high possibility of being a benign cyst. With this high probability, aspiration of the cyst may be all that is required. It is therefore advised that the cyst be aspirated under local anesthesia. First, the aspiration determines whether the mass is solid or cystic. If it is cystic, and clear, yellow or greenish fluid is obtained, it is most likely benign. In this setting, the cyst should be completely aspirated. On follow-up examination, if the cyst has completely disappeared and does not recur, no further therapy is advised. On the other hand, if the cyst fluid is bloody or if the mass does not completely resolve with aspiration, a formal excisional biopsy should be performed. If the cyst fluid is bloody, it should be submitted to the cytopathology laboratory for further cytologic evaluation. Fine-needle aspiration of a solid mass should be submitted for cytopathologic study also. If the diagnosis of carcinoma is made by fine-needle aspiration, a discussion as to therapeutic options might be carried out prior to definitive therapy. Any cyst or mass that reappears after being aspirated should be biopsied for formal diagnosis.

The postmenopausal patient is more likely to have breast cancer and less likely to have a cyst. The postmenopausal breast is usually more easily evaluated owing to the decrease in the glandular/fat ratio and the decrease in fibrocystic and glandular activity induced by menopausal levels of sex steroids. Hormone replacement therapy during menopause, however, may worsen the glandular pattern and the patient's

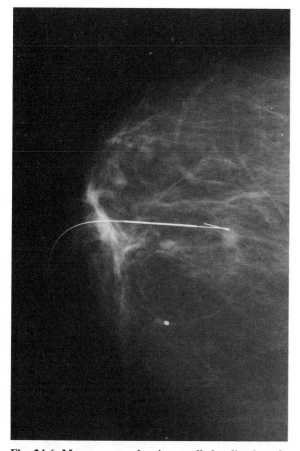

Fig. 24-6. Mammogram showing needle localization of a clinically occult lesion.

symptoms. Because masses in the menopausal breast are rarely cysts, fine-needle aspiration is usually used only for cytologic diagnosis. In the patient with a *dominant mass,* mammograms should be obtained of both breasts and then fine-needle aspiration performed, followed by open biopsy. For the patient who has no dominant mass but there is nodularity or thickening, mammography should be performed followed by biopsy if a suspicious lesion is noted.

Breast Biopsy

Breast biopsy is usually performed to clarify uncertain clinical or radiographic conditions. Because there is always the potential that a biopsy may not excise

the lesion of interest, even open biopsy is not 100 percent accurate. Attempts to more accurately localize a lesion preoperatively and the use of radiographic techniques to confirm the removal of the lesion of interest have helped to improve the accuracy of biopsy. In modern practice, biopsy is usually performed under local anesthesia or a light general anesthesia, most often in an outpatient surgical setting. After careful pathologic evaluation of the biopsy specimen, definitive therapy is recommended. In days past, attempts were made to obtain a biopsy specimen, determine frozen section pathology, and then provide definitive therapy for breast cancer under the same anesthetic. It has been clearly shown that the risks of delaying definitive therapy for breast cancer are not increased by awaiting a diagnosis based on the examination of the formalin-fixed specimen.

Most biopsies of breast lesions are *excisional* with the plan of completely removing the lesion. For lesions that are located away from the areola and that are considered possible cancer, a curvilinear incision is usually made over the lesion, observing Langer's lines to obtain the best cosmetic result. The dissection is carried down around the lesion, which is entirely excised. Hemostasis is achieved and the skin closed with fine sutures. For young women in whom fibroadenoma is the likely diagnosis, the mass may be excised through a circumareolar incision. Using this incision, a subcutaneous tunnel is made through the breast tissue to reach the lesion to be excised. This incision affords the best cosmetic results. The specimen should be inked to determine margins and adequacy of excision; and if cancer is suspected, a frozen section specimen should be obtained. If cancer is found on frozen section, some tissue should be preserved (frozen) for estrogen and progesterone receptor analysis of the tumor.

If a patient's breast mass is too large to be removed completely or if she has clinically inoperable malignancy, an *incisional biopsy* may be performed. A portion of the mass is excised, some of which should be submitted for estrogen and progesterone receptor analysis to guide subsequent palliative therapy.

In situations where a nonpalpable mass is found on mammographic examination, needle localization is required to ensure accurate removal of the lesion and

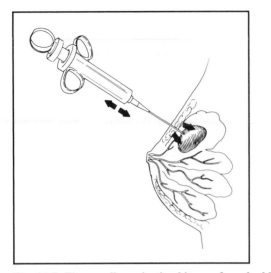

Fig. 24-7. Fine-needle aspiration biopsy of a palpable breast lesion. The same technique may be used to aspirate a breast cyst.

to minimize the amount of normal breast tissue removed. The needle is placed under mammographic guidance by the radiologist (see Fig. 24-6). In general, the biopsy specimen is obtained by incising along the needle tract and removing the tissue at the tip of the needle. Close communication between the radiologist, surgeon, and pathologist is mandatory to ensure that the specimen removed truly contains the lesion found on mammography. Radiopaque dyes are sometimes injected into the site and radiographs of the biopsy specimen obtained to ensure that the appropriate tissue has been removed.

Fine-Needle Aspiration

In the situation where a palpable mass is noted, whether interpreted as cystic or solid, fine-needle aspiration may be employed as an initial step of evaluation and, on occasion, is all that is necessary for adequate evaluation. The management of a breast cyst has been discussed previously (*vide supra*). When a solid mass or an area of thickening is noted, a fine-needle aspiration biopsy may be performed.

A 22- to 20-gauge needle with a syringe attached is inserted into the mass; then with fine inward and out-

ward movements and with negative pressure applied to the syringe, a small amount of tissue and cellular material is obtained in the needle tip (Fig. 24-7). Some of this material is smeared on a glass slide, and the remainder is placed in saline for cytopathologic evaluation. The accuracy of fine-needle aspiration is reasonably good. False-negative fine-needle aspiration results are reported to range between 5 and 20 percent. Therefore if the aspirate shows no evidence of malignancy, open biopsy must be performed. On the other hand, the false-positive rate is low, approaching 0 percent. With the knowledge of malignancy, more definite therapy may be planned.

EVALUATION OF NIPPLE DISCHARGE

Nipple discharge is a frequent complaint of women with both benign and malignant breast disease. Although most patients with nipple discharge have benign conditions, thorough evaluation (including mammography) and usually biopsy are necessary to establish the correct diagnosis. Cytologic study of the nipple discharge is easily performed but is falsely negative in up to 20 percent of patients with cancer. Cancer may be associated with a discharge of any consistency or nature, although some general comments may be made based on the character of the discharge. Intraductal papillomas and fibrocystic disease are the most common cause of nipple discharge. Overall, approximately 1 in 8 patients with a nipple discharge (not galactorrhea) are found to have a malignancy of the breast.

A milky discharge from the nipple, such as is encountered with galactorrhea, is usually bilateral. This discharge is most frequently associated with endocrine disturbances. The approach to the diagnosis and management of this problem is discussed in Chapter 11. However, if this type of nipple discharge should appear in a postmenopausal woman, especially if it is unilateral, careful investigation regarding possible local breast disease must be undertaken, including mammography, cytologic study of the discharge, and biopsy if the discharge can be demonstrated to originate in a focal area of the lobular system or if a mass is palpable.

Serous discharge is seen most often with benign intraductal lesions such as papillomatosis, small papillomas, or epithelial hyperplasia. Again, if no mass is palpable, mammography may be helpful. If a mass is detected or if the discharge can be shown to originate in a specific segment of the ductal system, excisional biopsy is indicated. Bloody nipple discharge is most often associated with intraductal papilloma, whereas serosanguineous discharge is more characteristic of intraductal carcinoma. In either situation, full evaluation with mammography and examination as well as local excision is advised for diagnosis and treatment. A dark green or multicolor discharge that is thick and sticky and almost always bilateral is characteristic of mammary duct ectasia. This discharge results from dilatation of the terminal ducts, with formation of an irritating lipid-containing fluid that produces an inflammatory reaction and hypersecretion in the nipple. Conservative treatment with cleansing soaps and gentle alcohol wipes plus avoidance of any further nipple chafing or irritation should aid in the resolution of this problem.

NIPPLE RETRACTION AND EROSION

Nipple inversion is a frequent normal anatomic variation that is usually bilateral but may be unilateral. On examination, the involved nipple can usually be manually everted and temporarily placed in the more usual erect position. True nipple retraction is usually of recent origin, is invariably unilateral, and implies an underlying disease process of potential malignant nature. However, subareolar fat necrosis, chronic intraductal infection, and plasma cell mastitis can also cause irreversible nipple retraction. Biopsy is therefore usually necessary to establish a definite diagnosis.

Simple erosions of the nipple occur most commonly in nursing mothers and usually respond to conservative local measures and temporary suspension of nursing. Erosions or ulcerations can be traumatic in origin in nonlactating women, but this situation occurs infrequently. When the nipple and surrounding areolar area is eroded or covered by an eczematoid, weeping lesion (or both), the possibility of Paget's disease of the nipple with an underlying intraductal adenocarcinoma should be strongly suspected. Mammography and biopsies of the skin lesion and any pal-

pable masses or abnormal breast areas seen on mammography should be performed in order to arrive at a definitive diagnosis. Benign nipple and areolar swelling sometimes appear when inspissated secretions cause plugging and obstruction, with resulting cystic dilatation of one of the nipple ducts (galactocele) or when a similar type of ductal obstruction occurs and results in cystic dilatation of one of the areolar glands of Montgomery. Sometimes these obstructions disappear, drain spontaneously, and subside; usually, however, they need to be opened and drained or completely excised.

RECOGNITION AND MANAGEMENT OF COMMON BREAST DISORDERS

Although carcinoma of the breast is the most significant breast disease from the standpoint of the patient's overall present and future health and well-being, patients come to the physician far more frequently because of a variety of other benign breast disorders. Many of these disorders require some form of evaluation and therapy for relief of symptoms; and in almost all cases the possibility of malignancy must be excluded. This section concentrates on the evaluation and management of such benign breast conditions.

The therapy of breast carcinoma is constantly undergoing evolution, and the student is referred to other current oncology textbooks for more detailed discussions as to the appropriate surgical, medical, and radiotherapeutic management of breast carcinoma. Because the gynecologist most frequently sees patients with benign conditions and usually does not manage patients once breast cancer is diagnosed, the benign conditions are discussed in more detail in this section.

Fibrocystic Changes

Fibrocystic changes of the breast are the most common benign breast conditions encountered in the premenopausal woman. The older terms fibrocystic breast disease, chronic cystic mastitis, and mammary dysplasia have been replaced by the term *fibrocystic changes*. This condition is not a true disease or pathologic condition; it is an exaggerated response of breast tissue to fluctuating hormone levels. Therefore these changes are found most frequently in women 20 to 50 years of age or, if estrogens are prescribed, during menopause. The exact incidence is difficult to establish in life, but pathologic findings suggest that at least 50 percent of autopsy breast specimens contain fibrocystic changes. Some studies have suggested that one in three premenopausal women have clinical evidence of fibrocystic changes, and approximately 50 percent of these women have significant symptoms.

The etiology of fibrocystic changes is not clear. Proliferation and hyperplasia of the lobular, ductal, and acinar epithelium is noted along with proliferation of fibrous tissue in the breast. Because these tissues are under the influence of estrogen and progesterone, it is hypothesized that this condition is an exaggerated response of these tissues.

Symptoms of fibrocystic disease are usually worst during the premenstrual days of the menstrual cycle. The patient usually experiences cyclic bilateral breast pain with engorgement, increased density, increased nodularity and tenderness, and occasionally a nipple discharge. Some patients note a dominant cyst that may increase during the premenstrual period.

Examination of the patient usually reveals a lumpy nodularity more prominent in the upper outer quadrants of the breasts. The breasts may feel rubbery with solid areas, microcysts, or macrocysts. The diagnosis is usually based on these clinical signs and symptoms, although it may also be established by biopsy findings. Biopsy may show adenosis and fibrosis, ductal ectasia, apocrine metaplasia, papillomatosis, and intraductal epithelial hyperplasia. These conditions are in general not associated with an increased risk of breast cancer. On the other hand, findings of ductal hyperplasia with atypia or apocrine metaplasia with atypia are associated with an approximately fivefold risk of developing subsequent breast cancer.

Treatment of fibrocystic breast disease depends on the severity of symptoms. Initial therapy should include good breast support with a firmly fitted brassiere worn both day and night. If a dominant mass is noted on palpation or on mammography, biopsy should be performed.

Premenstrual use of diuretics and salt restriction may be of some help in reducing edema and breast fullness and tenderness. The complete elimination of methylxanthines from the diet has been reported to reduce breast symptoms in some patients, although the results of this therapy are debated by others. If tried, caffeine (including colas, coffee, tea, and chocolates) must be eliminated from the diet. The use of oral contraceptives and progesterone helps some patients minimize their breast symptoms.

In patients with severe fibrocystic breast symptoms, danazol may be tried. The patient should take 100 to 400 mg per day for four to six months. Approximately 90 percent of patients experience a decrease in symptomatology and decreased palpable nodularity with this regimen. Unfortunately, danazol is costly, and this factor must be balanced against the benefits the patient may experience. Alternative methods of therapy for patients who have failed the above treatments include the use of bromocriptine 5 mg per day or the antiestrogen tamoxifen.

Finally, in patients with severe symptoms who are unresponsive to medical management, subcutaneous mastectomy with breast implant may be advised. Usually, these patients are experiencing severe pain and have undergone multiple biopsies of breast lesions. This therapy is also appropriate in patients who have been found on biopsy to have evidence of the premalignant conditions cited above.

Benign Breast Tumors

Fibroadenomas. Fibroadenomas are by far the most common breast tumor and, although they may occur at any age, are most frequently seen in women in their late teens and early twenties. They are rarely painful or symptomatic in any way; the patient simply discovers a lump. Fibroadenomas do not change during the menstrual cycle and are usually easily distinguished from fibrocystic changes. Usually the mass (with an average size of 2.5 cm) is a firm, nontender, rubbery-feeling, smoothly rounded, mobile, slippery nodule most often found in the periareolar area. Its characteristic "feel" on physical examination is almost diagnostic. It is most often solitary, although occasionally (15 to 20 percent of patients) multiple lesions are present in one or both breasts.

It is sometimes difficult to distinguish fibroadenomas from cysts. In these situations, needle aspiration is a reasonable first step of evaluation. If the mass cannot be aspirated, surgical removal is indicated. Because fibroadenomas persist and sometimes continue to enlarge, local excision of these well encapsulated tumors is the treatment of choice. Most often these procedures can be performed under local anesthesia.

Cystosarcoma Phylloides. Cystosarcoma phylloides has been firmly established as a giant, rapidly growing fibroadenoma, and approximately 25 percent of the lesions are malignant. They comprise the most common sarcoma of the breast. The correct diagnosis is usually suggested by a rapidly growing large, hard, lobulated mass in the breast, usually during the fifth decade, without evidence of adjacent soft tissue or axillary involvement. Wide local resection and sometimes mastectomy may be required because of the large size of the benign cystosarcoma phylloides. When a microscopically verified, truly malignant cystosarcoma phylloides is encountered, radical mastectomy is the indicated treatment because it may be accompanied by axillary lymph node metastases.

Intraductal Papilloma. Intraductal papilloma is the second most common benign breast tumor and the most frequent cause of bloody discharge from the nipple. A papilloma most often arises in the lactiferous sinus of the milk system, which is usually situated approximately at the areolar margin. Intraductal papillomas are most often found in perimenopausal women. The symptomatic intraductal papilloma may or may not be large enough to be palpable, but the lobular duct system containing it can usually be localized by the systematic periareolar point-by-point pressure maneuver. A mammogram can also be helpful when localization is difficult.

Proper treatment is removal of the breast segment from which the discharge has been demonstrated to arise or which contains the palpable mass. Removal is important both to exclude the possibility that a much less common intraductal papillary adenocarcinoma is responsible for the bloody discharge and to put an end to the symptoms, which are a nuisance to the patient.

Miscellaneous Breast Tumors. A variety of less common benign breast tumors include lipomas, fibromas, sweat gland adenomas, hamartomas, and hemangiomas. All of these lesions require local excision for definitive diagnosis and treatment. Granular cell myoblastoma of the breast, a rare benign tumor, is significant primarily because it sometimes presents all the clinical signs of early breast cancer; even on cut section of the breast specimen, it may grossly resemble a scirrhous carcinoma. As is true for solid breast masses, biopsy and microscopic examination are essential to establish a correct diagnosis and are usually the only way a granular cell myoblastoma can be recognized as a benign lesion.

Nonneoplastic Lesions of the Breast

The breast, by virtue of the fact that it is covered with skin, may develop any of the skin changes or diseases noted elsewhere on the body. Because these diseases are numerous, they are not discussed in this chapter, and the student is referred to comprehensive dermatology textbooks for descriptions and treatments of these diseases.

Conditions that on physical examination mimic carcinoma may be caused by local breast trauma or inflammation. Because they must be distinguished from malignancy, they are discussed in more detail. Trauma to the breast may cause local tissue swelling, subcutaneous bleeding, erythema, and pain. The collection of blood in the subcutaneous tissues (*hematoma*) may cause additional localized swelling, which ultimately becomes more apparent as an evolving ecchymotic area. Treatment can usually be expectant, with spontaneous and uncomplicated resorption usually occurring. Local application of heat and mild analgesics may be necessary. On rare occasions, evacuation of a large hematoma by aspiration or incision and drainage may be required.

Trauma may also cause *fat necrosis,* although the traumatic incident may not be noted or remembered by the patient. The evolution of tissue trauma with fat necrosis may ultimately lead to physical findings that closely simulate breast cancer. As the traumatized area heals and repairs, fibrosis of the subcutaneous tissue occurs, leading to fixation to the skin and ultimately skin retraction. Because breast trauma is usually superficial, fibrosis and fixation to the chest wall rarely occur. This subcutaneous scar may evolve into dense fibrosis and a palpable mass or into a cystic cavity with calcification of the walls. Even mammographic findings may be indistinguishable from those of malignancy, and therefore excisional biopsy is invariably necessary to establish the correct diagnosis.

Phlebitis of the thoracoepigastric vein (Mondor's disease) may also be caused by local trauma or occur after cosmetic or diagnostic breast surgery. The phlebitis of the superficial vein is progressive and painful, ultimately resulting in a tender, fibrous cord underneath the skin. Skin retraction and dimpling often occur, and the inexperienced clinician may mistake the condition for some of the changes associated with breast cancer. However, because of its superficial and linear nature, Mondor's disease must be included in the differential diagnosis. Most often, the phlebitis resolves with symptomatic therapy of heat and anti-inflammatory agents such as aspirin or ibuprofen. Surgical intervention or anticoagulation is not necessary.

Infections in the nonpuerperal state are infrequent; and when they do occur, the diagnosis of an inflammatory carcinoma must be considered. *Chronic subareolar abscesses* may occur in women in their thirties and forties. These recurrent abscesses often drain spontaneously and ultimately may cause areolar fistula. Obstruction of the ducts, leading to inflammation and secondary infection, may be initially treated with heat, analgesics, and broad-spectrum antibiotics. However, for chronic recurrent abscesses, surgical removal of the duct and fistula tract is advised. It should be kept in mind that inflammatory carcinoma of the breast may suggest the possibility of cellulitis and breast abscess, and vice versa. That is, a breast abscess with surrounding cellulitis may simulate inflammatory carcinoma, even to the cutaneous thickening and the characteristic peau d'orange of the breast skin infiltrated by an underlying carcinoma. Rarely, an ordinary noninflammatory type of breast carcinoma becomes infected with or without prior ulceration of the tumor and presents a confusing picture until biopsy clarifies the situation.

The most common causes of breast inflammation, cellulitis, and abscess are associated with postpartum events. During the first one to three days after delivery, *breast engorgement* is noted in most women, typified by swelling, edema, and breast discomfort. A low grade fever may be associated with this diffuse process in both breasts. With adequate, firm breast support and ice packs, the engorgement usually resolves within a few days. If the woman wishes to breast-feed, it should be encouraged to reduce engorgement. Obstruction of a duct during the postpartum period predisposes to infection. *Postpartum mastitis* is usually recognized as a localized, exquisitely tender, edematous, erythematous region, usually of one breast. Treatment goals are aimed at emptying the obstructed segment, which may be accomplished by nursing, manual breast expression, or breast pumping. Ice packs may reduce swelling, thereby allowing the duct better drainage. Antibiotic therapy should also be employed, using a broad-spectrum antibiotic aimed at the treatment of skin bacteria. Ampicillin and erythromycin are the drugs most frequently selected for initial therapy.

Approximately 10 percent of patients who develop postpartum mastitis progress to a frank *breast abscess*. In this situation, broad-spectrum antibiotics alone are ineffective, and incision and drainage must be accomplished. Because the abscesses are often multiloculated, anesthesia must be adequate so that the loculations can be broken up and drains inserted into the abscess cavity. Incision into the breast abscess should be placed directly over the abscess, with observation of Langer's lines so as to have the best cosmetic outcome. If a chronic infection in an old abscess cavity persists, excision of that portion of breast may be required.

SELECTED READINGS

Blichert-Toft, M., and Watt-Boolsen, S. Clinical approach to women with severe mastalgia and the therapeutic possibilities. *Acta Obstet. Gynecol. Scand. [Suppl.]* 123:185, 1984.

Cole, P., Elwood, J. M., and Kaplan, S. D. Incidence rates and risk factors of benign breast neoplasms. *Am. J. Epidemiol.* 108:112, 1978.

Dupont, W. D., and Page, D. L. Risk factors for breast cancer in women with proliferative breast disease. *N. Engl. J. Med.* 312:146, 1985.

Durning, P., and Sellwood, R. A. Bromocriptine in severe cyclical breast pain. *Br. J. Surg.* 69:248, 1982.

Foster, R. S., Jr., and Costanza, M. C. Breast self-examination practices and breast cancer survival. *Cancer* 53:999, 1984.

Goodson, W. H., Meilman, R., Jacobson, M., et al. What do breast symptoms mean? *Am. J. Surg.* 150:271, 1985.

Harris, J. R., Hellman, S., Henderson, I. C., and Kinne, D. W. *Breast Diseases.* Philadelphia: Lippincott, 1987.

Hislop, T. G., and Elwood, J. M. Risk factors for benign breast disease: a 30-year cohort study. *Can. Med. Assoc. J.* 124:283, 1981.

Hislop, T. G., and Threlfall, W. J. Oral contraceptives and benign breast disease. *Am. J. Epidemiol.* 120:273, 1984.

Homer, M. J. Breast imaging: pitfalls, controversies and some practical thoughts. *Radiol. Clin. North Am.* 23:459, 1985.

Hutter, R. V. P. Goodbye to "fibrocystic disease." *N. Engl. J. Med.* 312:179, 1985.

Leis, H. P., Jr., Cammarata, A., and LaRaja, R. D. Nipple discharge significance and treatment. *Breast* 11:6, 1985.

Lorenzen, J. R., and Gravdal, J. A. Bloody nipple discharge. *Am. Fam. Physician* 34:151, 1986.

Love, S. M., Gelman, R. S., and Sileu, W. S. Fibrocystic "disease" of the breast: a non-disease. *N. Engl. J. Med.* 307:1010, 1982.

Lubin, F., Ron, E., Wax, Y., et al. A case-control study of caffeine and methylxanthine in benign breast disease. *J.A.M.A.* 253:2388, 1985.

Meyer, J. E., Kopans, D. B., Stomper, P. C., et al. Occult breast abnormalities: percutaneous needle localization. *Radiology* 15:335, 1984.

Sattin, R. W., Rubin, G. L., Webster, L. A., et al. Family history and the risk of breast cancer. *J.A.M.A.* 253:1908, 1985.

Shapiro, S. Ten to fourteen-year effects of screening on breast cancer mortality. *J. Natl. Cancer Inst.* 69:349, 1982.

Sickles, E. A., Filly, R. A., and Callen, P. W. Breast cancer detection with sonography and mammography: comparison using state-of-the-art equipment. *A.J.R.* 140:843, 1983.

Tabar, I., Gad, A., Holmberg, L. H., et al. Reduction in mortality from breast cancer after mass screening with mammography. *Lancet* 1:829, 1985.

Tinnemans, J. G. M., Wobbes, T., Lubbers, E. C., et al. The significance of microcalcifications without palpable mass in the diagnosis of breast cancer. *Surgery* 99:652, 1986.

Wanebo, H. J., Feldman, P. G., Morton, C. W., et al. Fine needle aspiration cytology in lieu of open biopsy in management of primary breast disease. *Ann. Surg.* 199:569, 1984.

Wang, D. Y., and Fentiman, I. S. Epidemiology and endocrinology of benign breast disease. *Breast Cancer Res. Treat.* 6:5, 1985.

Young, J. O., Sadowsky, N. L., Young, J. W., et al. Mammography of women with suspicious breast lumps. *Arch. Surg.* 121:807, 1986.

The mammograms in this chapter kindly supplied by Daniel Sullivan, M.D., Department of Radiology, Duke University Medical Center.

IV

Gynecologic Oncology

25

Intraepithelial Diseases of the Lower Genital Tract

At the turn of the twentieth century, carcinoma of the cervix was the leading cause of cancer death in American women. Since the 1950s the incidence of, and the death rate from, cervical cancer have declined steadily. Although treatment modalities have improved, the primary reason for the reduction in the incidence of and mortality from cervical cancer is the Papanicolaou smear. This simple screening test allows early detection of invasive cervical cancer and detection of preinvasive intraepithelial neoplasia. During this same period, the number of cases diagnosed of intraepithelial neoplasia of the lower genital tract has steadily increased.

This chapter discusses the etiology and epidemiology of preinvasive diseases of the cervix, vagina, and vulva, as well as the appropriate evaluation and treatment of these diseases. It is clear that intraepithelial disease, if left untreated, may progress to invasive carcinoma. The concepts and principles of intraepithelial neoplasia of the lower genital tract squamous epithelium are based, in great part, on our knowledge of the disease of the cervix.

EPIDEMIOLOGY

Intraepithelial disease of the lower genital tract must be considered a venereal disease in most instances. We have known for decades that starting sexual intercourse at an early age, early childbearing, and multiple sexual partners increase the risk of cervical intraepithelial neoplasia and invasive carcinoma. Additional knowledge has suggested that one of the predominant epidemiologic factors is sexually transmitted viral genital disease, especially human papilloma virus and herpes simplex virus II infections. There also appear to be male factors associated with the development of

intraepithelial disease, as evidenced by the fact that men whose first wives developed cervical cancer carry a threefold risk of a subsequent wife having the disease. Conversely, celibate nuns rarely develop cervical cancer. The concept of a sexually transmitted disease(s) being a cause of intraepithelial disease of the lower genital tract has been further supported by basic research in virology pointing toward herpes simplex virus II and human papilloma virus as likely candidates as carcinogens or co-carcinogens. Another factor associated with the development of intraepithelial disease of the lower genital tract is a depressed immune response. This situation is particularly true in patients who are immunosuppressed (e.g., renal transplant patients). Smoking and decreased dietary intake of vitamin A have also been associated with an increased incidence of intraepithelial neoplasia.

Virology research strongly suggests virus-induced transformation of the squamous epithelium of the lower genital tract to intraepithelial neoplasia. Whereas herpes simplex virus II appeared to be a leading contender during the 1970s, human papilloma virus now seems to be a much more likely etiologic factor in intraepithelial disease and invasive carcinoma. Evidence supporting the herpes simplex virus (HSV) theory is primarily based on the identification of a high HSV antibody titer in the serum of women with cervical intraepithelial neoplasia and carcinoma compared to that in controls who did not have intraepithelial disease. Similar evidence, utilizing serum antibody titers, also suggested that cytomegalovirus may contribute to the development of intraepithelial disease. Furthermore, transformation of squamous cells in vitro and in animal models by exposure to herpes simplex virus suggested this virus as an etiologic factor.

With the advent of molecular hybridization of DNA, human papilloma virus (HPV) has been found incorporated in the DNA of the human cell that has either intraepithelial disease or invasive cancer. Increasing numbers of HPV subtypes are being identified, and at the present time it appears that some carry a greater malignant potential than others. For example, benign lower genital tract condylomas are caused by HPV types 6 and 11. The malignant transformation potential appears to be limited with these subtypes. On the other hand, HPV subtypes 16, 18, and 31 are much more frequently found in intraepithelial neoplasia and invasive squamous cell carcinoma. Some studies have indicated that HPV 16 can be identified in 90 percent of invasive squamous cell carcinoma and 70 percent of intraepithelial neoplasia of the cervix and lower genital tract. Much of the evidence related to the HPV appears to fit our previous understanding of intraepithelial neoplasia, including the fact that HPV infection is a sexually transmitted disease and that, if studied closely, at least 70 percent of male sexual partners of women infected with HPV are found to have a subclinical HPV infection of the penis, scrotum, or medial thighs.

All women who develop HPV infection (as evidenced by classic cellular changes on the Papanicolaou smear or grossly evident condyloma acuminatum of the lower genital tract) do not develop intraepithelial neoplasia or invasive carcinoma. A variety of factors may come into play leading to intraepithelial neoplasia and invasive cancer, including the type of virus infecting the squamous epithelium (types 16, 18, and 31 appear to be more malignant), the time in the woman's life when the virus exposure takes place (especially during the late teenage years and early twenties, when the cervix is undergoing active squamous metaplasia), and the presence of other cofactors such as immunologic depression and smoking.

Although the entire lower genital tract (vulva, vagina, and cervix) must be exposed to similar carcinogens, it appears that the cervix is much more apt to develop intraepithelial neoplasia. The hypothesis explaining the natural history of this disease proposes that during the periods when squamous metaplasia occurs on the cervix (late teenage years and after pregnancy) the cervix is most susceptible to the carcinogen. Squamous metaplasia begins at the onset of menarche with the change of vaginal pH. During this time, the junction between the squamous epithelium of the exocervix and the columnar epithelium of the endocervix (*squamocolumnar junction*) changes its location on the exocervix to a point closer to the external cervical os. This transformation, caused by squamous metaplasia appearing in areas of previous glandular epithelium, creates a new zone of metaplastic squamous epithelium (*transformation zone*). It

is in this transformation zone that most intraepithelial neoplasia and cervical carcinoma occur (Fig. 25-1). There is no other similar transformation zone in the vagina or vulva that may explain why the squamous epithelium of the vulva and vagina is more resistant to carcinogenic influence. The hypothesis, then, is that during "susceptible" times in the natural history of cervical squamous epithelium a carcinogen may attack these immature cells and become incorporated into the genome, ultimately leading to malignant transformation.

The Papanicolaou smear, a sensitive, accurate screening technique, provided us the opportunity to understand the natural history of cervical carcinoma and intraepithelial neoplasia. Most patients with invasive cancer have had preinvasive changes of the cervix (intraepithelial neoplasia), which can be detected months to years prior to the development of invasive cancer. It is therefore our goal to use the Papanicolaou smear to detect preinvasive changes and then apply appropriate therapy to reverse these preinvasive (intraepithelial neoplastic) changes, thereby eliminating most invasive cervical cancers. With the high level of medical care available in the United States, this goal should be achievable.

PAPANICOLAOU SMEAR

The Papanicolaou (Pap) smear, developed and championed by George Papanicolaou during the early 1940s, did not become widely available for cancer screening until the 1950s and 1960s. The Pap smear is one of the best methods available today for identifying preinvasive lesions of the cervix and for cancer screening and control. Although the Papanicolaou smear is not 100 percent sensitive or specific, it is an excellent screening test if applied and utilized appropriately.

The Pap smear relies on the collection of cells exfoliated from the genital tract (especially the cervix), which are then treated with a nuclear stain and studied individually. The concept of diagnosing carcinoma based on single-cell and nuclear morphology was not readily accepted by most pathologists but has gained acceptance over the past three decades. The accuracy of the Pap smear depends on many factors, including obtaining a smear from the appropriate patient, adequately sampling the epithelium at highest risk, carefully preparing the cytologic material, and applying accurate diagnostic methods in the cytopathology laboratory. Care must be taken throughout the entire chain of the diagnostic procedure to ensure accurate, optimal cancer screening.

Although easily and painlessly performed, the indications for obtaining a Papanicolaou smear have been widely debated in recent years. Initially, it was thought that a Pap smear should be performed annually in all women over age 18 (or younger if sexual intercourse had begun). When a cost-benefit analysis was performed, however, it appeared that an annual Pap smear is not cost-effective in women who are at low risk. The definition of the low-risk patient has included women who have had three consecutive annual Pap smears that were entirely normal, who had become sexually active after age 25, and who have a monogamous sexual relationship. In this group of women, it appears that a cost-effective approach to performing Pap smears might be to extend the interval between smears to approximately three years. The rationale for this extended interval is further supported by natural history evidence of intraepithelial and invasive carcinoma, which suggests a slow transformation of intraepithelial neoplasia to invasive carcinoma (see discussion later in this chapter).

Although statistically there is a slow transformation from intraepithelial neoplasia to invasive carcinoma, it is also clear that some patients with normal Pap smears may progress rapidly (over a matter of months) to invasive carcinoma. It has therefore been the contention of groups such as the American College of Obstetricians and Gynecologists that an annual Pap smear remains a cost-effective method for diagnosis of cervical intraepithelial neoplasia and invasive carcinoma and that it promotes general gynecologic health care because of the annual checkup. This recommendation for annual Pap smears is further supported by experience in England and Canada where longer intervals between Pap smears have resulted in an increasing mortality rate from cervical cancer. It is therefore the belief of most gynecologists that Pap smears should be performed annually on women over age 18 (or younger, if active sexually).

The Pap smear is an outpatient diagnostic modality

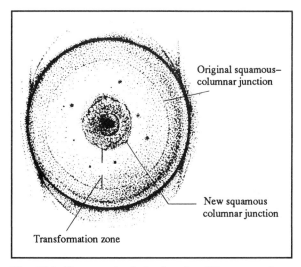

Fig. 25-1. Gross anatomic landmarks of the exocervix. Intraepithelial neoplasia and cervical carcinoma almost always arise in the transformation zone.

performed at the time of pelvic examination. With the cervix exposed using a bivalve speculum, the entire transformation zone of the cervix should be scraped using a wooden or plastic spatula. This single specimen has the highest yield of detection of intraepithelial and invasive disease, as this site is the area of highest risk (Fig. 25-1). Properly obtained, the cytologic specimen is not mixed with lubricating gel or other foreign materials. The cytologic specimen is smeared carefully but quickly onto a microscope slide and fixed immediately in 90% alcohol or with a spray fixative. Allowing the specimen to air-dry even 10 seconds may severely distort the cytologic preparation and lead to inaccurate diagnoses by the cytopathologist. A second sample is obtained from the endocervical canal using a saline-moistened Q-Tip, small brush, or aspirating bulb. This specimen is likewise smeared thinly on a microscopic slide and fixed immediately.

Papanicolaou smears may be obtained from other sites in the lower genital tract using similar methods. Pap smears obtained from vulvar lesions should be scraped directly from the lesion. If the lesion is not moist, saline is applied to the vulva so the keratin can be moistened and scraped away, obtaining a better cytologic preparation.

Care taken when obtaining and preparing a Pap smear provides the cytopathologist the best opportunity for accurate microscopic diagnosis. Specimens must be labeled carefully and an appropriate clinical history supplied to the cytopathologist, including the patient's age, menstrual history, and other coexisting conditions, e.g., pregnancy, presence of an intrauterine contraceptive device, previous radiation therapy, concurrent medications, and other significant medical diseases.

The slide is then stained with Papanicolaou stain (a nuclear stain) and screened by trained cytopathology technicians. After screening, abnormal or suspicious Pap smears are reviewed with a cytopathologist. Factors associated with the accurate diagnosis of Pap smear material include appropriate volume of screening material by the laboratory, the skill of the cytopathology technicians and the pathologist, and careful quality control in the laboratory. In high quality laboratories, Pap smears are falsely negative in 5 to 10 percent of cases of invasive cancer. In laboratories with poor quality control, the false-negative rate may approach 40 to 50 percent. This variation in the quality of Pap smear interpretation is worrisome and should be considered when the clinician chooses a laboratory to which to submit cytopathologic slides.

Interpretation of the Pap smear by the cytopathology laboratory may provide many pieces of information of clinical usefulness. There are several classification systems that have been used to report Pap smears. However, because of variations in the numbering systems, we have encouraged the abandonment of reporting Pap smears as a number in a classification system, preferring to rely on the description of the cytopathologic specimen (Table 25-1). Using this descriptive system, the clinician has a more uniform diagnosis on which to base therapeutic decisions.

Papanicolaou smears not only provide a diagnosis of normal-appearing cells, they can also be used to recognize inflammation caused by a variety of infective organisms such as *Trichomonas, Candida, Chlamydia,* and herpes simplex virus. Moreover, changes of the squamous cells caused by human papilloma virus (HPV) are usually recognized by the perinuclear cavitation, or "halo," of the squamous cells. These cells, called *koilocytes,* are usually diagnosed when a patient has an HPV infection that may be clinically obvious (condyloma acuminatum) or subclinical (flat warts) and may be associated with intraepithelial neoplasia or dysplasia.

When diagnosing intraepithelial neoplasia and invasive carcinoma, the cytopathologist relies on the identification of a variety of cellular morphologic features. These features include the nuclear/cytoplasmic ratio, the character of the nuclear chromatin, and the presence of nucleoli. It is beyond the scope of this book to present a detailed discussion of cytopathologic changes or criteria for diagnosis of the various intraepithelial and invasive lesions of the cervix. Currently, there are two sets of nomenclature used to

Table 25-1. General Papanicolaou Smear Classification

Classification	Criteria
Normal	Normal-appearing cellular material; endocervical cells are present*
Inflammatory	May be further identified as an infection due to a specific organism, e.g., *Trichomonas vaginalis* or *Candida*
Dysplastic	
Mild dysplasia CIN-I	
Moderate dysplasia CIN-II	
Severe dysplasia CIN-III	
Carcinoma in situ CIN-III	
Microinvasive carcinoma	
Invasive carcinoma	

*If endocervical cells are not present, the cytopathologist cannot be certain that the transformation zone and squamocolumnar junction have been adequately sampled.

describe the intraepithelial neoplasias. Neither is optimal because neither suggests the fact that intraepithelial neoplasia is a continuum and that there is not a clear or sharp demarcation between these grades of change.

NATURAL HISTORY OF INTRAEPITHELIAL NEOPLASIA

Experience gained from following patients with Pap smears that demonstrate cytologic changes of intraepithelial neoplasia has shown that some of the intraepithelial disease progresses to invasive carcinoma. Although at the present time we cannot predict which abnormality will progress to a worsening lesion or invasive carcinoma, some general estimates have been made. Of *all* of the intraepithelial neoplastic lesions, progression to carcinoma in situ may take, on average, 44 months. The lowest grade of CIN, mild dysplasia, takes longer to progress to carcinoma in situ (on the order of 86 months). Of all cases of mild dysplasia (CIN-I), it is estimated that 60 percent spontaneously regress, 22 percent remain stable, and 16 percent progress to worsening grades of intraepithelial disease or invasive carcinoma. Statistically, there appears to be, in some patients, a slow progression of intraepithelial neoplasia to worsening grades and then to invasive carcinoma.

The problem in terms of clinical management of this disease is that we have no way of predicting which patient will progress, which will regress, and which will remain stable. Fortunately, the modern evaluation and treatment of intraepithelial neoplasia is relatively simple, inexpensive, and effective. At the same time, fertility can be maintained in most patients, and therapy can be provided on an outpatient basis.

All patients with an abnormal Pap smear suggesting intraepithelial neoplasia or invasive carcinoma should be evaluated thoroughly and a treatment plan instituted to eradicate the lesion. (Evaluation and treatment of cervical carcinoma is discussed in Chapter 26.) The primary goal of evaluating the patient with an abnormal Pap smear is to identify patients with invasive carcinoma and to provide appropriate and timely treatment. For patients who are found to

have cervical intraepithelial neoplasia, a variety of treatment options are available. Most patients today can be evaluated and treated in the outpatient setting without incurring excessive medical bills or compromising the patient's subsequent fertility. This outpatient management scheme has been developed and tested and has demonstrated cost-effectiveness and safety. Key to this evaluation has been the availability of colposcopy and clear criteria for the diagnosis of CIN by colposcopic evaluation and biopsy.

COLPOSCOPY

Prior to the advent and widespread clinical use of colposcopy, all patients with abnormal Pap smears underwent cold-knife conization for diagnosis. Although the cold-knife cone biopsy supplies abundant tissue to the pathologist for thorough pathologic evaluation and determination of the extent of the lesion, the surgical procedure is not without hazard. First, this minor surgical procedure requires a general anesthetic, with its accompanying risks and expense. Significant complications include hemorrhage and infection. Finally, removal of cervical stroma and scarring of the cervix following conization may lead to an incompetent cervix or cervical stenosis. Although these major complications are relatively infrequent, they must be recognized and can be avoided in most patients. It is important to realize that most patients with CIN are young and have not fulfilled their childbearing wishes.

Colposcopy and biopsy in the outpatient setting have significantly reduced the need for cold-knife conization. The colposcope itself is nothing more than a dissecting microscope, providing magnification of approximately 15× (Fig. 25-2). With this magnification, vascular patterns associated with intraepithelial neoplasia may be identified. These lesions would not be apparent to the naked eye. With the aid of the colposcope, the gynecologist may then obtain a biopsy specimen of the most suspicious lesion to confirm the severity of the intraepithelial lesion and to exclude invasive carcinoma.

Colposcopy is performed in the office. A vaginal speculum is used to expose the cervix as when obtaining material for a Pap smear. The cervix is washed

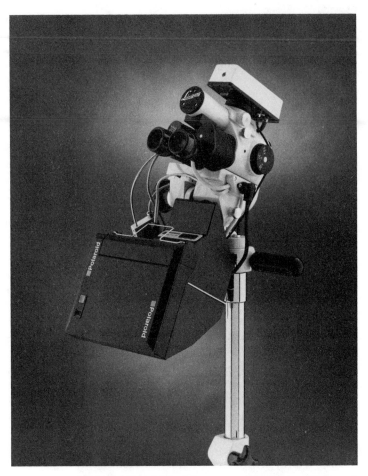

Fig. 25-2. Binocular colposcope. The colposcope is used to evaluate the cervix, vagina, and vulva in patients who are suspected of having intraepithelial neoplasia or carcinoma. Magnification of approximately 15× allows identification of abnormal epithelial coloration and vascular patterns.

with 3% acetic acid to remove mucus and debris and to slightly dehydrate the cells on the cervix. The cervix and upper vagina are then inspected with the colposcope, searching for specific lesions. Lesions of importance are usually discrete (focal) with vascular patterns described as punctation or mosaicism, or they are frankly abnormal vessels (associated with invasive carcinoma). Intraepithelial neoplasia is usually white, in contrast to the gray-pink of normal squamous epithelium in the transformation zone. The character of this epithelium may range from a faint white to a dense, "oyster shell" appearance. The whitened epithelium occurs because of the increased

nuclear/cytoplasmic ratio of intraepithelial neoplasia—thus more easily reflecting light and giving a white appearance.

During the colposcopic procedure the entire cervix and transformation zone should be studied. As previously discussed, it is this area that is most likely to harbor intraepithelial neoplasia or invasive carcinoma. In most premenopausal women the lower aspect of the endocervical canal can be inspected and the endocervical glands visualized. Endocervical glands appear as clefts and "grape-like" structures protruding through the external cervical os. In most cases the original squamocolumnar junction can be identified. The upper vaginal fornices may also be inspected on routine examination, although careful colposcopic evaluation of the entire vagina is time-consuming and is not usually indicated for a patient who has abnormal cervical cytology. A green filter on the light source of the colposcope helps augment vascular patterns.

On occasion a lesion cannot be visualized, and further investigation of the cervix may be aided by application of an iodine stain (Lugol's or Schiller's solution). Most areas containing dysplasia do not take up the Lugol's stain as well as the normal richly glycogenated squamous epithelium of the exocervix and vagina.

Although the clinician may suspect a degree of dysplasia based on colposcopic findings (e.g., white epithelium, punctation, or mosaicism), there is no specific correlation between colposcopic findings and the grade of the dysplasia. It is therefore necessary to obtain a biopsy specimen of the cervix from abnormal areas. Biopsy is usually performed at the time of colposcopy and can be easily done in the office without anesthesia. Directed biopsies obtain both squamous epithelium and a small amount of cervical stroma to exclude invasive carcinoma. Hemostasis is easily achieved with topical application of silver nitrate or Monsel's solution. To exclude disease residing in the endocervical canal, endocervical curettage should be performed and the specimen separately submitted for pathologic evaluation.

In patients who have no identifiable lesion or in whom there is no correlation between clinical examination, cervical cytology, colposcopy, and cervical biopsies, cold-knife conization is recommended for diagnosis (and usually treatment). As mentioned previously, cold-knife conization is an outpatient surgical procedure that requires general or regional anesthesia. A cone-shaped piece of the cervix is excised with a scalpel (Fig. 25-3). The carbon dioxide laser may also be used to excise a "cylinder" of the cervix. Properly performed, the conization should excise any lesion on the exocervix as well as lesions hidden in the endocervical canal. The cone specimen is usually made

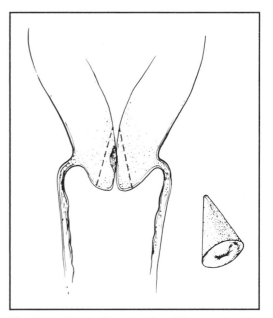

Fig. 25-3. Cold-knife conization. When performing cold-knife conization, a portion of the cervical canal and stroma are excised along with the exocervix. Preoperative colposcopy guides the surgeon as to the extent of the exocervical resection.

into 10 to 15 slides for detailed histologic study. The potential intraoperative and postoperative hazards and complications of cold-knife conization have been outlined above. Dilatation and curettage (D&C) of the endometrium is not necessarily performed in conjunction with a conization, especially for premenopausal women who have no abnormal uterine bleeding or menstrual dysfunction.

TREATMENT OF CERVICAL INTRAEPITHELIAL NEOPLASIA

Approximately 90 percent of patients with cervical intraepithelial neoplasia may be evaluated and treated in the outpatient setting. The advantages of this management schema include reduced expense, unaltered fertility, minimal discomfort, and effective therapy. To proceed with outpatient therapy, however, certain strict criteria must be fulfilled, most important of which is close correlation of all parameters of the evaluation. In a setting where any parameter does not correlate, or when there is any suspicion of micro-invasive or invasive carcinoma, cold-knife conization must be performed. Specifically, clinical evaluation of the cervix, cytologic findings, colposcopic impression, and cervical biopsies must correlate within one grade of dysplasia. That is, a patient who has a Pap smear suggesting CIN-III but whose lesion is called CIN-I on biopsy should not be treated in the out-patient setting without further study to exclude the possibility of a more advanced lesion that was missed on the initial evaluation.

The rationale for treatment of cervical intraepithe-lial neoplasia is to prevent the development of inva-sive carcinoma. The time of progression from one grade of dysplasia to another has been estimated in mathematic models and in long-term patient follow-up during the 1950s and 1960s. It is clear that some patients with cervical dysplasia ultimately develop invasive cancer if left untreated. What is unclear is how to predict which patient will develop invasive cancer. The odds are high that a patient with CIN-III will progress to invasive cancer. Likewise, it is im-possible to predict a time course of the progression. It is also clear that some patients have not progressed slowly through the various grades of cervical intraepi-thelial neoplasia before developing frankly invasive cancer. Therefore, because we are unable to predict which patients will progress to invasive carcinoma or the time course that will be taken, the eradication of cervical intraepithelial neoplasia is recommended for all patients.

The treatment of CIN in most patients should be di-rected to eradicating the dysplastic epithelium. The traditional treatment in the past was a cold-knife conization that not only excised the affected epithe-lium but also removed a considerable amount of cer-vical stroma. This procedure led to the subsequent problems of cervical stenosis and incompetent cervix once the cervix healed. There is no reason to remove normal cervical stroma, so our treatment plans should be directed at eradicating the affected epithelium with minimal stromal damage. Approximately 90 percent of patients can be managed with locally destructive techniques that can be performed in the office with minimal or no analgesia or anesthesia.

Cryotherapy

Eradication of CIN by cryotherapy is the most widely used technique in the United States. Using either liquid nitrogen or carbon dioxide, the cervical epithe-lium may be frozen (and thereby destroyed) by local application of a probe through which a refrigerant is circulated (Fig. 25-4). The usual cryotherapy session lasts a matter of a few minutes (usually freezing for 3 minutes, allowing the cervix to thaw, and then re-freezing for 3 minutes). During cryotherapy most patients note some uterine cramping, likened to mod-erate to severe menstrual cramps. Following cryo-therapy the patient has a watery vaginal discharge for approximately two to three weeks before the cervix is reepithelialized. Fertility after cryotherapy appears to be equal to that of untreated control patients.

Laser Vaporization

Carbon dioxide laser may be directed through an operating microscope or colposcope at the cervix to vaporize affected epithelium. The laser may precisely eradicate a specific lesion, but the most success has been achieved when the entire transformation zone has been vaporized. The depth of laser vaporization should be approximately 6 to 7 mm to eradicate endo-cervical glands that might harbor squamous intra-epithelial neoplasia (Fig. 25-5). Laser vaporization can also be performed in the office, usually without anesthesia. Some patients experience enough uterine cramping that a paracervical block of 1% lidocaine (Xylocaine) is recommended. Laser vaporization takes about 10 to 15 minutes to perform. The laser is asso-ciated with a slightly increased risk of bleeding during therapy and 2 to 3 percent of patients return with heavy cervical bleeding 7 to 10 days after laser therapy.

The advantage of laser therapy is the precision and control of the laser beam used to eradicate a specific area. This capability is particularly attractive for large lesions that extend onto the portio of the cervix or into the upper fornix of the vagina. To date, there are no

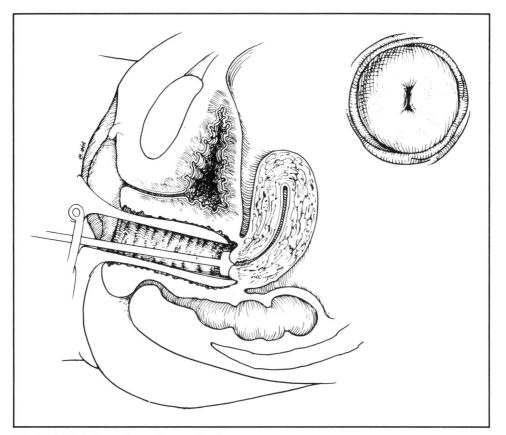

Fig. 25-4. Technique of cryotherapy for the treatment of cervical intraepithelial neoplasia. The cryotherapy probe is placed against the exocervix, and the refrigerant (nitrous oxide or carbon dioxide) circulates through the metal tip. The treatment usually involves freezing the cervix for 3 minutes, allowing a 5-minute thaw, and then refreezing for 3 minutes. An "ice ball" of approximately 4 mm should be achieved beyond the edge of the cryotherapy probe to ensure adequate cryotherapy.

clear improved treatment results with laser therapy versus cryotherapy. Because of the high cost of laser equipment, patient charges are usually higher for laser therapy than they are for cryotherapy.

Electrocautery

Electrocautery may be applied to the cervix to eradicate intraepithelial disease. Because of the severe pain associated with this procedure, general anesthesia is required. Electrocautery is not as popular in the United States as the two previously mentioned treatment techniques, and the final treatment results are no better than cryotherapy or laser vaporization.

Cold-Knife Conization

Cold-knife conization may be performed for treatment of cervical intraepithelial neoplasia. In the past, it was the standard therapy, although as previously mentioned it is not necessary to remove as much cervical stroma as the cold-knife cone requires. However, in a patient undergoing cold-knife conization for diagnostic purposes, the procedure may also be adequate therapy. The risk of subsequent infertility and incompetent cervix make conization less attractive,

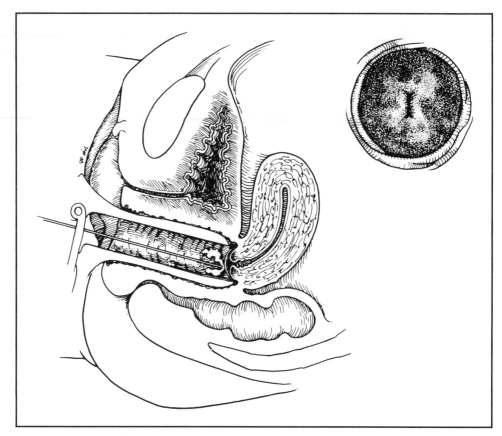

Fig. 25-5. Laser vaporization of the cervix. The carbon dioxide laser may be used to vaporize a lesion from the exocervix. When performing laser vaporization, a depth of 6 to 7 mm should be vaporized to eradicate intraepithelial neoplasia, which may be in the endocervical glands. The entire transformation zone should be vaporized. At the completion of the procedure, the cervix appears charred (inset). Healing is usually complete in approximately four weeks.

although the real risks are probably encountered by only 1 to 2 percent of patients. Occasionally, it is found that the cone margin is involved with dysplasia. The concern then is that dysplasia has been left behind, and further therapy may be necessary. In most instances, however, follow-up evaluation with Pap smear is all that is required, as most patients do not have subsequent recurrence of their dysplasia.

Hysterectomy

Obviously, removal of the uterus and cervix eliminates the focus of cervical dysplasia. In most patients, hysterectomy is excessive treatment for intraepithelial disease unless it is of a high grade (CIN-III). Even in patients with CIN-III disease, additional indications for hysterectomy should coexist, such as the need for sterilization or other gynecologic pathology (e.g.,

abnormal uterine bleeding from a benign source, leiomyoma uteri, severe dysmenorrhea).

Follow-up and Treatment Results

After locally destructive procedures such as cryotherapy or laser therapy, a Pap smear should be obtained four months later. This four-month interval allows complete healing of the cervix and elimination of the repair cells, which might be interpreted as abnormal by the cytopathologist. Provided the first Pap smear after treatment is normal, subsequent Pap smears are obtained approximately every four months to complete a year of follow-up. Thereafter, Pap smears are repeated at six-month intervals.

Patients with a history of cervical dysplasia are at increased risk to develop a recurrence and should be monitored more closely than the normal patient population. This fact is further emphasized by our understanding that cervical intraepithelial neoplasia is induced by human papilloma virus. The virus may have remained latent for years, or the patient may become reinfected.

Patients who have abnormal Pap smears after therapy should be reevaluated using the same steps of outpatient evaluation noted previously. Because the squamocolumnar junction is usually moved into the endocervical canal after cryotherapy, it is often necessary to perform a cold-knife conization to fully evaluate a patient with recurrent dysplasia. Laser therapy, on the other hand, usually leaves the squamocolumnar junction on the exocervix, which is then easily evaluated by colposcopy.

Treatment with cryotherapy, laser therapy, or electrocautery results in approximately 90 percent of patients having a normal Pap smear during follow-up. Of the approximate 10 percent of patients who have persistently abnormal Pap smears, one-half of them can be successfully reevaluated and retreated in an outpatient setting. Risk factors associated with a persistently abnormal Pap smear or a recurrence include those patients who have large lesions (lesions occupying more than two quadrants of the cervix) and those with high-grade lesions (CIN-III).

Even though cold-knife conization removes more of the cervix than the other procedures, success after conization is also only slightly in excess of 90 percent of cases. Most patients who have persistent disease after conization have disease far out on the portio of the cervix that was left behind, or the lesion is in the cervical canal, which was cut across.

It is interesting to point out that even after a hysterectomy intraepithelial neoplasia is detected in approximately 6 percent of patients. These patients either develop or have residual intraepithelial neoplasia in the upper vagina. Realizing that this neoplastic process is often a multifocal disease, it is therefore not surprising that patients who have had a hysterectomy for cervical intraepithelial neoplasia subsequently develop vaginal intraepithelial neoplasia. Therefore patients who have had a hysterectomy for cervical intraepithelial neoplasia should continue to be followed with Pap smears. Of the patients whose disease recurs after outpatient therapy, 75 percent demonstrate a recurrence within two years.

Invasive carcinoma has been reported after cryotherapy. In review of these unfortunate cases, it becomes clear that most could have been prevented by adequate outpatient evaluation. In most instances the evaluation criteria outlined earlier in the chapter were not fulfilled. The most frequent error in the management of these patients is not performing colposcopy plus directed biopsy or subjecting the patient to endocervical curettage. It must be emphasized that the clinical management of the patient with an abnormal Pap smear must be rigid, following specific criteria. Colposcopy and treatment should be performed by a well trained, qualified gynecologist.

VULVAR INTRAEPITHELIAL NEOPLASIA

Intraepithelial neoplasia of the vulva is actually two discrete disease processes: vulvar intraepithelial neoplasia of the squamous epithelium and Paget's disease. The incidence of either disease process is unknown; however, it appears that the frequency of carcinoma in situ is increasing and that the disease is being diagnosed in increasingly younger women.

Etiology

The etiology of vulvar intraepithelial neoplasia is poorly understood. An association with sexually transmitted diseases such as herpes or human papilloma virus (HPV) infection and condyloma acuminatum has been noted frequently. The hypothesis of a viral etiology for this disease is further supported by the association of squamous intraepithelial neoplasia and invasive carcinoma in the vagina and cervix. Furthermore, patients who are chronically immunosuppressed, such as patients with renal transplants or those receiving chronic steroid therapy, have a higher incidence of vulvar carcinoma in situ. The role of an intact immune system in combating a viral carcinogen is suggested by these findings.

The pathophysiology of vulvar intraepithelial neoplasia is also poorly understood, although it is generally thought to be similar to the process on the uterine cervix, i.e., variable progression from atypia (dysplasia) to carcinoma in situ and then further progression to invasive carcinoma of the vulva. The time course of the disease process and the frequency of progression from carcinoma in situ (VIN-III) to invasive carcinoma is not known. Spontaneous regression of carcinoma in situ, especially multifocal carcinoma in situ or bowenoid papulosis, has also been reported. Vulvar intraepithelial neoplasia may be associated with vulvar dystrophies (both hyperplastic and atrophic) as well as with other lower genital tract malignancies.

Diagnosis

The diagnosis of vulvar intraepithelial neoplasia is characterized by a delay in patient identification of lesions and a further delay in the patient seeking medical attention. Unfortunately, many cases, once brought to medical attention, have been treated symptomatically without a pathologic diagnosis. Therefore extended periods have passed with the use of ineffective therapies. Vulvar intraepithelial neoplasia generally occurs during the third to fourth decade of life but may also be diagnosed during the postmenopausal years.

Patients with vulvar intraepithelial neoplasia often complain of vulvar pruritus or a lump or thickening of the vulvar skin. Approximately 50 percent of patients with carcinoma in situ are asymptomatic and must be diagnosed by clinical recognition of a lesion on routine examination.

Vulvar intraepithelial neoplasia has a variety of clinical appearances, ranging from white, hyperkeratotic islands that are occasionally scaly to red lesions appearing as papules or macules. Ten to fifteen percent of carcinoma in situ lesions are hyperpigmented. Vulvar intraepithelial neoplasia may be a single lesion but more often is *multicentric,* involving several discrete areas of the vulva, perineum, and perianal skin. This disease process must be thought of as an *anogenital disease.*

Examination of the vulva is enhanced by adequate lighting and a careful inspection of the vulvar and perianal skin. The *colposcope* or other form of *magnification* is often helpful for identifying multifocal lesions. Colposcopic examination of the vulva, however, does *not* reveal the typical vascular patterns recognized on the cervix that are associated with cervical intraepithelial neoplasia. Vulvar colposcopic findings are usually those of raised white or hyperpigmented lesions. Evaluation of the perianal skin is often aided by the use of an anoscope, as carcinoma in situ frequently involves the anal canal.

The application of *3% acetic acid* to the vulva enhances the diagnostic capabilities and augments the recognition of white or hyperpigmented lesions. *Toluidine blue 1%* may also be used to identify vulvar intraepithelial neoplasia. Toluidine blue is a nuclear stain that concentrates in neoplastic areas with parakeratosis. It is applied liberally to the vulva and perianal skin and allowed to dry for 2 to 3 minutes. It is then washed off with 2% acetic acid, and the vulva is reinspected. Areas of increased nuclear activity stain deeply blue and are therefore considered abnormal. This test is often helpful in the identification of multifocal lesions. However, hyperkeratotic lesions, even though neoplastic, rarely stain deeply blue because increased amounts of superficial keratin prevent absorption of the dye. Excoriated or traumatic areas, despite their benign histology, often take up the toluidine blue stain, leading to a false-positive diagnosis.

Paramount to the accurate diagnosis of vulvar lesions is the liberal use of vulvar biopsy. A Pap smear of suspicious lesions is of little value and should not be considered a screening test of significant reliability. Biopsy of suspicious vulvar lesions may be easily accomplished under local anesthesia in the office. Discrete lesions may be widely excised with a scalpel and more diffuse lesions sampled using a *Key's skin punch* (Fig. 25-6).

Treatment

The malignant potential of vulvar intraepithelial neoplasia is uncertain, although the lesion may be found

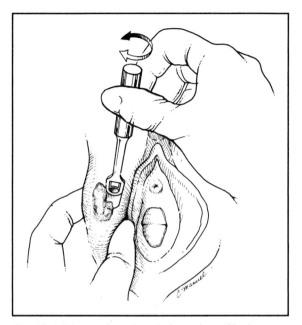

Fig. 25-6. Biopsy of a vulvar lesion using a Key's punch.

in association with invasive carcinoma. Therefore it is treated as if it might progress to a frankly invasive carcinoma.

The primary goal in the management of intraepithelial vulvar lesions is to excise or ablate the intraepithelial lesion. Several treatment choices are available and should be selected based on the extent of the lesion as well as the patient's desires and needs for cosmetic result and continued sexual function.

Discrete vulvar lesions may be widely excised under local, regional, or general anesthesia. Primary closure of the wound is usually possible, as the vulvar skin has significant elasticity and redundancy. The use of a rhomboid flap or split-thickness skin graft to cover a large area of excision is occasionally necessary.

Vulvar intraepithelial neoplasia is often a diffuse process involving multiple sites on the vulva, perineum, and perianal area. In these instances, more extensive therapy is required. Treatment options include simple vulvectomy, superficial ("skinning") vulvectomy with split-thickness skin graft, and laser vaporization. Electrocautery and cryotherapy have also been used but in general are discouraged because of

pain, slowness of healing, and poor cosmetic results compared to laser vaporization.

5-Fluorouracil ointment (Efudex 5%) may also be used as topical chemotherapy for carcinoma in situ. A success rate of 60 to 70 percent is achieved if the ointment is applied three times a day for four to six weeks. The success of this therapy depends on a cooperative patient who can tolerate the pain and discomfort as the skin becomes ulcerated by the therapy.

Results of the various treatments for vulvar intraepithelial neoplasia vary. In general, an 80 to 90 percent success rate is reported. Because of the relatively high recurrence rate, continued surveillance of the lower genital tract is recommended throughout the patient's life.

PAGET'S DISEASE

Paget's disease of the vulva is included in this chapter because it is also an intraepithelial neoplastic process. It is, however, entirely different than the squamous cell neoplastic processes. Paget's disease is an abnormal differentiation of the epidermal stem cell that would otherwise become a normal component of the skin or its appendages. This rare disease is typified by the unique, pathognomonic, large, pale cells of the epithelium and skin adnexa, called *Paget cells*. Paget cells are usually located just above the basal cell layer, often appearing as nests or clusters of cells.

Pain, burning, and pruritus are the most frequent symptoms of Paget's disease. In contrast to squamous cell vulvar intraepithelial neoplasia, Paget's disease is more likely to cause intense burning and pain. Clinically, the lesion is usually an intensely "brick red" color with islands of white epithelium. The sharp borders of the lesion suggest a discrete area of involvement. This finding, however, is misleading because the disease is usually multifocal and is typified by recurrences despite apparently adequate wide excision. Skin of the perirectal area, buttocks, inguinal region, and vagina may also be involved. White women are most often affected.

Biopsy of the lesion is encouraged because it may be clinically mistaken for vulvar candidiasis or severe reactive dermatitis. The incorrect clinical diagnosis delays proper treatment and detection of associated malignancies.

The proper treatment of Paget's disease is wide excision of all involved skin. The excision should extend into the superficial fat to remove all potentially involved skin appendages. Because of its multifocal nature and involvement well beyond the clinically apparent areas of involvement, *simple vulvectomy* is recommended. Surgical margins based on frozen sections are of little value and offer a false sense of security, as the disease is multifocal and not necessarily contiguous. Most less extensive procedures are likely to result in multiple recurrences and chronic disability for the patient.

The surgical specimen must be thoroughly sectioned to exclude the possibility of coexistent occult adenocarcinomas of the sweat glands, which are found in fewer than 20 percent of cases and are best treated by radical vulvectomy. Paget's disease may also be *associated with* coexisting or subsequent malignancies. Therefore, before treating Paget's disease, a search should be undertaken to exclude other adenocarcinomas, especially of the breast, colon, stomach, cervix, and vulva.

Follow-up of the patient previously treated for Paget's disease should include adequate cancer surveillance including mammography, cervical cytology, and stool examination for occult blood. Routine follow-up of patients is important because of the high risk of recurrence. Most recurrences should be treated by wide excision or local destruction with the carbon dioxide laser.

VAGINAL INTRAEPITHELIAL NEOPLASIA

Vaginal intraepithelial neoplasia is a rare condition that in most respects is similar to intraepithelial neoplasia of the cervix and vulva. In fact, it is often antecedent or coexistent with other intraepithelial or invasive neoplasias of the lower genital tract. Being essentially asymptomatic, the lesion is usually detected by Pap smear. The multifocal nature of these lesions should be investigated and treatment options exercised that preserve vaginal function.

The incidence of vaginal intraepithelial neoplasia is unknown, although it is much less common than intraepithelial neoplasia of the cervix or vulva. Its etiology seems to be similar to that of intraepithelial lesions of the cervix or vulva. Because of its frequent association with antecedent or coexistent squamous neoplasia of the cervix or vulva, the "field effect" of a carcinogen must be strongly considered. A viral etiology (human papilloma virus or herpes simplex virus) is most reasonable in view of current research.

One to two percent of patients who undergo hysterectomy for carcinoma in situ of the cervix ultimately develop carcinoma in situ in the upper vagina. Some of these lesions are persistent disease from direct extension of the carcinoma in situ from the cervix to the upper vagina, but other lesions develop in the vagina subsequent to the hysterectomy. Intraepithelial neoplasia of the vagina also has been reported after pelvic and vaginal irradiation for another gynecologic malignancy.

The clinical course of vaginal intraepithelial neoplasia is variable, but we assume that if left untreated carcinoma in situ may progress to invasive carcinoma. Dysplasia and carcinoma in situ of the vagina appear to be slowly progressive diseases. Therefore radical therapy (e.g., vaginectomy) should be withheld until conservative measures have failed. Twenty-five percent of the cases of carcinoma in situ of the vagina that follow radiation therapy progress to invasive carcinoma if left untreated.

Laboratory and Diagnostic Procedures

The *Papanicolaou smear* is usually the diagnostic method by which carcinoma in situ of the vagina is identified. Yearly Pap smears of the upper vagina should be obtained from all patients who have undergone hysterectomy for cervical intraepithelial neoplasia. Directed Pap smears from specific vaginal lesions may be obtained with a spatula. Vaginal discharge, pruritus, or postcoital spotting is sometimes associated with vaginal intraepithelial neoplasia.

Inspection and palpation of the vagina should be part of the routine pelvic examination. Unfortunately, the vagina is often inspected in only a cursory fashion, with much of the vaginal mucosa not visualized at all because it is hidden behind the blades of the speculum. The bimanual examination should also include palpation of the vaginal tube. Routine inspection and palpation of the vagina rarely reveal evidence of vaginal intraepithelial neoplasia. In few patients, a raised, white, hyperkeratotic lesion or an ulcerated lesion may be found to be vaginal intraepithelial neoplasia. Usually, however, examination must be aided by colposcopy and Schiller's staining to identify these subclinical lesions.

Colposcopy is an excellent method for identifying this disease when suspected by Pap smear or clinical examination. Colposcopic examination of the vagina is time-consuming and requires adequate exposure of all walls of the vagina. Colposcopy before and after application of 3% acetic acid, as well as the use of a green light filter, usually show white epithelium and punctation or mosaic vascular patterns similar to those recognized on the cervix. In patients who have had a hysterectomy, the upper apex of the vaginal vault should be closely inspected. Vaginal intraepithelial neoplasia is often multifocal, with lesions noted throughout the vagina. The entire vagina must therefore be carefully inspected and biopsy specimens obtained from all suspicious areas. The application of Schiller or Lugol solution to the vagina assists in identification of multifocal lesions.

Vaginal biopsy must be performed on all suspicious areas to rule out invasive carcinoma and to confirm the location and grade of the neoplasia. Biopsy can usually be performed in the outpatient setting without difficulty. Anesthesia is best achieved with a topical benzocaine gel or 1% lidocaine injection in the vaginal mucosa. Because of the pliability of the vaginal wall, traction and stabilization of the area to be biopsied with a skin hook or tenaculum is helpful.

Treatment

The primary goals in the management of vaginal intraepithelial neoplasia are to ablate the lesion and at the same time preserve vagina depth and caliber—and thus sexual function. As part of the treatment considerations, care must be taken to avoid injury to the

bladder, urethra, and rectum. Injury to adjacent viscera is especially likely when a lesion is located on the anterior or posterior vaginal wall.

The most common methods for treatment are local excision (partial colpectomy) and laser vaporization. Both procedures may cause pain or bleeding. Laser vaporization may be performed in the office if the lesion is not too extensive. Vaporization to a depth of 2 mm is sufficient to ablate the intraepithelial lesion in the vagina and avoids penetration of an adjacent viscus.

Cryotherapy, on the other hand, is a poor method for treating intraepithelial neoplasia of the vagina because of the inability to control the depth of freeze and the uneven contact of the cryotherapy probe to the undulating vaginal mucosa.

Extensive or multifocal vaginal intraepithelial neoplasia may be treated with *5-fluorouracil cream* (Efudex 5%). One gram is applied high in the vagina by vaginal applicator at bedtime for ten consecutive nights. The major hazard of this therapy is chemical irritation of the vulva, urethra, or anus.

Total or partial vaginectomy with application of a split-thickness skin graft over a vaginal mold or stint (McIndoe procedure) is usually reserved for treatment of carcinoma in situ of the vagina after the previously described treatments fail. Vaginectomy with split-thickness skin graft is a major surgical procedure requiring general anesthesia. After application of the skin graft, the vaginal mold must continue to be used for approximately six months to avoid frequent problems of vaginal stenosis, stricture, and scarring.

Irradiation with a vaginal cylinder has been used to treat carcinoma in situ. However, radiation therapy usually leads to vaginal fibrosis and stenosis, and it unduly exposes the patient to radiation therapy and secondary malignancies.

Untreated carcinoma in situ of the vagina usually progresses to invasive carcinoma over a long period. On the other hand, successful treatment with colpectomy, laser vaporization, 5-fluorouracil cream, or vaginectomy should result in an 80 to 95 percent cure rate. Certainly, all patients who have had vaginal intraepithelial neoplasia should remain under close surveillance, with inspection and Pap smears from all vaginal walls, for the remainder of their lives. The cervix and vulva must also be part of the careful surveillance, as intraepithelial and invasive lesions in these organs are often associated with vaginal intraepithelial neoplasia.

SELECTED READINGS

Andreasson, E. A., Bock, J. E., Bostofte, E., et al. Outpatient treatment of cervical intraepithelial neoplasia: the CO_2 laser versus cryotherapy; a randomized trial. *Acta Obstet. Gynecol. Scand.* 66:531, 1987.

Baggish, M. S. Management of cervical intraepithelial neoplasia by carbon dioxide laser. *Obstet. Gynecol.* 60:378, 1982.

Baggish, M. S., and Dorsey, J. H. CO_2 laser for treatment of vulvar carcinoma in situ. *Obstet. Gynecol.* 57:371, 1981.

Bjerre, B., Eliasson, G., Linell, F., et al. Conization as the only treatment of carcinoma in situ of the uterine cervix. *Am. J. Obstet. Gynecol.* 125:143, 1976.

Caglar, H., Hurtzog, R. W., and Hreshchyshyn, M. M. Topical 5-FU treatment of vaginal intraepithelial neoplasia. *Obstet. Gynecol.* 58:580, 1981.

Capen, C. V., Masterson, B. J., Magrina, J. F., et al. Laser therapy of vaginal intraepithelial neoplasia. *Am. J. Obstet. Gynecol.* 142:973, 1982.

Champion, M. J., McCance, D. J., Cuzick, J., et al. Progressive potential of mild cervical atypia: prospective cytological, colposcopic and virological study. *Lancet* 2:237, 1986.

Chanen, W., and Hollyock, V. E. Colposcopy and the conservative management of cervical dysplasias and carcinoma in situ. *Obstet. Gynecol.* 43:527, 1974.

Creasman, W. T., Clarke-Pearson, D. L., and Weed, J. C., Jr. Results of outpatient therapy of cervical intraepithelial neoplasia. *Gynecol. Oncol.* 12:306, 1981.

Creasman, W. T., Clarke-Pearson, D. L., Ashe, C. A., et al. The abnormal Pap smear: what to do next. *Cancer* 48:515, 1981.

Creasman, W. T., Hinshaw, W. M., and Clarke-Pearson, D. L. Cryosurgery in the management of cervical intraepithelial neoplasia. *Obstet. Gynecol.* 63:145, 1984.

Crum, C. P., Braun, L. A., Shah, K. V., et al. Vulvar intraepithelial neoplasia: correlation of nuclear DNA content and the presence of human papilloma virus (HPV) structural antigen. *Cancer* 49:468, 1982.

Kwikkel, H. J., Helmerhorst, T. J. M., Bezemer, P. D., et al. Laser or cryotherapy for cervical intraepithelial neoplasia: a randomized study to compare efficacy and side effects. *Gynecol. Oncol.* 22:23, 1985.

Lurain, J. R., and Gallup, D. G. Management of abnormal Papanicolaou smears in pregnancy. *Obstet. Gynecol.* 53:484, 1979.

Richart, R. M. Natural history of cervical intraepithelial neoplasia. *Clin. Obstet. Gynecol.* 10:748, 1968.

Richart, R. M., Townsend, D. E., Crisp, W., et al. An analysis of "long-term" follow-up results in patients with cervical intraepithelial neoplasia treated by cryotherapy. *Am. J. Obstet. Gynecol.* 137:823, 1980.

Rutledge, F. Cancer of the vagina. *Am. J. Obstet. Gynecol.* 97:635, 1967.

Rutledge, F., and Sinclair, M. Treatment of intraepithelial carcinoma of the vulva by skin excision and graft. *Am. J. Obstet. Gynecol.* 102:806, 1968.

26

Cervical Cancer

Fifty years ago cervical cancer was the leading cause of female death in the United States. Today it ranks behind five other malignancies. The decline in mortality caused by cervical cancer is in great part due to the advent of an effective screening test, the Papanicolaou smear. To a lesser extent, improved treatment modalities have increased survival from this malignancy. Because of the widespread availability of the Papanicolaou smear and its high sensitivity and specificity for the detection of invasive and preinvasive cervical cancer, it should be anticipated that cervical cancer may become close to extinct in the near future. Unfortunately, many women do not avail themselves of the opportunity to have a Papanicolaou smear examination on an annual basis, and some physicians do not perform this simple test as part of their health maintenance screening strategy. Because of the importance of this test, the quality control of cytopathology laboratories must be monitored; and appropriate treatment of preinvasive and invasive neoplasia of the cervix must be available if quality care is to be provided to all women.

There are approximately 16,000 cases of invasive cervical cancer diagnosed in the United States annually. Not only has the mortality rate from invasive cervical cancer declined, but there has been a parallel steady fall in the diagnosis of invasive cancer. During this same period of time the incidence of preinvasive disease, cervical intraepithelial neoplasia (CIN), has increased steadily. There are approximately 45,000 new cases of carcinoma in situ (CIN-III) diagnosed annually in the United States. As previously discussed (Chap. 25) carcinoma in situ, left untreated, progresses to invasive carcinoma in most cases. This chapter deals with the management of invasive cervical cancer.

Etiology

For many decades the etiology of most cervical cancers (squamous cell carcinoma) has been considered to be the sexually transmitted diseases. Historical case-control studies have shown that the earlier age of the onset of sexual intercourse, increasing numbers of sexual partners, age at first childbirth, and lower socioeconomic status are all associated with an increased incidence of invasive cervical cancer. On the other hand, celibacy, as in nuns in convents, is associated with rare occurrences of cervical cancer. The carcinogen that ultimately causes cervical cancer remains unknown, although current investigation points strongly toward human papilloma virus (HPV) as a likely etiologic factor in many cases. HPV DNA fragments have been identified in the human genome by DNA probing of invasive squamous cell carcinoma and CIN. Other theories that have been promoted include association with herpes simplex virus infections, and indeed there is a body of literature that supports this contention. Others have proposed a "male factor," which may be some chemical component of the sperm head. It may ultimately be found that several factors are necessary for the transformation of the cervical squamous epithelium to an invasive process.

Other epidemiologic factors are important to consider as well. The age of onset of sexual intercourse, i.e., the time of exposure to the carcinogen, is important. During the teenage years, with the onset of ovulation and the change in vaginal pH, active squamous metaplasia is taking place on the exocervix (the transformation zone). It seems that during this time of squamous metaplasia and cellular immaturity or vulnerability, the carcinogen is most likely to have its influence on the squamous epithelium. Finally, the integrity of the immune system probably plays an important role in the development of cervical cancer. Certainly, the occurrence of invasive cancer of the cervix, as well as CIN, is increased in patients who are immunosuppressed, e.g., patients who have received kidney transplants.

In general, invasive cervical cancer is preceded by CIN, with the gradual transformation in the grade of CIN to ultimately become invasive carcinoma. The usual transformation time is on the order of 10 to 20 years. Further evidence of a transformation period is supported by noting that the median age at the onset of cervical carcinoma in situ is approximately 35 years, and median age of onset of invasive cancer is 45 years. It must be emphasized, however, that for any individual patient this transformation time may be much less, is unpredictable, and *may not* be preceded by CIN.

Diagnosis

It would be ideal if all patients were diagnosed in an asymptomatic state by routine use of the Papanicolaou smear. Unfortunately, an alarming number of patients still present for medical evaluation with the classic signs and symptoms of cervical cancer. The signs and symptoms of invasive cervical cancer are abnormal uterine bleeding, often associated with or brought on by cervical trauma, e.g., sexual intercourse. Post-coital bleeding may have been preceded by months of a thin, blood-tinged, watery vaginal discharge. As the malignancy progresses, the patient may complain of pain or pelvic pressure, urinary tract frequency, or rectal pressure. In advanced cases, encroachment on the ureters or sacrum may cause flank or sciatic pain or uremic coma secondary to bilateral ureteral obstruction.

Patients who have cervical cancer detected by Pa-panicolaou smear usually have a lesion that is so small as to be considered clinically occult. These patients should be evaluated with colposcopy, directed biopsy, and endocervical curettage. If the diagnosis of cervical cancer cannot be established with these techniques, cold-knife conization of the cervix along with dilatation and curettage (D&C) should be performed to fully evaluate the exocervix and endocervix (Fig. 26-1). Clinically obvious cervical lesions may be biopsied in the office without the need for anesthesia or magnification provided by colposcopy. Unfortunately, we continue to see an occasional patient who does not have cervical cancer diagnosed until an abdominal or vaginal hysterectomy has been performed for some benign indication. Review of these cases usually shows that the patient was inadequately evaluated preoperatively. Many times a Papanicolaou smear was deleted from the preoperative evaluation or other

Fig. 26-1. Gross appearance of cervical cancer. A. Carcinoma of the cervix may appear grossly to be extending from the cervix and filling the upper vaginal canal. This exophytic cancer is the most typical type. B. Squamous cell carcinoma of the cervix may also invade the cervical stroma with little exophytic component (endophytic lesion). C. Adenocarcinoma of the endocervix often penetrates the cervical stroma and expands the cervix and lower uterine segment without an obvious lesion on the exocervix. This expanded lower uterine segment and cervix are designated a "barrel lesion."

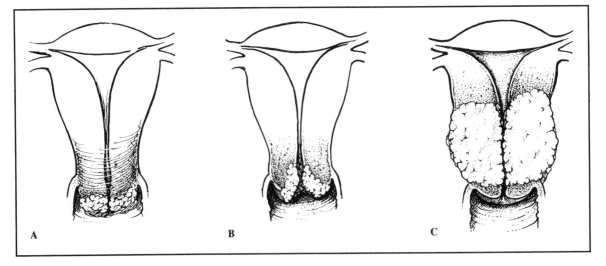

A   B   C

signs and symptoms (e.g., abnormal bleeding or vaginal discharge) were attributed to some benign cause and were not fully evaluated. The practice of incomplete evaluation of patients before undertaking gynecologic surgery, resulting in less than adequate management, should be condemned.

Approximately 90 percent of cervical cancer arises from the squamous epithelium in the transformation zone of the cervix. *Squamous cell carcinoma* is further subdivided into large cell nonkeratinizing, large cell keratinizing, and small cell carcinoma. *Adenocarcinoma* of the cervix, arising from endocervical glands, comprises approximately 10 percent of cases in most modern reports. In some institutions, adenocarcinoma of the cervix accounts for as many as 20 percent of all invasive cervical cancers. Whether this increased incidence of adenocarcinoma is due to a true increase in occurrence or to a decrease in the incidence of squamous cell carcinoma is not fully understood at the present time. Clear cell carcinoma of the cervix, a subtype of adenocarcinoma, has been associated with in utero exposure to diethylstilbestrol (DES). It appears, from the long-term follow-up of this patient population, that the peak incidence of clear cell carcinoma has passed; and as this cohort group of women who were exposed to DES in utero have aged, the incidence of clear cell carcinoma of the cervix has declined. Other, much rarer invasive malignancies of the cervix include *sarcomas* (sarcoma botryoides, see Chapter 29) and *lymphomas*. In general, squamous cell and adenocarcinomas of the cervix are managed in similar fashion, and discussion with regard to treatment encompasses both of the common histologic subtypes.

Spread Patterns

Squamous cell carcinoma of the cervix has two primary routes of spread (Fig. 26-2). First, it can spread *locally* through the cervical stroma and up the endocervical canal to involve the endometrium or distally to involve the vagina. It also spreads directly into the paracervical tissues (parametra) and, infrequently, penetrates anteriorly or posteriorly into the bladder or rectal mucosa. The second important route of spread for cervical cancer is along the *paracervical lym-*

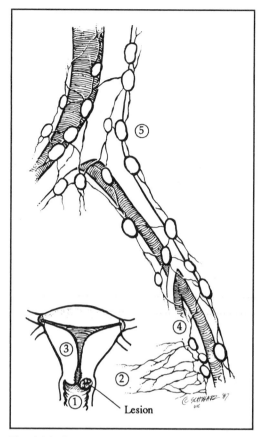

Fig. 26-2. Spread patterns of cervical cancer. Direct extension of cervical cancer may involve the vagina (1), parametria (2), and endometrial cavity (3). Lymphatic embolization by way of the paracervical lymphatics results in metastases in the pelvic lymph nodes—the obturator, hypogastric, and common iliac chains (4). From the pelvis, metastases can spread to the aortic lymph nodes (5).

phatics. Lymph channels draining the cervix spread through the parametria in which some lymph nodes exist but then drain further to the pelvic side wall. The lymph node groups at risk for metastases include the obturator, external iliac, and hypogastric lymph node chain. Further embolic spread along lymphatic channels allows extension to the common iliac and paraaortic lymph nodes. It should be noted, however, that cervical cancer cannot spread directly into the common iliac or paraaortic lymph nodes and bypass the pelvic lymphatics. *Hematogenous* spread of cervical cancer is infrequent and is usually seen only in advanced cases. To plan treatment appropriately, survey should be made to establish as well as possible the extent of spread of the cervical cancer.

By agreement of the International Federation of Gynecology and Obstetrics (FIGO), a clinical staging system has evolved that has been used worldwide since the mid-1970s. This staging system relies on careful clinical examination as well as elementary radiographic techniques. Although more sophisticated radiographic techniques such as lymphangiography, computed tomography, and magnetic resonance imaging are not included in the staging system, they are often utilized in the United States for more accurate staging methods.

The FIGO staging system, outlined in Table 26-1, requires a careful history and physical examination, with particular attention to palpation of inguinal and supraclavicular lymph nodes, abdominal examination, and thorough pelvic examination including bimanual and rectovaginal assessments. On pelvic examination, evaluation should include inspection and palpation for metastases in the vagina and parametria and an evaluation of spread of disease through the parametria to the pelvic side wall.

Cystoscopy and proctosigmoidoscopy aid the evaluation of potential involvement of the bladder or rectal mucosa. Intravenous pyelography is done routinely to assess the integrity of the renal units as well as the course of the ureters. Cervical cancer can cause abnormalities in the intravenous pyelogram in two frequent locations. First, as the ureter passes through the parametria in the last 5 cm of its course before entering the bladder trigone, paracervical tumor involvement may encroach on the ureter, leading to distal ureteral obstruction. Second, metastases in lymph nodes in the hypogastric or lower common iliac chain

Table 26-1. FIGO Staging of Cervical Cancer: Invasive Carcinoma (1985)

Stage I:	Carcinoma strictly confined to the cervix (extension to the corpus should be disregarded).
	Stage I-A: Preclinical carcinomas of the cervix, i.e., those diagnosed only by microscopy.
	Stage I-A1: Minimal microscopically evident stromal invasion.
	Stage I-A2: Lesions detected microscopically that can be measured. The upper limit of the measurement should not show a depth of invasion of more than 5 mm taken from the base of the epithelium, either surface or glandular, from which it originates; and a second dimension, the horizontal spread, must not exceed 7 mm. Larger lesions should be staged as I-B.
	Stage I-B: Lesions of dimensions greater than those of Stage I-A2 whether seen clinically or not. Preformed space involvement should not alter the staging but should be specifically recorded so as to determine if it should affect treatment decisions in the future.
Stage II:	Carcinoma extends beyond the cervix but has not extended onto the pelvic wall. The carcinoma involves the vagina but not the lower third.
	Stage II-A: No obvious parametrial involvement.
	Stage II-B: Obvious parametrial involvement.
Stage III:	Carcinoma has extended onto the pelvic wall. On rectal examination, there is no cancer-free space between the tumor and the pelvic wall. The tumor involves the lower third of the vagina. All patients have hydronephrosis or a nonfunctioning kidney.
	Stage III-A: No extension onto the pelvic wall.
	Stage III-B: Extension onto the pelvic wall and/or hydronephrosis or a nonfunctioning kidney.
Stage IV:	Carcinoma has extended beyond the true pelvis or has clinically involved the mucosa of the bladder or rectum. Bullous edema as such does not permit a case to be allotted to Stage IV.
	Stage IV-A: Spread of the growth to adjacent organs (bladder or rectum).
	Stage IV-B: Spread to distant organs.

may cause ureteral deviation or encroachment of the ureter at this point close to the pelvic brim. Ureteral obstruction allows upstaging the tumor to Stage III-B.

Barium enema, liver scan, and bone scan are of little value for evaluating patients with early-stage cervical cancer and are of minimal additional value unless the patient has signs or symptoms specifically pointing toward distant metastases. On the other hand, a more careful search for metastatic disease in pelvic and paraaortic lymph nodes is suggested prior to undertaking therapy. Clearly the patient who has metastatic disease in the paraaortic lymph nodes but receives treatment only to the pelvis will not have the opportunity to enjoy long-term survival. At present, computed tomography of the pelvic and paraaortic lymph nodes has been shown to be reasonably accurate for detecting enlarged lymph nodes with potential metastatic deposits. Enlarged lymph nodes can then be confirmed by fine-needle aspiration and cytologic study of the aspirated material. In some institutions, bipedal lymphangiography has played an important role in detecting lymphatic metastases, although the interpretation of the lymphangiogram is subjective and is greatly dependent on the skill of the radiologist.

Finally, in some study protocols and in some cancer centers, surgical evaluation of the retroperitoneal lymph nodes is undertaken. The safest strategy is to use a retroperitoneal approach, thereby avoiding intraperitoneal or pelvic adhesions, which might lead to complications of radiation therapy. The value of retroperitoneal lymphadenectomy for staging cervical cancer remains debatable, especially concerning an honest assessment of the number of patients who benefit from this surgical staging. At the present time staging laparotomy for cervical cancer must be considered an investigational tool.

Treatment

Microinvasive Carcinoma. As squamous cell carcinoma in situ begins to invade beyond the basement membrane, an early state of invasion exists that has little potential to metastasize. The definition of microinvasive carcinoma is not uniformly agreed upon. In the United States most gynecologic oncologists consider invasion to less than 3 mm as microinvasive. This definition is further modified to exclude lesions that are found to be confluent or anaplastic or that invade vascular or lymphatic channels. Cold-knife conization of the cervix is required to fully evaluate the lesion and to exclude cases of frankly invasive carcinoma.

Because the probability of lymphatic metastasis is less than 1 percent with microinvasive carcinoma, treatment is aimed at excising the primary lesion on the cervix. In general, microinvasive carcinoma is treated by extrafascial vaginal or abdominal hysterectomy. Individualized therapy for patients who wish to preserve fertility may be possible if the conization margins are free of disease.

Invasive Carcinoma. The general goals of treatment of cervical cancer are directed at eliminating the central disease (in the cervix, vagina, and parametria), as well as eradicating metastases in lymph nodes. Primary therapy for cervical cancer at the present time is radiation therapy. Radical surgery is reserved for patients with Stage I-B and occasional Stage II-A disease who are in good medical condition and would tolerate radical pelvic surgery.

RADIATION THERAPY. Cervical cancer can be treated successfully with radiation therapy, especially if it is early-stage disease. Surprisingly, even with advanced-stage disease (Stage III-B) with extension to the pelvic side wall, approximately 30 percent of patients can be cured with radiation therapy. The reason that radiation therapy can be so successful in treating a large volume of advanced disease is because of our ability to direct high doses of radiation to the pelvis in the form of external irradiation and intracavitary irradiation (brachytherapy). High doses in this region may be achieved because of anatomic access to the cervix and upper vagina, allowing intracavitary cesium application. Additionally, the adjacent pelvic viscera (bladder, vagina, and rectum) tolerate reasonably high doses of radiation before complications are encountered.

The specific treatment plan for the various stages of cervical cancer are outlined in Table 26-2. In general, external beam radiation is delivered, preferably

Table 26-2. Therapy Options for Carcinoma of the Cervix

Stage	Surgery	Radiation therapy	
		External whole pelvis (cGy)	Brachytherapy (mg-hr)
0	Extrafascial hysterectomy *or* Cold-knife conization *or* Local destruction: laser, cryotherapy		
I-A	Extrafascial hysterectomy		
I-B	Radical hysterectomy *and* pelvic lymphadenectomy	4000	6000 (2 applications)
II-A	Radical hysterectomy *and* pelvic lymphadenectomy		6000 (2 applications)
II-B	None	4000–5000	5000–6000 (2 applications)
III-A	None	5000–6000	2000–3000 (1–2 applications or interstitial implant)
III-B	None	5000–6000	4000–5000 (1–2 applications or interstitial implant)
IV-A	None	6000	4000–5000 (1–2 applications or interstitial implant)
IV-B	None	1000 pulse, repeat × 2 (palliation only)	

by a linear accelerator of 2 to 20 meV; or cobalt is given to encompass the whole pelvis through antero-posterior and posteroanterior ports or through four fields including two lateral fields (Fig. 26-3). This technique delivers equal doses of radiation to the central tumor, parametria, and lymph nodes. If the common iliac or paraaortic chain appear to be involved with metastatic disease, the radiation port can be extended to encompass the common iliac and paraaortic chain to the diaphragm (extended field technique). Initiating therapy with external beam radiation allows shrinkage of the central tumor and in advanced cases hopefully allows the anatomy to return closer to normal to achieve a more optimal intracavitary cesium application.

At this juncture, it is optimal to proceed with brachytherapy. The most frequently used technique in the United States today is through Fletcher-Suit intra-uterine tandem and colpostats, which allow loading of radium or cesium after the patient has left the operating room (afterloading technique) (Fig. 26-4).

The application of intracavitary cesium achieves high doses of radiation centrally. The dose of radiation to the pelvic lymph nodes is diminished significantly owing to the falloff in radiation described by the inverse square law.

Combined doses of external and intracavitary radiation therapy are calculated at specific points in the pelvis (dosimetry). Point A is an arbitrary point found by measuring 2 cm up the cervical canal and 2 cm lateral to the cervix. In general, this site is at the parametria at approximately the point where the ureter crosses under the uterine artery. An arbitrary point 3 cm lateral to point A is designated point B, which approximates the position of the pelvic lymph nodes (Fig. 26-4). Calculations of dosimetry by radiotherapists today are individualized to the patient's pelvis, and measurements of doses specifically to the pelvic side wall are calculated from a pelvic radiograph. Doses are also calculated to the vaginal mucosa, bladder, and rectum, and a limit is set to minimize the potential for long-term complications.

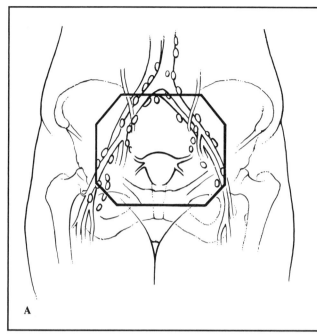
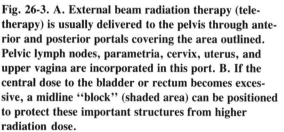
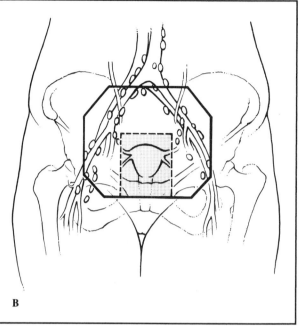

A

B

Fig. 26-3. A. External beam radiation therapy (tele-therapy) is usually delivered to the pelvis through anterior and posterior portals covering the area outlined. Pelvic lymph nodes, parametria, cervix, uterus, and upper vagina are incorporated in this port. B. If the central dose to the bladder or rectum becomes excessive, a midline "block" (shaded area) can be positioned to protect these important structures from higher radiation dose.

The overall survival of patients with cervical cancer treated by radiation therapy are listed in Table 26-3. Attempts to improve results of radiation therapy have been directed primarily at evaluating radiation sensitizers, which augment the effect of radiation therapy, or radioprotectors, which protect normal tissue from radiation therapy, thereby allowing higher doses of radiation therapy to be delivered to the tumor. Finally, the adjunctive use of hyperthermia remains investigational but, on theoretical and experimental grounds, seems to improve the ability of radiation therapy to achieve tumor cell kill.

Radiation therapy is generally well tolerated by most patients, no matter what their medical condi-

tion. External beam radiation therapy is an outpatient modality, delivered in fractions of 160 to 200 cGy per day over a four- to six-week course. Acute side effects such as nausea and diarrhea, cystitis, or neutropenia secondary to bone marrow suppression are usually easily managed and reverse at the completion of radiation therapy. Intracavitary brachytherapy has minimal acute hazard aside from that associated with a general anesthetic and 48 to 72 hours of strict bed rest while the cesium is in place. Long-term complications of radiation therapy are infrequent, occurring in approximately 5 to 10 percent of patients. On occasion these complications are life-threatening (Chap. 5).

Severe complications include urinary or gastrointestinal fistulas, small bowel obstruction, and hemorrhagic cystitis or proctitis. These complications may not become apparent for months or years after therapy because the radiation damages small blood vessels leading to endarteritis with tissue hypoxia and subsequent fibrosis. The vicious cycle of continued tissue hypoxia and fibrosis progresses over a period of years and may be further aggravated by coexisting vascular

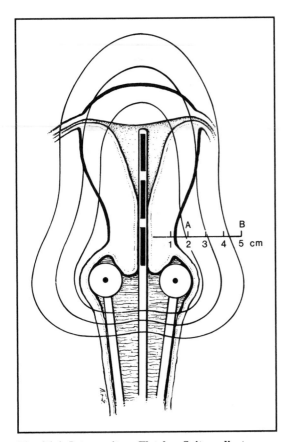

Fig. 26-4. Intracavitary Fletcher-Suit applicator system. Intracavitary radiation therapy (brachytherapy) is usually given by placing cesium in an intrauterine tandem and contracervical applicators. The cesium sources are placed in a tandem fashion in the uterus, and a single source of cesium is placed in each vaginal applicator. The isodose curve from this application is depicted as three concentric lines. The dose to various pelvic sites is calculated (dosimetry) and depends on the strength of the cesium sources placed, the duration the sources remain in place, and the distance from the sources to the tissue in question. Two arbitrary points are usually calculated. Point A is found 2 cm cephalad and 2 cm lateral from the external cervical os. This point is where the ureter crosses underneath the uterine artery. Point B, which is 3 cm more lateral to point A, represents approximately the pelvic side wall and pelvic lymph nodes.

Table 26-3. Survival After Treatment for Carcinoma of the Cervix

Stage	5-Year survival (%)
0	100
I-A	99
I-B	85–90 (surgery or irradiation)
II-A	73–80
II-B	68
III-A	45
III-B	36
IV-A	15
IV-B	2

diseases such as diabetes or atherosclerotic vascular disease. Ultimately, tissue hypoxia progresses to the point of tissue necrosis and either fistulization or hemorrhage.

Surgical repair of irradiated tissues is difficult. It usually is most successful when nonirradiated tissues can be brought into the operating field, thereby introducing a new blood supply to the damaged tissues.

RADICAL SURGERY. Radical surgery for the primary treatment of cervical cancer is limited to patients with Stage I-B or early Stage II-A cervical carcinoma. The surgical concept of radical hysterectomy (*Wertheim hysterectomy*) is complete resection of the uterus, cervix, and parametrial tissue as well as an adequate vaginal cuff. This surgery is designed to encompass the entire cervical cancer, including adequate surgical margins, as well as to resect the paracervical lymphatics. In addition to the radical hysterectomy, *pelvic lymphadenectomy* is performed for both staging and treatment purposes. The radical nature of this surgical procedure includes extensive dissection of the base of the bladder and terminal ureter as well as deep pelvic dissection. Intraoperative hemorrhage and injury to the bladder, ureter, or rectum are hazards of the surgical procedure. Postoperative hemorrhage, infection, and venous thrombosis or pulmonary embolism are potential complications, as are the complications associated with general anesthesia and the general physiologic stress of a radical surgical procedure. The surgical technique, goals, and management of complications are discussed in Chap. 5.

Treatment results of radical hysterectomy are well

established. For Stage I-B cervical carcinoma treated by radical hysterectomy, survival is nearly identical to that achieved with radiation therapy. Approximately 85 to 90 percent of patients should enjoy disease-free survival of five years or more.

Advantages of radical hysterectomy over radiation therapy are several: preservation of ovarian function in young women, improved vaginal function and subsequent sexual satisfaction, and mimimal long-term or delayed morbidity. The down side of radical surgery includes the acute intraoperative and postoperative complications that may ensue and that some patients cannot tolerate physiologically. Therefore radical hysterectomy with pelvic lymphadenectomy is usually recommended to women who are in good medical condition. Some gynecologic oncologists recommend radical hysterectomy only in patients with lesions 3 cm or less in diameter based on the premise that these patients have minimal risk for lymph node metastases. Although this presumption is true, the survival of patients with larger lesions is not necessarily improved by the use of radiation therapy.

Follow-up

Careful surveillance of patients who have been treated for cervical cancer is important, as an occasional patient with recurrence might still be treated for cure by secondary means. In addition, it is important to follow patients so as to minimize and manage any treatment-related morbidity. Follow-up routines vary from one institution to another, but in general patients are seen at intervals of approximately three months for the first one to two years after therapy. In approximately 75 percent of patients who do develop a recurrence, it becomes apparent during the first two years of follow-up. Furthermore, more than 90 percent of patients whose disease recurs experience the recurrence during the first five years of follow-up.

The most frequent site of recurrence of cervical cancer is the pelvis, so careful pelvic examination and a Papanicolaou smear are advised. Progressive obstruction of one or both ureters is highly suggestive of recurrent cancer and warrants further investigation. On rare occasion, radiation therapy or scarring after radical surgery leads to ureteral obstruction, and

therefore patients with ureteral obstruction must not be presumed to have recurrence of their carcinoma until it is proved histologically. The value of a screening follow-up of patients with serial computed tomography has not been established, although it might be an effective strategy for detection of enlarging pelvic or paraaortic lymph nodes. Chest radiographs at 6- to 12-month intervals is also reasonable for the detection of early pulmonary metastases. A suspicious lesion in a patient thought to have a recurrence should be evaluated and confirmed by cytology or histology. Technology utilizing fine-needle biopsies directed by clinical palpation or by radiographic methods has greatly augmented our ability to diagnose deep-seated recurrences yet avoid major surgery to obtain a tissue biopsy.

Recurrent Disease

Unfortunately, most patients who develop recurrence after primary treatment for cervical cancer cannot be cured by secondary treatment. Most of our efforts to date are aimed at achieving partial remission of the progressive recurrent disease and providing effective palliation. In situations where radiation therapy might be delivered to previously nonirradiated regions, it is a reasonable approach to secondary treatment. On rare occasion, a lesion that recurs in the central pelvis after radical hysterectomy may be treated and cured by radiation therapy. More frequently, the recurrence develops outside a previous radiation port in a paraaortic or supraclavicular lymph node. These regions may be irradiated to achieve local control of the cancer, although the location of the recurrence usually represents systemic disease that cannot be cured by radiation therapy.

In other instances—pulmonary, hepatic, or bony metastases, or recurrence in a previously irradiated field—the only treatment that can be offered is systemic chemotherapy. Currently, the efficacy of systemic chemotherapy is limited to a few drugs, which can achieve clinical responses approximately 30 percent of the time. The cornerstone to most therapy today is cis-platinum given by intravenous infusion. Other active drugs include vinblastine, bleomycin, and mitomycin-C. It must be emphasized that patients

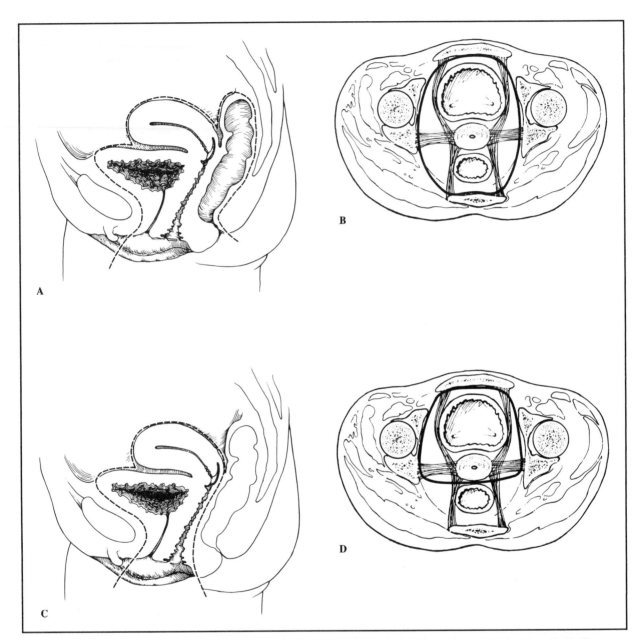

Fig. 26-5. Pelvic exenteration for the treatment of recurrent cervical carcinoma after radiation therapy. A, B. The extent of resection is depicted here for total pelvic exenteration. C, D. When lesions are located on the anterior wall, an anterior exenteration may be performed, thereby saving rectal function. E, F. Conversely, if the recurrent carcinoma is located on the posterior aspect of the vagina, a posterior exenteration may be performed, thereby attempting to save bladder function.

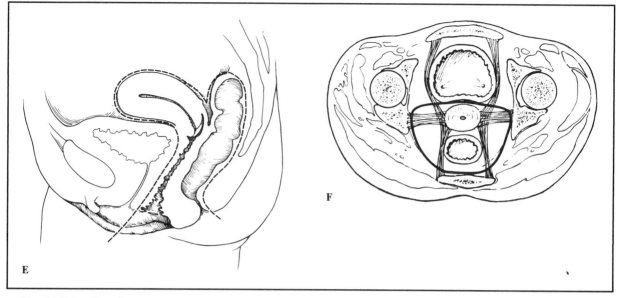

Fig. 26-5 (continued).

are not cured by systemic chemotherapy but may have regression of the tumor and on rare occasions complete elimination of clinical tumor for a period of time. Until more effective drugs or drug regimens are found, chemotherapy must be considered palliative; and the benefits of palliative therapy must be weighed against the toxicity of the drugs used.

In approximately 2 to 5 percent of patients with recurrent cervical cancer, the disease is found to be in the central pelvis if the patient was previously treated by radiation therapy. This selected subgroup of patients may benefit from ultraradical surgical resection of the pelvic tumor and can expect to be cured in approximately 40 to 50 percent of cases. Care must be taken when evaluating these patients to exclude those who are found to have distant metastases that are not amenable to surgical resection. Thorough workup with radiographic imaging, physical examination, and general evaluation of medical and psychological status is important.

In the patient who is thought to have disease confined to the central pelvis that a gynecologic oncologist believes might be surgically resected, the patient should be given the opportunity to undergo pelvic exenteration (Fig. 26-5). This procedure is de-

signed to resect en bloc the central pelvic tumor, including tissue margins free of disease. Most frequently, total pelvic exenteration is performed, resecting the bladder, uterus and cervix, vagina, and rectum; the lateral margins of the surgical resection are the pelvic side walls. Clearly it is an extended radical procedure with considerable potential for intraoperative and postoperative complications. It is also a deforming procedure that in most cases leaves a patient with a urinary conduit and colostomy. More recently, with the circular intestinal stapling techniques, low rectal reanastomosis has been accomplished, thus saving the patient a colostomy stoma. Further reconstruction of the pelvis utilizing gracilis myocutaneous flaps to construct a new vagina have aided considerably in the sexual rehabilitation of some patients. Careful selection occasionally allows preservation of the rectum or the bladder by performing either an anterior or a posterior exenteration. Although it is laudable to attempt to preserve as much normal bowel or bladder function as possible, the surgeon must be vigilant to not cut across tumor, thus compromising the patient's only chance of cure.

As the technique of pelvic exenteration has been refined, the indications have been clearly established;

the surgical and medical management of these patients has been optimized, reducing the operative mortality rate to a reasonable 5 percent in most modern series. Long-term disease-free survival is achieved in approximately 40 to 50 percent of patients.

SELECTED READINGS

Averette, H. E., Lichtinser, M., Sevin, B. U., et al. Pelvic exenteration: a 15-year experience in a general metropolitan hospital. *Am. J. Obstet. Gynecol.* 150:179, 1984.

Bandy, L. C., Clarke-Pearson, D. L., Soper, J. T., et al. Long-term effects on bladder function following radical hysterectomy with and without postoperative radiation. *Gynecol. Oncol.* 26:160, 1987.

Berek, J. S., Castaldo, T. W., Hacker, N. F., et al. Adenocarcinoma of the uterine cervix. *Cancer* 48:2734, 1981.

Berman, M. L., Keys, H., Creasman, W. T., et al. Survival and patterns of recurrence in cervical cancer metastatic to periaortic lymph nodes (a Gynecologic Oncology Group study). *Gynecol. Oncol.* 19:8, 1984.

Brinton, L. A., Schairer, C., Haenszel, W., et al. Cigarette smoking and invasive cervical cancer. *J.A.M.A.* 255:3265, 1986.

Burke, T. W., Hoskins, W. J., Heller, P. B., et al. Prognostic factors associated with radical hysterectomy failure. *Gynecol. Oncol.* 26:153, 1987.

Choo, Y. C. Chemotherapy in advanced primary and recurrent cervical carcinoma. *Int. J. Gynaecol. Obstet.* 20:417, 1982.

Creasman, W. T., Fetter, B. F., Clarke-Pearson, D. L., et al. Management of stage I-A carcinoma of the cervix. *Am. J. Obstet. Gynecol.* 153:164, 1985.

Creasman, W. T., Soper, J. T., and Clarke-Pearson, D. Radical hysterectomy as therapy for early carcinoma of the cervix. *Am. J. Obstet. Gynecol.* 155:964, 1986.

Gallion, H. H., van-Nagell, J. R., Jr., Donaldson, E. S., et al. Combined radiation therapy and extrafascial hysterectomy in the treatment of stage IB barrel-shaped cervical cancer. *Cancer* 56:262, 1985.

Henriksen, E. Distribution of metastases in stage I carcinoma of the cervix. *Am. J. Obstet. Gynecol.* 80:919, 1960.

Herbst, A. L. An analysis of 346 cases of clear cell adenocarcinoma of the vagina and cervix with emphasis on recurrence and survival. *Gynecol. Oncol.* 7:11, 1979.

Hreschyshn, M. M., Aron, B. S., Boronow, R. C., et al. Hydroxyurea or placebo combined with radiation to treat stages IIIB and IV cervical cancer confined to the pelvis. *Int. J. Radiat. Oncol. Biol. Phys.* 5:317, 1979.

Ketchan, A. S., Deckers, P. J., Sugarbaker, E. V., et al. Pelvic exenteration for carcinoma of the uterine cervix: a 15-year experience. *Cancer* 26:513, 1970.

Lynge, E., and Poll, P. Incidence of cervical cancer following negative smear: a cohort study. *Am. J. Epidemiol.* 124:345, 1986.

Montag, R. W., D'Abaing, G., and Schlaerth, J. B. Embryonal rhabdomyosarcoma of the uterine corpus and cervix. *Gynecol. Oncol.* 25:171, 1986.

Montana, G. S., Fowler, W. G., Varia, M. A., et al. Carcinoma of the cervix, stage III. *Cancer* 57:148, 1986.

Morrow, C. P. Is pelvic radiation beneficial in the postoperative management of stage IB squamous cell carcinoma of the cervix with pelvic node metastasis treated by radical hysterectomy and pelvic lymphadenectomy? *Gynecol. Oncol.* 10:105, 1980.

Perez, C. A., Breaux, S., Madoc-Jones, H., et al. Correlation between radiation dose and tumor recurrence and complications in carcinoma of the uterine cervix: stages I and IIA. *Int. J. Radiat. Oncol. Biol. Phys.* 5:373, 1979.

Potish, R. A. Radiation therapy of periaortic node metastases in cancer of the uterine cervix and endometrium. *Radiology* 164:567, 1987.

Rutledge, E. N., Smith, J. P., Wharton, J. T., et al. Pelvic exenteration: analysis of 296 patients. *Am. J. Obstet. Gynecol.* 129:881, 1977.

Thigpen, T., Shingleton, H., Homesley, H., et al. cis-Platinum in the treatment of advanced or recurrent squamous cell carcinoma of the cervix: a phase II study of the Gynecologic Oncology Group. *Cancer* 48:899, 1981.

27

Endometrial Cancer and Uterine Sarcoma

Malignancies arising in the uterine corpus are composed primarily of endometrial carcinoma and uterine sarcomas. Adenocarcinoma arising in the endometrium is the leading invasive gynecologic malignancy encountered in the United States, with approximately 37,000 women developing it annually.

ENDOMETRIAL CANCER

Endometrial carcinoma is generally a disease of postmenopausal women, with three-fourths of cases diagnosed after the onset of menopause. Only 3 percent of patients are younger than age 40 at the time of initial diagnosis. Endometrial cancer may be more difficult to diagnose in the woman between age 40 and 50 because of the difficulty determining whether abnormal bleeding is due to uterine neoplasia or irregular ovulation, which occurs at this point of menstrual life.

Risk factors associated with the development of endometrial carcinoma are recognized as obesity, nulliparity, menopause after age 53, and diabetes mellitus. Endogenous sources of unopposed estrogen, as in the polycystic ovarian disease patient or due to functioning ovarian tumors such as granulosa cell tumors, are also associated with an increased incidence of endometrial carcinoma, as is the exogenous use of estrogen for the treatment of menopausal symptoms. Case-controlled cohort studies during the early 1970s demonstrated that the risk of developing endometrial carcinoma in patients taking estrogen was increased from 3-fold to 12-fold. Further investigation of the role of exogenous estrogens has shown this risk factor to be closely tied to the dosage and duration of use of estrogen therapy. Modern management of menopause with the combined use of estrogens and progestins (Chap. 23) is not associated with an increased incidence of endometrial cancer.

Diagnosis

The most frequent sign (and symptom) of endometrial carcinoma is abnormal uterine bleeding. It is an obvious factor in the postmenopausal patient, in whom any bleeding must be considered abnormal and should be further evaluated with endometrial sampling. As alluded to previously, the etiology of irregular perimenopausal bleeding is sometimes difficult to determine, but with any suspicion of abnormality the patient should also be evaluated by endometrial biopsy or curettage. Occasionally the patient presents during menopause with an abnormal vaginal or uterine discharge, which should raise suspicion of a uterine malignancy. Rarely, in advanced stages of endometrial cancer, pelvic pain or pressure or ascites may be recognized as the first symptom.

Patients with abnormal uterine bleeding should be evaluated by careful physical examination and pelvic examination. Attention should be directed at potential sites of metastasis: palpation of supraclavicular and inguinal lymph nodes; abdominal examination searching for masses, ascites, hepatomegaly, or any evidence of vaginal or cervical metastases; assessment of uterine size by palpation and sounding the uterus; and bimanual and rectovaginal examination searching for adnexal or parametrial disease. In most cases, aside from uterine bleeding and possibly a slightly enlarged uterus, the remainder of the physical examination is normal.

Further evaluation of abnormal uterine bleeding should include Papanicolaou smear and endometrial and endocervical biopsy. Whereas the Papanicolaou smear is relatively sensitive for the detection of invasive cervical cancer, it suggests adenocarcinoma of the endometrium in only approximately 50 percent of patients. Therefore the Papanicolaou smear is not an adequate evaluation of a patient with abnormal bleeding. Direct biopsy of the endocervix and the endometrium should be performed. Most of the time it can be done in the office setting with minimal analgesia.

A variety of biopsy techniques are available, including use of small curets and suction aspiration devices. In general, these instruments provide sufficient tissue for the pathologist to evaluate the histology of the endocervix and the endometrium.

In situations where the patient has a cervical os so stenotic that office instruments cannot be passed into the uterus or where a clear diagnosis by outpatient biopsy has not been established, a fractional dilatation and curettage (D&C) should be performed. Fractional curettage is performed under general or spinal anesthesia so that the cervix may be dilated adequately to obtain tissue from the endometrial cavity. Before dilating the cervix, the cervical canal should be curetted and this tissue submitted separately. The cervix is then dilated and the endometrial cavity curetted, and that specimen is sent separately to the pathologist. These two specimens help to determine whether a malignancy is arising from the endometrium or the endocervix and if the endometrial carcinoma might be extending into the endocervix. Prior to 1988, endocervical curettage was also required to accurately stage the patient with endometrial carcinoma. However, because of the lack of accuracy of endocervical curettage for detecting endocervical involvement by endometrial cancer, we now determine cervical involvement by pathologic evaluation of the hysterectomy specimen.

Histology

Most endometrial carcinomas arise from endometrial glands and are therefore adenocarcinomas. There are three degrees of differentiation of the adenocarcinoma.

Grade 1, well differentiated: adenocarcinoma composed predominantly of glandular elements without intervening endometrial stroma

Grade 2, moderately differentiated: adenocarcinoma composed of a mixture of glandular elements and areas of sheets of carcinoma cells that are not further differentiated

Grade 3, poorly differentiated: adenocarcinoma composed of sheets of anaplastic cells without any glandular epithelium

The malignant potential and prognosis is linked to the differentiation of adenocarcinoma. The most poorly differentiated (grade 3) portends an unfavorable overall prognosis.

Endometrial adenocarcinoma may also contain squamous elements. In the past, benign squamous elements combined with adenocarcinoma were designated *adenoacanthoma.* If the squamous elements were malignant, the histologic diagnosis was called *adenosquamous carcinoma.* In general, adenoacanthoma was considered a relatively good-prognosis histology, whereas adenosquamous carcinoma was considered a poor-prognosis lesion. More recently, prospective pathologic studies have found that the significant prognostic factor depends on the degree of differentiation of the adenocarcinoma element. Current nomenclature therefore calls these endometrial carcinomas *"adenocarcinoma with squamous differentiation"* and clearly assigns the grade of the adenocarcinoma portion. The designation of "benign" or "malignant" squamous elements has been deleted.

The other rare endometrial carcinomas are *papillary serous* and *clear cell carcinoma.* The papillary serous lesion has a histologic pattern similar to that of serous cystadenocarcinoma of the ovary. Both have a much worse overall prognosis than the common adenocarcinomas of the endometrium.

Spread Patterns

Studies have shown that endometrial carcinoma may spread through several pathways and is somewhat unpredictable (Fig. 27-1). Initially, adenocarcinoma arising in the endometrium progresses locally to invade the myometrium, sometimes extending through the entire myometrial wall to involve the uterine serosa. Endometrial carcinoma may also extend directly into the endocervix. Lymphatic metastases are clearly demonstrated with endometrial carcinoma.

There are two lymphatic drainage systems of the uterus. First, endometrial carcinoma may travel through the lymphatics draining the cervix and spread to the pelvic lymph nodes in the hypogastric, obturator, and external iliac chains. Additionally, endometrial carcinoma may spread through the rich anastomosis of collateral lymphatics in the uterine cornua and travel to the paraaortic chain directly along the infundibulopelvic ligament (ovarian ves-

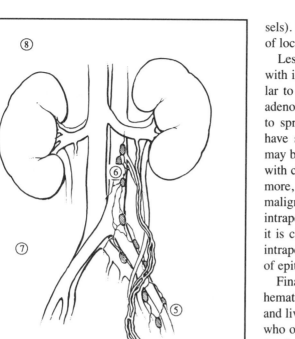

Fig. 27-1. Spread patterns of endometrial cancer. Endometrial cancer arises in the endometrial cavity and may initially spread by direct extension into the myometrium (1) or the endocervix (2). Metastases may also appear in the vagina (3), arising by either "drop metastases" or lymphatic spread. The adnexal structures—fallopian tubes and ovaries (4)—may be involved by direct extension or metastatic disease. Endometrial cancer may also spread to the pelvic lymph nodes draining the cervix (5) or to the paraaortic lymph nodes (6). The rich collateral circulation from the uterine cornua allows direct metastases along the ovarian vessels to the paraaortic chain. Intraperitoneal implants (7) are also occasionally found, along with malignant cells in peritoneal fluid. Finally, hematogenous spread to distant sites such as the lung (8) may be encountered.

sels). Endometrial cancer can also metastasize by way of local lymphatics to the vaginal vault.

Less frequently, endometrial carcinoma presents with intraperitoneal carcinomatosis and ascites, similar to advanced ovarian carcinoma. Papillary serous adenocarcinoma of the endometrium seems frequently to spread as intraperitoneal carcinomatosis. Studies have shown that malignant cells in peritoneal fluid may be found in approximately 15 percent of patients with clinical Stage I endometrial carcinoma. Furthermore, we have noted that in some of these patients the malignant cells ultimately transform into a picture of intraperitoneal carcinomatosis and ascites. Therefore it is clear that endometrial carcinoma can spread by intraperitoneal implantation in a pattern similar to that of epithelial ovarian cancer.

Finally, endometrial cancer can spread by way of hematogenous dissemination. Metastases to the lung and liver may be a first site of recurrence for a patient who otherwise was thought to have a carcinoma confined to the uterus.

Clinical Staging

Having made the diagnosis of endometrial carcinoma, distant metastases must be sought and the extent of the cancer evaluated. A clinical staging system adopted by the International Federation of Gynecology and Obstetrics (FIGO) in 1971 (Table 27-1) limited our evaluation of the extent of spread to clinical examination combined with routine radiography. Because of the significant inaccuracy of this clinical staging system, FIGO staging was changed to a surgical staging system in 1988 (Table 27-2). Many data concerned with the management of endometrial carcinoma are based on the former clinical staging system, and there are few prospective long-term data regarding the surgical staging system; therefore both staging systems are discussed here. It is hoped that the increased accuracy of the surgical staging system will lead to improved individualized treatment and improved survival so that the next edition of this text will consider clinical staging as a historical issue.

Approximately 75 percent of endometrial cancer patients have disease that is clinically confined to the uterus (clinical Stage I). Ten percent have malig-

Table 27-1. FIGO Clinical Staging of Endometrial Carcinoma (1971)

Stage I: Carcinoma is confined to the corpus.
    Stage IA: Length of the uterine cavity is 8 cm or less.
    Stage IB: Length of the uterine cavity is more than 8 cm.
    Stage I cases should be subgrouped with regard to the histologic type of adenocarcinoma as follows.
        G1: Highly differentiated adenomatous carcinoma.
        G2: Differentiated adenomatous carcinoma with partly solid areas.
        G3: Predominantly solid or entirely undifferentiated carcinoma.
Stage II: Carcinoma involves the corpus and cervix.
Stage III: Carcinoma extends outside the corpus but not outside the true pelvis. (It may involve the vaginal wall or para-metrium but not the bladder or rectum.)
Stage IV: Carcinoma involves the bladder or rectum or extends outside the pelvis.

Table 27-2. FIGO Surgical Staging of Endometrial Carcinoma (1988)

Stage IA G123:	Tumor limited to endometrium
IB G123:	Invasion to less than one-half of the myometrium
IC G123:	Invasion to more than one-half of the myometrium
Stage IIA G123:	Endocervical glandular involvement only
IIB G123:	Cervical stromal invasion
Stage IIIA G123:	Tumor invading serosa, adnexa, or both; and/or positive peritoneal cytology
IIIB G123:	Vaginal metastases
IIIC G123:	Metastases to pelvic and/or paraaortic lymph nodes
Stage IVA G123:	Tumor invades bladder, bowel mucosa, or both
IVB:	Distant metastases including intraabdominal and/or inguinal lymph node

Rules related to staging
1. Because corpus cancer is now surgically staged, procedures previously used for differentiation of stages are no longer applicable, e.g., the findings of D&C to differentiate between Stage I and Stage II.
    It is appreciated that there may be a small number of patients with corpus cancer who are treated primarily with radiation therapy. If that is the case, the clinical staging adopted by FIGO in 1971 would still apply but use of that staging system would be noted.
2. Ideally, the width of the myometrium is measured along with the width of tumor invasion.

nancy found to involve the cervix (Stage II), and a few patients have disease spread beyond the uterus and cervix discovered by clinical examination. The histologic differentiation (tumor grade) is included in the staging system. Therefore for clinical Stage I disease (a malignancy thought to be confined to the uterus), there are actually six substages. The reason for incorporating histologic grade is that it is an important prognostic factor. For example, patients with clinical Stage Ia, grade 1 adenocarcinoma of the endometrium have an approximately 95 percent chance of survival at five years. On the other hand, patients with clinical Stage Ib, grade 3 adenocarcinoma of the endometrium have less than 50 percent chance of being alive five years after the primary diagnosis and therapy. The FIGO clinical staging classification essentially considered the clinical stage and histologic grade as the only prognostic features significant to the patient.

Surgical Staging and Treatment

Prior to initiating treatment, it is important to establish the extent of spread an individual patient might harbor and its prognostic features. The FIGO clinical staging system considered only clinical stage and histologic grade of malignancy. Using these features, treatment schemas were developed that recognized that advanced stage or more poorly differentiated malignancies had a higher recurrence rate and therefore required more aggressive initial therapy. Unfortunately, with these treatment plans the overall survival for clinical Stage I endometrial carcinoma patients is only approximately 75 percent (Table 27-3).

During the 1980s many gynecologic oncologists sought to improve survival and to individualize patient treatment by obtaining information regarding prognostic factors not included in the clinical stage and grade of tumor. Treatment based on the surgically determined extent of spread offers the potential to more precisely individualize treatment, thereby avoiding unnecessary radiation therapy in patients with good prognosis disease and using more effective adjunctive treatment modalities for patients with high risk lesions.

Because most patients with endometrial carcinoma have clinical Stage I disease, the major effort to improve treatment plans has been directed to this group of patients. Findings at surgery have expanded our knowledge of this tumor and allow us to define more precisely individual risk factors. The surgical findings in clinical Stage I endometrial cancer are summarized in Table 27-4.

As might be expected, the more poorly differentiated lesions tend to be more deeply invasive in the myometrium and to have a higher incidence of pelvic and paraaortic lymph node metastases. In other words, many poor risk factors are interrelated, although for

Table 27-3. Distribution of and Survival After Endometrial Carcinoma

Clinical stage*	Percent of total cases	Survival at 5 years (%)
I	74	72
II	14	56
III	6	31
IV	3	9
No stage total	4	65

*FIGO Clinical Staging System, 1971.
Source: FIGO Annual Report, Volume 20. F. Pettersson (ed.). International Federation of Gynecology and Obstetrics Stockholm, 1988.

Table 27-4. Surgical Findings in FIGO Clinical Stage I Endometrial Carcinoma

Prognostic factor	Percent of Cases
Deep myometrial invasion	15
Occult invasion of cervix	8
Occult metastases to adnexa	7
Pelvic lymph node metastases	10
Paraaortic lymph node metastases	11
Peritoneal implants	3
Malignant peritoneal cytology	15

an individual patient it may not be true. For example, most patients with well differentiated adenocarcinoma carry a favorable prognosis. However, we occasionally find a patient who has deep myometrial invasion even though her tumor is well differentiated. It is this patient who is more likely to have nodal metastases and to die of recurrent disease if not given adjunctive therapy. Therefore, although prognostic factors are often interrelated, we believe they cannot be predicted with certainty based on clinical stage and grade alone and that surgical evaluation should be the first step in the treatment of most patients with endometrial carcinoma.

In 1988 FIGO recognized the significant inadequacies in the clinical staging system and changed to a surgical staging system (Table 27-2). This new staging system allows all clinical, radiographic, surgical, and pathologic information to be used for determining the extent of spread (stage) of disease. Because surgery (hysterectomy) is the cornerstone of treatment for endometrial carcinoma, the initial surgical approach provides detailed surgical-pathologic information regarding extent of spread and at the same time serves as definitive therapy for most patients. With improved medical and anesthetic management of the endometrial cancer patient, in excess of 95 percent should be medically fit to undergo major surgery. (In years past, as many as 20 percent of endometrial cancer patients were thought to be inoperable because of medical problems.) If a patient cannot undergo surgical staging, the clinical staging system should be employed.

Surgical staging and the treatment of endometrial

Table 27-5. Steps in Surgical Treatment, Staging, and Pathologic Review of Early Endometrial Carcinoma

1. Through intraabdominal exploration
2. Peritoneal fluid sent to cytopathology for study
3. Total abdominal hysterectomy and bilateral salpingo-oophorectomy
4. Selective pelvic and paraaortic lymphadenectomy
5. Careful pathologic study
   a. Malignant cells in peritoneal fluid
   b. Histologic grade of carcinoma
   c. Depth of invasion in corpus
   d. Extension to cervix, fallopian tubes, or ovaries
   e. Lymph node metastases
   f. Metastasis to other sites
   g. Estrogen and progesterone receptor content

cancer are summarized in Table 27-5. First, the abdomen is carefully explored and washings obtained from the pelvis to ascertain if malignant cells are floating in the peritoneal cavity. Total abdominal hysterectomy and bilateral salpingo-oophorectomy, the cornerstone for treatment of endometrial carcinoma, are then performed. Patients with deeply invasive well differentiated carcinoma, all patients with moderately differentiated and poorly differentiated adenocarcinoma, and those with papillary or clear cell histology should undergo selective pelvic and paraaortic lymphadenectomy as well. Any other suspicious areas or lesions should also be removed or biopsied. After careful pathologic evaluation the additional prognostic features listed in Table 27-4 may be ascertained and the surgical stage assigned (Table 27-2).

Surgical treatment and staging of patients with endometrial carcinoma must be undertaken with caution in many patients because of underlying medical diseases and advanced age. Excessive obesity, which is often noted in patients with endometrial carcinoma, may further complicate surgery by limiting exposure in the operating field as well as contributing to postoperative complications. On the other hand, it is a rare patient who is so medically infirm that she cannot undergo surgery.

Patients with early stage endometrial adenocarcinoma who are not medical candidates may be treated successfully with radiation therapy alone. Such treatment should include external beam radiation therapy to the whole pelvis (covering the uterus, cervix, and pelvic lymph nodes) followed by intracavitary cesium or radium application. Intracavitary therapy seems to be optimally applied by the use of Heymann capsules packed into the uterus to distend the myometrium and achieve a more favorable isodose curve in the fundus of the uterus (Fig. 27-2). Treatment results using radiation therapy alone are not as good, however, as for patients treated with total abdominal hysterectomy and bilateral salpingo-oophorectomy.

Adjuvant Therapy

Adjuvant therapy for endometrial carcinoma must be aimed at improved survival by eliminating clinically occult disease in areas at high risk. Traditionally, radiation therapy was given to the whole pelvis in high risk patients. Often radiation therapy was applied preoperatively to patients who were considered at high risk based on their clinical stage or poor prognosis histology. The general clinical impression has been that pelvic irradiation reduces (local) pelvic recurrences, although it has never been proved by a prospective study.

With the advent of surgical staging, adjuvant therapy is reserved for patients with proved high risk factors. Some factors portend a higher risk of localized recurrence, whereas other risk factors are associated with widespread intraperitoneal or systemic (e.g., lung or brain) metastases.

If the malignancy is found to be confined to the uterus (surgical Stage I), there is probably no value to adding adjuvant therapy. Some oncologists believe that additional pelvic radiation therapy for a Stage Ic, grade 1 lesion is advisable, but the value of this regimen is yet to be proved. Patients with surgical Stage IIb disease have a higher risk of occult parametrial or vaginal involvement than those with Stage I disease and therefore may benefit from pelvic radiation therapy.

Positive peritoneal cytology (Stage IIIa) has been associated with a high recurrence rate, especially intraperitoneal carcinomatosis. Although not all studies have agreed that positive cytology is a poor prognostic factor, we believe that it is and that such patients may be treated with either postoperative intraperitoneal

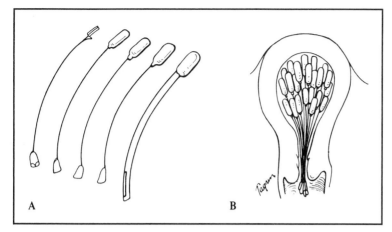

Fig. 27-2. Heymann capsules employed for intra-cavitary radiation therapy of endometrial carcinoma. A. Capsules of various sizes, the one on the right shown in position on a curved intrauterine applicator. B. Capsules in place within the uterine cavity. The use of multiple small radium sources rather than a single large radium applicator provides a more uniform distribution of radiation to all areas of the uterus.

chromic phosphate (^{32}P) or whole abdominal and pelvic irradiation.

Patients with documented metastases in the vagina (Stage IIIb) or the pelvic or paraaortic lymph nodes (Stage IIIc) should undergo radiation therapy to these areas of known spread. Even when patients are found to have aortic nodal metastases, up to 40 percent may be long-term survivors after radiation therapy.

Some patients, especially those with Stage III or Stage IV disease, are likely to suffer recurrences beyond the pelvis. The value of adjuvant therapy in this situation is unproved. Options might include hormonal therapy (progestins or antiestrogens) or chemotherapy. Prospective randomized trials of adjuvant therapy for the prevention of distant metastases are in progress, but none has yet demonstrated an effective regimen.

Treatment of Advanced Endometrial Carcinoma

Fortunately, clinically advanced endometrial adenocarcinoma is relatively rare. Treatment of these pa-

tients should also be individualized and is occasionally successful in achieving long-term survival.

Patients with clinical Stage III disease with gross metastases in the vaginal vault may be treated by combining external beam radiation therapy to the pelvis with vaginal application of cesium followed by total abdominal hysterectomy and bilateral salpingo-oophorectomy. Likewise, a patient with metastases to the ovary (Stage III) may be successfully treated by surgical excision followed by radiation therapy or intraperitoneal chromic phosphate (^{32}P).

Patients with distant metastases may benefit from surgical excision of a bleeding, potentially infected uterus despite the fact that metastases are left in the peritoneal cavity or elsewhere. Additional therapy with progestins, tamoxifen, or chemotherapy may be guided by the knowledge of estrogen and progesterone receptor content of the primary tumor. The combination chemotherapy regimen of adriamycin/cyclophosphamide/cisplatin has been reported to have a 50 percent response rate in patients with metastatic disease.

Follow-up

After primary therapy for endometrial carcinoma the patient should be seen at approximately three- to four-month intervals for the first two years after therapy. Approximately 80 percent of patients who develop a recurrence manifest it within two years of the primary therapy. Careful physical examination, pelvic examination, and Papanicolaou smear of the vaginal vault are reasonable clinical screening tests. Chest radiographic screening for pulmonary metastases is also advised in high risk patients. The serum marker CA-125 may be useful for detecting recurrent endometrial carcinoma, although large prospective studies have not been completed.

Treatment of Recurrent Disease

Patients with recurrent endometrial carcinoma may be treated with a variety of modalities individualized to the site of recurrence. Patients who have recurrence in the pelvis and who have not undergone previous irradiation may be treated with whole-pelvis or intra-vaginal irradiation (or both). In some instances, especially with vaginal vault recurrences, radiation therapy may achieve a cure. More distant metastases, e.g., lung metastases, are usually best treated with hormonal therapy. For several decades we have known that patients with metastatic endometrial cancer may show a significant response, and some patients go into remission with the use of progestin therapy (Fig. 27-3). The antiestrogen drug tamoxifen may also be active against recurrent endometrial carcinoma. Laboratory evidence has demonstrated that some endometrial carcinomas are rich in estrogen and pro-gesterone receptors. Preliminary studies confirm that the tumors that are receptor-rich are most likely to respond to hormonal therapy. Because hormonal therapy is nontoxic, relatively inexpensive, and active against endometrial cancer, it is usually our first choice for treating distant metastases. Chemotherapy is also a reasonable choice for distant widespread metastases. Unfortunately, significantly active chemotherapy regimens are yet to be found. Currently the most popular regimen is adriamycin/cisplatin/cyclophosphamide (Cytoxan) given intravenously every four weeks. Chemotherapy at the present time is considered palliative, with sustained remissions after chemotherapy rare.

Fig. 27-3. Progesterone therapy of pulmonary metastases in a patient with endometrial carcinoma. A persistent cough developed in a 55-year-old woman 4½ years after hysterectomy for endometrial cancer. Although there was no sign of local recurrence, a chest radiograph (at left) revealed multiple pulmonary metastases. Progesterone therapy employing 17α-hydroxy-progesterone caproate (Delalutin) in a dosage of 500 mg twice weekly produced a dramatic response, with almost complete disappearance of the pulmonary lesions (the film on the right was obtained two months after instituting progesterone therapy). On continuation of treatment the patient remained in complete remission for more than ten years.

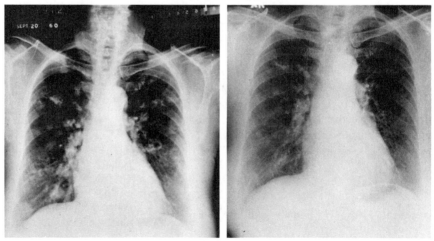

UTERINE SARCOMAS

Sarcomas arising from the uterus are rare gynecologic malignancies that carry a poor prognosis. Sarcomas account for approximately 3 percent of all malignancies of the uterine corpus and, like endometrial adenocarcinoma, usually present in the postmenopausal age woman.

The symptoms of uterine sarcomas may be similar to those of endometrial cancer, with postmenopausal bleeding, vaginal discharge, pelvic pain, and pelvic pressure. In addition, uterine sarcomas should be included in the differential diagnosis of the patient with an enlarging uterus or pelvic mass. The diagnosis of uterine sarcomas may be made by endometrial sampling or D&C. However, sarcomas arising in the myometrium may not protrude into the endometrial cavity and therefore may not be detected by uterine curettage. Leiomyosarcoma (smooth muscle sarcoma arising from the myometrium) may not be detected until the enlarged uterus is surgically removed. The clinical and surgical staging of uterine sarcomas is similar to that of endometrial adenocarcinoma (Tables 27-1 and 27-2).

Histology

Uterine sarcomas are a family of uterine malignancies of varying histologic appearance. Because they can represent myriad cell types and combinations, the classification is often confused. A simple approach to uterine sarcomas subdivides these tumors into those of the single-cell type (*pure sarcomas*) and those of two or more cell types (*mixed sarcomas*). Mixed sarcomas may be subdivided into those containing elements found in the uterus (*homologous mixed müllerian tumors*) and those containing one or more elements not found in the uterus (*heterologous mixed müllerian tumors*). The most common types of pure uterine sarcoma are *leiomyosarcoma* and *endometrial stromal sarcoma*. Mixed homologous müllerian tumors, called *carcinosarcomas* in the older literature, represent a mixture of adenocarcinoma elements combined with other sarcomatous elements in the same tumor. Heterologous mixed tumors may contain elements such as rhabdomyosarcoma, chondrosarcoma,

osteosarcoma, or any other sarcomatous tissue not found in the uterus. For a leiomyosarcoma, the prognosis is clearly tied to mitotic count and tumor anaplasia. More than ten mitoses per ten high-power microscopic fields augers a poor prognosis even for Stage I lesions.

Spread Patterns and Treatment

Uterine sarcomas are virulent tumors that appear to metastasize early in their course. In contrast to endometrial adenocarcinoma, they have a much higher propensity to metastasize hematogenously. Lungs, liver, and bony metastases are found with reasonable frequency. Intraperitoneal metastases to the omentum and bowel are not uncommon. Uterine sarcomas can also metastasize to pelvic lymph nodes and invade locally through the wall of the uterus and to adjacent pelvic organs. The staging system for uterine sarcomas is the same as that for endometrial carcinoma.

Treatment

Treatment of uterine sarcomas is based on surgical excision. To date, preoperative or postoperative radiation therapy or adjunctive chemotherapy has been of little value. Total abdominal hysterectomy with bilateral salpingo-oophorectomy appears to be the only treatment modality that can effect cure with some consistency. Nonetheless, the overall survival for patients with Stage I uterine sarcoma is only approximately 50 percent. Postoperative radiation therapy may be of some benefit in preventing pelvic recurrences, although data from retrospective studies suggest that it does not improve overall survival. It is even more frustrating to realize that systemic chemotherapy, to date, has had little impact as the primary or secondary treatment of uterine sarcomas. The combination of adriamycin/cisplatin/cyclophosphamide has been reported to have some effect on advanced sarcomas, especially the mixed müllerian tumors. Methotrexate, DTIC, dactinomycin, ifosfamide, and VP-16 (etoposide) all have limited activity against uterine sarcomas, although complete responses are exceedingly rare. Active research is under way to evaluate new systemic chemotherapeutic agents in hopes of achieving improved survival of patients with this disease.

SELECTED READINGS

Anderson, B. Diagnosis of endometrial cancer. *Clin. Obstet. Gynecol.* 13:739, 1986.

Antunes, C. M., Strolley, P. D., and Rosenshein, N. B. Endometrial cancer and estrogen use (report of a large case-control study). *N. Engl. J. Med.* 300:9, 1979.

Berchuck, A., Rubin, S. C., Hoskins, W. J., et al. Treatment of uterine leiomyosarcoma. *Obstet. Gynecol.* 71: 845, 1988.

Boronow, R. C., Morrow, C. P., Creasman, W. T., et al. Surgical staging in endometrial cancer: clinical pathologic findings of a prospective study. *Obstet. Gynecol.* 63:825, 1985.

Bruchner, H. W., and Deppe, G. Combination chemotherapy of advanced endometrial adenocarcinoma and adriamycin, cyclophosphamide, 5-fluorouracil, and medroxyprogesterone acetate. *Obstet. Gynecol.* 50:105, 1977.

Christopherson, W. N., Alberhasky, R. C., and Connely, P. J. Carcinoma of the endometrium. II. Papillary adenocarcinoma: a clinico-pathological study of 46 patients. *Am. J. Clin. Pathol.* 77:534, 1982.

Creasman, W. T., DiSaia, P. J., and Blessing, J. Prognostic significance of peritoneal cytology in patients with endometrial cancer and preliminary data concerning therapy with intraperitoneal radiopharmaceuticals. *Am. J. Obstet. Gynecol.* 141:921, 1981.

Creasman, W. T., Morrow, C. P., and Bundy, L. Surgical pathological spread patterns of endometrial cancer. *Cancer* 60:2035, 1987.

Creasman, W. T., Soper, J. R., McCarty, K. S., Jr., et al. Influence of cytoplasmic steroid receptor content on prognosis of early stage endometrial carcinoma. *Am. J. Obstet. Gynecol.* 151:922, 1985.

Dinh, T. V., and Woodruff, J. D. Leiomyosarcoma of the uterus. *Am. J. Obstet. Gynecol.* 144:817, 1982.

DiSaia, P. J., Creasman, W. T., Boronow, R. C., et al. Risk factors and recurrence patterns in stage I endometrial cancer. *Am. J. Obstet. Gynecol.* 151:1009, 1985.

Frauenhoffer, E. E., Zaino, R. J., Wolff, T. V., et al. Value of endocervical curettage in the staging of endometrial carcinoma. *Int. J. Gynecol. Pathol.* 6:195, 1987.

Hendrickson, M., Ross, J., Eifel, P. J., et al. Adenocarcinoma of the endometrium: analysis of 256 cases of carcinoma limited to the uterine corpus: pathology review and analysis of prognostic variables. *Gynecol. Oncol.* 13:373, 1982.

Heyman, J. The so-called Stockholm method and the results of treatment of uterine cancer at the radiumhemmet. *Acta Radiol. (Stockh.)* 16:129, 1935.

Hricak, H., Stern, J. L., Fisher, M. R., et al. Endometrial carcinoma staging by MR imaging. *Radiology* 162:297, 1987.

Jones, H. W. Treatment of adenocarcinoma of the endometrium. *Obstet. Gynecol. Surv.* 30:147, 1975.

Kempson, R. L., and Bari, W. Uterine sarcomas: classification, diagnosis, and prognosis. *Hum. Pathol.* 1:331, 1970.

Meredith, R. F., Eisert, D. R., Kaka, Z., et al. An excess of uterine sarcomas after pelvic irradiation. *Cancer* 58:2003, 1986.

Norris, H. F., and Taylor, H. B. Mesenchymal tumors of the uterus. I. A clinical and pathological study of 53 endometrial stromal tumors. *Cancer* 19:755, 1966.

Onsrud, M., Kolstad, P., and Normann, T. Postoperative external pelvic irradiation in carcinoma of the corpus stage I: a controlled clinical trial. *Gynecol. Oncol.* 4: 222, 1976.

Perez, C. A., Askin, F., Baslan, R. J., et al. Effects of irradiation on mixed müllerian tumors of the uterus. *Cancer* 43:1274, 1979.

Peters, W. A., Kumar, N. B., and Fleming, W. P. Prognostic features of sarcomas and mixed tumors of the endometrium. *Obstet. Gynecol.* 63:550, 1984.

Salazar, O. M., Bonfislio, T. A., Patten, S. F., et al. Uterine sarcomas: natural history, treatment and prognosis. *Cancer* 42:1152, 1978.

Soper, J. T., Creasman, W. T., Clarke-Pearson, D. L., et al. Intraperitoneal chromic phosphate P^{32} suspension therapy of malignant peritoneal cytology in endometrial carcinoma. *Am. J. Obstet. Gynecol.* 153:191, 1985.

Sutton, G. O., Brill, L., Michael, H., et al. Malignant papillary lesions of the endometrium. *Gynecol. Oncol.* 27:294, 1987.

Varia, M., Rosenman, J., Halle, J., et al. Primary radiation therapy for medically inoperable patients with endometrial carcinoma: stages I–II. *Int. J. Radiat. Biol. Phys.* 13:11, 1987.

28

Ovarian and Fallopian Tubal Cancer

OVARIAN CANCER

Ovarian cancer is the leading cause of death from gynecologic malignancy and the fifth leading cause of cancer mortality in American women. About 19,000 new cases of ovarian cancer are diagnosed annually in the United States, and approximately 11,000 women die from the disease. One of seventy newborn female infants ultimately develops ovarian cancer, with the probability rising in women over the age of 40 to approximately 1 in 10.

Unfortunately, ovarian cancer is often detected only when it has spread widely throughout the abdominal cavity. Despite aggressive surgical resection and improved chemotherapy, most patients ultimately die from malnutrition and small bowel obstruction caused by intraperitoneal tumor burden. There has been no significant change in survival over the past five decades, which is most likely due to the lack of any means for early detection of ovarian cancer.

Ovarian cancer is actually several different malignancies arising from the ovary (Table 28-1). These cancers have different characteristics, treatments, and survival rates and therefore are addressed under separate headings in this chapter. Epithelial ovarian cancer, arising from the germinal epithelium of the ovary, comprises nearly 80 percent of the ovarian cancer treated today. Other malignancies of the ovary include those of germ cell origin, stromal and sex cord tumors, mesenchymal tumors of the ovary, and cancer metastatic to the ovary from another primary site. The age at onset varies for different tumors, as does the overall incidence. Epithelial ovarian cancer is primarily a disease of women over age 35. On the other hand, germ cell cancers of the ovary occur predominantly during childhood and the adolescent years.

Gonadal, stromal, and sex cord tumors and mesenchymal malignancies are relatively infrequent and can occur throughout a woman's lifetime.

Etiology

The epidemiology and etiology of the ovarian cancers are poorly understood, particularly for germ cell, mesenchymal, and stromal sex cord tumors. The primary etiology of epithelial ovarian cancer is thought to be linked to ovulation. This hypothesis is supported by several facts, including the recognition that epithelial ovarian carcinoma is rarely found in prepubertal girls or during early reproductive life. Furthermore, the risk of developing epithelial ovarian carcinoma is increased in nulliparous women and diminished in women who have had two or more pregnancies.

The suppression of ovulation during pregnancy and lactation appears to be an important preventive characteristic. Evidence has shown that women who have used oral contraceptives (and therefore have had prolonged periods of suppression of ovulation) are also at approximately one-half the risk to develop ovarian cancer compared with women who have never used oral contraceptives.

Other investigators have proposed that a carcinogen in the peritoneal cavity may lead to the malignant transformation of ovarian epithelium. Case-control studies have shown that women who use talcum powder as part of their perineal hygiene are at increased risk to develop ovarian carcinoma. The malignant transformation of the peritoneum in women has been likened histologically to the mesothelioma of the pleural cavity that results from asbestos exposure. Other environmental factors may play a role in the etiology of ovarian cancer, as the incidence of ovarian cancer appears to be higher in all industrialized countries except Japan, where its incidence is one of the lowest in the world. It is of interest to note that as Japanese women move to the United States their incidence of ovarian carcinoma increases to eventually approach that of the United States Caucasian population. Other environmental, dietary, or personal customs contributing to an increased incidence of ovarian cancer in industrialized countries are unknown.

A viral etiology of ovarian cancer has also been

Table 28-1. Histologic Classification of Ovarian Cancers

Epithelial ovarian carcinoma
    Serous cystadenocarcinoma
    Mucinous cystadenocarcinoma
    Endometrioid cystadenocarcinoma
    Mesonephroid carcinoma (clear cell)
    Brenner tumor
    Undifferentiated carcinoma
Germ cell ovarian carcinoma
    Dysgerminoma
    Immature teratoma
    Endodermal sinus tumor
    Choriocarcinoma
    Embryonal carcinoma
    Polyembryoma
    Gonadoblastoma
Malignancies of gonadal stroma
    Granulosa cell cancer
    Arrhenoblastoma
    Sertoli tumor
    Gynandroblastoma
    Lipid cell tumors
Malignancy of nonspecific mesenchyme
    Sarcoma
    Lymphoma
Metastatic to ovary
    Colorectal carcinoma
    Breast carcinoma
    Endometrial carcinoma
    Lymphoma

suggested, with mumps virus a leading contender; but to date this hypothesis remains speculative. Finally, a genetic basis for ovarian cancer has been noted in isolated reports of families in which two or three generations of women have developed ovarian cancer.

Clearly, with only these shreds of epidemiologic and etiologic evidence, much work needs to be done to further define the cause of ovarian cancer. The hope is to identify factors that may be eliminated from our environment and to recognize women who are at high risk to develop ovarian cancer, thereby affording them more careful surveillance or prophylaxis.

Diagnosis

The definitive diagnosis of ovarian cancer is based on the results of surgical exploration and pathologic review. In most cases the patient has been found to have a pelvic or abdominal mass and occasionally ascites. As discussed in Chapter 18, any woman with a pelvic mass must be considered to possibly have ovarian cancer. The evaluation and a decision to proceed with surgery has been outlined in Chapter 18. Only with prompt surgical exploration can ovarian cancer be diagnosed early, thereby reversing the current situation where most epithelial ovarian cancers are diagnosed only when the disease is disseminated throughout the peritoneal cavity.

The symptoms of epithelial ovarian cancer are often vague and nonspecific. Close questioning of patients with ovarian cancer reveals that many have had months of gastrointestinal symptoms, including belching, early satiety, abdominal fullness, or dyspepsia. Abdominal pain and pressure may have been noted to be transient. As the disease progresses, symptoms become more specific and constant, related to pain and pressure caused by an enlarging pelvic abdominal mass or increased abdominal girth secondary to intraperitoneal tumor or ascites. Uterine bleeding is occasionally noted. Children and adolescents who develop germ cell ovarian cancers are often found to have an abdominal mass that appears to be rapidly expanding. The acute pain caused by torsion or hemorrhage into the ovarian tumor are infrequent presenting symptoms.

Key to the diagnosis of ovarian cancer is a high index of suspicion in patients with these vague symptoms, combined with careful abdominal and pelvic examination. At the present time, the mainstay to the diagnosis of ovarian cancer is finding an adnexal mass on bimanual and rectovaginal examination. Of special note is the postmenopausal patient who has a palpable ovary. The ovary during the menstrual years is approximately 2.5×3.5 cm and is frequently palpated on routine pelvic examination. Within the first year or two of the onset of menopause, ovarian atrophy ensues and the size of the ovary gradually shrinks to approximately 1.5×2.0 cm. This small postmenopausal ovary is nearly impossible to palpate, even in a relaxed, cooperative, slender patient. An ovary that can be palpated in a postmenopausal patient therefore must be considered enlarged and abnormal, warranting further investigation including surgical exploration, removal, and histologic study. Further evaluation of a pelvic mass with ultrasonography or computed tomography (CT) is of little benefit.

If the pelvic mass is of clinical significance and warrants surgical exploration, the surgeon must always be prepared to manage ovarian cancer. Therefore radiographic findings suggesting the mass to be solid or of mixed solid or cystic components, bilateral masses, or associated with ascites are of little assistance to the surgeon or the patient. If the surgeon is unsure as to the management of a suspicious or unsuspected ovarian cancer, the patient should be immediately referred to a gynecologic oncologist capable of managing the patient appropriately.

The identification of an ovarian carcinoma-associated antigen (CA-125) has been introduced into our diagnostic armamentarium. CA-125 appears to be elevated in approximately 80 percent of patients with nonmucinous epithelial ovarian cancers. Unfortunately, this antigen is also elevated in patients with other malignancies and with such benign conditions as endometriosis, pregnancy, and pelvic inflammatory disease. Nonetheless, a CA-125 assay may provide some guidance as to whether an adnexal mass is of benign or malignant nature. Studies to date suggest that more than 80 percent of menopausal women with an adnexal mass who also have an elevated CA-125 level are found to have ovarian malignancy. On the other hand, fewer than 10 percent of patients with a normal CA-125 level and an adnexal mass are found to have ovarian cancer. With the rapid development of immunodiagnostic techniques, it is hoped that in the near future a diagnostic serum marker(s) will be found to more specifically identify ovarian cancer and possibly diagnose ovarian cancer at an early stage. Germ cell tumors (especially endodermal sinus tumors) and ovarian choriocarcinoma frequently secrete specific tumor markers: α-fetoprotein and human chorionic gonadotropin (hCG), respectively. In patients who are in the age group to have an ovarian germ cell tumor, assays for these markers should be performed preoperatively.

Preoperative Evaluation

The workup of a woman with suspected ovarian cancer should be aimed at a general assessment of medical status as well as an evaluation of other potential causes for an abdominal pelvic mass or ascites (Chap. 18). Plain abdominal radiographs may identify calcifications more often associated with uterine myomas or rudimentary teeth associated with benign cystic teratomas (dermoid). Papillary serous cystadenocarcinomas may contain psammoma bodies, which appear on radiographs as calcified flecks. An intravenous pyelogram is of value for identifying obstruction and deviation of the ureters due to a pelvic mass or disease metastatic to pelvic or paraaortic lymph nodes. A barium enema should also be performed and may detect extrinsic compressions, obstruction, or a primary carcinoma of the colon that may be metastatic to the ovary. An upper gastrointestinal series with small bowel follow-through is usuallly reserved for patients with upper gastrointestinal symptoms and need not be part of a routine workup.

Paracentesis is to be discouraged. Ascites from other causes such as congestive heart failure, liver failure, or pancreatitis may be excluded in nearly all cases based on a general medical evaluation. It should be noted that despite the presence of ascites, cytologic evaluation of the ascitic fluid may be negative in 50 percent of patients with ovarian carcinoma, and therefore a negative paracentesis must not delay exploratory surgery. Similarly, Meigs' syndrome must be managed by surgical removal of the benign ovarian neoplasm. Paracentesis therefore is of no value for determining the need for surgery. Most important, however, is the occasional patient who has a large encapsulated ovarian cyst that might be ruptured by the paracentesis trocar, thus worsening the patient's cancer prognosis or causing pseudomyoma peritonei. Metastatic carcinoma may also be seeded into the paracentesis tract. Because the diagnosis of ovarian cancer ultimately rests on exploratory laparotomy, we have found no value in carrying out preoperative paracentesis except in the rare patient with such respiratory compromise that, to safely induce anesthesia, several liters of ascitic fluid must be removed.

Preoperative preparation should include the usual medical assessment and correction of any underlying medical problems to optimize intraoperative and postoperative recovery. In particular, the patient with suspected ovarian carcinoma should undergo a mechanical bowel preparation prior to surgery. If colonic resection or colostomy is anticipated, antibiotic bowel preparation with neomycin and erythromycin is recommended. In patients with pleural effusion, thoracentesis should be carried out not only for diagnosis and staging but also to optimize respiratory function intraoperatively and postoperatively. Some patients reaccumulate a pleural effusion rapidly, and placement of a chest tube preoperatively may be necessary. Patients with intermittent or a complete small bowel obstruction benefit from a long intestinal tube placed preoperatively for decompression. Finally, many patients are nutritionally depleted, and consideration should be given to the use of total parenteral nutrition preoperatively and postoperatively.

Spread Patterns of Epithelial Ovarian Cancer

The natural history of ovarian carcinoma initially is direct capsular extension of the tumor leading to seeding of tumor into the peritoneal cavity (Fig. 28-1). Bilateral ovarian involvement is common even in early stage disease. Implants of tumor may cover peritoneal surfaces on the adjacent pelvic viscera and the peritoneum and then spread by flow of the peritoneal fluid along the pericolic gutters and to the leaves of the diaphragm. The diaphragm and omentum, with their rich lymphatic channels exiting from the peritoneal cavity, are often prime sites for metastatic disease. Ovarian cancer also may metastasize through retroperitoneal lymphatics and in particular along the ovarian vessels with direct metastases to the paraaortic lymph nodes at the level of the renal vessels. Pelvic lymph nodes may also be involved through collateral lymphatic flow from the uterus and cervix. In more advanced cases, malignant pleural effusion or metastasis to the parenchyma of the liver is found.

Staging Criteria

The staging of ovarian carcinoma is based on the findings at the time of surgery and pathologic review.

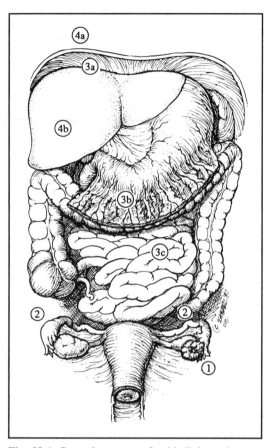

Fig. 28-1. Spread patterns of epithelial ovarian cancer. Once ovarian carcinoma penetrates the ovarian capsule (1) the malignancy has direct access to the remainder of the peritoneal cavity. Implants may be found on the pelvic viscera and peritoneum (2) or anywhere else in the peritoneal cavity. Common sites of metastases include the diaphragm and liver capsule (3a), the omentum (3b), and other peritoneal surfaces of the bowel serosa and mesentery (3c). Lymphatic drainage to the paraaortic lymph node chain along the ovarian vessels is also common (not shown). In more advanced cases there may be malignant effusions in the pleura (4a), as seen on a chest radiograph, or in the liver parenchyma (4b).

Because of the clinically occult nature of spread, surgical exploration is mandatory. It is therefore imperative for the surgeon to be familiar with the staging criteria so that an accurate and adequate operative procedure clearly defines the stage of disease. Ultimately, accurate staging is of utmost importance for the patient's further therapy and for discussing prognosis. The staging classification shown in Table 28-2 reflects the natural history of ovarian carcinoma as well as many of the prognostic factors important to overall survival.

Surgery for Ovarian Cancer: Staging and Tumor Resection

With knowledge of the natural history and staging of ovarian carcinoma, a systematic operative procedure should be undertaken. There are two goals of the operative procedure: (1) accurate staging and (2) removal of as much tumor as is technically and prudently possible (*cytoreduction*).

The abdomen should be opened through a midline or paramedian incision, which affords the opportunity to extend the incision to the xiphoid if necessary for exploration or tumor resection in the upper abdomen. With the potential for early upper abdominal spread, a low transverse incision that does not allow adequate upper abdominal evaluation and surgery must be condemned. Should the surgeon have entered the abdomen through a small transverse incision (e.g., in a young woman who was strongly suspected of having a benign neoplasm) accommodation must be made with an extended J incision or a new vertical incision so that the patient may benefit from an adequate operative procedure.

Upon entry into the peritoneal cavity, ascitic fluid is aspirated. If no ascites is present, 50 to 100 ml of saline is instilled and aspirated separately from the pelvis, pericolic gutters, and diaphragm. The ascitic or aspirated fluid is submitted for cytologic evaluation. All peritoneal surfaces are inspected and palpated, including both leaves of the diaphragm, the liver, omentum, and pericolic gutters. The large and small bowels are inspected in their entirety including the root of the mesentery. The pelvis is evaluated including the anterior and posterior cul-de-sac and the ovaries and uterus.

Table 28-2. FIGO Staging for Primary Carcinoma of the Ovary

Stage I: Growth limited to the ovaries.
Stage Ia: Growth limited to one ovary; no ascites. No tumor on the external surface; capsule intact.
Stage Ib: Growth limited to both ovaries; no ascites. No tumor on external surfaces; capsules intact.
Stage Ic: Tumor either Stage Ia or Ib but with tumor on surface of one or both ovaries; or with capsule ruptured; or with ascites present containing malignant cells or with positive peritoneal washings.

Stage II: Growth involving one or both ovaries with pelvic extension.
Stage IIa: Extension and/or metastases to the uterus and/or tubes.
Stage IIb: Extension to other pelvic tissues.
Stage IIc: Tumor either Stage IIa or IIb but with tumor on surface of one or both ovaries; or with capsule(s) ruptured; or with ascites present containing malignant cells or with positive peritoneal washings.

Stage III: Tumor involving one or both ovaries with peritoneal implants outside the pelvis and/or positive retroperitoneal or inguinal nodes. Superficial liver metastasis equals Stage III. Tumor is limited to the true pelvis but with histologically proved malignant extension to small bowel or omentum.
Stage IIIa: Tumor grossly limited to the true pelvis with negative nodes but with histologically confirmed microscopic seeding of abdominal peritoneal surfaces.
Stage IIIb: Tumor of one or both ovaries with histologically confirmed implants of abdominal peritoneal surfaces, none exceeding 2 cm in diameter. Nodes are negative.
Stage IIIc: Abdominal implants more than 2 cm in diameter and/or positive retroperitoneal or inguinal nodes.

Stage IV: Growth involving one or both ovaries, with distant metastases. If pleural effusion is present, there must be positive cytology to allot a case to Stage IV. Parenchymal liver metastases equal Stage IV.

In cases apparently confined to one or both ovaries, efforts are made to detect occult peritoneal metastasis with peritoneal cytology, biopsies of peritoneum from the pericolic gutters and diaphragm, and resection of the greater omentum. Additionally, selective pelvic and paraaortic lymphadenectomy to evaluate potential retroperitoneal spread is carried out at this operation. In one study of patients initially thought to have Stage I or II disease, reexploration found that occult disease resided in the retroperitoneal nodes in approximately 10 percent of patients, 15 percent of patients had occult metastasis in the omentum, and 10 percent of patients had microscopic disease on the diaphragm. Any of these findings would advance the disease to Stage III.

Specific comments relevant to the diagnosis and treatment of the individual ovarian cancer groups are detailed in the following sections.

Clinical Management of Epithelial Ovarian Carcinoma

The clinical management of the patient with ovarian carcinoma may be divided into the surgical aspects of the patient's care and adjunctive therapy. The two goals of surgical intervention are (1) accurate surgical staging and (2) tumor resection. Adjunctive therapy is required for most patients to improve their chances of survival and provide effective palliation. The choices of adjunctive therapy in large part depend on the surgical stage of the disease as well as the amount and location of residual disease. The management of ovarian carcinoma may also be divided into the management of patients with early stage disease and that for most other patients, who have advanced-stage of disease.

Early Stage Ovarian Carcinoma. The patient with early stage ovarian carcinoma most often has a relatively asymptomatic pelvic or adnexal mass. Frequently, ovarian carcinoma is not the leading preoperative diagnosis, and therefore ovarian carcinoma is somewhat of a surprise to the surgeon. Because of these circumstances, all surgeons who operate on women with an undiagnosed pelvic mass should have

the knowledge and skills capable of providing optimal surgical care for the patient with early ovarian cancer. The skills, simply stated, include the ability to perform strict surgical staging procedures and resect as much disease as is technically feasible. In the case of patients with Stage I or II ovarian carcinoma, it should be a rare patient in whom not all of the gross disease is completely resected.

The surgical staging of early ovarian carcinoma must include the factors listed in Table 28-2. The surgical procedure outlined for thorough staging of early ovarian carcinoma is rarely accomplished in practice today. This circumstance is unfortunate and leaves the physician with inadequate information for prognosis and for correctly selecting adjuvant therapy. This state of affairs is most likely due to the fact that most gynecologists and general surgeons are not aware of the surgical procedures required (e.g., paraaortic lymphadenectomy) or are unable to perform them.

Surgical resection of early stage ovarian carcinoma should not be difficult. It is usually accomplished by performing a total abdominal hysterectomy and bilateral salpingo-oophorectomy. Patients with Stage II disease (spread to pelvic peritoneum) should also have all tumor resected, although it may require additional care to protect the ureter, bladder, or rectum as the peritoneal implants are excised. Patients with grossly apparent Stage II disease should be thoroughly explored using multiple upper abdominal and omental biopsies to exclude the possibility of upper abdominal spread. In most cases, occult metastases have spread to the upper abdomen and can be documented if the surgeon's exploration is thorough.

Prior to the era of adjuvant therapy, surgery alone for patients with Stage I ovarian carcinoma resulted in approximately 50 to 60 percent five-year survival. Of the patients whose disease recurred, most of the lesions were in the peritoneal cavity or in the retroperitoneal lymph nodes. Based on this information, it became clear that despite the fact that the surgical procedure resected all apparent disease, in actuality microscopic disease or tumor cells had already spread beyond the ovary (or pelvis) and had seeded the peritoneal cavity or lymph nodes with occult lesions. For this reason, additional postoperative therapy has been tried and investigated in hopes of improving survival. Today the overall survival for patients with Stage I ovarian carcinoma is in the range of 85 to 90 percent with appropriate surgical staging and adjuvant therapy.

Surgical staging and therapy alone are adequate for a select subgroup of patients with early stage ovarian cancer. Specifically, those patients with Stage Ia ovarian carcinoma who have either a low malignant potential tumor or a tumor that is well differentiated (grade 1) have an excellent prognosis with surgery alone (95 to 100 percent long-term survival) and therefore do not benefit from adjuvant therapy. In fact, in this setting, if a woman wishes to retain the other normal ovary and uterus for reproductive function, it should be allowed. Because it is sometimes difficult to ascertain the grade of disease at the time of initial surgical exploration, the surgeon operating on a woman of reproductive age should ascertain preoperatively if further reproductive capability is desired and if so respect the patient's wishes until all pathology has been thoroughly reviewed. To make an intraoperative decision based on frozen section histology may unnecessarily castrate a patient who might have preserved fertility and at the same time had an excellent prognosis. In general, the surgeon should be conservative and await final pathology reports. If the reports show a higher grade tumor or metastases to extraovarian sites, a second operation may be necessary to more thoroughly stage the patient and remove the other ovary and uterus.

With all other cases of early ovarian carcinoma, survival is compromised if surgery alone is performed. Adjunctive therapy has been investigated intensely in this setting. Prior to the era of chemotherapy, external beam radiation therapy was used in an attempt to sterilize residual tumor cells in the pelvis. Whole-pelvis irradiation is usually well tolerated and may be delivered effectively beginning a few weeks after surgical staging and resection. Unfortunately, whole-pelvis irradiation is of no benefit to the patient with early stage ovarian cancer. Randomized trials have shown that patients undergoing whole-pelvis irradiation have no better long-term survival than patients who have surgery alone. The reason for this finding is clear: Ovarian cancer is not a locally pro-

gressive disease that can be encompassed in a pelvic field. The basic principle to be remembered is that epithelial ovarian cancer spreads throughout the peritoneal cavity, and therefore the entire peritoneal cavity is at risk for metastases. Others have attempted to irradiate the whole abdomen so as to cover all peritoneal surfaces with an effective radiation dose. Although this method may seem to have some theoretical justification, problems are encountered when one attempts to irradiate the upper abdomen, particularly because the upper abdominal organs (especially the liver and kidneys) do not tolerate tumoricidal doses of radiation. It has therefore been necessary when irradiating the abdomen to place lead shields over the liver and kidneys to protect them. However, the lead shields also protect peritoneal surfaces and the diaphragm, which are at high risk to harbor occult metastases. Additionally, whole-abdomen radiation therapy irradiates all of the small intestines and colon as well as the stomach and is associated with high morbidity and injury to normal organs.

Historically, chemotherapy became available after the use of radiation therapy had become established and was investigated for the treatment of ovarian cancer. Alkylating agents in particular (melphalan, chlorambucil, and cyclophosphamide) have been found to have activity against epithelial ovarian cancer and could offer significant palliation and an occasional cure of patients with advanced ovarian cancer. Clinical studies have evaluated the activity of these active agents for reducing recurrence after surgical removal of early stage ovarian cancer. In most studies, clear benefit was noted when an alkylating agent was given to the patient for 12 to 18 months after surgical resection. In this group of patients, 85 to 90 percent five-year survival was reported by many investigators. Alkylating agent (especially melphalan) therapy is relatively easy to administer and has minimal acute toxicity. Unfortunately, the long-term side effects of alkylating chemotherapy include the development of leukemia in approximately 5 percent of patients, and this second malignancy is often fatal. The occurrence of leukemia after alkylating therapy is directly dependent on the total dose of the alkylating agent and the duration of its administration. More recently, other chemotherapeutic agents, e.g., cis-platin and adriamycin, have been shown to have activity against ovarian carcinoma. To date, however, these agents have not been investigated for treatment of patients with early stage ovarian cancer.

Another approach to the treatment of ovarian cancer is the use of intraperitoneal radiocolloids. Theoretically, the intraperitoneal administration of a radiocolloid (e.g., chromic phosphate, or ^{32}P) "coats" the peritoneal surfaces and delivers radiation therapy to microscopic tumor or tumor cell clusters on peritoneal surfaces. Dosimetry studies of ^{32}P show that its effective dose penetrates only about 2 mm. On peritoneal surfaces, a standard dose of ^{32}P delivers approximately 7000 rads, which is clearly tumoricidal. Moreover, because of its low tissue penetration, it does not appear to significantly injure bowel, liver, or other abdominal organs. ^{32}P does not penetrate retroperitoneal lymph nodes or tumor nodules. Therefore the role of ^{32}P might lie in the setting of early stage ovarian cancer where there is no gross residual disease and no metastases to lymph nodes. Alkylating chemotherapy (melphalan) has been compared in a randomized trial with the intraperitoneal administration of ^{32}P in patients with early stage ovarian carcinoma. This trial demonstrated that both treatments offered a higher survival rate than surgery alone; and in fact, both afforded approximately 90 percent survival for patients with Stage I ovarian cancer. Because of the low risk of complications from intraperitoneal ^{32}P, the therapeutic index suggests that ^{32}P is the better therapy for patients with early stage ovarian cancer.

Ovarian Tumors of Low Malignant Potential. There is a group of epithelial ovarian cancers that histologically do not invade the ovarian cyst capsule or adjacent tissues, yet they do not act entirely benignly. Histologically, these tumors have been found to spread throughout the peritoneal cavity, appearing grossly identical to the more common epithelial ovarian cancers. Approximately 10 percent of all epithelial ovarian cancers may be classified as *tumors of low malignant potential (borderline ovarian carcinoma)*. Most of these borderline tumors are clinically Stage I and tend to occur in menstrual age women.

As noted previously, the tumors that are Stage Ia may be adequately managed by unilateral salpingo-oophorectomy. Surgical resection affords a nearly 100 percent survival for patients with Stage Ia epithelial ovarian cancer of borderline malignant potential. On the other hand, an occasional patient is found to have widespread intraperitoneal disease that appears grossly to be epithelial ovarian carcinoma. As many as 50 percent of patients with Stage III low malignant potential tumors ultimately succumb to their disease, running a prolonged clinical course but ultimately dying of intestinal obstruction. Responses to chemotherapy or radiation therapy are not well documented, and a definite treatment plan for patients with advanced low malignant potential tumors has not been established. At the present time, aggressive surgical resection may offer the patient the best opportunity for prolonged palliation and long-term survival. The addition of chemotherapeutic agents commonly used for the treatment of epithelial ovarian carcinoma seems reasonable, although response rates are not yet established.

Advanced Ovarian Cancer. Unfortunately, most patients with ovarian cancer have metastases to the upper abdomen or beyond at the time of initial diagnosis and surgical exploration. It will only be with new technologies for the early detection of ovarian cancer or identification of ways to prevent ovarian cancer that we will make a major impact on the stage at initial diagnosis. The advanced stage of most patients with ovarian cancer is probably the single most important determinant of long-term survival. Other prognostic features of advanced stage ovarian cancer include (1) the amount of residual disease at the completion of the surgical procedure, (2) the patient's age, (3) the patient's functional status, and (4) the response of tumor to adjunctive therapy.

The surgical management of advanced ovarian cancer is aimed at documenting the stage of disease (which is usually apparent) and aggressive tumor resection (cytoreductive surgery, or *debulking*). Surgical staging of advanced ovarian carcinoma includes the steps of the surgical procedure outlined in Table 28-3. The only modification of this procedure would be the lack of need for pelvic and paraaortic lymphadenectomy in the patient in whom gross disease will

Table 28-3. Surgical Procedures Required for Accurate Staging of Ovarian Carcinoma

1. Thorough intraabdominal exploration including inspection and palpation of all peritoneal, mesenteric, and serosal surfaces.
2. Careful exploration of the diaphragm with random biopsies.
3. Peritoneal washings (or aspiration of frank ascites). Washings should be obtained from the pelvis, pericolic gutters, and diaphragm.
4. Total abdominal hysterectomy and bilateral salpingo-oophorectomy (in selected cases, unilateral salpingo-oophorectomy may provide adequate therapy and staging).
5. Selective pelvic and paraaortic lymphadenectomy.
6. Omentectomy.
7. Random peritoneal biopsies from the pelvic peritoneum: cul-de-sac, pelvic side walls, anterior cul-de-sac, pericolic gutter biopsies.

be left at the completion of the surgical procedure. The addition of lymphadenectomy in this situation probably serves to increase morbidity and does not change the patient's stage or ultimate therapy.

The surgeon who operates on the patient with advanced ovarian cancer should have the skills and capabilities to perform aggressive surgical debulking. The value of debulking has been shown in nearly all retrospective studies. That is, the median as well as the long-term survival and response to multiagent chemotherapy are related inversely to the volume of residual disease at the completion of the surgical procedure. The diameter of residual tumor nodules is critically important. The term "optimal debulking" has entered discussions, although it is not clearly defined. In general, at the time of this writing, an "optimal" tumor nodule size is less than 1 cm in diameter. It is therefore important for the surgeon to attempt to resect as much tumor as possible and to leave the patient with the smallest tumor nodules as is technically feasible. When adopting this aggressive approach in the patient with advanced ovarian carcinoma, the surgeon must temper the surgical attack to avoid excessive morbidity or operative mortality. Surgical procedures that often significantly reduce tumor burden include omentectomy, intestinal resection,

total abdominal hysterectomy with bilateral salpingo-oophorectomy, and rectosigmoid resection. With the advent of intestinal stapling devices, most patients may have their tumor aggressively resected without incurring excessive morbidity. Intestinal resections with reanastomoses are easily accomplished, thereby avoiding colostomy or ileostomy in most cases. Not only does aggressive surgical resection put the patient into a position of benefiting maximally from adjunctive therapy, tumor resection provides significant palliation and relief of ascites and the pelvic pressure and pain due to an enlarging tumor mass.

Advanced ovarian carcinoma requires postoperative therapy in all cases with the hope of achieving an occasional cure and, more often, providing a lengthened median survival time. The overall survival of patients with Stage III ovarian carcinoma is only 15 percent. At the present time we do not have methods to determine or select which patient will benefit from adjunctive therapy. Therefore adjunctive therapy is offered and suggested for almost all patients with advanced ovarian carcinoma unless they are so medically infirm as to not be able to tolerate additional therapy.

Options for treatment of advanced ovarian carcinoma include (1) whole-abdomen radiation therapy, (2) intraperitoneal chromic phosphate (^{32}P), and (3) multiagent chemotherapy. Whole-abdomen radiation therapy and intraperitoneal ^{32}P may both be effective treatment for the patient with Stage III ovarian carcinoma who has had all gross disease resected. Because ^{32}P does not effectively irradiate the retroperitoneal lymph nodes, its use should be reserved for patients who had a lymphadenectomy that showed no evidence of metastases. Whole-abdomen radiation therapy is fraught with some of the same difficulties outlined previously in the treatment of early ovarian carcinoma. That is, effective doses to the upper abdomen are limited by the lack of tolerance of the liver, kidneys, and small bowel. A few randomized trials have shown that whole-abdomen irradiation may be effective in patients with minimal or no gross residual disease.

For most patients with advanced ovarian carcinoma, chemotherapy is the mainstay of postoperative care. Initially, alkylating agents such as melphalan and cyclophosphamide were used and were found to have reasonable activity and provided ascites control and tumor response in up to 40 percent of patients. The addition of more than one agent to the chemotherapeutic regimen came during the 1970s with the development of other chemotherapeutic agents that have activity against ovarian cancer. The most promising of these drugs, cis-platin, is now part of the standard chemotherapeutic regimen for ovarian cancer. Other drugs with activity include adriamycin, cyclophosphamide, hexamethylmelamine, and 5-fluorouracil.

Current standard therapy of ovarian carcinoma includes the administration of cis-platin, an alkylating agent (e.g., cyclophosphamide), and adriamycin. These drugs are administered intravenously and repeated at an every three- to four-week interval for approximately six months. Prior to each treatment the patient is reassessed with complete physical examination and pelvic examination with attention paid to any residual disease that can be measured (e.g., pelvic mass). The response to chemotherapy may also be semiquantitatively assessed by measuring the serum CA-125 level. So long as there is no evidence of progressive disease, chemotherapy is continued for at least six months. Should progressive disease be noted or severe toxicity be encountered, alternative therapies might be considered. Unfortunately, alternative therapies in terms of other chemotherapeutic agents are limited and in general provide no expectation of long-term cure or prolonged survival.

The multiagent regimen of cisplatin/cytoxan/ adriamycin has been found to achieve a significant increase in response rates compared with patients previously treated with alkylating chemotherapy. The definition of responses are outlined in Table 28-4. The *total response rate* is the number of patients demonstrating a partial response plus those with complete clinical response. It should be obvious that only patients who have a complete clinical response have any hope of prolonged survival and cure. Nonetheless, the increased complete response rate and the increased number of patients who are found to be free of disease at second-look laparotomy have encouraged gynecologic oncologists to pursue this course of therapy. Unfortunately, recurrences are high, and the overall five-

Table 28-4. Definitions of Criteria Used to Designate Response to Chemotherapy

Status	Definition
Complete response	Complete disappearance of all evidence of disease for at least 1 month.
Partial response	Reduction of the product of the greatest diameter of a lesion and its perpendicular by at least 50% for at least 1 month; these criteria must be exhibited by each measurable lesion.
Stable disease	Maintenance for each lesion of criteria less than those required for either a partial response or increasing disease.
Increasing disease	Increase of the product of the greatest diameter of a lesion and its perpendicular by at least 50% or the appearance of a new lesion within 1 month.

year survival rate has not been significantly affected by multiagent chemotherapy. In other words, patients are living an average of two years, which is probably 6 to 12 months longer than might have been expected with alkylating chemotherapy, yet they are dying of disease progression before they can be counted as five-year survivors. Clearly, new and better postoperative treatments for advanced ovarian carcinoma are required to change the poor survival rate currently achieved.

An alternative approach for delivery of chemotherapeutic agents is intraperitoneal administration. The basic premise on which this treatment is based is that a higher dose of chemotherapy may be delivered to the tumor yet at the same time systemic toxicity to the patient is minimized. This investigational technique has been shown to be effective for treating patients with advanced ovarian carcinoma, especially those with minimal residual disease. Whether intraperitoneal chemotherapy is more effective than intravenous chemotherapy has yet to be proved. Other strategies for the treatment of ovarian carcinoma with ultra high dose chemotherapy and autologous bone marrow transplant, immunotherapy, or immunotherapy conjugated with radioisotopes or toxins are investigational and warrant careful evaluation before being brought into standard clinical practice.

Second-Look Laparotomy. Many patients with ovarian carcinoma are rendered clinically free of disease at the completion of the initial surgical procedure, or their tumors have shrunk to a point where they cannot be detected clinically during chemotherapy. This situation occurs in up to 50 percent of patients with Stage III and Stage IV ovarian carcinoma.

For patients who have no measurable disease at the completion of a standard course of chemotherapy, certain questions arise that require answers: Does the patient have any remaining ovarian carcinoma? If not, can chemotherapy be safely discontinued? If the patient does have residual disease, is the amount less than was previously noted? (That is, has the chemotherapy regimen been partially effective?) If the patient has residual disease, where is it located and are there alternative treatments that might be employed? Could some or all of the residual disease be surgically resected, thereby affording the patient a slightly improved chance at longer survival and palliation? These questions should be asked prior to the administration of each course of chemotherapy; and they are definitively important issues at some later juncture, usually after six months of chemotherapy.

They may be answered in part by careful physical examination or radiographic examinations such as abdominopelvic CT scan. The serum CA-125 level may also indicate if tumor is present. However, physical examination, radiographic studies, and the CA-125 assay lack significant sensitivity and specificity for small volumes of ovarian carcinoma. In the setting where patients have a normal physical examination, normal CT scan, and normal CA-125 level, persistent ovarian carcinoma is seen in up to 50 percent of patients if they undergo surgical exploration. It is for this reason that second-look laparotomy has been advocated as a sensitive, specific diagnostic technique to ascertain the status of ovarian cancer after completion of a course of therapy.

The second-look laparotomy, then, is surgical reexploration to allow thorough reassessment of the status of a patient's ovarian cancer. To avoid a major surgical procedure, diagnostic laparoscopy has been used in many patients for initial assessment of tumor status. Because laparoscopy does not allow visualization of all peritoneal surfaces, however, it is of limited value. The value of laparoscopy is demonstrated in the patient who has obvious intraperitoneal implants that may be biopsied via the laparoscope. Thus in this situation the status of the disease is documented to be persistent, and continued therapy is usually advocated. For these patients, a full laparotomy may have been of no value. On the other hand, if laparoscopy is performed and no disease is found it is not adequate reassurance that no disease persists. In fact, when patients are surgically explored through a laparotomy incision, metastatic implants are detected in up to 50 percent of patients who had a negative laparoscopy. Exploratory laparotomy therefore is the "gold standard" for assessing the status of patients with ovarian cancer.

The possibility of having no evidence of disease is influenced greatly by the following factors: initial stage of disease, the size of residual tumor deposits at the completion of the initial operation, the histologic grade of the ovarian carcinoma, the number of courses of chemotherapy administered prior to second-look laparotomy, the clinical response to chemotherapy, and the completeness of second-look laparotomy. In patients who have no gross evidence of disease at laparotomy, a thorough "restaging" procedure should be performed that includes careful exploration of all peritoneal surfaces, biopsy of any suspicious nodules or adhesions, and random biopsies of pelvic, pericolic, and diaphragm peritoneum. Washings from the pelvis, pericolic gutters, and diaphragms are also obtained in a search for malignant cells floating in the peritoneal cavity. Biopsy specimens should also be obtained from any sites where ovarian carcinoma was known to reside at the completion of the first operation.

Decisions regarding further management in the patient who has had a complete clinical response and has undergone second-look laparotomy depend on the pathologic findings at second-look laparotomy. For patients who are fortunate enough to have an entirely normal second-look laparotomy, chemotherapy is usually discontinued and the patient followed with clinical examinations and CA-125 levels. Most of these patients remain free of recurrent disease and enjoy long-term survival. Unfortunately, a number of patients who have Stage III and Stage IV ovarian carcinoma and who ultimately achieve complete resolution of the disease as documented by second-look laparotomy ultimately have recurrences (up to 30 to 40 percent of patients). One of the most vexing problems to date is identifying the patient who will have a recurrence after a negative second-look laparotomy and, then, finding effecting therapy to prevent these recurrences.

For patients who have not had complete disease resolution at the time of second-look laparotomy, therapeutic choices are difficult. As previously noted, second-line chemotherapy for ovarian carcinoma is notoriously ineffective. In selected patients a variety of therapeutic choices are available that, in a few patients, provide a chance at prolonged remission. These choices range from whole-abdomen radiation therapy, to different chemotherapy, to chemotherapy administered in the peritoneal cavity, to intraperitoneal chromic phosphate, to experimental therapies. Because there is no clear-cut standard therapy, these therapy modalities should be individualized and may be guided significantly by the findings at second-look laparotomy.

Palliation of Ovarian Cancer. With only 15 percent of patients with Stage III ovarian carcinoma surviving five years and only 30 percent of all ovarian carcinomas achieving long-term survival, it is apparent that most patients with ovarian carcinoma succumb from their disease. The clinician caring for the patient with ovarian carcinoma must be capable therefore of managing the patient who will ultimately die of her disease and be skilled in offering effective palliation and supportive care for the terminally ill patient.

As ovarian carcinoma progresses, small bowel obstruction is the most common problem. Often progression of the ovarian carcinoma involving intestinal mesentery and serosa does not lead to complete intestinal obstruction, yet the patient has poor bowel function with decreased appetite, nausea and vomiting, and crampy abdominal pain. Progression of ascites may further distend the abdomen, causing increased intraabdominal pressure and decreased appetite. Attempts at palliation including frequent small feedings and the use of metoclopramide to improve intestinal motility. Gastric decompression by nasogastric tube or gastrostomy may offer some benefit to the patient who develops intractable nausea, vomiting, and abdominal distention. On rare occasion, exploratory laparotomy with attempts at intestinal bypass or resection to relieve intestinal obstruction may offer several more months of prolonged quality survival. These women form a select group of patients who must be considered seriously by the surgeon before performing a major surgical procedure during the last weeks or months of their lives.

Malignant effusions (ascites and pleural effusion) are frequently encountered in patients with advanced ovarian carcinoma resistant to adjuvant therapy. Progressive ascites leads to abdominal distention, intermittent bowel obstruction and ileus, abdominal pain and pressure, and elevation of the diaphragm. Many patients experience gradually increasing discomfort and respiratory compromise. Relief of this increasing pressure from the ascites can often be achieved by performing paracentesis and drawing off as much ascitic fluid as possible. In contrast to the patient with ascites associated with hepatic cirrhosis, massive fluid shifts and hypotension are not encountered when a large amount of ascites is removed from the patient with ovarian cancer. Therefore it is reasonably safe to remove as much fluid as possible and thereby achieve maximal palliation. The rate of reaccumulation of ascites varies. In some terminally ill patients ascitic fluid may need to be removed on a weekly basis, whereas others may enjoy several weeks of comfort before it reaccumulates. Instillation of a variety of chemotherapeutic agents occasionally offers some control of the ascites.

Malignant pleural effusion is also a problem in patients with advanced ovarian carcinoma. Respiratory compromise may be temporarily alleviated by thoracentesis. However, in most patients fluid reaccumulates rapidly, and respiratory embarrassment recurs. More definitive relief of the pleural effusion requires placement of a chest tube (tube thoracostomy) with drainage of the pleural effusion. Once the effusion is reduced to a volume of less than 200 ml per day, a variety of caustic agents may be instilled to sclerose the pleural space and prevent reaccumulation of the effusion. Tetracycline is the drug of choice for sclerosis of the pleura.

Overall, the goals of palliation of the ovarian cancer patient who has failed standard therapy are aimed at providing maximal comfort and quality of life. It is frustrating for the physician to stand by watching the patient slowly succumb to malnutrition from extensive intraperitoneal disease while she remains fully cognizant of her status.

Germ Cell Ovarian Tumors

Malignancies arising from the germ cells of the ovary are rare tumors most frequently encountered in young women. Germ cell tumors account for 15 to 20 percent of all ovarian neoplasms. The most common germ cell tumor is the dermoid cyst (benign teratoma), found most frequently in women in their reproductive years. This benign tumor is discussed in Chapter 18.

In young women the most common malignancy of the ovary is the ovarian germ cell tumor. In the past, these tumors were notoriously aggressive with rapid progression even after surgical resection of apparent Stage I disease, and for many patients the prognosis was grim. However, with the advent of multiagent chemotherapy, the prognosis has improved, and the disease should be nearly completely curable for patients with Stage I disease; this regimen also offers a reasonably high survival rate even for patients with advanced stage disease.

Tumors of the germ cell arising in the ovary may differentiate along several lines. A schema for germ cell tumor differentiation is shown in Figure 28-2. In decreasing order of frequency, ovarian germ cell tumors are the mature teratoma (dermoid cyst), dysgerminoma, endodermal sinus tumor, immature teratoma, embryonal carcinoma, choriocarcinoma, and polyembryoma. Careful pathologic study of germ cell tumors reveals that 10 to 15 percent are a mixture of more than one cell type.

Germ cell tumors are usually discovered in children or young women, with a median age of onset of 19 years. The usual presenting symptom is abdominal pain and distention from an apparently rapidly enlarg-

Fig. 28-2. Derivation of ovarian germ cell tumors. (Germ cell tumors may also be mixed—composed of any possible combination of germ cell elements.)

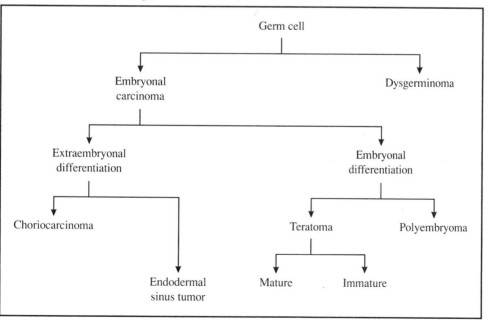

ing abdominal pelvic mass. The mass is occasionally associated with aberration of menstrual periods, and it may present as an acute abdomen due to ovarian tumor torsion. The surgeon operating on a young woman or child with an abdominal pelvic mass should be aware of the possibility of a germ cell tumor and its optimal management. In many cases the tumor is grossly confined to one ovary, and fertility may be conserved. Even though disease appears to be confined to one ovary (except for the pure dysgerminoma) adjuvant chemotherapy has clearly been demonstrated to improve long-term survival.

Dysgerminoma. The dysgerminoma is the most common malignant germ cell tumor of the ovary, comprising approximately 40 percent of all germ cell tumors reported. Histologically, this tumor appears similar to the seminoma in the male testes: It metastasizes in a similar fashion (to retroperitoneal lymph nodes) and is sensitive to radiation therapy. Ten to fifteen percent of dysgerminomas are found to have other malignant germ cell elements (mixed tumors) and should be treated as aggressive tumors.

Most dysgerminomas are found as a large abdominal pelvic mass and at surgical exploration appear to be confined to one ovary. Because of the young age of most of these patients, conservative surgical resection of the involved ovary and careful surgical staging are required. However, aggressive surgical resection of an apparently normal contralateral ovary and the uterus is not necessary to have a successful outcome. The contralateral ovary should be carefully inspected, as approximately 10 percent of patients have bilateral disease. However, bivalving or wedge biopsy of the contralateral ovary is not advocated, as it may reduce the patient's fertility potential and is rarely useful for detecting occult disease.

Human chorionic gonadotropin (hCG) is detected in the serum of some patients with dysgerminomas, likely secreted by the syncytiotrophoblast-like giant cells contained in many of these tumors. The hCG may serve as a tumor marker in these cases. On the other hand, patients with elevated serum α-fetoprotein are most likely to have a mixed germ cell tumor with endodermal sinus tumor elements. Lactate de-

hydrogenose may also be elevated in patients with dysgerminoma.

In general, dysgerminomas are large, gray-white, and lobulated with firm and soft areas within the solid tumor. The spread pattern of dysgerminoma tends to be predominantly in retroperitoneal lymph nodes, especially the paraaortic nodes. It seems that dysgerminomas are more likely than other germ cell tumors to spread to lymph nodes. The ovarian capsule may rupture, and spread may also occur through an intraperitoneal metastasis much like epithelial ovarian carcinoma.

Management of the dysgerminoma is slightly different from that of the other germ cell malignancies. For patients with Stage Ia disease no additional therapy is necessary. For patients who wish to maintain fertility, unilateral salpingo-oophorectomy provides adequate therapy. Patients with more advanced disease metastatic to lymph nodes may be treated with either radiation therapy or chemotherapy. For the patient with disease that has spread beyond the primary ovary but who does not have metastases in the contralateral ovary, conservative surgery preserving the contralateral ovary and uterus might still be considered. In this setting, multiagent chemotherapy should be initiated in hopes of preserving ovarian function. In the patient for whom fertility is no longer a concern, radiation therapy may be administered to the lymph node-bearing areas or the whole abdomen. Dysgerminomas are radiosensitive tumors with adequate therapy achieved at approximately 3000 rad. Dysgerminomas containing mixtures of other germ cell elements should be treated aggressively with multiagent chemotherapy as discussed under the general management for other germ cell tumors. Approximately 10 percent of patients with Stage IA dysgerminoma are found to have recurrent disease many years after their primary surgery. In most instances, surgical resection and treatment with either chemotherapy or radiation therapy can achieve secondary response and cures in most patients.

Teratomas. The most common germ cell neoplasm is the benign cystic teratoma (dermoid cyst). The management of these benign neoplasms is discussed in

Chapter 18. Approximately 1 to 2 percent of dermoid cysts ultimately develop a malignant focus. In most instances it is a squamous cell carcinoma, occurring most frequently in postmenopausal women. Rare malignancies arising in dermoid cysts include carcinoid, adenocarcinoma, sarcoma, melanoma, and thyroid carcinoma.

Immature teratomas are the second most frequent germ cell malignancy, accounting for approximately 20 percent of all malignant ovarian germ cell tumors. These tumors arise in young women of the same age group as the other germ cell tumors and may achieve a large size before being detected. These tumors tend to be solid and cystic in nature with bosselation of the surface. Grossly, areas of hemorrhage and necrosis are noted on cut section. Histologically, these tumors contain immature tissue normally found in the human embryo, most frequently neuroepithelium, glia, neuroblastoma, cartilage, and respiratory and gut epithelium. The malignant potential of these tumors, which is determined histologically, is inversely related to the degree of differentiation of the tumor.

Immature teratomas tend to achieve large size (up to 18 cm in diameter) and are often found as unilateral ovarian tumors. They spread beyond the ovary to peritoneal surfaces as well as the retroperitoneal lymph nodes. Careful histologic study may reveal that the immature teratoma has other germ cell elements in it. Pure immature teratomas may secrete α-fetoprotein from the glial cells, and it may be detected in the patient's serum and serve as a tumor marker. Immature teratomas that are histologically Grade II or III should be treated with multiagent chemotherapy after surgical resection (see discussion of the management of germ cell tumors, above). Intraperitoneal implants may dedifferentiate to mature elements after a course of chemotherapy. Most often, they are mature glial elements that may remain in the peritoneal cavity causing no particular symptoms and requiring no further therapy.

Endodermal Sinus Tumor. The endodermal sinus tumor is probably the most aggressive of the germ cell malignancies. Prior to the advent of multiagent chemotherapy, a 20 percent two-year survival rate was noted for patients with Stage I endodermal sinus tumors. Endodermal sinus tumors occur in children and young women (average age 20). Most are detected as clinical Stage I but often are ruptured at the time of surgical exploration. The spread pattern is similar to that of immature teratoma, with intraperitoneal metastases and metastases to retroperitoneal lymph nodes. Surgical staging should be complete, but it should conserve the contralateral ovary and uterus in patients with apparent Stage Ia disease. Histologically, the endodermal sinus tumor is similar to the endodermal sinus of Duval in the rodent placenta. Therefore these tumors have been termed yolk sac tumors by many authors. Endodermal sinus tumors often secrete α-fetoprotein, which may be detected in the serum of patients. Patients who have elevated serum hCG levels should be suspected of having a mixed germ cell tumor rather than a pure endodermal sinus tumor. Management of the endodermal sinus tumor is discussed more fully under general considerations of management of germ cell tumors.

Rare Germ Cell Tumors. Approximately 10 to 15 percent of germ cell tumors contain *mixed elements* of more than one distinctive germ cell tumor. The most frequent mixtures include dysgerminoma, immature teratomas, and endodermal sinus tumors. Because of these mixed elements, serum α-fetoprotein or hCG is elevated in many of these cases. The treatment and management of mixed germ cell tumors is similar to that of pure germ cell tumors, although their prognosis may be slightly worse.

Choriocarcinoma rising primarily as a germ cell tumor of the ovary is distinct from gestational trophoblastic disease. These primary tumors of the ovary are usually part of a mixed ovarian tumor, although some are pure choriocarcinoma. In contrast to gestational trophoblastic disease, which always secretes hCG, choriocarcinoma of the ovary is not nearly as consistent and the levels of hCG are not quite as reliable as a tumor marker. Treatment with surgical resection followed by multiagent chemotherapy is standard and similar to that for other germ cell ovarian carcinomas. Compared to gestational trophoblastic disease, primary ovarian choriocarcinoma appears to be more resistant to chemotherapy, and the prognosis is worse.

Embryonal ovarian carcinoma and *polyembryoma* are rare ovarian germ cell tumors, with approximately 20 cases reported in the world's literature. The clinical management of these tumors and the clinical characteristics are similar to those for other germ cell tumors.

Gonadoblastoma. The gonadoblastoma is a rare ovarian tumor usually found in genetically abnormal individuals with gonadal dysgenesis, nearly all of them with chromatin-negative nuclear patterns and virilization but with female internal genital tracts. The most common karyotype is 46,XY and 45,X/46,XY. One-fourth of these patients are phenotypically male, with many also having ambiguous external genitalia.

The gonadoblastoma is composed of mixed elements of both germ cells (dysgerminoma) combined with indifferent sex cord elements (immature granulosa, Sertoli, and Leydig cells). The tumors are usually small, and approximately one-third are bilateral. On abdominal radiograph the gonadoblastoma is frequently seen to be calcified. Although the gonadoblastoma itself is usually benign, it is often associated with malignant germ cell elements. Therefore surgical resection of the primary tumor as well as the contralateral ovary is advised. The malignant component of gonadoblastomas is the germ cell element, which is frequently dysgerminoma, though occasionally choriocarcinoma, embryonal carcinoma, or a mixture of germ cell elements may be apparent. Treatment of gonadoblastomas that have malignant germ cell elements is in general similar to that of other germ cell tumors.

Treatment. Prior to the advent of multiagent chemotherapy, patients with germ cell cancers had a dismal outlook. Even apparent Stage Ia disease frequently recurred after surgical resection. Attempts at radiation therapy (except for dysgerminoma) were futile, and the patients ultimately died of advanced ovarian germ cell malignancy. The modern era of multiagent chemotherapy has had a dramatic impact on the long-term survival of young women with germ cell ovarian tumors, allowing most of the patients to retain fertility and yet at the same time be cured of their aggressive

malignancy. Initially, multiagent chemotherapy found to be effective as an adjuvant for patients with Stage Ia disease incorporated a combination of vincristine, dactinomycin (Adriamycin), and cyclophosphamide, the so-called *VAC regimen*. The duration of therapy remained somewhat controversial for patients with Stage I disease. Because of the poor prognosis, patients were given two years of chemotherapy but encountered significant toxicity in many instances. Other investigators have used the multiagent chemotherapy for only three cycles in patients with no residual disease. The long-term survival of Stage I patients receiving three courses of chemotherapy has been reported to be 90 percent.

Advanced ovarian germ cell tumors also should be treated with multiagent chemotherapy, although the duration of treatment is poorly defined. If the patient's tumor produces a tumor marker, e.g., α-fetoprotein or hCG, therapy should be continued until the marker is absent. Because these tumor markers are not as sensitive for detecting residual disease, second-look laparotomy is advised to fully document the patient's disease status prior to discontinuing chemotherapy. More recently, the combinations vinblastine/bleomycin/cisplatin or VP-16/bleomycin/cisplatin have been found to have significant activity against widely metastatic ovarian germ cell tumors resistant to the VAC regimen. These chemotherapy regimens are intense, and many patients encounter significant toxicity. Fortunately, most patients with germ cell tumors are otherwise young healthy women with significant hematologic, cardiopulmonary, renal, and hepatic reserve.

Complications of these multiagent chemotherapy regimens include pancytopenia, sepsis, alopecia, hepatic toxicity, nephrotoxicity, neurotoxicity, and pulmonary toxicity. Most of the complications and side effects of chemotherapy are transient but may require significant supportive medical care until the patient has recovered. Long-term complications of multiagent chemotherapy include potential for ovarian failure and pulmonary fibrosis due to bleomycin. In addition, leukemia has been encountered in a small percentage of patients receiving prolonged courses of alkylating chemotherapy agents. Because of these severe, acute, and potentially long-term side effects of chemotherapy, it is desirable to discontinue chemotherapy at a point when the patient has developed complete clinical remission from the cancer. Second-look laparotomy is strongly advised for making this assessment and substantiating the need for continued therapy or its discontinuation.

As previously noted, dysgerminoma is the one ovarian germ cell tumor that is exquisitely sensitive to radiation therapy. A total dose of 3000 rad of radiation therapy is usually adequate to achieve tumor regression. Therefore patients with dysgerminomas with metastases to lymph nodes or the peritoneal cavity may be adequately treated with radiation therapy. If the patient wishes to retain fertility, however, radiation therapy is avoided and systemic chemotherapy prescribed. Systemic multiagent chemotherapy is also advised for patients with dysgerminomas that have mixed germ cell elements.

At the present time, in excess of 70 percent of patients with Stage III ovarian germ cell tumors should enjoy a complete remission following treatment with surgical resection and multiagent chemotherapy.

Stromal Sex Cord Tumors of the Ovary

In most cases, neoplasms arising from stromal or sex cord cells of the ovary are benign neoplasms. Many of these lesions are functional hormone-producing tumors and are discussed in Chapter 18. On rare occasion, each of these tumors is found to be malignant, requiring aggressive therapy (both surgery and adjuvant therapy).

Granulosa Cell Tumors. Most malignant granulosa cell tumors occur in postmenopausal women. In contrast, most granulosa cell tumors in children and young women are unilateral (Stage Ia), are histologically benign, and have a benign clinical course.

Granulosa cell tumors found in older women are often ruptured, demonstrating infarction and necrosis. In this setting, careful surgical exploration should be performed to search for other intraperitoneal or retroperitoneal metastases. The involved ovary should be surgically removed, as should the contralateral ovary and uterus in menopausal women and in menstrual-age women who no longer wish to maintain fertility.

The overall survival for patients with Stage Ia granulosa cell tumors is more than 95 percent at five years. On the other hand, patients with Stage II and III disease have a five-year survival of 55 percent and a 10-year survival of 25 percent. It is clear, then, that surgical staging is important in the prognostic evaluation of these patients and to identify patients with Stage II and III disease who might benefit from adjuvant therapy.

Survival statistics showing continued mortality from granulosa cell tumors between five and ten years after diagnosis also points out the fact that granulosa cell tumors often are late to recur. Long-term surveillance of women who had a previous diagnosis of granulosa cell tumors is therefore warranted. The size of the primary granulosa cell tumor is also important with regard to recurrence and survival. Rarely does a patient who has a tumor less than 5 cm in diameter develop recurrent disease. Among patients with Stage Ia granulosa cell tumors that are 5 to 15 cm in diameter, fewer than 20 percent of the tumors recur. On the other hand, patients with tumors larger than 15 cm have a 30 percent recurrence rate.

Ruptured granulosa cell tumors also have worse prognosis than those removed with the capsule intact. Finally, histologic study of granulosa cell tumors may identify the tumors with a high mitotic count and cellular atypia. Those tumors with a mitotic count of more than two mitoses per ten high power fields or containing atypical cells have a worse prognosis and may benefit from adjuvant therapy.

Careful histologic study of a presumed malignant granulosa cell tumor should be performed, as undifferentiated carcinomas, adenocarcinomas, and carcinoids may be mistaken for a granulosa cell tumor on cursory evaluation. Clearly, this diagnosis, based on misinterpretation of histology, could result in inadequate treatment.

The estrogenic stimulation of a granulosa cell tumor often leads to endometrial proliferation, hyperplasia, polyp formation, and endometrial carcinoma. About 10 to 20 percent of patients with granulosa cell tumors, most of them postmenopausal, have an associated carcinoma of the endometrium. It is therefore imperative to evaluate the endometrium of patients with granulosa cell tumors to identify patients with endometrial hyperplasia or carcinoma. Conversely, postmenopausal patients showing increasing estrogenization or who have endometrial hyperplasia or carcinoma should also be evaluated for the possibility of having a concurrent granulosa cell tumor.

Fibromas and *thecomas* of the ovary are generally considered to be benign neoplasms and may be managed by surgical resection alone. On rare occasion, malignancy is demonstrated in these stromal tumors. *Fibrosarcomas* and *malignant thecomas* account for fewer than 1 percent of all stromal tumors. These malignant neoplasms are usually much larger than their benign counterparts. At surgical exploration, a malignancy should be suspected if adhesions, hemorrhage, necrosis, and rupture of the ovarian tumor are noted. The diagnosis of malignancy is based on histologic findings. Fibrosarcomas are designated truly malignant if more than three mitoses per ten high power fields are found.

Arrhenoblastoma (*Sertoli-Leydig cell tumor*) and *lipid cell tumors* are also malignant on rare occasion. Similar to their benign counterparts, these malignancies may produce excessive amounts of testosterone, and the patient may manifest hirsutism. Pathologic evaluation of the arrhenoblastoma may identify it as malignant based on the lack of differentiation of the tumor, increased mitotic activity, or finding heterologous elements in the tumor (most commonly skeletal muscle and cartilage).

Management of Malignant Stromal-Sex Cord Tumors. Surgical management of patients with malignant stromal sex cord tumors may be based on two considerations: surgical stage of the tumor and the patient's desire to retain reproductive capacity. For patients with apparent Stage Ia tumors who wish to retain fertility, unilateral salpingo-oophorectomy with careful surgical exploration is usually adequate surgical therapy. Careful exploration of all peritoneal surfaces, omentectomy, and evaluation of the contralateral ovary is mandatory. If on final histologic review the malignancy appears to be only a Stage Ia stromal malignancy, there is no indication that adjuvant therapy (chemotherapy or irradiation) offers improved survival. Surgical management of the Stage I stromal

malignancy patient who does not desire preservation of fertility or who is perimenopausal or postmenopausal should include bilateral salpingo-oophorectomy with total abdominal hysterectomy and complete surgical staging. In this setting, preservation of the contralateral ovary is of no value and in fact should be removed to eliminate the site of potential recurrence. Careful and prolonged follow-up of patients with stromal malignancies is important, as it has been noted that many of these tumors (especially granulosa cell tumors) may not recur for 10 to 20 years after the initial diagnosis. Serial serum estradiol levels may be used to predict recurrent granulosa cell tumors prior to their clinical reappearance.

Management of advanced stage (II, III, and IV) stromal malignancy should include complete surgical resection of the tumor if possible. There are no randomized trials comparing treatment modalities for stromal sex cord malignancies, and therefore recommendations for appropriate therapy may vary from one institution to another. Combination chemotherapy has been shown to be effective in some cases of advanced stromal tumors. In particular, the combinations vincristine/actinomycin D/cyclophosphamide (VAC), vinblastine (Velban)/cis-platin/bleomycin, and cis-platinum/adriamycin/cyclophosphamide (PAC) have been shown to have activity against these tumors. Whole-abdomen radiation therapy has been advocated for the primary treatment of patients with no residual disease in the peritoneal cavity at the completion of surgical debulking. In addition, whole-pelvis radiation therapy has been recommended for local recurrences in the pelvis, especially granulosa cell tumors that have recurred late in the course and appear to be localized to the pelvis only.

Lymphoma

The ovary may be the initial site of a lymphoma. Although some authors believe that primary ovarian lymphoma can occur, nearly all cases of ovarian lymphoma have been found either to have concurrent generalized lymphoma or eventually to manifest as generalized lymphoma. Because the ovary ordinarily does not contain lymphocytes, the possibility of developing a primary ovarian lymphoma remains somewhat controversial. Nonetheless, the first sign of lymphoma may be the development of a pelvic mass leading to exploratory surgery to establish the etiology of an ovarian neoplasm. Lymphoma should be suspected when a patient is found to have ovarian masses (many times bilateral) and enlarged lymph nodes. Frozen section should be obtained from these solid tumors from which the diagnosis is usually easily made.

Salpingo-oophorectomy for diagnosis and removal of the enlarging lymphomatous ovary is appropriate. Histologically, lymphomas may be mistaken for granulosa cell tumor or dysgerminoma, and therefore care should be exercised with the pathologic evaluation. At the same laparotomy, additional surgical staging of lymphoma should be carried out, which involves selective lymphadenectomy of the pelvic and aortic lymph nodes, liver biopsy, assessment of the spleen, and complete intraabdominal exploration. In addition, bone marrow biopsy and CT scan of the abdomen, pelvis, and chest should be performed postoperatively. Chemotherapy or irradiation for lymphoma should be undertaken based on the type of lymphoma and stage of disease.

Sarcomas

Mixed mesodermal sarcoma of the ovary is another rare ovarian tumor that has an aggressive natural history. Most sarcomas are diagnosed as Stage III disease and may appear initially to be similar to other advanced epithelial or germ cell tumors of the ovary. Because experience with these rare tumors is limited, our approach to therapy is generalized, based on the management of other, more common ovarian tumors. Surgical debulking and postoperative chemotherapy appear to offer the best chance of prolonged survival and palliation. Combination chemotherapy with the VAC or PAC regimen has been reported to have some activity in treating these advanced malignancies.

Cancer Metastatic to the Ovary

Approximately 5 to 10 percent of ovarian malignancies are metastatic from another site. The most common malignancies to metastasize to the ovary are breast carcinoma, malignancies of the gastrointestinal tract (especially stomach and colorectum), and endometrial carcinoma. Most patients who have cancer metastatic to the ovary have bilateral ovarian involvement and are found to have metastases of the primary malignancy at other sites as well.

In 1896 Krukenberg described an ovarian tumor he thought was a primary malignancy of sarcoma origin. Further investigation showed that the "Krukenberg tumor" was actually a metastatic tumor to the ovary. Nonetheless, we continue to describe tumors that meet the criteria set forth by Krukenberg as *Krukenberg tumors*. Most often, the primary malignancy is in the stomach, although other sites, including colon and breast, may meet the criteria of a Krukenberg tumor. Grossly, Krukenberg tumors are solid masses with an average size of 10 to 15 cm, and most are bilateral. On cut section, the tumor has characteristic gelatinous and necrotic areas. Microscopic study of the tumor shows exuberant stromal hyperplasia with mucous-secreting malignant signet ring cells.

No extraovarian primary site can be demonstrated in 10 to 20 percent of patients with histologically bona fide Krukenberg tumors, and some patients have apparently been cured by removal of the uterus and adnexa. For this reason, this small group of lesions are sometimes classified as primary ovarian Krukenberg tumors. These tumors are presumed to arise in small preexisting teratomas, although the possibility that the initial microscopic primary focus remained dormant or underwent spontaneous regression cannot be completely excluded.

When metastatic disease to the ovary is encountered, it should be surgically resected if possible. Although such resection may not have any bearing on the patient's long-term survival, palliation can be achieved by removing an enlarging pelvic mass, thereby preventing the pain, pressure, and colonic obstructive symptoms of an enlarging pelvic mass. In patients with known breast carcinoma, the ovarian tumor should be submitted for estrogen and progesterone receptor analysis, as these results may have some bearing on subsequent adjuvant therapy. After surgical resection, appropriate therapy for the particular metastatic lesion should be instituted.

MALIGNANCIES OF THE FALLOPIAN TUBE

Carcinoma of the fallopian tube is the rarest gynecologic malignancy. Overall, tubal cancer accounts for

0.1 to 0.5 percent of all gynecologic cancers. Because of the rarity of this malignancy, information regarding epidemiology and treatment results are limited. Adenocarcinoma is the most common fallopian tube carcinoma, arising from the epithelium of the fallopian tube. Although a variety of adenocarcinoma cell types (e.g., endometrioid, clear cell, adenosquamous) have been reported, by far the most frequent is the serous adenocarcinoma. Histologically, the malignancy looks identical to serous cystadenocarcinoma of the ovary. Fallopian tube carcinoma appears to have a predilection for women of low parity, with the average age at diagnosis 55 years.

The signs and symptoms of fallopian tube carcinoma are often vague, with the patient giving a history of lower abdominal and pelvic pain that has been mild but chronic in nature. As the disease progresses, intraperitoneal metastases lead to other gastrointestinal symptoms and, with progression, abdominal distention and ascites. Some patients have vaginal bleeding, and many report an amber-yellow discharge prior to diagnosis. Some authors have suggested that abdominal pain relieved by the rapid release of a "tea-colored" vaginal discharge (hydrops tubae profluens) is pathognomonic for fallopian tube cancer. In truth, however, this symptom complex is rarely reported by patients with fallopian tube carcinoma. Cervical and vaginal cyptopathology are positive for adenocarcinoma in only 5 to 10 percent of cases. On the physical examination, the most frequently detected finding is an adnexal mass. although many cases of fallopian tube cancer are not suspected until exploratory laparotomy. Certainly, because of the rarity of this disease, it is not high on the list of the differential diagnosis of an adnexal mass. Fallopian tube cancer might be suspected in a patient with a Papanicolaou smear showing adenocarcinoma with a negative fractional D&C.

Fallopian tube carcinoma behaves like ovarian cancer in many aspects. Initially, adenocarcinoma arising from the tubal epithelium penetrates the wall of the fallopian tube or protrudes out the fimbriated end of the fallopian tube (Fig. 28-3). From there, it may spread locally to the ovary, uterus, and pelvic peritoneum, but at the same time there is diffuse intraperitoneal spreading of malignant cells. Adenocar-

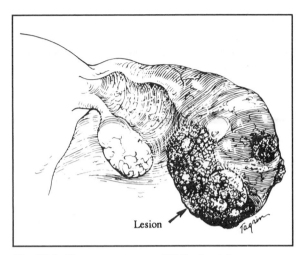

Fig. 28-3. Gross appearance of fallopian tube carcinoma.

cinoma is therefore sometimes difficult to distinguish between fallopian tube carcinoma and ovarian carcinoma. Fallopian tube carcinoma also spreads by way of retroperitoneal lymphatics, especially along the lymphatics draining the ovary to the paraaortic region. There is no official staging system for fallopian tube carcinoma, although most oncologists use the staging system proposed for ovarian carcinoma (Table 28-2).

Treatment of fallopian tube carcinoma is also similar to that proposed for epithelial ovarian cancer. Complete surgical staging is important, including total abdominal hysterectomy with bilateral salpingo-oophorectomy, omentectomy, peritoneal cytology, biopsy of suspicious peritoneal implants, and selective pelvic and paraaortic lymphadenectomy. Cytoreductive surgery of large masses should be attempted, as this tumor appears to have a sensitivity to multiagent chemotherapy similar to that of ovarian cancer.

Patients with Stage I or Stage II disease who have had complete surgical resection of their carcinoma should be treated with adjuvant therapy because of the reasonably high risk of recurrence if surgery alone is used. Intraperitoneal instillation of chromic phosphate (^{32}P) or whole-abdomen radiation therapy might be considered in this setting. Patients with advanced-stage disease, including those with metastases to lymph nodes, should be treated with multiagent chemotherapy. The combination cisplatin/cyclophosphamide/adriamycin appears to have reasonably good activity and is currently used as first-line therapy. Some authors have suggested that use of progestins might also be effective in achieving some palliation.

Overall treatment results gathered from the literature suggest that patients with Stage I ovarian cancer have a 65 to 75 percent five-year survival; patients with Stage II disease have a 40 to 60 percent five-year survival; and patients with Stage III disease have an 18 percent five-year survival. Because the therapy for fallopian tube carcinoma parallels that for ovarian cancer, and because its spread patterns are similar to those of ovarian cancer, with occult disease being highly probable in advanced stages, second-look laparotomy is recommended for patients with advanced-stage disease after a course of chemotherapy.

Rarer than adenocarcinoma of the fallopian tube is *fallopian tube sarcoma*. Most of these lesions are mixed müllerian tumors that are usually of advanced stage when initially diagnosed. Overall, these malignancies have a poor prognosis and should be treated aggressively with surgical resection and chemotherapy. Cooperative group treatment protocols are necessary to evaluate treatment modalities for this rare malignancy.

SELECTED READINGS

Asadourian, L. A. and Taylor, H. B. Dysgerminoma: an analysis of 105 cases. *Obstet. Gynecol.* 33:370, 1969.

Aure, J. B., Hoeg, K., and Kolstad, P. Clinical and histologic studies of ovarian carcinoma: long-term follow-up of 990 cases. *Obstet. Gynecol.* 37:1, 1971.

Bast, R. C., Klug, T. L., Schaetzl, E., et al. Monitoring human ovarian carcinoma with a combination of CA 125, CA 19-9, and carcinoembryonic antigen. *Am. J. Obstet. Gynecol.* 149:553, 1984.

Braly, P., Doroshaw, J., and Hoff, S. Technical aspects of intraperitoneal chemotherapy in abdominal carcinomatosis. *Gynecol. Oncol.* 25:319, 1986.

Breen, J. L., Bonamo, J. F., and Maxson, W. S. Genital tract tumors in children. *Pediatr. Clin. North Am.* 28:355, 1981.

Bruckner, H. W., Cohen, C. J., Goldberg, J. D., et al. Improved chemotherapy for ovarian cancer with cis-diamminedichloroplatinum and adriamycin. *Cancer* 47:2288, 1981.

Clarke-Pearson, D. L., Delong, E. R., Chin, N., et al. Intestinal obstruction in patients with ovarian cancer: variables associated with surgical complications and survival. *Arch. Surg.* 123:42, 1988.

Copeland, L. J. Second-look laparotomy for ovarian carcinoma. *Clin. Obstet. Gynecol.* 28:816, 1985.

Cramer, D. W., Welch, W. R., Scully, R. E., et al. Ovarian cancer and talc: a case-control study. *Cancer* 50:372, 1982.

Creasman, W. T., and Soper, J. T. Assessment of contemporary management of germ cell malignancies of the ovary. *Am. J. Obstet. Gynecol.* 153:828, 1985.

Creasman, W. T., Park, R., Norris, H., et al. Stage I borderline ovarian tumors. *Obstet. Gynecol.* 59:93, 1982.

Delgado, G., Aram, D. H., and Petrilli, E. S. Stage III epithelial ovarian cancer: the role of maximal surgical reduction. *Gynecol. Oncol.* 18:293, 1984.

Dembo, A. J. Abdominopelvic radiotherapy in ovarian cancer: a 10 year experience. *Cancer* 55:2285, 1985.

Deppe, G., Bruckner, H. W., and Cohen, C. J. Combination chemotherapy for advanced carcinoma of the fallopian tube. *Obstet. Gynecol.* 56:530, 1980.

Eddy, G. L., Copeland, L. J., Gershenson, D. M., et al. Fallopian tube carcinoma. *Obstet. Gynecol.* 64:546, 1984.

Ehrlich, C. E., Einhorn, L., Stehman, F. B., et al. Treatment of advanced epithelial ovarian cancer using cisplatin, adriamycin and Cytoxan—The Indiana University experience. *Clin. Obstet. Gynecol.* 10:325, 1983.

Gershenson, D. M., Del-Junco, G., Herson, J., et al. Endodermal sinus tumor of the ovary. *Obstet. Gynecol.* 61:194, 1983.

Greene, M. H., Boice, J. D., Jr., Greer, B. E., et al. Acute nonlymphocytic leukemia after therapy with alkylating agents for ovarian cancer: a study of five randomized clinical trials. *N. Engl. J. Med.* 307:1416, 1982.

Hacker, N. F., Berek, J. S., Pretorius, R. G., et al. Intraperitoneal cisplatin as salvage therapy for refractory epithelial ovarian cancer. *Obstet. Gynecol.* 70:759, 1987.

Hart, W. R., and Norris, H. J. Borderline and mucinous tumors of the ovary: histologic criteria and clinical behavior. *Cancer* 31:3031, 1973.

Heintz, A. P. M., Hacker, N. F., and Lagasse, L. D. Epidemiology and etiology of ovarian cancer: a review. *Obstet. Gynecol.* 66:127, 1985.

Holtz, F., and Hart, W. R. Krukenberg tumors of the ovary: a clinicopathologic analysis of 27 cases. *Cancer* 50:2438, 1982.

Hoskins, W. J., Lichter, A. S. Whittington, R., et al. Whole abdominal and pelvic irradiation in patients with minimal disease at second-look surgical reassessment for ovarian carcinoma. *Gynecol. Oncol.* 20:271, 1985.

Hreshchyshyn, M. M., Park, R. C., Blessing, J. A., et al. The role of adjuvant therapy in stage I ovarian cancer. *Am. J. Obstet. Gynecol.* 138:139, 1980.

Lavin, P. T., Knapp, R. C., Malkasian, G., et al. CA 125 for the monitoring of ovarian carcinoma during primary therapy. *Obstet. Gynecol.* 69:223, 1987.

Lucas, W. E., Markman, M., and Howell, S. B. Intraperitoneal chemotherapy for advanced ovarian cancer. *Am. J. Obstet. Gynecol.* 152:474, 1985.

Lynch, H. T., Albano, W. A., Lynch, J. F., et al. Surveillance and management of patients at high genetic risk for ovarian carcinoma. *Obstet. Gynecol.* 59:589, 1982.

Meigs, J. V., and Cass, J. W. Fibroma of the ovary with ascites and hydrothorax with a report of 7 cases. *Am. J. Obstet. Gynecol.* 33:249, 1937.

Omura, G., Blessing, J. A., Ehrlich, C. E., et al. A randomized trial of cyclophosphamide and doxorubicin with or without cisplatin in advanced ovarian carcinoma. *Cancer* 57:1725, 1986.

Piver, M., Mettlin, C. J., Tsukada, Y. S., et al. Familial ovarian cancer registry. *Obstet. Gynecol.* 64:195, 1984.

Piver, M. S., Barlow, J. J., and Lele, S. B. Incidence of subclinical metastasis in stage I and II ovarian carcinoma. *Obstet. Gynecol.* 52:100, 1978.

Podratz, K. C., Podczaski, E. S., Gaffey, T. A., et al. Primary carcinoma of the fallopian tube. *Am. J. Obstet. Gynecol.* 154:1319, 1986.

Rosenburg, L., Shapiro, S., Slone, D., et al. Epithelial ovarian cancer and combination oral contraceptives. *J.A.M.A.* 247:3210, 1982.

Soper, J. T., Wilkinson, R. H., Bandy, L. C., et al. Intraperitoneal chromic phosphate (P-32) as salvage therapy for persistent carcinoma of the ovary after surgical restaging. *Am. J. Obstet. Gynecol.* 156:1153, 1987.

Stenwig, J. T., Hazekamp, J., and Beecham, J. Granulosa cell tumors of the ovary: a clinicopathological study of 118 cases with long term follow-up. *Gynecol. Oncol.* 7:136, 1979.

Tazelaar, H. D., Bostwick, D. G., Ballon, S. C., et al. Conservative treatment of borderline ovarian tumors. *Obstet. Gynecol.* 66:417, 1985.

Thigpen, T., and Blessing, J. A. Current therapy of ovarian carcinoma: an overview. *Semin. Oncol.* 12:47, 1985.

29

Vulvar and Vaginal Cancer

Malignancy of the vulva and vagina is relatively rare. Most cancers in the lower genital tract are derived from squamous epithelium and should be easily detected by pelvic examination, Papanicolaou smear, and direct biopsy. Nonetheless, many lesions are found late in their course owing to patient and physician delay. Despite their anatomic proximity, the treatment of vulvar and vaginal cancers is significantly different. Radical surgery is most often used to treat the vulva, whereas radiation therapy is generally used for vaginal carcinoma.

VULVAR CARCINOMA

Vulvar cancer accounts for 3 to 4 percent of gynecologic malignancies. Eighty-five to ninety percent of all vulvar cancer is squamous cell carcinoma and occurs in women with a median age of 65 years. Many patients are in their eighth to ninth decade of life, and concurrent medical conditions often complicate therapy. In recent years, however, younger women have been reported with invasive vulvar carcinoma. *Melanoma* arising primarily on the vulva accounts for 5 percent of vulvar malignancies and has the same characteristics as other cutaneous melanomas. Other malignancies of the vulva include basal cell carcinoma (1.4 percent), adenocarcinoma (1.2 percent), and sarcoma (2 percent). Basal cell carcinoma and adenocarcinoma affect an elderly age group, whereas melanomas and sarcomas often arise in premenopausal women.

Etiology

The etiologic agent(s) or carcinogen(s) for vulvar carcinoma has not been identified. Early studies associ-

ated vulvar carcinoma with previous granulomatous or venereal disease and condylomas. More recent studies have suggested that carcinoma of the vulva is associated with human papilloma virus or herpesvirus (Chap. 25).

Pathophysiology

Carcinoma of the vulva is usually localized and well demarcated, with 70 percent arising on the labia. In contrast to carcinoma in situ, invasive carcinoma is rarely multifocal except for the "kissing lesion" found on an abutting portion of the contralateral labia.

Squamous cell carcinoma tends to be a slowly growing malignancy with local extension and late lymphatic metastases (Fig. 29-1). Key to the successful treatment of squamous cell carcinoma is an understanding of the lymphatic drainage of the vulva. Lymphatic vessels drain the labia minora and majora anteriorly to the upper vulva and mons. The lymphatics then turn laterally and terminate in the inguinal and femoral lymph nodes (primarily the medial upper quadrant of the femoral nodes). The inguinal-femoral nodes are comprised of a superficial and deep set of nodes that are separated by the cribriform fascia. The superficial nodes are the first chain to be exposed to metastatic tumor emboli. Subsequently, the malignancy may metastasize to the deep femoral nodes and then to the pelvic nodes. The last deep femoral node, which lies just underneath Poupart's ligament and is considered the sentinel node prior to the beginning of the pelvic lymph node chain, is designated *Cloquet's node*. Direct drainage from the vulva to the pelvic nodes has been demonstrated anatomically especially from the clitoral region. However, it does not appear to be clinically significant. In most cases when a clitoral lesion has been found to be metastatic to pelvic nodes, metastases were also noted in inguinal lymph nodes. The collateral flow of lymphatics across the anterior vulva also allows contralateral inguinal metastasis. However, lateral lesions nearly always metastasize to the ipsilateral lymphatic chain, and it is highly unusual to have contralateral metastasis without concurrent ipsilateral metastasis. Tumor extension to the vagina, urethra, or anus allows lymphatic

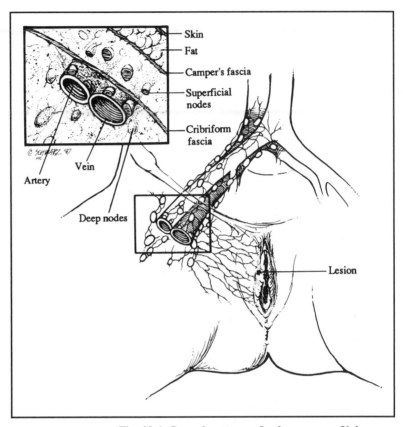

Skin
Fat
Camper's fascia
Superficial nodes
Cribriform fascia
Vein
Artery
Deep nodes
Lesion

Fig. 29-1. Spread patterns of vulvar cancer. Vulvar cancer can spread by local extension to adjacent structures such as the vagina, urethra, perineum, or anus. Because of the rich lymphatic supply to the vulva, metastases appear in the ipsilateral inguinal lymph nodes. The inguinal lymph node chain is subdivided (inset) into a superficial chain and a deeper chain. The progression is stepwise from the superficial to the deeper inguinal chain and then to the pelvic lymph nodes. Direct spread to pelvic lymph nodes, bypassing the inguinal lymph nodes, is not found in clinical practice.

drainage directly to the associated pelvic lymphatic chains.

Melanoma, adenocarcinoma, and *sarcoma* of the vulva also spread to the inguinal-femoral lymphatics. On the other hand, *basal cell carcinoma* tends to be locally progressive and rarely metastasizes to pelvic lymph nodes.

Diagnosis

Symptoms. Symptoms of *squamous cell carcinoma* of the vulva are usually reported to be pruritus, pain, bleeding, discharge, or the recognition of a mass or a "lump." Patients may also complain of dysuria or dyspareunia. *Melanomas* of the vulva may cause pruritus or pain or may be recognized only as a raised or dark lesion. *Adenocarcinoma,* especially that arising

in Bartholin's gland, may cause significant pain, a palpable mass, and dyspareunia.

Examination. Clinical examination of the vulva is part of every routine pelvic examination. Certainly in patients with vulvar symptoms, treatment by telephone diagnosis is inappropriate. The examiner may find an ulcerated endophytic lesion or a raised exophytic lesion arising on the labia or perineum. Palpation of the vulva may identify a mass especially near Bartholin's gland. Careful palpation should also be performed to ascertain fixation to underlying muscle or bone.

Melanoma of the vulva usually is pigmented and raised, although it may present as an ulcerated bleeding lesion.

The location and size of the vulvar lesion as well as any involvement of adjacent structures such as urethra, vagina, or the anus should be noted. Because the primary route of spread is to inguinal-femoral lymphatics, the inguinal lymph nodes should be palpated carefully. In cases where adenocarcinoma or melanoma is found, other sites of primary disease should be sought.

Laboratory Evaluation. The cornerstone of the diagnosis of vulvar cancers is a biopsy, which usually can be obtained in the office under local anesthesia. An incisional biopsy from the lateral margin of an ulcerated lesion is often helpful for identifying the invasive component and avoiding necrotic tissue in the center of a tumor. Small lesions may be completely excised in the office, allowing thorough evaluation of the depth of invasion. Rarely is colposcopy or toluidine blue or acetic acid staining of significant assistance when evaluating sites to biopsy in frankly invasive carcinoma.

The staging of vulvar carcinoma was established by the International Federation of Gynecology and Obstetrics (FIGO) in 1971 and was revised significantly in 1988 (Table 29-1). The former (1971) clinical staging system was fraught with error, especially in the evaluation of inguinal lymph nodes. Because assessment of lymph nodes was based on clinical evaluation rather than histology, a 15 percent false-positive rate and a nearly 40 percent false-negative rate were encountered. The revised staging system (1988) requires surgical removal and pathologic study of the nodes.

Staging studies should include a chest radiograph and an intravenous pyelogram as well as complete blood count, liver function tests, and renal function tests. Cystoscopy and proctoscopy are usually reserved for patients who have specific symptoms or disease located near the anus or urethra.

Management

Standard treatment of squamous cell carcinoma, melanoma, adenocarcinoma, and sarcoma of the vulva is by radical vulvectomy with inguinal and femoral lymphadenectomy (Fig. 29-2). The extent of surgical excision of the mons and inguinal skin and fat varies from one surgeon to another. For obvious reasons, the more radical excision is associated with a higher complication rate. Morbidity from radical vulvectomy includes significant changes in body image and sexual function. Inguinal and vulvar wound infection and disruption are reported in approximately 50 percent of the patients, and some degree of leg lymphedema follows inguinal lymphadenectomy in approximately 50 percent. Deep venous thrombosis and pulmonary embolism, inguinal lymphocyst, and stress urinary incontinence are other frequently associated complications of radical vulvectomy.

Advanced vulvar carcinoma involving the urethra, vagina, or anus has usually been managed by pelvic examination combined with radical vulvectomy. Careful patient selection is obviously necessary, and this ultraradical surgery is usually limited to young patients with advanced disease.

In the past, many surgeons performed an extraperitoneal pelvic lymphadenectomy in combination with inguinal lymphadenectomy, especially if inguinal lymph nodes were found to contain metastasis. Others have advised whole-pelvis radiation therapy in this setting, thereby avoiding the morbidity of the pelvic lymphadenectomy. One randomized trial has clearly demonstrated that whole-pelvis radiation therapy is significantly more successful than extensive surgery for treating potential disease in pelvic lymph nodes.

Alternative Management

EARLY INVASIVE VULVAR CARCINOMA. Several gynecologic oncologists have questioned the need for radical vulvectomy and inguinal lymphadenectomy for

Table 29-1. FIGO Classification and Staging of Carcinoma of the Vulva (1988 Revision)

Stage 0: Carcinoma in situ, intraepithelial carcinoma.
  Tis
Stage I: Tumor confined to the vulva and/or perineum; 2 cm or less in greatest dimension. No nodal metastasis.
  T1 N0 M0
Stage II: Tumor confined to the vulva and/or perineum; more than 2 cm in greatest dimension. No nodal metastasis.
  T2 N0 M0
Stage III: Tumor of any size with (1) adjacent spread to the lower urethra and/or the vagina or the anus, and/or (2) unilateral regional lymph node metastasis.
  T3 N0 M0
  T3 N1 M0
  T1 N1 M0
  T2 N1 M0
Stage IVA: Tumor invades any of the following: upper urethra, bladder mucosa, rectal mucosa, pelvic bone; and/or bilateral regional node metastasis.
  T1 N2 M0
  T2 N2 M0
  T3 N2 M0
  T4, any N, M0
Stage IVB (any T, any N, M1): Any distant metastasis including pelvic lymph nodes.

   T (primary tumor)
     T1:   Tumor confined to vulva and/or perineum; 2 cm or less in greatest dimension.
     T2:   Tumor confined to vulva and/or perineum; >2 cm in greatest dimension.
     T3:   Tumor of any size with adjacent spread to the lower urethra and/or the vagina and/or the anus.
     T4:   Tumor invades any of the following: upper urethra, bladder mucosa, rectal mucosa, pelvic bone.
   N (regional lymph nodes)
     N0:   No nodal metastasis (surgically proved).
     N1:   Unilateral regional lymph node metastasis.
     N2:   Bilateral regional lymph node metastasis.
   M (distant metastasis)
     M0:   No distant metastasis.
     M1A: Pelvic lymph node metastasis.
     M1B: Other distant metastasis.

early invasive vulvar carcinoma. Although the term "microinvasive carcinoma" of the vulva has not been widely accepted, *early invasive vulvar carcinoma* is usually considered to be squamous cell carcinoma invading less than 5 mm and a lesion which is less than 2 cm in diameter. Using this criterion, only 5 to 10 percent of patients have metastatic disease in inguinal lymph nodes. In addition, the local recurrence rate is low. Because of this favorable prognosis, it has been suggested that these small lesions can be treated with an excellent chance of cure and preservation of significant vulvar anatomy. Moreover, the morbidity associ-

ated with complete inguinal lymphadenectomy is avoided.

The surgical procedure suggested is a modified radical vulvectomy: radical excision of unilateral disease while leaving the contralateral vulva intact (Fig. 29-3). Because the prognosis for vulvar cancer is highly correlated with metastatic disease in the lymph nodes, the superficial inguinal nodes are completely excised and studied. If there is no metastasis in the superficial nodes, deeper inguinal node dissection seems to be unnecessary. On the other hand, if metastatic disease is in the inguinal nodes, a complete

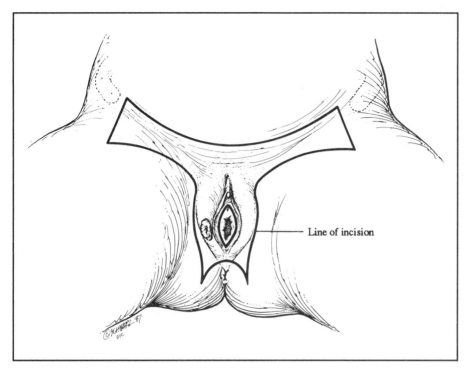

Line of incision

Fig. 29-2. Radical vulvectomy with bilateral inguinal lymphadenectomy. The lines of excision of vulvar and inguinal skin are shown by the heavy outline. The inner incision allows an adequate surgical margin and usually is made at the introitus. With this resection the mons, clitoris, and labia are entirely excised to the depth of the pelvic floor fascia and pubic symphysis.

inguinal-femoral lymphadenectomy as well as radical vulvectomy is recommended. Although this therapeutic alternative is based on sound anatomic and clinical premises, it has been applied to a limited number of patients and therefore must still be considered investigational.

ADVANCED VULVAR CARCINOMA. Radiation therapy is generally poorly tolerated by the vulva and cannot be considered as primary therapy in most cases. However, some investigators have shown excellent treatment results for locally advanced vulvovaginal carcinoma by combining preoperative radiation therapy with wide excision of the remaining malignancy. With such an approach, exenterative surgery has been avoided. Preoperative radiation therapy does lead to increased operative complications, however, especially poor wound healing of the groin and vulvar incisions.

Management of Metastatic Disease in Inguinal Lymph Nodes. The best management of metastatic disease in inguinal lymph nodes is yet to be established, although it is clear that these metastases worsen the individual's prognosis, especially if the patient has more than three lymph nodes involved with metastatic tumor. In this setting inguinal and whole-pelvis radiation therapy can effectively improve survival.

Sexual rehabilitation of the patient following radical vulvectomy may be augmented by plastic surgery procedures such as vulvar reconstruction with gracilis flaps or coverage of the inguinal region with tensor fascia lata flaps or skin grafts. Attention must be directed to the continued sexual rehabilitation of these patients and emotional support offered as necessary.

Management of Rare Vulvar Cancers. Basal cell carcinoma can usually be adequately managed by

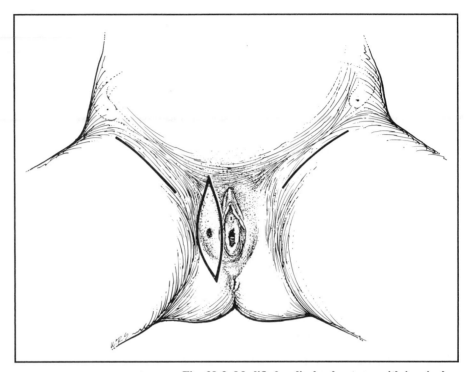

Fig. 29-3. Modified radical vulvectomy with inguinal lymphadenectomy. Small unilateral (Stage I) lesions may be adequately treated by a modified radical vulvectomy. Shown here are the lines of incision. The depth of the excision is carried down to the pelvic floor fascia and pubic ramus, as for a complete radical vulvectomy. The inguinal incisions shown allow inguinal lymphadenectomy through separate incisions.

wide local excision, as this malignancy has a low propensity to metastasize to inguinal lymph nodes.

Vulvar melanoma has traditionally been treated with radical vulvectomy and inguinal lymphadenectomy, although more recently wide local excision of the melanoma has been advocated. The need for inguinal lymphadenectomy also must be debated as to whether it serves only as a prognostic staging tool or it is therapeutic. In most patients with metastatic disease to inguinal lymph nodes, long-term survival is minimal.

Recurrent Disease. Approximately 80 percent of recurrent disease is noted within the first two years of follow-up. One-half of recurrences are local—on the vulva or inguinal regions—and are usually found in patients who had large primary malignancies or positive inguinal lymph nodes. Occasionally, a vulvar recurrence can be treated successfully by wide resection or interstitial radiation therapy. Recurrent disease in inguinal lymph nodes is much more difficult to treat. Wide local excision (if possible) followed by radia-

tion therapy is recommended. The remainder of recurrences are at distant sites in pelvic and paraaortic lymph nodes, or they appear as bony metastases; they are usually only palliated with chemotherapy regimens such as cis-platinum.

Prognosis

The overall survival for patients with vulvar carcinoma is approximately 75 percent at five years (corrected survival). Prognostic features significantly associated with survival include primary tumor size, metastatic disease in inguinal lymph nodes, grade of tumor, depth of invasion, and invasion of lymphatic channels. Patients with Stage I and II squamous cell carcinoma of the vulva enjoy an approximately 90 percent corrected five-year survival. Irrespective of stage of disease, if the patient has negative inguinal lymph nodes the survival rate is approximately 90 percent. On the other hand, if the patient has a metastasis in inguinal lymph nodes, the overall survival plummets to approximately 35 percent at five years. The number of inguinal nodes affected also seems to be important, as those patients with three or fewer lymph nodes involved have approximately 69 percent five-year survival, whereas those with more than three lymph nodes involved in the inguinal femoral region rarely survive. Patients with known pelvic lymph node metastases have an approximately 20 percent five-year survival.

VAGINAL CARCINOMA

Only 1 to 2 percent of gynecologic malignancies arise in the vagina. Squamous cell carcinomas comprise approximately 95 percent of these malignancies and generally occur in women 55 to 65 years of age. The incidence of vaginal squamous cell carcinoma is increased in patients who have been previously treated with pelvic irradiation, and the diagnosis should be strongly considered in patients who develop abnormal genital cytology after radiotherapy.

Adenocarcinoma of the vagina accounts for only 2 percent of vaginal carcinomas. The identification of a cluster of young women with clear cell adenocarcinoma of the vagina led to studies that demonstrated in utero exposure to diethylstilbestrol (DES) as the etiologic factor. The incidence of adenocarcinoma following DES exposure has been calculated to be 0.14 to 1.40 per 1000 female fetuses exposed. The median age of onset of clear cell adenocarcinoma of the vagina is 19 years.

Melanoma of the vagina accounts for approximately 2 percent of vaginal malignancies. Rarer still are leiomyosarcoma, fibrosarcoma, and rhabdomyosarcoma (sarcoma botryoides) arising primarily in the vagina. The possibility of a vaginal lesion being metastatic from another primary malignancy should be considered. Frequently encountered metastases to the vagina include carcinoma of the cervix, endometrium, vulva, colorectal carcinoma, ovarian carcinoma, choriocarcinoma, and urethral carcinoma.

Etiology

The etiology of squamous cell carcinoma of the vagina is unknown. Because of its close association with malignancies arising in the cervix or vulva, a "field" effect has been suggested; and the possibility of a viral etiology has been entertained. Some authors have shown an association between squamous cell carcinoma of the vagina and vaginal prolapse, pessary use, and prior pelvic irradiation.

Clear cell adenocarcinoma of the vagina arising in young women was described in 1971 by Herbst, who demonstrated a link with in utero exposure to DES. These women who developed clear cell adenocarcinoma were exposed to DES before the eighteenth week of gestation. Duration of therapy and dosage of DES exposure were not necessarily proportional to the subsequent development of adenocarcinoma of the vagina in these young women.

The etiologies of melanoma, sarcoma, and sarcoma botryoides are unknown.

Pathophysiology

Squamous cell carcinoma of the vagina spreads by local extension and lymphatic metastasis. Because the vesicovaginal and rectovaginal septum are relatively thin, local extension directly into the bladder or rectum is frequently encountered. Invasion into the paravaginal tissues and extension to the pelvic side wall is seen in advanced cases (Fig. 29-4). The incidence of lymph node metastasis is unknown, although it is assumed to be approximately the same as that of squamous cell carcinoma arising on the cervix.

The lymphatic drainage of the vagina is complex and must be considered when planning treatment (Fig. 29-5). The location of the carcinoma in the vaginal tube predicts the groups of regional nodes that may be at risk. The upper one-half of the vagina drains into the pelvic lymph nodes, including the external iliac, obturator, hypogastric, and common iliac lymph nodes. Lesions located in the lower portion of the vagina may drain into lymphatic channels in a

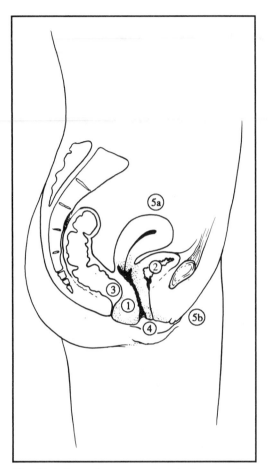

Fig. 29-4. Spread patterns of vaginal cancer. Vaginal carcinoma can spread through direct extension to submucosa and paravaginal tissues (1), into the bladder (2), into the rectum (3), and to the vulva or urethra (4). Metastasis to pelvic lymph nodes (5a) and inguinal lymph nodes (5b) is by embolization and is related to the location of the carcinoma in the vagina.

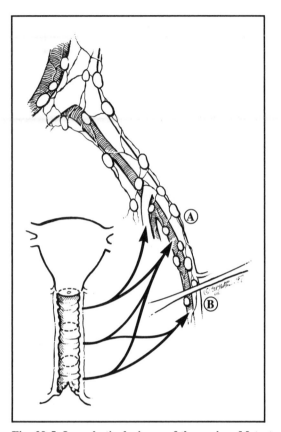

Fig. 29-5. Lymphatic drainage of the vagina. Metastases from vaginal carcinoma may spread to the pelvic (A) and inguinal lymph nodes (B). The pattern is contingent on the location of the cancer in the vagina. Disease in the lower two-thirds of the vagina can spread by way of the pelvic or inguinal lymph nodes. Upper vaginal disease is more likely to metastasize only to pelvic lymph nodes.

fashion similar to vulvar carcinoma, i.e., the inguinal femoral lymphatics. Treatment of the lymphatic groups at risk for metastasis is crucial to achieve therapeutic success. Fifty-four percent of vaginal squamous cell carcinoma is located in the upper one-third of the vagina, most often on the posterior wall. Fourteen percent of vaginal carcinomas are located in the middle third, whereas 32 percent are located in the lower one-third of the vagina.

Clear cell adenocarcinoma following DES exposure usually occurs in the upper one-half of the vagina and may be associated with adenocarcinoma of the cervix. Local extension and nodal metastasis are the primary means of spread of this carcinoma. Eighteen percent of patients with Stage I disease and 30 percent of those with Stage II disease have metastasis to the pelvic lymph nodes.

Sarcoma botryoides usually arises from the anterior

vaginal wall and is often multicentric. The disease tends to be locally recurring, although it may spread to distant sites by hematogenous routes.

Diagnosis

Optimally, vaginal cancer is diagnosed by Papanicolaou smear screening. However, most patients present with bleeding or vaginal discharge. As the lesion progresses, and depending on its location, the patient may also develop urinary tract symptoms, rectal pain or pressure, or lower extremity pain or edema. These signs and symptoms may also be found in patients with melanoma or adenocarcinoma, although it appears that screening programs for young women exposed to DES have been successful in identifying a large proportion of patients who are asymptomatic but have early stage clear cell carcinoma. Biopsy of obvious lesions or biopsy directed by colposcopy is necessary to confirm the diagnosis.

Vaginal sarcomas often present with symptoms of a mass lesion, pressure, or pain. Bleeding may also occur if the sarcoma becomes necrotic. Sarcoma botryoides usually presents as a bloody vaginal discharge or protruding masses of "grape-like" polyps noted at the introitus of a young child.

Staging

The staging procedures for carcinoma of the vagina include investigation of local as well as distant metastasis in a fashion similar to that of carcinoma of the cervix. Complete physical and pelvic examinations assess the extent of pelvic disease and search for distant metastases. Laboratory studies include assessment of renal and hepatic function. Radiographic studies advised include a chest radiograph and intravenous pyelogram. Cystoscopy and proctosigmoidoscopy should be performed to assess possible extension into the bladder or rectum. Lymphangiography and computed tomography may be of assistance in identifying metastasis to pelvic lymph nodes. The clinical staging system for carcinoma of the vagina is shown in Table 29-2.

In patients with adenocarcinoma, especially the older patient, metastasis from another primary site

Table 29-2. Clinical Staging of Vaginal Cancer (FIGO)

Stage 0: Carcinoma in situ
Stage I: Carcinoma is limited to the vaginal mucosa
Stage II: Carcinoma has involved the subvaginal tissue but has not extended onto the pelvic wall
Stage III: Carcinoma has extended onto the pelvic wall
Stage IV: Carcinoma has extended beyond the true pelvis or has involved the mucosa of the bladder or rectum

should be excluded, and therefore endocervical and endometrial biopsy specimens must be obtained. In addition, the gastrointestinal tract, especially stomach and colon, should be surveyed for the possibility of primary adenocarcinoma. Melanoma may also be metastatic to the vagina from another primary site.

Therapy

Squamous cell carcinoma of the vagina may be treated by either surgery or radiotherapy. Surgical resection is usually reserved for lesions in the upper vagina. When performing this surgery, resection of the paravaginal tissues and pelvic lymph nodes requires a radical hysterectomy and upper vaginectomy combined with pelvic lymphadenectomy. Lesions in the lower vagina, especially those involving the vulva, may be successfully treated with pelvic exenteration and radical vulvectomy. Ultraradical surgical resection obviously does not allow conservation of the bladder or rectum and may not be appropriate for many patients who are not medically fit to undergo such extensive surgery.

To conserve bladder and rectal function, most patients with vaginal squamous cell carcinoma are treated with radiation therapy. Small lesions (less than 2 cm) may be successfully treated with interstitial implants (radium or irridium 192 afterloading needles) or with a vaginal cylinder loaded with cesium or radium. Larger lesions are treated with a combination of external beam radiotherapy delivered to the whole pelvis covering the primary lesion as well as the lymph nodes on the pelvic side wall. External beam therapy of 4000 to 5000 rad is delivered first to optimize shrinkage of the primary tumor. After external radiation therapy, interstitial or intracavitary brachytherapy is usually given. Lesions located in the upper vagina are often treated like cervical carcinoma with Fletcher-Suit tandem-and-ovoids (see Fig. 26-4). Lesions located in the lower one-third of the vagina may metastasize to the inguinal lymph nodes, and therefore inguinal lymphadenectomy is recommended prior to instituting radiation therapy.

Young women with clear cell adenocarcinoma usually have a lesion located in the upper one-half of the vagina and may be treated by radical hysterectomy with upper vaginectomy combined with pelvic lymphadenectomy. Advantages of this therapeutic approach include preservation of ovarian function and vaginal pliability as well as prevention of long-term radiation therapy complications. For large lesions, advanced stage lesions, or those located in the lower one-half of the vagina, adenocarcinoma should also be treated with radiation therapy or an exenterative surgical procedure.

Melanoma of the vagina is treated with radical surgery if possible. Radiation therapy and chemotherapy have had little effect on these lesions.

In the past, sarcoma botryoides was treated by pelvic exenteration. It is an unpalatable procedure to consider in any patient but especially so in the young child. More recent reports suggest that excision combined with multiagent chemotherapy can lead to sustained remissions and at the same time preserve the bladder and rectum.

Leiomyosarcoma in the vagina should be treated by wide excision if anatomy allows. Many of these lesions are sensitive to radiation therapy and therefore may be amenable to therapy schemas similar to those recommended for squamous cell carcinoma.

Morbidity

The morbidity associated with vaginal cancers is usually secondary to treatment modalities. Cancers arising in the vagina are difficult to treat, and high morbidity is encountered because of the close anatomic association of the bladder and rectum. Radiation therapy, the primary treatment modality for most patients, leads to reasonably high complication rates associated with urinary tract or rectovaginal fistulas,

vaginal radionecrosis, and vaginal stenosis and fibrosis. Morbidity and mortality from radical surgical treatment can also be significant.

Prognosis

Because of the varying treatment modalities for squamous cell carcinoma of the vagina, it is difficult to evaluate whether surgery or radiation therapy achieves a higher cure rate. Most survival statistics are presented as combined survival of both irradiated and surgically treated patients. Representative survival statistics for squamous cell carcinoma and adenocarcinoma are shown in Table 29-3. The overall survival for melanoma of the vagina is approximately 5 percent. As with melanoma elsewhere in the body, survival is directly related to depth of invasion and whether metastasis to lymph nodes has occurred. Reliable statistics for survival of leiomyosarcoma, fibrosarcoma, and rhabdomyosarcoma are difficult to present as they are rare tumors that have been treated in a variety of ways.

Recurrence of squamous cell carcinoma of the vagina is similar to cervical cancer in its behavior, with most recurrences seen within two years of primary therapy and usually localized in the pelvis. Treatment of a recurrence after radiation therapy must be ultraradical surgery if the patient's medical condition and location of the tumor are favorable. Recurrence after surgical treatment, especially in the DES-exposed fe-

Table 29-3. Survival Rates for Squamous Cell Carcinoma and Clear Cell Adenocarcinoma of the Vagina (DES Exposure)

| FIGO stage* | Survival rate (%) | |
	Squamous cell	Clear cell adenocarcinoma
I	65	90
II	60	80
III	35	37
IV	39	—
Overall	51	80

* 1971 Staging system. Data are not available for revised staging system reported in 1988.

male, may be treated with radiation therapy or more radical exenterative procedures.

Distant metastasis from squamous cell carcinoma or adenocarcinoma have occasionally responded to chemotherapeutic agents such as cis-platinum, methotrexate, bleomycin, mitomycin C, and vincristine, although the optimal drug or treatment regimen has yet to be identified.

SELECTED READINGS

Andreasson, B., and Nyboe, J. Value of prognostic parameters in squamous cell carcinoma of the vulva. *Gynecol. Oncol.* 22:341, 1985.

Ball, H. G., and Berman, M. L. Management of primary vaginal carcinoma. *Gynecol. Oncol.* 14:154, 1982.

Boyce, J., Fruchter, R. G., Kasambilides, E., et al. Prognostic factors in carcinoma of the vulva. *Gynecol. Oncol.* 20:364, 1985.

Cavanagh, D., and Shepherd, J. H. The place of pelvic exenteration in the primary management of advanced carcinoma of the vulva. *Gynecol. Oncol.* 13:318, 1982.

Copeland, L. J., Gershenson, D. M., Saul, P. B., et al. Sarcoma botryoides of the female genital tract. *Obstet. Gynecol.* 66:262, 1985.

Copeland, L. J. Sneise, N. Gershenson, D.M. et al. Bartholin gland carcinoma. *Obstet. Gynecol.* 67:794, 1986.

Curry, S. L., Wharton, J. T., and Rutledge, F. Positive lymph nodes in vulvar squamous carcinoma. *Gynecol. Oncol.* 9:63, 1980.

DiSaia, P. J., Creasman, W. T., and Rich, W. M. An alternate approach to early cancer of the vulva. *Am. J. Obstet. Gynecol.* 133:825, 1979.

Gallup, D. G., Talledo, O. E., Shah, K. J., et al. Invasive squamous cell carcinoma of the vagina: a 14 year study. *Obstet. Gynecol.* 69:782, 1987.

Herbst, A. L., Ulfelder, H., and Poskanzer, D. C. Adenocarcinoma of the vagina; association of maternal stilbestrol therapy with tumor appearance in young women. *N. Engl. J. Med.* 284:878, 1971.

Hoffman, J. S., Kumar, N. B., and Morley, G. W. Microinvasive squamous carcinoma of the vulva: search for a definition. *Obstet. Gynecol.* 61:615, 1983.

Homesley, H. B., Bundy, B. N., Sedlis, A., et al. Radiation therapy versus pelvic node resection for carcinoma of the vulva with positive groin nodes. *Obstet. Gynecol.* 68:733, 1986.

Kucera, H., Langer, M., Smekal, G., et al. Radiotherapy of primary carcinoma of the vagina: management and results of different therapy schemes. *Gynecol. Oncol.* 21:87, 1985.

Melnick, S., Cole, P., Anderson, D., et al. Rates and risks of diethylstilbestrol-related clear cell adenocarcinoma of the vagina and cervix. *N. Eng. J. Med.* 316:514, 1987.

Morrow, C. P., and Rutledge, F. N. Melanoma of the vulva. *Obstet. Gynecol.* 39:745, 1972.

Parker, R. T., Duncan, I., Rampone, J., et al. Operative management of early invasive epidermoid carcinoma of the vulva. *Am. J. Obstet. Gynecol.* 123:349, 1975.

Peters, W. A., Kumar, N. B., and Morley, G. W. Carcinoma of the vagina: factors influencing treatment outcome. *Cancer* 55:892, 1985.

Podratz, K. C., Gaffey, T. A. Symmonds, R. E., et al. Melanoma of the vulva: an update. *Gynecol. Oncol.* 16:153, 1983.

Podratz, K. C., Symmonds, R. E., and Taylor, W. F. Carcinoma of the vulva: analysis of treatment failures. *Am. J. Obstet. Gynecol.* 143:340, 1982.

Stacy, D., Burrell, M. O., and Franklin, E. W. Extramammary Paget's disease of the vulva and anus: use of intraoperative frozen-section margins. *Am. J. Obstet. Gynecol.* 155:519, 1986.

Way, S. The surgery of vulvar carcinoma: an appraisal. *Clin. Obstet. Gynecol.* 5:623, 1978.

Wharton, J. T., Gallager, S., and Rutledge, F. N. Microinvasive carcinoma of the vulva. *Am. J. Obstet. Gynecol.* 118:159, 1974.

30

Gestational Trophoblastic Disease

John T. Soper

Gestational trophoblastic disease (GTD) is a generic term for a group of benign and malignant neoplasms derived from the human placenta. Patients afflicted with GTD tend to be young women in the peak years of their childbearing and child-caring years. Histologically, the forms of GTD include hydatidiform mole (complete and partial), invasive mole (chorioadenoma destruens), choriocarcinoma, and placental site tumors. Despite the apparent histologic diversity of these entities, the various forms of GTD share several features: derivation from the human placenta, paternal genome contribution, and secretion of human chorionic gonadotropin (hCG).

Malignant forms of GTD are rapidly growing and, if improperly treated, rapidly fatal. However, they are among the most sensitive human solid malignancies and respond to a wide variety of chemotherapeutic regimens. Most patients with benign and malignant forms of GTD can be cured of their neoplasm and retain the potential for future childbearing. Therefore it is important to understand the current management of these potentially devastating but relatively rare diseases.

HYDATIDIFORM MOLE: COMPLETE AND PARTIAL

Two distinct types of molar gestation have been described—partial and complete hydatidiform moles—that have distinct cytogenetic origins, pathologic features, and clinical behavior (Table 30-1). Until a larger number of patients with partial molar pregnancies are studied, they should be considered as being at risk for malignant sequelae. Most patients with molar gestations do not require chemotherapy and after evacuation can safely be monitored with serial hCG

level determinations until spontaneous regression occurs or until the patient develops criteria for beginning chemotherapy.

Hydatidiform moles are pregnancies characterized by replacement of a large portion of the placenta by hydropic (edematous) swelling of placental villi. With complete moles the fetus and membranes are absent and generalized hydropic changes are present, resulting in the characteristic gross appearance of a mass of grape-like tissue replacing the placenta. Variable amounts of trophoblastic proliferation are present, and fetal vessels are not identified microscopically. Partial moles are characterized by focal hydropic placental changes that may not be identified grossly and are more frequently associated with a fetus or amnionic membranes. Histologically, there is focal trophoblastic proliferation and evidence of fetal vessels in placental villi.

The cytogenetic origin of complete and partial hydatidiform moles are distinct. Partial moles have complete trisomy with one haploid set of maternal chromosomes and two haploid sets of paternal chromosomes resulting from either dispermic fertilization or reduplication of the haploid genome from a single sperm. Most complete moles have a 46,XX karyotype resulting from fertilization of an empty egg by a haploid sperm that reduplicates. Rare complete moles have a 46,XY karyotype; all of the genome in complete hydatidiform moles are derived from paternal chromosomes.

Epidemiology

Hydatidiform moles are identified in approximately 1 of 1500 to 2000 pregnancies in the United States. There is marked geographic variation in the incidence of hydatidiform mole, with the incidence increased 5 to 15 times higher in Central America, the Far East, and Southeast Asia than in Western industrialized nations. Racial and dietary factors may account for some of the difference in incidence. Both teenage and elderly maternal age appear to increase the risk of hydatidiform mole, suggesting that a defective ovum may be important in the etiology; the effects of paternal age are uncertain. The incidence of partial hydatidiform mole is unknown, but approximately 10 per-

Table 30-1. Complete and Partial Hydatidiform Moles

Feature	Partial hydatidiform mole	Complete hydatidiform mole
Karyotype	Triploid, paternal and maternal origin	Most 46,XX, paternal origin
Pathology		
Fetus/amnion, fetal vessels	Present	Absent
Hydropic villi	Variable, often focal	Pronounced, generalized
Trophoblast proliferation	Focal	Variable, often marked
Clinical parameters		
"Mole" clinical diagnosis	Rare	Common
Uterus large for dates	Rare	30–50%
Malignant sequelae	<10%	6–36%

cent of all molar pregnancies have histologic features of partial hydatidiform mole.

Clinical Features and Diagnosis

Partial hydatidiform moles are generally diagnosed at the time of a spontaneous or induced abortion. A fetus is frequently identified. The uterus is usually small for dates, and malignant sequelae are uncommon. In contrast, approximately one-third to one-half of patients with complete hydatidiform mole have uterine enlargement more than expected for gestational dates. Patients often present with vaginal hemorrhage and spontaneous abortion of atypical hydropic vesicles. Benign ovarian cysts (theca-lutein cysts) are caused by ovarian stimulation by hCG and are detected in approximately 20 percent of patients with complete moles. Pulmonary decompensation, pregnancy-induced hypertension, hyperemesis, and hyperthyroidism are occasionally observed. Fetal heart tones are usually absent.

The clinical diagnosis of molar gestation is supported by characteristic ultrasonographic findings consisting of a "snow storm" pattern of mixed echogenic foci, reflecting the edematous hydropic villi and intrauterine hemorrhage (Fig. 30-1). Ultrasonography has largely replaced other radiographic techniques for diagnosis of hydatidiform mole. Although serum hCG levels are markedly elevated in patients with hydatidiform mole, a single serum hCG level is not a reliable diagnostic test to establish the diagnosis of hydatidiform mole.

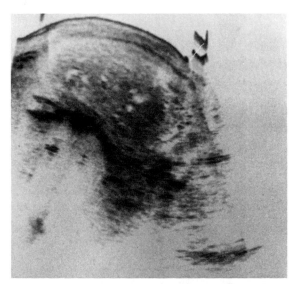

Fig. 30-1. Longitudinal ultrasonographic scan of the pelvis demonstrating a typical hydatidiform mole. Note the mixed echogenic foci caused by edematous villi and focal intrauterine hemorrhage.

Management and Evacuation

Evaluation of the patient with hydatidiform mole is directed toward preparation for evacuation, obtaining baseline hCG level information and screening for occult metastatic disease and associated hyperthyroidism. The following studies are recommended.

1. Complete physical and pelvic examination
2. Complete blood count

3. Blood chemistries, including renal, hepatic, and thyroid function tests
4. Baseline serum hCG level
5. Chest radiograph
6. Pelvic ultrasonography

Uterine evacuation is most safely performed using suction curettage (dilatation and curettage; D&C) followed by sharp uterine curettage. Suction D&C is safe and effective even if the uterus is markedly enlarged. Oxytocic agents are given after cervical dilatation and partial uterine evacuation to aid in postoperative hemostasis. Patients with excessive uterine enlargement have a high risk of pulmonary complications associated with D&C that may be related to trophoblastic deportation, fluid overload, anemia, hyperthyroidism, and preeclampsia. In these patients, baseline arterial blood gases should be assayed preoperatively and the evacuation performed with facilities for central hemodynamic monitoring.

Hysterectomy reduces the incidence of malignant sequelae after evacuation of hydatidiform mole and is the method of choice for treatment of patients who desire concurrent sterilization. However, these patients need to be followed with hCG level determinations after hysterectomy, as a small number develop malignant GTD. Hysterotomy and induction of labor with oxytocic agents or prostaglandins are *not* recommended, as complete uterine evacuation may not occur and blood loss is greater than with D&C or hysterectomy. The incidence of malignant GTD following these methods of uterine evacuation is higher than that observed after D&C or hysterectomy.

Ovarian theca lutein cysts are thin-walled, multiple, simple cysts that result from ovarian hyperstimulation caused by high levels of hCG. Occasionally, they achieve massive size, but most resolve spontaneously after molar evacuation. Rarely, torsion or hemorrhage from theca lutein cysts requires operative intervention. Malignant sequelae of hydatidiform moles are increased in the presence of theca lutein cysts but do not result from the cysts. Therefore oophorectomy or cystectomy are not indicated in uncomplicated theca lutein cysts.

Management After Molar Evacuation

Before the development of sensitive hCG assays, a variety of histologic and clinical criteria were used to define groups of patients at high risk and low risk for malignant GTD after molar evacuation. Patients with histologic features of marked trophoblastic proliferation and anaplasia identified in the mole are at higher risk than those who have only focal trophoblastic proliferation. Likewise, patients with excessive uterine enlargement beyond 12 to 14 weeks' gestational size, theca lutein cysts, hyperthyroidism, pulmonary complications, or hemorrhage requiring transfusion at the time of uterine evacuation are at increased risk compared to those who lack these clinical features. However, none of these histologic or clinical features has sufficient sensitivity to accurately predict the development of malignant sequelae for individual patients.

Older semiquantitative bioassays and latex agglutination tests used to measure hCG lack the ability to discriminate between normal luteinizing hormone (LH) levels and minimal elevations of hCG. Since the early 1970s, polyclonal and monoclonal antibodies against the beta subunit of hCG have allowed the development of radioimmunoassays and other immunoassays that can detect and quantify minimal elevations of serum hCG levels. Because production of hCG is the hallmark for lesions of GTD, these assays should be used for surveillance after molar evacuation and during therapy of malignant GTD.

Prophylactic chemotherapy has been used in an attempt to decrease the risk of subsequent malignant GTD after molar evacuation. Although the use of methotrexate or dactinomycin decreases this risk, it does not eliminate postmolar malignant GTD. Also, even short courses of chemotherapy are associated with toxicity and the chance of toxicity-related death. Currently, studies are attempting to define the role for prophylactic chemotherapy in patients at high risk for postmolar malignant GTD. However, if sensitive hCG assays are available and the patient is compliant, there appears to be no place for routine administration of prophylactic chemotherapy. Followup as suggested below virtually eliminates the possibility of mortality caused by malignant GTD developing after evacuation of a hydatidiform mole. Recommendations for postmolar followup include the following measures.

1. Baseline physical examination, pelvic examination, and chest radiograph
2. Serum hCG level every one to two weeks after evacuation until the hCG level is normal
3. Assay of hCG level two to four weeks after the first normal level to confirm spontaneous hCG regression
4. Surveillance of hCG level every one to two months for 6 to 12 months after the first negative hCG level

Intercurrent pregnancies should be prevented during hCG level surveillance, so that an hCG level elevation caused by pregnancy does not raise the specter of malignant GTD or obscure an hCG elevation caused by malignant GTD. Low to intermediate dose oral contraceptives are safe and do not increase the incidence of postmolar GTD. After completion of 6 to 12 months of negative hCG level surveillance, patients are allowed to become pregnant if desired. Because these women are at a four- to fivefold increased risk for recurrent molar pregnancy, it is recommended that they undergo early screening of future pregnancies with ultrasonography to exclude recurrent molar gestation.

Malignant GTD After Molar Evacuation

The purpose of hCG level surveillance after evacuation of hydatidiform mole is early detection of malignant GTD before the development of complications related to local proliferation, uterine invasion, or distant metastasis. Prior to the advent of chemotherapy, approximately 9 percent of women required hysterectomy for malignant GTD after evacuation of a hydatidiform mole. Studies of patients since the development of chemotherapy have reported diverse figures regarding the frequency of patients who require therapy after molar evacuation, the figures ranging from 6 percent to 36 percent. These observed differences likely reflect inclusion of patients with partial hydatidiform moles in some studies, a different incidence of metastatic disease among patient popula-

tions, or different hCG level regression criteria used to define malignant GTD.

As previously discussed, histologic and clinical features can be used to assign high and low risk groups of patients after molar evacuation but are of little value for determining the need for therapy in individual patients. Conservative criteria for institution of chemotherapy include the following.

1. hCG level rise
2. hCG level plateau for three or more consecutive weekly hCG levels (x, $x + 7$ days, $x + 14$ days)
3. Appearance of metastases
4. Histologic evidence of invasive mole or choriocarcinoma

On the basis of these criteria, the incidence for therapy of postmolar malignant GTD is approximately 20 percent. Patients who are treated for malignant GTD that is identified promptly after evacuation of hydatidiform mole have an excellent prognosis.

MALIGNANT GTD

Diagnosis

Approximately 50 to 70 percent of women treated for malignant GTD are identified after evacuation of a hydatidiform mole. Many of these patients probably have only local uterine proliferation of molar tissue confined to the endometrial cavity or with direct invasion of the myometrium (invasive mole or chorioadenoma destruens). A few of these patients have histologic evidence of choriocarcinoma. The remaining patients with malignant GTD have choriocarcinoma that develops after a normal pregnancy or after a nonmolar spontaneous abortion or ectopic pregnancy. Because a precise histologic diagnosis is often lacking, the clinical entities are usually referred to as *malignant GTD*.

Choriocarcinoma is an anaplastic malignancy composed histologically of sheets of malignant syncytioblastic and cytotrophoblastic cells. Malignant nodules rapidly outgrow the vascular supply, resulting in a tendency to central necrosis and hemorrhage.

Choriocarcinoma directly invades small blood vessels, resulting in the potential for rapid hematogenous dissemination of malignant arterial and venous emboli. Before the development of effective chemotherapy, surgical approaches to metastatic choriocarcinoma resulted in dismal survival rates, reflecting the highly malignant behavior of this neoplasm. Choriocarcinoma retains the ability to secrete hCG and is sensitive to a variety of chemotherapeutic agents.

It has been estimated that the incidence of choriocarcinoma is approximately 1:5000 to 1:10,000 pregnancies overall. The incidence increases with abnormalities of pregnancy: Whereas the incidence is 1:160,000 after normal pregnancy, it is between 1:5000 and 1:15,000 after spontaneous abortion or ectopic pregnancy and as high as 1:40 after hydatidiform mole. Fortunately, patients with hydatidiform moles usually have identification of malignant GTD promptly after evacuation through serial hCG level monitoring, as discussed previously. These patients are usually treated successfully with simple chemotherapy.

In contrast, patients who develop malignant GTD after normal pregnancies, spontaneous or induced abortions, or nonmolar ectopic pregnancies often have a delay in diagnosis or present with unusual clinical features such as postpartum bleeding, hyperthyroidism, or manifestations of distant metastases, which obscure the diagnosis. It should be stressed that any woman in the reproductive age group presenting with cerebral hemorrhage, pulmonary nodule, or metastases from an unknown primary site of malignancy should be screened for GTD with a serum hCG level.

Pretherapy Evaluation

Successful management of patients with malignant GTD depends on recognizing patients with high risk disease who require intensive initial therapy. The pretherapy evaluation is directed toward recognition of these factors. The following studies are recommended prior to therapy of the patient with malignant GTD.

1. Physical and pelvic examinations
2. Baseline hCG level
3. Complete blood count and baseline chemistries
4. Chest radiograph
5. Pelvic ultrasonography
6. Computed tomography (CT) or radionuclide brain scan
7. Abdominopelvic CT scan or combination of radionuclide liver scan and intravenous pyelography

When treating a patient for malignant GTD after evacuation of a hydatidiform mole or in any situation where pregnancy is suspected, it is essential to exclude the possibility of intrauterine pregnancy using pelvic ultrasonography before subjecting the patient to multiple radiographic scans and chemotherapy.

Approximately 50 percent of patients with malignant GTD have pulmonary metastases detected by a routine chest radiograph (Fig. 30-2), but the clinical significance of small pulmonary metastases detected

Fig. 30-2. Isolated pulmonary metastasis (arrow) in a woman with poor prognosis metastatic GTD. Note the left subclavian line for administration of chemotherapy. This patient ultimately required multiple courses of chemotherapy and thoracotomy with resection of the pulmonary metastasis to achieve cure.

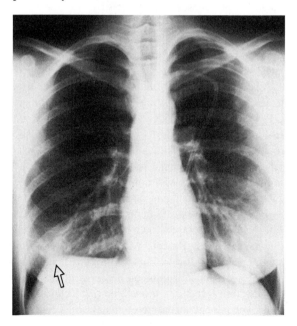

only by whole-lung tomography or CT scans of the lung is unknown. Because high risk metastases have occasionally been encountered without clinical or radiographic evidence of pulmonary or vaginal metastases, other radiographic studies are strongly recommended regardless of whether abnormalities are detected by physical examination or a chest radiograph.

A histologic diagnosis is *not* required before beginning therapy for malignant GTD. Radiographic evidence of metastases coupled with an elevated hCG level are sufficient to justify therapy in a woman of reproductive age. In these settings, there is no justification for thoracotomy, craniotomy, or hysterectomy *solely* for the purpose of histologic confirmation.

Staging and Classification

The International Federation of Obstetrics and Gynecology (FIGO) has adopted a staging system for malignant GTD that is similar to staging systems used for malignancies at other sites.

Stage I: GTD confined to the uterus
Stage II: metastases to pelvis and vagina
Stage III: pulmonary metastases
Stage IV: metastases to other sites

Experience with the FIGO staging system has been limited, and it is not clear if this staging system correlates with survival.

A simple clinical classification system is often used to assign initial therapy for patients with malignant GTD (Table 30-2). This system takes into account factors that predict failure of initial single-agent chemotherapy and allows identification of patients who would benefit from initial aggressive multiagent chemotherapy. Patients with nonmetastatic GTD are not subdivided into good and poor prognosis groups, as essentially all of these patients can be cured successfully using single-agent chemotherapy as part of initial management. Patients with metastatic GTD are subdivided into low risk/good prognosis and high risk/poor prognosis groups on the basis of easily definable clinical features: If one high risk factor is identified, the patient is considered to have high risk/poor prognosis metastatic GTD (Table 30-2).

Table 30-2. Clinical Classification of Malignant GTD

Nonmetastatic GTD (not defined in terms of good versus poor prognosis—see text)
Metastatic GTD
    Good prognosis—absence of high risk factors
        Pretreatment hCG level <40,000 mIU/ml serum β-hCG
        < Four months' duration of disease
        No evidence of brain or liver metastasis
        No significant prior chemotherapy
        No antecedent term pregnancy
    Poor prognosis—any single high risk factor
        Pretreatment hCG level >40,000 mIU/ml serum β-hCG
        > Four months' duration of disease
        Brain and/or liver metastasis
        Failed prior chemotherapy
        Antecedent term pregnancy

These risk factors were originally derived by analyzing the experience of early investigators using single-agent methotrexate and actinomycin D as the initial therapy for patients with metastatic GTD. Patients with a high pretherapy hCG level, duration of disease of more than four months, brain or liver metastases, or failed prior chemotherapy had a much worse outcome than those who lacked these features. Nonmolar gestation has been found to correlate with poor survival as well.

Since the 1970s, investigators have used more elaborate prognostic scoring systems in an attempt to more clearly define risk in patients with malignant GTD. The World Health Organization has formalized a prognostic index (Table 30-3) that incorporates many of these features. In addition to using a weighted scale for risk factors analyzed by the clinical classification system, e.g., hCG level and duration of disease, this system utilizes a weighted scale for additional risk factors. For example, ectopic pregnancies and abortions are considered to have a risk intermediate between molar and term pregnancy. Blood types and age contribute to the score. Tumor burden is evaluated on the basis of hCG level, the largest tumor mass, number of metastatic sites, and anatomic site of metastases. After computation of total score for all risk factors, a patient is considered to be at low risk if

Table 30-3. WHO Prognostic Scoring System for GTD

Prognostic factor	Score[a]			
	0	1	2	4
Age	≤39	>39		
Antecedent pregnancy	HM	Abortion; ectopic	Term	
Interval (months)[b]	<4	4–6	7–12	>12
hCG level (IU/liter)	$<10^3$	$10^3–10^4$	$10^4–10^5$	$>10^5$
ABO blood groups (female × male)		O × A	B	
		A × O	AB	
Largest tumor (cm)	<3	3–5	>5	
Site of metastasis		Spleen, kidney	GI tract, liver	Brain
No. of metastases		1–3	4–8	>8
Prior chemotherapy			Single drug	Multiple drugs

Key: WHO = World Health Organization; HM = hydatidiform mole; GI = gastrointestinal.
[a]Low risk ≤4; intermediate risk 5–7, high risk ≥8.
[b]Interval: time between antecedent pregnancy and start of chemotherapy.

Table 30-4. Chemotherapy for Malignant GTD

GTD status	Initial	Salvage
Nonmetastatic	Single agent (methotrexate or MTX/FA)	Single agent (dactinomycin) Combination chemotherapy
Good-prognosis metastatic	Single agent (methotrexate)	Single agent (dactinomycin) Combination chemotherapy
Poor-prognosis metastatic	Triple therapy (MAC)	Other combination chemotherapy (see text)

Key: MTX/FA = methotrexate-folinic acid; MAC = methotrexate/dactinomycin/chlorambucil.

the score if 4 or less, intermediate risk with a score of 5 to 7, and high risk with a score of 8 or more. This scoring system has been found to correlate well with survival after conventional approaches to chemotherapy, but not all of the factors have been critically evaluated to determine if the graded scoring used to generate the prognostic score is valid.

Therapy

Since the development of the antimetabolite methotrexate during the 1950s, chemotherapy has been successfully used to treat malignant GTD. Other agents active against malignant GTD include dactinomycin, alkylators, and vinca alkaloids. More recently cisplatinum and 5-fluorouracil have been shown to have activity. Etoposide (VP-16) is perhaps the most active

new agent to be used for therapy of GTD. Although chemotherapy has revolutionized successful therapy of malignant GTD, surgery and radiation therapy continue to have roles in the therapy of these women.

Nonmetastatic GTD. Single-agent chemotherapy using methotrexate or dactinomycin is the cornerstone of therapy for nonmetastatic GTD (Table 30-4). Essentially, 80 to 95 percent of patients can be cured with the initial agent using several treatment regimens. Patients who fail primary therapy are almost always salvaged with alternative single-agent chemotherapy. In an effort to increase the dose of methotrexate and reduce toxicity, methotrexate with folinic acid rescue has been used. Methotrexate 1 mg per kilogram IM is administered on days 1, 3, 5, and 7 with folinic acid 0.1 mg per kilogram IM given on days 2, 4, 6, and 8 of each cycle. Chemotherapy is recycled every 14 days, and one cycle of therapy is administered after the first normal hCG level is obtained. One Gynecologic Oncology Group (GOG) study has suggested that methotrexate 30 mg per square meter administered as a single intramuscular dose on a weekly basis yields similar results with minimal cost and toxicity to the patient. Most patients who fail initial therapy with these treatment regimens are salvaged with actinomycin D.

Simple hysterectomy can be incorporated into therapy; hysterectomy performed during the first cycle of chemotherapy reduces the length of chemotherapy required to achieve remission and can be used as salvage for patients who have failed primary therapy with single agents. However, most patients with nonmetastatic GTD can be successfully treated using chemotherapy alone, thereby avoiding hysterectomy. This issue is important, as most of these women wish to retain the potential for childbearing.

Metastatic GTD

GOOD PROGNOSIS METASTATIC GTD. Single-agent chemotherapy with methotrexate 0.4 mg per kilogram IM on days 1 to 5 recycled every 14 days or dactinomycin 500 μg IV on days 1 to 5 recycled every 14 days are standard chemotherapeutic regimens for patients with good prognosis metastatic GTD (Table 30-4). Approximately 40 percent of patients fail therapy with the initial agent and require salvage with the alternative single agent, but more than 90 percent can be cured using single-agent chemotherapy alone. It is of note that patients with "micrometastatic" pulmonary involvement detected only with CT scans of the lungs have a similar failure rate with initial methotrexate/folinic acid regimens, suggesting that these patients behave similarly to patients with good prognosis metastatic GTD. Most of these patients can also be cured without resorting to surgical intervention.

POOR PROGNOSIS METASTATIC GTD. The basic principles of therapy for patients with poor prognosis metastatic GTD consist in initially recognizing patients with high risk disease and treating them aggressively with multiagent chemotherapy (Table 30-4). Patients with poor prognosis metastatic GTD who are

initially treated with single-agent methotrexate have a poor outcome. Single-agent therapy is rarely successful, and efforts to salvage these women are hampered by accumulated toxicity.

Standard initial therapy consists of "triple therapy" with methotrexate/dactinomycin/chlorambucil (or cyclophosphamide), commonly referred to as MAC. Other examples of currently used combinations include the modified Bagshawe regimen (hydroxyurea/methotrexate / vincistine / cyclophosphamide / dactinomycin/adriamycin), and EMA/CO (VP-16 with methotrexate/folinic acid rescue, dactinomycin, vincristine, and cyclophosphamide). In general, cycles of chemotherapy are administered as soon as toxicity from the previous cycle has cleared. Although toxicity may be marked with these combinations, aggressive initial chemotherapy is necessary to ensure optimal survival for women in this disease category. Approximately 80 percent of patients with poor prognosis metastatic GTD treated initially at a trophoblastic disease center survive, compared to 40 to 50 percent who are referred for therapy after failed initial therapy. Therefore it is imperative that these patients be identified and referred promptly for therapy at centers that specialize in the treatment of patients with GTD.

Surgery and Radiation Therapy

HYSTERECTOMY. Before the development of effective chemotherapy, hysterectomy rarely resulted in the cure of patients with even nonmetastatic GTD. Owing to refinements in chemotherapy, hysterectomy is rarely indicated as the initial therapy of women with nonmetastatic or good prognosis metastatic GTD who do not desire sterilization. However, in these patients it appears to decrease the duration of hospital stay and number of courses of chemotherapy required to achieve remission. Therefore initial hysterectomy should be considered in a woman who desires sterilization. Delayed hysterectomy is required for approximately 10 percent of patients in these categories, but it should be reemphasized that chemotherapy alone successfully cures approximately 85 percent of patients with nonmetastatic and good prognosis metastatic GTD.

Occasionally, hysterectomy is integrated into the therapy of women with poor prognosis metastatic

GTD. In general, these patients have an extrauterine tumor burden that is too large to benefit from routine hysterectomy. However, carefully selected individual patients may be rendered disease-free with salvage hysterectomy.

THORACOTOMY. Segmental pulmonary resection is the most frequently performed procedure other than hysterectomy aimed at excision of foci of drug-resistant disease. Because most patients with lung metastases are cured using chemotherapy alone, there is no place for routine thoracotomy as primary therapy for metastatic GTD. It should be emphasized that resolution of radiographic changes may lag far behind hCG level response to chemotherapy. It is not unusual to observe chest radiographic changes that persist for months or years beyond hCG level remission in individual patients. Therefore thoracotomy should be reserved for therapy of patients with drug-resistant GTD. Women with solitary pulmonary nodules who have drug-resistant disease (Fig. 30-2) can often be cured when thoracotomy is combined with salvage chemotherapy.

MISCELLANEOUS SURGICAL PROCEDURES. Craniotomy is usually performed only in situations where there is acute neurologic decompensation caused by hemorrhage into central nervous system metastases. Exploratory laparotomy is sometimes performed for catastrophic intraabdominal hemorrhage from peritoneal or hepatic metastasis or for drainage of abscesses related to disease or complications of therapy. Tunneled multiport central venous (Hickman or Broviac) catheters are invaluable for treating patients with poor prognosis GTD who often require prolonged chemotherapy and support with blood products, antibiotics, and total parenteral nutrition during therapy.

Usually extirpative procedures (hysterectomy, pulmonary resections) are performed under coverage of chemotherapy. Theoretically, this method decreases the chance of metastasis through embolization of malignant cells caused by manipulation of tissues during surgery. Complications related to wound healing and infection are not increased significantly when surgery and chemotherapy are combined.

RADIATION THERAPY. Whole-brain and whole-liver irradiation have been used to treat brain and liver me-

tastases in an attempt to decrease hemorrhage from metastases at these sites. Approximately 50 percent of patients with brain metastases are cured using the combination of multiagent chemotherapy and whole-organ irradiation. Patients with liver metastases often have multiple other high risk factors and require aggressive therapy. Hepatic irradiation does not seem to compromise tolerance of therapy.

Prevention of Recurrent GTD. Chemotherapy is routinely administered beyond hCG level remission in an attempt to reduce the frequency of recurrent or persistent GTD. It is known that a sensitive hCG assay can detect subclinical tumor burden but a tumor burden of fewer than 10^4 cells may not be detected. In general, recurrence rates correlate with disease status. Patients with nonmetastatic or good prognosis metastatic GTD have a less than 5 percent chance of recurrence versus 10 to 15 percent for patients with poor prognosis metastatic GTD. Maintenance chemotherapy delivered after hCG level remission appears to reduce the risk of recurrence. In general, patients with nonmetastatic or good prognosis metastatic GTD are given one or two cycles of maintenance therapy depending on the amount of chemotherapy required to achieve remission. Patients with poor prognosis GTD are given three or more cycles of maintenance chemotherapy.

Surveillance and Reproduction
After Therapy for Malignant GTD

During therapy, the hCG levels are followed on at least a weekly basis; therapy is changed if there is not a steady decline in hCG levels during the interval following a cycle of chemotherapy. Complete remission is defined as three consecutive hCG levels in the normal range. After remission has been achieved, hCG levels should be followed every one to two weeks for the first three months after completion of therapy, every two to four weeks for the next three months, and every one to two months to complete the first year of surveillance. Recurrent episodes of GTD usually develop within a few months after completion of therapy, but late recurrences develop in a few cases. Therefore hCG levels should be repeated at three- to six-month intervals indefinitely. Patients are counseled to avoid pregnancy throughout the first year of hCG surveillance.

Pregnancy After Therapy for GTD

Most women with malignant GTD are successfully cured by chemotherapy without resorting to hysterectomy. There is little, if any, increased risk of congenital malformation in infants from subsequent pregnancies in these women. There may be a slight increase in the incidence of spontaneous abortions, but this apparent increase may be due to increased intensity of hCG level surveillance in this patient population. Obstetric complications, particularly the incidence of placenta accreta, are increased in pregnancies that occur after therapy of malignant GTD. There is also an increased incidence of repeat molar gestation in patients who have had a previous hydatidiform mole. Ultrasonography should be performed early in subsequent pregnancies to exclude the possibility of recurrent molar gestation. A chest radiograph should be obtained and serum hCG levels assayed six to eight weeks after delivery to screen for the rare case of recurrent choriocarcinoma developing after an intercurrent normal pregnancy. Despite these concerns, most women who are successfully treated for malignant GTD have normal reproductive capacity and should be encouraged in this regard after they have completed at least one year of negative hCG level surveillance.

PLACENTAL SITE TUMOR

Placental site tumors are rare, locally invasive neoplasms of placental origin. A dimorphic cellular population is not observed as in choriocarcinoma. These lesions are composed of intermediate cytotrophoblast cells only. Because syncytiotrophoblastic elements are absent, there is minimal secretion of hCG. Sometimes human placental lactogen (hPL) is actively secreted by placental site tumors and can serve as a tumor marker in individual patients. In contrast to other forms of malignant GTD, placental site tumors are not sensitive to chemotherapy. Although most of these tumors have an indolent, locally invasive course and can be cured by hysterectomy, an occasional patient develops widely metastatic and rapidly progressive disease.

SELECTED READINGS

Azab, M. B., Pejovic, M. H., Theodore, C., et al. Prognostic factors in gestational trophoblastic tumors: a multivariate analysis. *Cancer* 62:585, 1988.

Bagshawe, K. D. Risk and prognostic factors in trophoblastic neoplasia. *Cancer* 38:1373, 1976.

Berkowitz, R. (ed.), Symposium on trophoblastic disease. *J. Reprod. Med.* 32:1, 1987.

Curry, S. L., Hammond, C. B., Tyrey, L., et al. Hydatidiform mole: diagnosis, management and longterm followup of 347 patients. *Obstet. Gynecol.* 45:1, 1975.

DuBeshter, B., Berkowitz, R. S., Goldstein, D. P., et al. Metastatic gestational trophoblastic disease: experience at the New England Trophoblastic Disease Center, 1965 to 1985. *Obstet. Gynecol.* 69:390, 1987.

Hammond, C. B., Borchert, L., Tyrey, L., et al. Treatment of metastatic trophoblastic disease: good and poor prognosis. *Am. J. Obstet. Gynecol.* 115:451, 1973.

Hammond, C. B., Weed, J. C., Jr., and Currie, J. L. The role of operation in the current therapy of gestational trophoblastic disease. *Am. J. Obstet. Gynecol.* 136:844, 1980.

Lurain, J. R., Brewer, J. I., Torok, E. E., et al. Gestational trophoblastic disease: treatment results at the Brewer Trophoblastic Disease Center. *Obstet. Gynecol.* 60:354, 1982.

Lurain, J. R., Brewer, J. I., Torok, E. E., et al. Natural history of hydatidiform mole after primary evacuation. *Am. J. Obstet. Gynecol.* 145:591, 1983.

Soper, J. T., and Hammond, C. B. Gestational trophoblastic disease and gestational choriocarcinoma. In Gusberg, S. B., Shingleton, H. M., and Deppe, G. (eds.), *Female Genital Cancer.* New York: Churchill Livingstone, 1988. Pp. 435–458.

Soper, J. T., and Hammond, C. B. Role of surgical therapy and radiotherapy in gestational trophoblastic disease. *J. Reprod. Med.* 32:663, 1987.

Soper, J. T., Clarke-Pearson, D. L., and Hammond, C. B. Metastatic gestational trophoblastic disease: prognostic factors in previously untreated patients. *Obstet. Gynecol.* 71:338, 1988.

Szulman, A. E., and Buchsbaum, H. T. (eds.), *Gestational Trophoblastic Disease.* New York: Springer-Verlag, 1987.

Weed, J. C., Jr., and Hammond, C. B. Cerebral metastatic choriocarcinoma: intensive therapy and prognosis. *Obstet. Gynecol.* 55:89, 1980.

Index

Index

Gonorrhea (*continued*)
syphilis with, 305
Graafian follicle, 129–130
Grafenberg spot, 423–424
Granuloma inguinale, 329–330
of vulva, 286
Granulomatous disease, vulvar cancer
and, 553
Granulosa cell tumor, 385, 547–548
endometrial cancer and, 521
Graves speculum, 6, 7
Gravlee Jet Washer, 17
Gravindex Slide Test for Preg-
nancy, 26
Groove sign, 286
Growth hormone, menstrual cycle
and, 167–168
G-spot, 423–424
GTD. *See* Gestastional trophoblastic
disease (GTD)
Gynecography, 59
Gynecologic cancer, early detection
program for, 11–13
Gynecologic history, 4–5
in pelvic mass, 374

Halo sign, 339
Hashimoto's thyroiditis, 36
hCG. *See* Human chorionic gonado-
tropin (hCG)
Hegar's sign, of pregnancy, 335
Hemangioma, 292
Hematocolpos, 145
Hematoma, of vulva, 293
Hematometrium, 145, 149
Hematosalpinx, 145, 149, 309
Hemodialysis, in septic pelvis, 322
Hemophilus ducreyi infection, in
chancroid, 286–287
Hemophilus vaginalis infection, 327
Hemorrhage
hysterectomy and, 104
postoperative, 78, 91–92
Hemosiderin, in uterine adenomyo-
sis, 366
Heparin
in deep venous thrombosis, 79
postoperative, 101
Hermaphrodite, 137
Hernia
incisional, 99

Hernia (*continued*)
inguinal, 292
pudendal, 292
ventral, 99
Herpes simplex virus
intraepithelial disease and, 501
of vulva, 283–285
vulvar cancer and, 553
Herpes simplex virus I, 283
Herpes simplex virus II, 283
diagnosis of, 331–332
treatment of, 332
Heymann capsules, for radiotherapy,
527
Hickman catheter, in malignant
GTD, 572
Hidradenitis suppurativa
partial vulvectomy in, 287
of vulva, 287
Hidradenoma, 291–292
Hilar cell tumor, 32
Hirsutism, 212–213
anovulation and, 212–213
in polycystic ovarian syndrome,
203, 207
testosterone and, 32
HIV antibody test
premarital, 13
in sexual assault, 417, 419
Homan's sign, 101
Hormone therapy
in endometrial cancer, 527
in endometriosis, 237
Hot flushes, 460–461
Human chorionic gonadotropin (hCG)
in contraception, 455
corpus luteum cyst and, 379
in ectopic pregnancy, 353
in germ cell tumor, 376
in hydatidiform mole, 566, 567
in malignant GTD, 573–574
in placental site tumor, 574
in pregnancy testing, 25–26
theca lutein cyst and, 379
in threatened abortion, 337
vs. ultrasound, 67–68
Human immunodeficiency virus
(HIV), 332
Human menopausal gonadotropin
in amenorrhea, 218–219
in polycystic ovarian syndrome, 207

Human papilloma virus (HPV)
cervical cancer and, 279, 509
condyloma acuminata and, 278
in intraepithelial neoplasia, 493–
494
cervical, 494
vaginal, 506
vulvar, 503
vulvar cancer and, 553
Human placental lactogen, in placental site tumor, 574
HY antigen, amenorrhea and, 132
Hydatid cyst of Morgagni, 389–390
fetal, 139
Hydatidiform mole, 365–368
Hydrocolpos, 145
Hydrocortisone, in vulvar pruritis, 291
Hydrosalpinx, 309
Hydrothorax, Meigs' syndrome
and, 386
17-Hydroxycorticosteroids, 32
21-Hydroxylase deficiency, in
congenital adrenal hyperplasia,
159
17-Hydroxyprogesterone, 30–31
Hydroxyzine, in vulvar lichen sclerosus, 290
Hymen
embryology of, 139
imperforate, 145
cryptic menstruation and, 131
microperforate, 145
Hymenectomy, 14, 145
Hyperbaric oxygen, in pelvic sepsis,
322
Hypercapnia, laparoscopy and, 103
Hyperpigmentation, of vulva, 293
Hypertension
estrogen therapy and, 466
oral contraceptives and, 441
preoperative evaluation for, 77
Hyperthyroidism, anovulation and,
209
Hypogastric artery, 92
embolism of, 59
Hypoglycemia, in premenstrual
syndrome, 188
Hypospadia
in females, 247
infertility and, 256
perineoscrotal, 158